Advances in Cancer Research

Advances in Cancer Research

Edited by **Eden Dennis**

hayle medical

New York

Published by Hayle Medical,
30 West, 37th Street, Suite 612,
New York, NY 10018, USA
www.haylemedical.com

Advances in Cancer Research
Edited by Eden Dennis

International Standard Book Number: 978-1-63241-422-9 (Hardback)

The publisher's policy is to use permanent paper from mills that operate a sustainable forestry policy. Furthermore, the publisher ensures that the text paper and cover boards used have met acceptable environmental accreditation standards.

Trademark Notice: Registered trademark of products or corporate names are used only for explanation and identification without intent to infringe.

Printed in the United States of America.

Contents

Preface

Cancer is the nomenclature used for a set of diseases that occur due to excessive cell growth in any body part and may infest other parts of the body. It is generally characterized by formation of malignant tumors. These are caused due to various factors such as chemical pollutants, radiations, obesity, genetic inheritance, infections, etc. Classification of cancer can be done on the basis of origin of the tumor. This book aims to shed light on some of the unexplored aspects related to cancer and the recent researches in this field. The extensive content of this book provides the readers with a thorough understanding of the subject. It is a collective contribution of a renowned group of international experts. It will serve as a resource guide for oncologists, researchers, professionals and students.

The information contained in this book is the result of intensive hard work done by researchers in this field. All due efforts have been made to make this book serve as a complete guiding source for students and researchers. The topics in this book have been comprehensively explained to help readers understand the growing trends in the field.

I would like to thank the entire group of writers who made sincere efforts in this book and my family who supported me in my efforts of working on this book. I take this opportunity to thank all those who have been a guiding force throughout my life.

Editor

Dissecting the Potential Interplay of DEK Functions in Inflammation and Cancer

Nicholas A. Pease,[1] Trisha Wise-Draper,[2] and Lisa Privette Vinnedge[1]

[1]Division of Oncology, Cincinnati Children's Hospital Medical Center, Cincinnati, OH 45229, USA
[2]Department of Internal Medicine, Division of Hematology/Oncology, University of Cincinnati College of Medicine, Cincinnati, OH 45267, USA

Correspondence should be addressed to Lisa Privette Vinnedge; lisa.privette@cchmc.org

Academic Editor: Valentina Di caro

There is a long-standing correlation between inflammation, inflammatory cell signaling pathways, and tumor formation. Understanding the mechanisms behind inflammation-driven tumorigenesis is of great research and clinical importance. Although not entirely understood, these mechanisms include a complex interaction between the immune system and the damaged epithelium that is mediated by an array of molecular signals of inflammation—including reactive oxygen species (ROS), cytokines, and NFκB signaling—that are also oncogenic. Here, we discuss the association of the unique DEK protein with these processes. Specifically, we address the role of DEK in chronic inflammation via viral infections and autoimmune diseases, the overexpression and oncogenic activity of DEK in cancers, and DEK-mediated regulation of NFκB signaling. Combined, evidence suggests that DEK may play a complex, multidimensional role in chronic inflammation and subsequent tumorigenesis.

1. Introduction

Chronic inflammation has been linked to cancer for decades with several epidemiologic reports suggesting causation. In fact, several infectious and noninfectious known causes of cancer, such as viral infection (human papilloma virus, HPV, and Epstein Barr virus, EBV), *Helicobacter pylori* infection, smoking, and asbestos exposure to name a few, can induce inflammation prior to tumor formation. Additionally, upregulation through polymorphisms of the proinflammatory cytokines, tumor necrosis factor (TNF), and interleukin-1 (IL-1) has been associated with poor prognoses and disease severity in non-Hodgkin's lymphoma and gastric cancer, respectively [1, 2]. Conversely, administration of known anti-inflammatory medications and herbs such as nonsteroidal anti-inflammatory drugs (NSAIDs), curcumin, and ginseng has been associated with a decreased risk of cancer, leading to several clinical studies investigating these agents as possible adjunct treatments [3–5]. However, the exact mechanisms of causation have remained unclear and in some instances, anti-inflammatory medications have been associated with a higher risk of cancer, making the association more complicated than initially proposed [6].

In general, inflammation and innate immunity are felt to be protumorigenic whereas adaptive immunity is antitumorigenic. In fact, tumor associated macrophages (TAMs), which are recruited during the inflammatory response, are indicators of a poor prognosis when identified in tumor tissue [7] while high levels of cytotoxic T (CD8+) cells, as part of adaptive immunity, correlate with a good prognosis [8, 9]. However, the presence of T cells in the microenvironment of tumors alone may not be sufficient to confer an immune response as they often are not active in recognizing the tumor as nonself. Therefore, a focus on negative regulators of the immune system, such as T regulatory (Treg) cells and other inhibitory molecules, is under investigation as a possible explanation for tumor immune escape. Multiple immune checkpoint molecules such as cytotoxic T lymphocyte antigen-4 (CTLA-4) and "programmed death-1" (PD-1) and its ligands (PD-L1 and PD-L2) are upregulated during the immune response in an attempt to prevent autoimmune damage to normal tissue. However, PD-1 is also induced on T cells after activation by immune stimulation, either by infection or by tumor progression and, therefore, is felt to be a mechanism of immune resistance. Additionally, high levels of PD-1 in the tumor microenvironment and PD-1 ligand (PD-L1) expression have been found in many tumors and are correlated with poor prognoses in multiple tumor types [10–13]. Targeting of these pathways has proved to be exciting and effective, resulting in FDA approval of several agents (ipilimumab, nivolumab, and pembrolizumab) for melanoma with expectations for approval for other tumors in the near future [14–16]. However, not all tumors respond to these immune therapies, requiring a better understanding of the mechanism of failure and the complex interactions of the immune response to tumors.

Several proinflammatory cytokines and chemokines such as IL-1, IL-6, TNF, and IL-8 are often upregulated in response to cancer and are associated with tumor development and progression in mice [17]. Interestingly, it has been demonstrated that the classical IKK-β-dependent NFκB pathway may be the link to inflammation and cancer as activation results in upregulation of proinflammatory cytokines as well as several antiapoptotic factors [18]. Targeting the NFκB pathway may, therefore, be another promising approach to antitumor therapy either alone or in combination with traditional therapies or checkpoint blockade.

2. DEK Structure and Functions

One protein recently found to control NFκB activity is the DEK oncogene. DEK is a highly conserved chromatin-associated, nonhistone phosphoprotein (43 kDa) that was originally identified as part of a fusion protein (DEK-CAN) in an acute myeloid leukemia (AML) subtype with translocation t(6;9), a balanced translocation, which confers a poor prognosis [19–21]. The presence of DEK *in vitro* was originally noted for its ability to partially correct cell sensitivity to mutagens and radiation in ATM-deficient fibroblasts [22]. Although it has no known enzymatic activity nor known homologs, it dynamically interacts with RNA, DNA, chromatin, and associated proteins to alter transcription, mRNA processing, DNA replication and repair, and chromatin topology [23–27]. DEK has three DNA binding domains: a central SAF-box, pseudo-SAF/SAP-box, and a C-terminal unique binding domain. The SAF-box domain enables DEK to preferentially bind cruciform and four-way junction structures and induce positive supercoiling; however, the C-terminal binding domain can facilitate DNA-DEK-DEK interactions that may facilitate regulatory processes [20, 28–30].

Nonetheless, other DEK domains participate in important molecular functions. Specifically, the acidic domains of DEK bind chromatin-bound histones and prevent optimal PCAF and p300-mediated histone acetyltransferase activity (HAT). This causes hypoacetylation of DEK-bound regions of nucleosomes and can result in inhibition of HAT-mediated transcriptional activation [31]. Also, the physical interaction between DEK with Daxx and HDACII can assist in transcriptional repression by promoting histone deacetylation [25]. Additional structure-function studies have identified

the SAP domain for its importance in DEK function. When the SAP domain of DEK interacts with casein kinase 2 (CK2) in the presence of ATP, DEK is phosphorylated. This DEK-CK2 complex displays an affinity for histone H3.3, a histone variant associated with active chromatin, and limits its placement on chromatin by protecting it from other potential histone chaperones that redistribute H3.3 in a DAAX/ATRX-dependent manner from PML nuclear bodies [32, 33]. Furthermore, DEK is also necessary for optimal binding of heterochromatin protein 1-α (HP1-α) to the repressive chromatin mark, H3K9me3. This interaction facilitates silencing loops that prevent histone acetylation and protect heterochromatin integrity [34]. Finally, DEK binding to chromatin was found to limit access of the transcriptional machinery to chromatin, which could be disrupted by PARP1 and another histone chaperone, SET [35]. These functions suggest that DEK has the capacity to modify chromatin, via regulating histone acetylation and placement, in a manner that silences the expression of particular regions while also promoting general genomic stability.

However, it is also worth mentioning that some reports indicate that DEK can function as a positive transcriptional cofactor to induce gene expression [33, 36, 37]. In *Drosophila*, DEK was associated with more transcriptionally active regions of chromatin and coactivated the nuclear ecdysone receptor, promoting its functions as a transcriptional activator [33]. In murine breast tumor models, DEK also drives expression of Wnt ligands, resulting in the promotion of β-catenin transcriptional activity, which has also been noted in human breast cancer cells [38, 39]. Chromatin immunoprecipitation sequencing (ChIP-Seq) results have also revealed that DEK preferentially binds areas of euchromatin near transcription start sites of highly expressed genes, many of which include motifs for common transcriptional regulators such as SP1 and RNA polymerase II [37].

Although the specific physical interactions are unknown, the molecular functions of DEK also extend to roles in DNA damage and stress response. DEK expression is necessary for proper DNA-PK mediated recruitment of DNA damage repair proteins Ku70/80 during nonhomologous end-joining (NHEJ) and prevents DNA damage accumulation that results in ATM mediated apoptosis [40]. This also supports evidence of DEK complementation in ataxia-telangiectasia cells, in which DEK fragments remedied the DNA damage phenotypes of ATM deficient fibroblasts [22]. DEK overexpression can also cause the destabilization of p53, resulting in the inhibition of normal p53-dependent apoptosis in cancer cells [41]. DEK also has a role in preventing p53-independent apoptosis by promoting the transcription of *MCL-1*, an antiapoptotic member of the BCL-2 family [42].

The molecular functions of DEK can be regulated by an array of protein modifications. Phosphorylation of DEK by CK2 weakens DEK-DNA binding [43] and has been linked to the secretion of DEK [44]. Other modifications that change DEK localization and function include acetylation by p300 [45], poly(ADP-ribosyl)ation by PARP1 [46], and truncation by DPP4 [47]. These posttranslational modifications of DEK are crucial for understanding the molecular functions that could contribute to pathogenesis. Phosphorylation by CK2 and poly(ADP-ribosyl)ation by PARP1 can induce the release of DEK from chromatin, enabling it to function beyond chromatin remodeling [35]. Nonchromatin bound DEK can contribute to mRNA splicing events by interacting with the serine/arginine repeats of splicing complexes, while phosphorylation of DEK serines enables it to associate with U2AF and facilitate intron excision; there is evidence that the role of DEK in mRNA splicing may play a role in alternative splicing events of transcripts from genes such as tropomyosin *TPM1* [48–51]. The function of DEK in the cytoplasm, if present, has not been determined; however, there are several different functions for DEK as a secretory molecule. These include inducing white blood cell migration as a chemoattractant [36], interacting with anti-DEK antibodies that trigger autoimmune responses [52], and possibly promoting chromatin remodeling and prosurvival functions by being taken up by neighboring cells [53]. Interestingly, it is currently unknown what conditions induce the posttranslational modifications of DEK that result in its delocalization from chromatin and secretion, resulting in pathological activities.

The ubiquitous and pleiotropic nature of DEK mandates that the expression and modification of DEK are tightly regulated in order to avoid pathology. The dysregulation of DEK can disturb normal cell functions and potentiate pathogenesis resulting in transformation, chemoresistance, inflammation, and tumor development. In this review, we postulate that DEK may be a crucial link between inflammation and tumorigenesis. We will discuss the role of DEK in viral infection and epitope presentation, which may provide mechanisms for both promoting intracellular viral oncogenesis and for eliciting T cell mediated immune responses that induce proinflammatory cytokines. These cytokines, such as IL-8, can further contribute to chronic inflammation, promote growth signaling in neighboring cells, and stimulate DEK secretion by macrophages. As a secretory molecule, DEK can be recognized by anti-DEK antibodies or be taken up as a functional exogenous protein by neighboring cells. The first function can exacerbate chronic inflammation and induce more proinflammatory factors that create favorable tumor microenvironments. The second secretory DEK function allows for excess DEK to amplify its normal intracellular, often prooncogenic, functions such as chromatin remodeling, transcriptional repression/activation, DNA damage repair, promoting cell proliferation, and silencing apoptotic pathways. These cellular consequences also have been observed when DEK expression is transcriptionally upregulated within a cell by other mechanisms. One potentially intracellular oncogenic function of DEK is its role as a transcription cofactor for NFκB activity. This regulation of the NFκB signaling pathway, as well as the other chromatin modifying and cell signaling roles of DEK, may provide a mechanistic link between inflammation and tumorigenesis.

3. DEK Expression and Function during Tumorigenesis and Inflammation

As a well-established oncogene, DEK overexpression has been documented in a continually expanding list of malignant neoplasms, including hepatocellular carcinoma, brain cancer, bladder cancer, retinoblastoma, T cell large granular lymphocytic leukemia, breast cancer, cervical cancer, melanoma, chronic lymphocytic leukemia, colon cancer, head and neck squamous cell carcinomas, and prostate cancer [42, 54–65]. *DEK* overexpression is most frequently caused by aberrant transcription via E2F [66], YY1, NF-Y [67], and ER-α transcription factors [68]. Increased *DEK* copy number as a result of gains on 6p22 is also observed in bladder cancer and retinoblastoma [57, 69]. DEK protein degradation can be induced by SPOP and FBXW7-alpha ubiquitin ligases, both of which are tumor suppressors and frequently experience loss-of-function mutations in cancers [49, 65, 70]. High DEK expression, and the presence of the DEK-CAN fusion gene, often correlates with higher grade, aggressive tumors [42, 71], chemoresistance [42, 60, 68, 72, 73], invasion [38, 39, 60], and poor patient prognosis [74–78]. DEK may contribute to these oncogenic activities by an array of different molecular mechanisms. In keratinocytes, DEK overexpression can inhibit senescence and apoptosis by promoting p53 destabilization [41, 79]. DEK overexpression also promotes keratinocyte proliferation while delaying differentiation and can contribute to keratinocyte transformation whereas the DEK-CAN fusion also induces transformation in hematopoietic stem cells [80–82]. In breast cancer cell lines, DEK overexpression promotes cell growth and mobility by inducing β-catenin nuclear translocation and enhances tumor growth and metastasis by activating Wnt/β-catenin autocrine and paracrine signaling loops [38, 39]. DEK depletion in transformed epithelial cells results in DNA damage, senescence, and apoptosis and can reduce ΔNp63 mediated cell growth [38, 41, 64, 82]. $Dek^{-/-}$ mice also demonstrate greatly diminished tumor formation, growth, and metastasis in both genetic and chemically induced tumorigenesis models [39, 64, 82]. Given its numerous functions in cancer cells, it is no surprise that DEK expression could be used as a biomarker for colorectal and bladder cancers and possibly other solid tumors as well [63, 83]. Of future clinical importance, RNA interference-mediated loss of DEK expression causes dramatic apoptosis or senescence of cancer cells whereas differentiated and nontransformed cells remain relatively unharmed [41, 79, 82].

In addition to gene amplification and overexpression in cancers, DEK expression and secretion are also induced in response to inflammation. In BEAS-2B human bronchial epithelial cells, *DEK* mRNA was upregulated in response to exposure to TiO_2 particles, which are fine particles found in industrial workplaces that are known to cause airway inflammation and respiratory symptoms in both acute and chronic exposure situations [84]. In addition, microarray analyses of livers from rats fed crude fish oil, which contained high levels of persistent organic pollutants, showed moderately elevated *DEK* expression [85]. In rodents, prolonged exposure to persistent organic pollutants has been shown to cause insulin resistance and was associated with chronic low-grade inflammation [85, 86]. Although the molecular mechanism for this transcriptional regulation is unknown,

DEK upregulation in response to inflammatory signals is supported by the presence of multiple putative AP-1 (c-Fos/c-Jun), Ets-1, NF-AT, NFκB, STAT4, and C/EBP-*β* transcription factor consensus binding sites in the *DEK* promoter, which are known downstream transcription factors induced by proinflammatory signals (data not shown) [87–89]. Furthermore, secretion of phosphorylated DEK by monocyte-derived macrophages (MDM) is induced by the proinflammatory chemokine interleukin-8 (IL-8) where it becomes a chemotactic factor, attracting neutrophils, CD8+ T lymphocytes, and natural killer cells [44]. Immunosuppressive agents, such as dexamethasone and cyclosporine A, could block the secretion of DEK in MDM cells. This suggests that *DEK* expression, modification, and secretion are induced during inflammation, possibly to mediate cell survival, transcriptional responses, and/or migration of immune cells, which can ultimately result in transformation due to the intracellular oncogenic functions of DEK.

4. The Role of DEK during Infection with Cancer-Associated Viruses

Viral infection results in an inflammatory response and many cancers are known to be driven by oncogenic viruses. Examples of cancers linked to viral infection include cervical and other anogenital cancers, oropharyngeal carcinomas, hepatocellular carcinomas, Kaposi's sarcomas, lymphomas, and T cell leukemia. In many instances, oncogenesis is thought to result from persistent, latent infections in which cell signaling processes are perturbed by either viral proteins or the chronic activation of inflammatory processes.

Cervical cancer and, more recently, head and neck cancer have been found to be associated with human papillomavirus (HPV) infection [90, 91]. Although HPV infection is quite common, in many individuals, the immune system clears the virus. However, in a select few, viral infection becomes persistent likely through the inability of infected cells to present antigenic epitopes to the host's adaptive immune system [92]. Upon additional multiple mutations and carcinogenic events often linked to the viral life cycle, some of these chronically infected individuals will develop epithelial carcinomas. Although in normal HPV infection viral DNA remains episomal, in cancer, HPV is often found to be integrated into the host DNA. Integration leads to loss of the normal viral repressor HPV E2 resulting in uninhibited expression of the viral oncogenes E6 and E7. HPV E6 causes degradation of the tumor suppressor p53 while HPV E7 causes inhibition of the retinoblastoma (Rb) family of proteins, effectively halting major tumor suppressor pathways. Expression of HPV E6 and HPV E7 is required for maintenance of the malignant phenotype. Interestingly, DEK was found to be upregulated by HPV E7 and the suppression of DEK in HPV infected cells resulted in senescence [79, 93]. Additional studies demonstrated that *DEK* was an E2F transcription factor target gene, explaining its upregulation in response to retinoblastoma protein inhibition by E7 [66]. *Dek* knockout (*Dek$^{-/-}$*) mice are resistant to HPV E6 and HPV E7 driven squamous cell carcinomas, supporting a critical role for DEK

function in HPV-induced tumors [64]. Furthermore, DEK mRNA and protein upregulation are present in both cervical and head and neck cancer specimens, further supporting the importance of continued DEK expression in these cancers [59, 79, 94]. Even more intriguing is that although HPV tumors often carry a higher metastatic potential, HPV+ head and neck cancers confer a better prognosis than their HPV− counterparts, due to enhanced responses to treatment [95, 96]. Some have argued that the adaptive immune response associated with HPV infection is the reason for better responses to therapy [97].

Similar to HPV infection, *DEK* expression is also differentially regulated during EBV infections [98]. *DEK* was one of three genes differentially regulated across two EBV+ tumor types and also differentially regulated between nasopharyngeal carcinoma cells with latent and recurrent EBV infections. *DEK* expression was downregulated in recurrent EBV-infected cells but upregulated in latent EBV-infected nasopharyngeal carcinoma (NPC) cells. This provides evidence for *DEK* as a potential viral oncogenic mediator that links EBV latency-reactivation dynamics and cell transformation [98]. This may be the result of a well-documented latent infection response mediated by the Rb-controlled activity of E2F, a known activator of *DEK* expression [66, 99]. This CDK2-Rb/E2F-*DEK* pathway may be a crucial step in EBV-associated transformation of epithelial cells as seen in EBV+ NPC. Furthermore, small DNA tumor viruses, like HPV and EBV, exhibit a common molecular mechanism to inhibit the Rb family of proteins, especially pRb, to drive cellular proliferation, viral replication, and eventually oncogenesis. Therefore, *DEK* upregulation is likely a common event in virally induced tumors.

In addition to being transcriptionally regulated in response to viral infection, DEK also controls the use and maintenance of viral genetic material during human immunodeficiency virus (HIV) and Kaposi's sarcoma-associated herpesvirus (KSHV) infections. Although HIV is not oncogenic, the immune suppression and chronic inflammation it causes dramatically increases the risk of cancer due to coinfection with oncogenic viruses like KSHV, EBV, Hepatitis B and C viruses, and HPV. In addition to binding eukaryotic chromatin, DEK also has unique binding properties that facilitate the use or maintenance of viral genetic material. In the case of HIV, DEK can bind to specific sequences of HIV-2 enhancer regions. These sequences, peri-ets (*pets*) sites, are one of several different *cis*-acting elements of the HIV-2 enhancer that stimulates transcription of viral genes in activated T lymphocytes. Within the HIV-2 enhancer region, the *pets* site contains a TTGGTCAGGG sequence that is found between the two Elf-1 binding sites, PuB1 and PuB2 [100]. DEK specifically binds these *pets* sites in human T lymphocytes, suggesting that DEK can regulate HIV-2 transcription and may be a downstream effector of T cell receptor activation [24]. Further investigation revealed that, upon phorbol ester 12-O-tetradecanoylphorbol-13-acetate (TPA) treatment to activate T cells, DEK is replaced on the *pets* site, in a protein phosphatase-2A (PP2A) dependent manner, with another factor to induce HIV-2 promoter activation.

The process is stymied by PKC inhibitors and/or PP2A inhibitors (such as Okadaic acid), suggesting that PKC mediates the catalytic activity of PP2A, which alters the stability or DNA-binding activity of DEK, possibly via dephosphorylation. This change activated HIV-2 LTR and promotes HIV-2 transcription, assisting in the maintenance of HIV-2 infections [101]. However, it is unclear if the same mechanism exists in HIV-1 infected cells because Okadaic acid, which permits DEK retention on the *pets* sites and inhibits HIV-2 transcription, actually activates HIV-1 transcription.

While the presence of DEK in HIV-infected cells primarily controls viral transcriptional activity in T lymphocytes, the presence of DEK in two herpesvirus family infections (EBV and KSHV) has more implications on the occurrence of viral oncogenesis. In both cases, the virus must maintain genetic material during latency but also ensure that viral genomes are passed during mitosis. In KSHV infections, the latency-associated nuclear antigen (LANA) facilitates the association between mitotic chromosomes and viral genomes so that viral genomes are distributed to host daughter cells during latent infections [102]. Two studies have documented LANA-DEK binding that could have implications on KSHV infections and associated oncogenesis. Verma et al. demonstrated that DEK interacts with LANA *in vitro* [103]. Through GST affinity and immunoprecipitation assays, Krithivas et al. determined that DEK binds to the C-terminus of LANA and that a GFP-DEK fusion protein can be seen specifically localized to chromosomes of mouse cells [102]. These studies suggest that DEK-LANA interactions provide a secondary tethering opportunity for KSHV genomes that enable KSHV latency and DEK-driven oncogenesis. Combined, DEK is an important cellular protein that can regulate the transcription and retention of viral genomes while promoting proliferation to facilitate the viral life cycle. Nonetheless, it is unclear what links these persistent viral infections that require or increase DEK expression and the host's inflammatory responses to the viruses.

5. DEK Is an Autoantigen in Inflammatory Autoimmune Diseases and Cancer

Nearly two dozen autoimmune diseases have been correlated with increased risk for cancer [104]. DEK autoantibodies have been found in the serum and synovial fluid of patients with many different autoimmune disorders including juvenile idiopathic arthritis (JIA), systemic lupus erythematosus (SLE), sarcoidosis, and rheumatoid arthritis [52]. JIA, formerly juvenile rheumatoid arthritis, is characterized by chronic inflammation in one or more joints and is the most common childhood rheumatoid-related condition [105]. SLE primarily affects women and is characterized by severe inflammation that is believed to be caused by a type I interferon mediated positive feedback loop with active B and T lymphocytes [106]. Sarcoidosis usually occurs in the lungs of patients suffering with this systemic granulomatous disease that is characterized by noncaseating granulomas that result from persistent inflammation of unknown origins [107].

DEK was first described as an autoantigen in JIA patients when the presence of DEK specific antibodies correlated with different subtypes of the condition, most frequently seen in pauciarticular onset JIA in 77% of tested patients. The presence of DEK antibodies in JIA patient serum and synovial fluid was later confirmed by several other groups; one revealed a similar percentage of anti-DEK(+) JIA patients at 57% [108, 109]. In addition to anti-DEK autoantibodies, which are produced by B cells, T cells may also become falsely activated in autoimmune diseases through the presentation of DEK peptides by HLA-A molecules. Specific DEK amino acid sequences (72–80, 163–171, and 155–153) can bind the HLA-A*0201 subclass associated with the pauciarticular subtype of JIA. This suggests that DEK may form complexes with class I MHC molecules which may provide a mechanism by which antigen presenting cells induce CD8+ stimulation to elicit inflammation events seen in JIA patients [110]. This is further supported in patients with the correlation between positivity for DEK antibodies and the presence of the class I HLA-A2 allele [108]. Furthermore, DEK can also be secreted by synovial macrophages, further compounding inflammatory pathogenesis. The C-terminal region of the secreted form of DEK, which is often acetylated, is recognized by IgG2 antibody complexes. These interactions demonstrate a second potential role for DEK in IgG-complement activation in the mediation of immune responses [111]. Additionally, multiallelic marker genotyping and SNP genotyping revealed that the $3'$ UTR of *DEK* was associated with rheumatoid arthritis susceptibility, further supporting evidence that DEK may be a crucial component of arthritis related chronic inflammation [112].

Several early studies discovered anti-DEK antibodies in the serum of patients with SLE and/or sarcoidosis [108, 113, 114]. Wichmann et al. found that 10.4% of tested SLE patients had DEK specific autoantibodies in their serum. The presence of the anti-DEK antibodies was associated with older patients and fewer cutaneous manifestations [115]. Dong et al. provided a broad screening of sera from patients with an array of inflammation-related conditions. They identified elevated frequency of anti-DEK positivity not only in JIA, SLE, sarcoidosis, and rheumatoid arthritis patient sera but also in systemic sclerosis, polymyositis, and tuberculosis patient sera [52]. These studies illuminate the potentially broad role of DEK in inflammation-related functions and interactions during infection and immune responses. However, the role of DEK in these interactions can also have substantial implications in cancer biology and tumor microenvironments.

The multifunctionality of DEK in immune cells and cancer cells suggests a paradoxical outcome in tumor biology. As previously discussed, elevated DEK can promote oncogenic activities in infected and uninfected cells; however, DEK also displays an affinity for inducing immune responses in local areas of expression. There are several mechanisms by which DEK may mediate inflammation and tumor immunity responses in tumor microenvironments. These include (1) transcriptional regulation of antigen presenting molecules [116], (2) stimulation of T cells by epitope presentation [117, 118], and (3) secretion into extracellular matrix [44, 53]. First,

DEK has the potential to regulate class II MHC expression by interacting with NF-Y and binding Y-box promoter elements unique to MHC class II alleles [116]. This role as a transcriptional regulator could influence the presentation of tumor-related antigens to CD4+ T cells and thus contribute to adaptive immune responses targeting tumor cells. Second, DEK may be a tumor-associated antigen. Dendritic cells loaded with DEK-CAN AML associated fusion proteins can present DEK epitopes via class II MHC molecules and stimulate specific CD4+ T-cells in coculture [118]. The capacity of DEK to stimulate CD8+ T cells was also documented *in vivo* and *in vitro* [117]. In this study, *DEK* was the only oncogenic transcript identified multiple times in a screening of genes possibly involved in an immune response against neuroblastoma. In subsequent experiments, mice received a T cell stimulant and a Treg inhibitor to enable self-antigen specific immune responses. *In vivo*, this combination increases DEK-specific IgG antibodies found in the serum. *In vitro*, CD8+ T cells from these mice showed elevated activity when cocultured with DEK-loaded macrophages or neuroblastoma cells. Together these three studies implicate DEK as a tumor-associated antigen that may mediate interactions between lymphocytes and tumor cells. Third, and finally, DEK secretion by macrophages also has two major implications on potential tumor microenvironments. As a proinflammatory chemoattractant, secreted DEK can stimulate white blood cell migration, including neutrophils, CD8+ lymphocytes, and natural killer (NK) cells [44]. The implications for this activity in the context of tumorigenic microenvironments are poorly understood. While tumor-associated macrophages and neutrophils are primarily known to promote tumorigenesis [119], CD8+ T cells and NK cells are likely antitumorigenic [120, 121]. Secreted DEK can also be internalized by DEK-deficient HeLa cells, in a heparan sulfate-dependent process, where it can function as a nuclear oncoprotein and rescue DEK depletion-induced DNA-damage repair and heterochromatin integrity [53]. Interestingly, macrophages are not the only cells to secrete DEK; conditioned media from HepG2 hepatocellular carcinoma cells were also found to contain DEK peptides [122, 123]. These results illuminate the potential role for extracellular DEK to stimulate tumor-associated immunological responses and promote intracellular oncogenic activity in neighboring epithelial cells within the tumor microenvironment.

6. DEK Regulates NFκB Transcriptional Activity

Through multiple mechanisms, DEK can regulate the activity of numerous oncogenic signal transduction pathways. These include p53 family members, p53 and ΔNp63, to inhibit apoptosis and promote proliferation, respectively, Wnt/β-catenin signaling to drive proliferation and invasion, Rho signaling to promote migration, mTOR activity to enhance cellular proliferation, and the NFκB pathway [38, 39, 41, 64, 124–127]. The nuclear factor kappa-light-chain-enhancer of activated B cells (NFκB) family of transcription factors regulates gene expression in response to a variety of external stress and inflammatory stimuli. The NFκB family includes RelA (p65), RelB, c-Rel, p100/p52 (NFκB2), and p105/p50 (NFκB1). These transcription factors are activated as a result of environmental stimuli that include cytokines like tumor necrosis factor alpha (TNFα), markers of microbial infection like lipopolysaccharide (LPS), T cell and B cell antigen receptors, and genotoxic stress including radiation and reactive oxygen species. The acute presence of these stress signals rapidly activates cell surface receptors, which eventually result in the activation of IκB kinase (IKK2) in a NEMO-dependent mechanism. IKK then phosphorylates IκB, which triggers its ubiquitination and degradation. The degradation of IκB thus releases its inhibitory binding of NFκB/RelA, permitting the nuclear translocation of the transcription factor complex, where it then binds to transcription cofactors to direct gene expression. In response to these acute stress stimuli, NFκB/Rel family members transcribe genes such as growth factors, inhibitors of apoptosis, and cytokines, primarily through RelA:RelA, c-Rel:p50, and RelA:p50 dimers [128]. This canonical NFκB pathway thus promotes cellular proliferation, inflammation, and immunity to survive the environmental stress. In contrast, the noncanonical NFκB pathway utilizes a NEMO-independent kinase complex that includes IKK1 and NFκB-inducing kinase (NIK) to respond to sustained developmental signals. This noncanonical pathway primarily utilizes RelB:p50 or RelB:p52 complexes, although RelA:p50 dimers may also be involved, to cause cell differentiation during development [129].

NFκB signaling is a crucial pathway involved in both inflammation and tumorigenesis, which is underscored by the finding that patients with chronic inflammatory conditions have an increased risk for developing cancer. The prosurvival functions of NFκB signaling promote tumor cell viability whereas the cytokines that are produced by NFκB transcriptional activity will alter the antitumor immune response. Furthermore, NFκB activity can promote angiogenesis and metastasis and has implications for genome stability [130]. Thus, the proproliferative and prosurvival canonical NFκB signaling pathway may be oncogenic if constitutively activated, which can occur through either activating mutations within the pathway or chronic exposure to cytokines from tumor associated macrophages within the microenvironment [130, 131]. However, the prodifferentiation function of NFκB signaling may be tumor suppressive. In fact, the oncogenic versus tumor suppressive functions of NFκB signaling may be context- and tissue-specific. For example, activated NFκB signaling has been documented in lymphoid malignancies and inflammation-associated colon cancer and other solid tumors. However, inactivated NFκB signaling through the loss of IKK proteins has also been linked to tumorigenesis, suggesting some tumor suppressive functions. These include genetic and chemically induced mouse tumor models and studies of squamous cell carcinomas of the skin, lungs, and head and neck [132, 133]. Interestingly, a recent report by Wang et al. suggests that NFκB signaling may begin as a tumor suppressive pathway in mouse embryonic fibroblasts (MEFs), by promoting cell senescence and maintaining genome stability, as determined using $p65^{-/-}$ MEFs.

NFκB signaling can then switch to a tumor promoting pathway as cells undergo transformation, such as the introduction of mutant Ras^{G12V} into the MEFs, by allowing the transformed cells to avoid macrophage-induced cell death and evading other antitumor immunity activities *in vivo* [134]. Thus, the role of NFκB signaling in tumorigenesis is complex and dynamic.

DEK has been identified as a downstream target of noncanonical NFκB signaling. In normal human dermal fibroblasts, the loss of noncanonical pathway members NFκB2 and RelB by siRNA resulted in decreased *DEK* mRNA and protein levels, which was associated with cellular senescence, in a p53-dependent mechanism [135]. The loss of p53 by shRNA restored DEK expression in NFκB2 and RelB-deficient cells and prevented senescence induced by the DEK depletion [135]. This suggests that p53 and noncanonical NFκB signaling converge on the *DEK* promoter to decide cell fate.

Previous reports have demonstrated that DEK can function as both transcription factor coactivator and corepressor [33, 125, 136–138]. Sammons et al. were the first to report on DEK-mediated regulation of canonical NFκB signaling using MEFs, HEK293T, and HeLa cells. It was found that *Dek*$^{-/-}$ MEFs had elevated baseline and TNFα-induced levels of the NFκB inhibitor, IκBα, although the phosphorylation status of IκBα was not investigated. *Dek*$^{-/-}$ MEFs also had increased luciferase expression from a NFκB-reporter construct and enhanced TNFα-induced transcription of the NFκB target gene and inflammatory chemokine *monocyte chemoattractant protein-1* (*MCP-1/CCL-2*). Furthermore, *Dek*$^{-/-}$ MEFs demonstrated increased TNFα-induced p65 (RelA) localization to the *MCP-1* and *IκBα* promoters [125].

In transformed cells, including Caski and HeLa cervical carcinomas, the loss of DEK by shRNA caused increased phosphorylation of IκBα. This was accompanied by the subsequent nuclear translocation and DNA-binding of p65 and increased luciferase reporter activity [124, 139]. Furthermore, in HeLa cells, DEK and p65 colocalized to multiple NFκB target gene promoters, including *1-cys-peroxiredoxin*, *c-IAP2*, and *IL-8* [125, 139]. Interestingly, TNFα treatment induced endogenous DEK-p65 colocalization at *c-IAP2* and *IL-8* promoters. This was accompanied by an increase in *c-IAP2* and *IL-8* mRNA levels [125]. However, when DEK was overexpressed in HeLa cells, there was a gradual dose-dependent inhibition of p65 transcriptional activity [125, 139]. In particular, overexpression of the C-terminal DEK DNA binding domain demonstrated inhibitory activity based on *1-cys-peroxiredoxin* luciferase reporter activity. In contrast, overexpression of the N-terminal 200 amino acids of DEK, which includes the SAP/ΨSAP DNA binding domains, were capable of activating reporter expression [139]. It is worth mentioning that there is a dose-effect observed with DEK expression and cell viability. Optimal cellular proliferation is observed at DEK levels slightly (2–5 fold) over those observed in normal cells, similar to the endogenous levels of DEK in HeLa cells. Both the loss of DEK by shRNA and the gross overexpression of DEK are detrimental and cause caspase-dependent apoptosis [38, 40–42, 140, 141] (and data not shown). Since the mechanism of apoptosis induced

by extreme changes in DEK expression is unclear, studies regarding the activity of specific transcription factors in response to DEK expression levels should be approached with caution. However, the data still supports a role for DEK in modulating RelA transcriptional activity in canonical NFκB signaling.

Combined, the data suggest that DEK may provide a dose-dependent mechanism for controlling p65/RelA transcriptional activity in the canonical NFκB pathway (Figure 1). In extreme excess, DEK inhibits NFκB signaling, which may lead to decreased survival. However, tumorigenic (modestly upregulated) levels of DEK may promote NFκB transcriptional activity through direct interactions with p65/RelA on gene promoters to induce expression of antiapoptotic genes like *c-IAP2* and prometastasis genes like *IL-8*. In contrast, the loss of DEK can upregulate NFκB activity through upstream regulation of IκBα, which may correlate with an inflammatory or immune response as suggested by *MCP-1* expression. Taken together, DEK is an important regulator of NFκB signaling to direct expression of both tumorigenic and proinflammatory target genes.

7. Summary

There is a growing understanding of the complex relationship between the immune system, inflammation, and tumorigenesis. Chronic inflammation is a well-known risk factor for tumor development, especially with epithelial tissues. This is likely due to either the highly oxidative environment during inflammation that can cause DNA damage and/or the creation of a highly vascularized growth factor-rich microenvironment resulting in a tumor-promoting stroma [142]. Various factors induce chronic inflammation including persistent bacterial and viral infections, exposure to environmental pollutants, and inflammatory autoimmune diseases. In addition to the creation of the tumor-promoting environment due to the immune response described above, the molecules produced by the immune system, like ROS and TNFα, can activate intracellular signaling pathways in the neighboring epithelial cells. One such example is the NFκB pathway, which responds to inflammatory signals and promotes cell survival. When constitutively activated, such as what may occur with chronic inflammation, NFκB signaling can promote tumorigenesis.

Here, we describe an oncogenic protein that is critically involved in infection, inflammation, and tumorigenesis. The chromatin modeling DEK protein has numerous roles that promote inflammation. These include (1) promoting the life cycles and latent infection with oncogenic viruses like HPV and EBV, (2) increased expression upon exposure to environmental pollutants, potentially to promote DNA repair or cell survival, (3) being a potent self-antigen in chronic inflammatory autoimmune diseases like arthritis and lupus, and (4) functioning as a proinflammatory chemoattractant to promote the migration of white blood cells when secreted by activated macrophages. These functions, whether they result in DEK overexpression or the internalization of excess

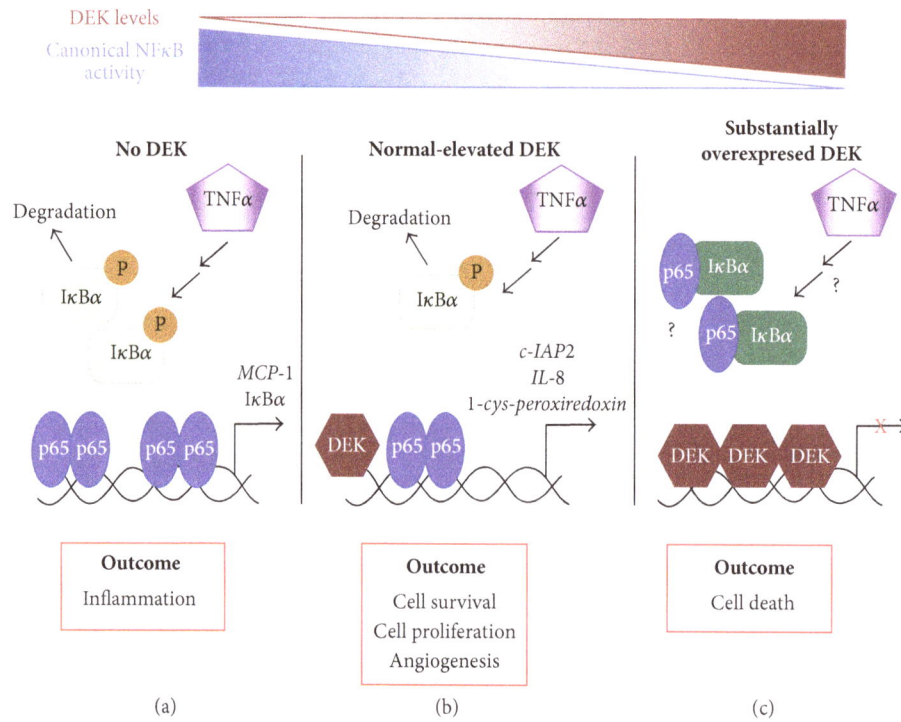

FIGURE 1: DEK-mediated regulation of NFκB pathway activity in a dose-dependent manner. As DEK expression increases (red), canonical NFκB transcriptional activity decreases (blue). (a) In the absence of DEK, there is increased phosphorylation of IκBa, which leads to its degradation and the translocation of p65/RelA to the nucleus where it is transcribes proinflammatory target genes like *MCP-1*. (b) In cells with endogenous levels of DEK, possibly in both normal and transformed cells, DEK colocalization with p65 on target gene promoters is induced by TNFα treatment. This results in the expression of potentially oncogenic, prosurvival target genes like *c-IAP2*. However, it is unknown how variations in DEK levels within this group, such as the difference between normal and transformed cells, may impact NFκB activity and the subsequent expression of various target genes. (c) When DEK is substantially overexpressed beyond physiological levels, such as what may occur when overexpressing DEK in already high-expressing transformed cell lines, NFκB activity is inhibited, which may trigger cell death.

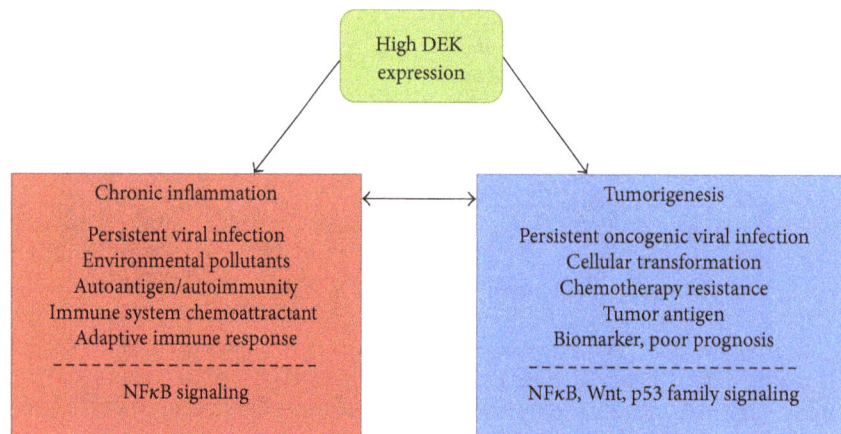

FIGURE 2: A summary of the roles of DEK in inflammation and tumorigenesis. DEK promotes inflammatory processes like persistent viral infection and autoimmune diseases, possibly through NFκB signaling (left). High DEK levels also promote tumor growth, metastasis, chemotherapeutic response, and an overall poor prognosis, which correlates with the activity of many oncogenic molecular mechanisms including Wnt/β-catenin, mTOR, Rho, and NFκB signaling as well as regulating expression of p53 family members (right). Chronic inflammation, supported by DEK expression, may promote tumorigenesis.

secreted DEK by neighboring epithelial cells, can promote DEK-induced tumorigenesis (Figure 2). Elevated intracellular DEK levels are oncogenic, resulting in increased proliferation, migration, and resistance to genotoxic agents via the perturbation of several signal transduction pathways. It is unclear how DEK mediates these pathogenic and oncogenic cellular and molecular functions, although it is likely due, in part, to its ability to alter chromatin accessibility and transcription factor function, thus deregulating the expression of numerous target genes. The downstream pathways that are affected by DEK protein levels and DEK-induced transcriptional deregulation include p53, Wnt/β-catenin, mTor, Rho, and NFκB signaling. Importantly, DEK can modulate the transcriptional activity of the NFκB pathway in response to proinflammatory signals like TNFα in what may be a dose- or context-specific mechanism. Combined, DEK can promote both chronic inflammation and tumorigenesis in a multifaceted manner and has been implicated in numerous disease processes. This suggests that limiting DEK levels may be a desirable way to treat both chronic inflammation, due to viral infection or autoimmune disease, and cancer.

Conflict of Interests

The authors declare that there is no conflict of interests regarding the publication of this paper.

References

[1] K. Warzocha, P. Ribeiro, J. Bienvenu et al., "Genetic polymorphisms in the tumor necrosis factor locus influence non-Hodgkin's lymphoma outcome," *Blood*, vol. 91, no. 10, pp. 3574–3581, 1998.

[2] E. M. El-Omar, M. Carrington, W. H. Chow et al., "Interleukin-1 polymorphisms associated with increased risk of gastric cancer," *Nature*, vol. 404, no. 6776, pp. 398–402, 2000.

[3] W. H. Wang, J. Q. Huang, G. F. Zheng, S. K. Lam, J. Karlberg, and B. C.-Y. Wong, "Non-steroidal anti-inflammatory drug use and the risk of gastric cancer: a systematic review and meta-analysis," *Journal of the National Cancer Institute*, vol. 95, no. 23, pp. 1784–1791, 2003.

[4] C. Hur, N. S. Nishioka, and G. S. Gazelle, "Cost-effectiveness of aspirin chemoprevention for Barrett's esophagus," *Journal of the National Cancer Institute*, vol. 96, no. 4, pp. 316–325, 2004.

[5] E. T. Chang, T. Zheng, E. G. Weir et al., "Aspirin and the risk of Hodgkin's lymphoma in a population-based case-control study," *Journal of the National Cancer Institute*, vol. 96, no. 4, pp. 305–315, 2004.

[6] E. S. Schernhammer, J.-H. Kang, A. T. Chan et al., "A prospective study of aspirin use and the risk of pancreatic cancer in women," *Journal of the National Cancer Institute*, vol. 96, no. 1, pp. 22–28, 2004.

[7] L. M. Duncan, L. A. Richards, and M. C. Mihm Jr., "Increased mast cell density in invasive melanoma," *Journal of Cutaneous Pathology*, vol. 25, no. 1, pp. 11–15, 1998.

[8] A. Näsman, M. Romanitan, C. Nordfors et al., "Tumor infiltrating CD8$^+$ and Foxp3$^+$ lymphocytes correlate to clinical outcome and human papillomavirus (HPV) status in tonsillar cancer," *PLoS ONE*, vol. 7, no. 6, Article ID e38711, 2012.

[9] X. Guo, Y. Fan, R. Lang et al., "Tumor infiltrating lymphocytes differ in invasive micropapillary carcinoma and medullary carcinoma of breast," *Modern Pathology*, vol. 21, no. 9, pp. 1101–1107, 2008.

[10] J. R. Kim, Y. J. Moon, K. S. Kwon et al., "Tumor infiltrating PD1-positive lymphocytes and the expression of PD-L1 predict poor prognosis of soft tissue sarcomas," *PLoS ONE*, vol. 8, no. 12, Article ID e82870, 2013.

[11] M. J. Kang, K. M. Kim, J. S. Bae et al., "Tumor-infiltrating PD1-positive lymphocytes and FoxP3-positive regulatory T cells predict distant metastatic relapse and survival of clear cell renal cell carcinoma," *Translational Oncology*, vol. 6, no. 3, pp. 282–289, 2013.

[12] T. S. Malaspina, T. H. Gasparoto, M. R. S. N. Costa et al., "Enhanced programmed death 1 (PD-1) and PD-1 ligand (PD-L1) expression in patients with actinic cheilitis and oral squamous cell carcinoma," *Cancer Immunology, Immunotherapy*, vol. 60, no. 7, pp. 965–974, 2011.

[13] R. Hino, K. Kabashima, Y. Kato et al., "Tumor cell expression of programmed cell death-1 ligand 1 is a prognostic factor for malignant melanoma," *Cancer*, vol. 116, no. 7, pp. 1757–1766, 2010.

[14] C. Robert, G. V. Long, B. Brady et al., "Nivolumab in previously untreated melanoma without BRAF mutation," *The New England Journal of Medicine*, vol. 372, pp. 320–330, 2015.

[15] R. M. Poole and R. T. Dungo, "Ipragliflozin: first global approval," *Drugs*, vol. 74, no. 5, pp. 611–617, 2014.

[16] F. S. Hodi, S. J. O'Day, D. F. McDermott et al., "Improved survival with ipilimumab in patients with metastatic melanoma," *The New England Journal of Medicine*, vol. 363, no. 8, pp. 711–723, 2010.

[17] F. Balkwill and A. Mantovani, "Inflammation and cancer: back to Virchow?" *Lancet*, vol. 357, no. 9255, pp. 539–545, 2001.

[18] M. Karin and F. R. Greten, "NF-κB: linking inflammation and immunity to cancer development and progression," *Nature Reviews Immunology*, vol. 5, no. 10, pp. 749–759, 2005.

[19] M. Fornerod, J. Boer, S. van Baal et al., "Relocation of the carboxyterminal part of CAN from the nuclear envelope to the nucleus as a result of leukemia-specific chromosome rearrangements," *Oncogene*, vol. 10, no. 9, pp. 1739–1748, 1995.

[20] F. Kappes, I. Scholten, N. Richter, C. Gruss, and T. Waldmann, "Functional domains of the ubiquitous chromatin protein DEK," *Molecular and Cellular Biology*, vol. 24, no. 13, pp. 6000–6010, 2004.

[21] M. von Lindern, M. Fornerod, S. van Baal et al., "The translocation (6;9), associated with a specific subtype of acute myeloid leukemia, results in the fusion of two genes, dek and can, and the expression of a chimeric, leukemia-specific dek-can mRNA," *Molecular and Cellular Biology*, vol. 12, no. 4, pp. 1687–1697, 1992.

[22] M. S. Meyn, J. M. Lu-Kuo, and L. B. K. Herzing, "Expression cloning of multiple human cDNAs that complement the phenotypic defects of ataxia-telangiectasia group D fibroblasts," *The American Journal of Human Genetics*, vol. 53, no. 6, pp. 1206–1216, 1993.

[23] V. Alexiadis, T. Waldmann, J. Andersen, M. Mann, R. Knippers, and C. Gruss, "The protein encoded by the proto-oncogene DEK changes the topology of chromatin and reduces the efficiency of DNA replication in a chromatin-specific manner," *Genes & Development*, vol. 14, no. 11, pp. 1308–1312, 2000.

[24] G. K. Fu, G. Grosveld, and D. M. Markovitz, "DEK, an autoantigen involved in a chromosomal translocation in acute myelogenous leukemia, binds to the HIV-2 enhancer," *Proceedings of the National Academy of Sciences of the United States of America*, vol. 94, no. 5, pp. 1811–1815, 1997.

[25] A. D. Hollenbach, C. J. McPherson, E. J. Mientjes, R. Iyengar, and G. Grosveld, "Daxx and histone deacetylase II associate with chromatin through an interaction with core histones and the chromatin-associated protein Dek," *Journal of Cell Science*, vol. 115, no. 16, pp. 3319–3330, 2002.

[26] F. Kappes, K. Burger, M. Baack, F. O. Fackelmayer, and C. Gruss, "Subcellular localization of the human proto-oncogene protein DEK," *Journal of Biological Chemistry*, vol. 276, no. 28, pp. 26317–26323, 2001.

[27] T. Waldmann, C. Eckerich, M. Baack, and C. Gruss, "The ubiquitous chromatin protein DEK alters the structure of DNA by introducing positive supercoils," *Journal of Biological Chemistry*, vol. 277, no. 28, pp. 24988–24994, 2002.

[28] F. Böhm, F. Kappes, I. Scholten et al., "The SAF-box domain of chromatin protein DEK," *Nucleic Acids Research*, vol. 33, no. 3, pp. 1101–1110, 2005.

[29] H.-G. Hu, H. Illges, C. Gruss, and R. Knippers, "Distribution of the chromatin protein DEK distinguishes active and inactive CD21/CR2 gene in pre- and mature B lymphocytes," *International Immunology*, vol. 17, no. 6, pp. 789–796, 2005.

[30] T. Waldmann, M. Baack, N. Richter, and C. Gruss, "Structure-specific binding of the proto-oncogene protein DEK to DNA," *Nucleic Acids Research*, vol. 31, no. 23, pp. 7003–7010, 2003.

[31] S.-I. Ko, I.-S. Lee, J.-Y. Kim et al., "Regulation of histone acetyltransferase activity of p300 and PCAF by proto-oncogene protein DEK," *FEBS Letters*, vol. 580, no. 13, pp. 3217–3222, 2006.

[32] K. Ivanauskiene, E. Delbarre, J. D. McGhie, T. Küntziger, L. H. Wong, and P. Collas, "The PML-associated protein DEK regulates the balance of H3.3 loading on chromatin and is important for telomere integrity," *Genome Research*, vol. 24, no. 10, pp. 1584–1594, 2014.

[33] S. Sawatsubashi, T. Murata, J. Lim et al., "A histone chaperone, DEK, transcriptionally coactivates a nuclear receptor," *Genes & Development*, vol. 24, no. 2, pp. 159–170, 2010.

[34] F. Kappes, T. Waldmann, V. Mathew et al., "The DEK oncoprotein is a Su(var) that is essential to heterochromatin integrity," *Genes & Development*, vol. 25, no. 7, pp. 673–678, 2011.

[35] M. J. Gamble and R. P. Fisher, "SET and PARP1 remove DEK from chromatin to permit access by the transcription machinery," *Nature Structural and Molecular Biology*, vol. 14, no. 6, pp. 548–555, 2007.

[36] H.-G. Hu, I. Scholten, C. Gruss, and R. Knippers, "The distribution of the DEK protein in mammalian chromatin," *Biochemical and Biophysical Research Communications*, vol. 358, no. 4, pp. 1008–1014, 2007.

[37] C. Sandén, L. Järvstråt, A. Lennartsson, P. Brattås, B. Nilsson, and U. Gullberg, "The DEK oncoprotein binds to highly and ubiquitously expressed genes with a dual role in their transcriptional regulation," *Molecular Cancer*, vol. 13, no. 1, article 215, 2014.

[38] L. M. Privette Vinnedge, R. McClaine, P. K. Wagh, K. A. Wikenheiser-Brokamp, S. E. Waltz, and S. I. Wells, "The human DEK oncogene stimulates B-catenin signaling, invasion and mammosphere formation in breast cancer," *Oncogene*, vol. 30, no. 24, pp. 2741–2752, 2011.

[39] L. M. Privette Vinnedge, N. M. Benight, P. K. Wagh et al., "The DEK oncogene promotes cellular proliferation through paracrine Wnt signaling in Ron receptor-positive breast cancers," *Oncogene*, 2014.

[40] G. M. Kavanaugh, T. M. Wise-Draper, R. J. Morreale et al., "The human DEK oncogene regulates DNA damage response

signaling and repair," *Nucleic Acids Research*, vol. 39, no. 17, pp. 7465–7476, 2011.

[41] T. M. Wise-Draper, H. V. Allen, E. E. Jones, K. B. Habash, H. Matsuo, and S. I. Wells, "Apoptosis inhibition by the human DEK oncoprotein involves interference with p53 functions," *Molecular and Cellular Biology*, vol. 26, no. 20, pp. 7506–7519, 2006.

[42] M. S. Khodadoust, M. Verhaegen, F. Kappes et al., "Melanoma proliferation and chemoresistance controlled by the DEK oncogene," *Cancer Research*, vol. 69, no. 16, pp. 6405–6413, 2009.

[43] F. Kappes, C. Damoc, R. Knippers, M. Przybylski, L. A. Pinna, and C. Gruss, "Phosphorylation by protein kinase CK2 changes the DNA binding properties of the human chromatin protein DEK," *Molecular and Cellular Biology*, vol. 24, no. 13, pp. 6011–6020, 2004.

[44] N. Mor-Vaknin, A. Punturieri, K. Sitwala et al., "The DEK nuclear autoantigen is a secreted chemotactic factor," *Molecular and Cellular Biology*, vol. 26, no. 24, pp. 9484–9496, 2006.

[45] J. Cleary, K. V. Sitwala, M. S. Khodadoust et al., "p300/CBP-associated factor drives DEK into interchromatin granule clusters," *The Journal of Biological Chemistry*, vol. 280, no. 36, pp. 31760–31767, 2005.

[46] F. Kappes, J. Fahrer, M. S. Khodadoust et al., "DEK is a poly(ADP-ribose) acceptor in apoptosis and mediates resistance to genotoxic stress," *Molecular and Cellular Biology*, vol. 28, no. 10, pp. 3245–3257, 2008.

[47] H. E. Broxmeyer, N. Mor-Vaknin, F. Kappes et al., "Concise review: role of DEK in stem/progenitor cell biology," *Stem Cells*, vol. 31, no. 8, pp. 1447–1453, 2013.

[48] T. McGarvey, E. Rosonina, S. McCracken et al., "The acute myeloid leukemia-associated protein, DEK, forms a splicing-dependent interaction with exon-product complexes," *Journal of Cell Biology*, vol. 150, no. 2, pp. 309–320, 2000.

[49] R. Babaei-Jadidi, N. Li, A. Saadeddin et al., "FBXW7 influences murine intestinal homeostasis and cancer, targeting Notch, Jun, and DEK for degradation," *The Journal of Experimental Medicine*, vol. 208, no. 2, pp. 295–312, 2011.

[50] H. le Hir, D. Gatfield, E. Izaurralde, and M. J. Moore, "The exon-exon junction complex provides a binding platform for factors involved in mRNA export and nonsense-mediated mRNA decay," *The EMBO Journal*, vol. 20, no. 17, pp. 4987–4997, 2001.

[51] L. M. M. Soares, K. Zanier, C. Mackereth, M. Sattler, and J. Valcárcel, "Intron removal requires proofreading of U2AF/3′ splice site recognition by DEK," *Science*, vol. 312, no. 5782, pp. 1961–1965, 2006.

[52] X. Dong, J. Wang, F. N. Kabir et al., "Autoantibodies to DEK oncoprotein in human inflammatory disease," *Arthritis & Rheumatology*, vol. 43, no. 1, pp. 85–93, 2000.

[53] A. K. Saha, F. Kappes, A. Mundade et al., "Intercellular trafficking of the nuclear oncoprotein DEK," *Proceedings of the National Academy of Sciences of the United States of America*, vol. 110, no. 17, pp. 6847–6852, 2013.

[54] N. Kondoh, T. Wakatsuki, R. Akihide et al., "Identification and characterization of genes associated with human hepatocellular carcinogenesis," *Cancer Research*, vol. 59, no. 19, pp. 4990–4996, 1999.

[55] R. A. Kroes, A. Jastrow, M. G. McLone et al., "The identification of novel therapeutic targets for the treatment of malignant brain tumors," *Cancer Letters*, vol. 156, no. 2, pp. 191–198, 2000.

[56] M. Sanchez-Carbayo, N. D. Socci, J. J. Lozano et al., "Gene discovery in bladder cancer progression using cDNA microarrays,"

The American Journal of Pathology, vol. 163, no. 2, pp. 505–516, 2003.

[57] C. Grasemann, S. Gratias, H. Stephan et al., "Gains and overexpression identify *DEK* and *E2F3* as targets of chromosome 6p gains in retinoblastoma," *Oncogene*, vol. 24, no. 42, pp. 6441–6449, 2005.

[58] M. C. Abba, H. Sun, K. A. Hawkins et al., "Breast cancer molecular signatures as determined by SAGE: correlation with lymph node status," *Molecular Cancer Research*, vol. 5, no. 9, pp. 881–890, 2007.

[59] Q. Wu, Z. Li, H. Lin, L. Han, S. Liu, and Z. Lin, "DEK overexpression in uterine cervical cancers," *Pathology International*, vol. 58, no. 6, pp. 378–382, 2008.

[60] H. A. Sansing, A. Sarkeshik, J. R. Yates et al., "Integrin $\alpha\beta1$, $\alpha_v\beta$, $\alpha_6\beta$ effectors p130Cas, Src and talin regulate carcinoma invasion and chemoresistance," *Biochemical and Biophysical Research Communications*, vol. 406, no. 2, pp. 171–176, 2011.

[61] F. Kappes, M. S. Khodadoust, L. Yu et al., "DEK expression in melanocytic lesions," *Human Pathology*, vol. 42, no. 7, pp. 932–938, 2011.

[62] Y. Aalto, W. El-Rifai, L. Vilpo et al., "Distinct gene expression profiling in chronic lymphocytic leukemia with 11q23 deletion," *Leukemia*, vol. 15, no. 11, pp. 1721–1728, 2001.

[63] L. Lin, J. Piao, W. Gao et al., "DEK over expression as an independent biomarker for poor prognosis in colorectal cancer," *BMC Cancer*, vol. 13, article 366, 2013.

[64] A. K. Adams, G. E. Hallenbeck, K. A. Casper et al., "DEK promotes HPV-positive and -negative head and neck cancer cell proliferation," *Oncogene*, vol. 34, pp. 868–877, 2015.

[65] J.-P. P. Theurillat, N. D. Udeshi, W. J. Errington et al., "Ubiquitylome analysis identifies dysregulation of effector substrates in SPOP-mutant prostate cancer," *Science*, vol. 346, no. 6205, pp. 85–89, 2014.

[66] M. S. Carro, F. M. Spiga, M. Quarto et al., "DEK expression is controlled by E2F and deregulated in diverse tumor types," *Cell Cycle*, vol. 5, no. 11, pp. 1202–1207, 2006.

[67] K. V. Sitwala, K. Adams, and D. M. Markovitz, "YY1 and NF-Y binding sites regulate the transcriptional activity of the *dek* and *dek*-can promoter," *Oncogene*, vol. 21, no. 57, pp. 8862–8870, 2002.

[68] L. M. Privette Vinnedge, S. M. Ho, K. A. Wikenheiser-Brokamp, and S. I. Wells, "The DEK oncogene is a target of steroid hormone receptor signaling in breast cancer," *PLoS ONE*, vol. 7, no. 10, Article ID e46985, 2012.

[69] A. J. Evans, B. L. Gallie, M. A. S. Jewett et al., "Defining a 0.5-mb region of genomic gain on chromosome 6p22 in bladder cancer by quantitative-multiplex polymerase chain reaction," *The American Journal of Pathology*, vol. 164, no. 1, pp. 285–293, 2004.

[70] C. C. Chang, H. H. Lin, J. K. Lin et al., "FBXW7 mutation analysis and its correlation with clinicopathological features and prognosis in colorectal cancer patients," *The International Journal of Biological Markers*, vol. 30, no. 1, pp. e88–e95, 2015.

[71] S. Liu, X. Wang, F. Sun, J. Kong, Z. Li, and Z. Lin, "DEK overexpression is correlated with the clinical features of breast cancer," *Pathology International*, vol. 62, no. 3, pp. 176–181, 2012.

[72] A. Deutzmann, M. Ganz, F. Schönenberger, J. Vervoorts, F. Kappes, and E. Ferrando-May, "The human oncoprotein and chromatin architectural factor DEK counteracts DNA replication stress," *Oncogene*, 2014.

[73] E. Riveiro-Falkenbach and M. S. Soengas, "Control of tumorigenesis and chemoresistance by the DEK oncogene," *Clinical Cancer Research*, vol. 16, no. 11, pp. 2932–2938, 2010.

[74] J. Piao, Y. Shang, S. Liu et al., "High expression of DEK predicts poor prognosis of gastric adenocarcinoma," *Diagnostic Pathology*, vol. 9, no. 1, article 67, 2014.

[75] X. Wang, L. Lin, X. Ren et al., "High expression of oncoprotein DEK predicts poor prognosis of small cell lung cancer," *International Journal of Clinical and Experimental Pathology*, vol. 7, pp. 5016–5023, 2014.

[76] H. C. Yi, Y. L. Liu, P. You et al., "Overexpression of DEK gene is correlated with poor prognosis in hepatocellular carcinoma," *Molecular Medicine Reports*, vol. 11, no. 2, pp. 1318–1323, 2015.

[77] L. Garçon, M. Libura, E. Delabesse et al., "DEK-CAN molecular monitoring of myeloid malignancies could aid therapeutic stratification," *Leukemia*, vol. 19, no. 8, pp. 1338–1344, 2005.

[78] T. Shibata, A. Kokubu, M. Miyamoto et al., "DEK oncoprotein regulates transcriptional modifiers and sustains tumor initiation activity in high-grade neuroendocrine carcinoma of the lung," *Oncogene*, vol. 29, no. 33, pp. 4671–4681, 2010.

[79] T. M. Wise-Draper, H. V. Allen, M. N. Thobe et al., "The human DEK proto-oncogene is a senescence inhibitor and an upregulated target of high-risk human papillomavirus E7," *Journal of Virology*, vol. 79, no. 22, pp. 14309–14317, 2005.

[80] T. M. Wise-Draper, R. J. Morreale, T. A. Morris et al., "DEK proto-oncogene expression interferes with the normal epithelial differentiation program," *The American Journal of Pathology*, vol. 174, no. 1, pp. 71–81, 2009.

[81] C. Oancea, B. Rüster, R. Henschler, E. Puccetti, and M. Ruthardt, "The t(6;9) associated DEK/CAN fusion protein targets a population of long-term repopulating hematopoietic stem cells for leukemogenic transformation," *Leukemia*, vol. 24, no. 11, pp. 1910–1919, 2010.

[82] T. M. Wise-Draper, A. R. Mintz-Cole, A. T. Morris et al., "Overexpression of the cellular DEK protein promotes epithelial transformation in vitro and in vivo," *Cancer Research*, vol. 69, no. 5, pp. 1792–1799, 2009.

[83] A. Datta, M. E. Adelson, Y. Mogilevkin, E. Mordechai, A. A. Sidi, and J. P. Trama, "Oncoprotein DEK as a tissue and urinary biomarker for bladder cancer," *BMC Cancer*, vol. 11, article 234, 2011.

[84] T.-H. Kim, S.-W. Shin, J.-S. Park, and C.-S. Park, "Genome wide identification and expression profile in epithelial cells exposed to TiO$_2$ particles," *Environmental Toxicology*, vol. 30, no. 3, pp. 293–300, 2015.

[85] J. Ruzzin, R. Petersen, E. Meugnier et al., "Persistent organic pollutant exposure leads to insulin resistance syndrome," *Environmental Health Perspectives*, vol. 118, no. 4, pp. 465–471, 2010.

[86] M. M. Ibrahim, E. Fjære, E.-J. Lock et al., "Chronic consumption of farmed salmon containing persistent organic pollutants causes insulin resistance and obesity in mice," *PLoS ONE*, vol. 6, no. 9, Article ID e25170, 2011.

[87] V. Poli, "The role of C/EBP isoforms in the control of inflammatory and native immunity functions," *The Journal of Biological Chemistry*, vol. 273, no. 45, pp. 29279–29282, 1998.

[88] D. A. Brenner, M. O'Hara, P. Angel, M. Chojkier, and M. Karin, "Prolonged activation of jun and collagenase genes by tumour necrosis factor-alpha," *Nature*, vol. 337, no. 6208, pp. 661–663, 1989.

[89] R. Grenningloh, B. Y. Kang, and I.-C. Ho, "Ets-1, a functional cofactor of T-bet, is essential for Th1 inflammatory responses,"

Journal of Experimental Medicine, vol. 201, no. 4, pp. 615–626, 2005.

[90] E.-M. de Villiers, L. Gissmann, and H. Z. Hausen, "Molecular cloning of viral DNA from human genital warts," *Journal of Virology*, vol. 40, no. 3, pp. 932–935, 1981.

[91] M. L. Gillison, W. M. Koch, R. B. Capone et al., "Evidence for a causal association between human papillomavirus and a subset of head and neck cancers," *Journal of the National Cancer Institute*, vol. 92, no. 9, pp. 709–720, 2000.

[92] C. B. J. Woodman, S. I. Collins, and L. S. Young, "The natural history of cervical HPV infection: unresolved issues," *Nature Reviews Cancer*, vol. 7, no. 1, pp. 11–22, 2007.

[93] K. Johung, E. C. Goodwin, and D. DiMaio, "Human papillomavirus E7 repression in cervical carcinoma cells initiates a transcriptional cascade driven by the retinoblastoma family, resulting in senescence," *Journal of Virology*, vol. 81, no. 5, pp. 2102–2116, 2007.

[94] T. M. Wise-Draper, D. J. Draper, J. S. Gutkind, A. A. Molinolo, K. A. Wikenheiser-Brokamp, and S. I. Wells, "Future directions and treatment strategies for head and neck squamous cell carcinomas," *Translational Research*, vol. 160, no. 3, pp. 167–177, 2012.

[95] M. L. Gillison, Q. Zhang, R. Jordan et al., "Tobacco smoking and increased risk of death and progression for patients with p16-positive and p16-negative oropharyngeal cancer," *Journal of Clinical Oncology*, vol. 30, no. 17, pp. 2102–2111, 2012.

[96] K. K. Ang and E. M. Sturgis, "Human papillomavirus as a marker of the natural history and response to therapy of head and neck squamous cell carcinoma," *Seminars in Radiation Oncology*, vol. 22, no. 2, pp. 128–142, 2012.

[97] A. S. Andersen, A. S. K. Sølling, T. Ovesen, and M. Rusan, "The interplay between HPV and host immunity in head and neck squamous cell carcinoma," *International Journal of Cancer*, vol. 134, no. 12, pp. 2755–2763, 2014.

[98] X. Chen, S. Liang, W. L. Zheng, Z. J. Liao, T. Shang, and W. L. Ma, "Meta-analysis of nasopharyngeal carcinoma microarray data explores mechanism of EBV-regulated neoplastic transformation," *BMC Genomics*, vol. 9, article 322, 2008.

[99] J. S. Knight, N. Sharma, and E. S. Robertson, "Epstein-Barr virus latent antigen 3C can mediate the degradation of the retinoblastoma protein through an SCF cellular ubiquitin ligase," *Proceedings of the National Academy of Sciences of the United States of America*, vol. 102, no. 51, pp. 18562–18566, 2005.

[100] J. M. Hilfinger, N. Clark, M. Smith, K. Robinson, and D. M. Markovitz, "Differential regulation of the human immunodeficiency virus type 2 enhancer in monocytes at various stages of differentiation," *Journal of Virology*, vol. 67, no. 7, pp. 4448–4453, 1993.

[101] N. E. Faulkner, J. M. Hilfinger, and D. M. Markovitz, "Protein phosphatase 2A activates the HIV-2 promoter through enhancer elements that include the pets site," *The Journal of Biological Chemistry*, vol. 276, no. 28, pp. 25804–25812, 2001.

[102] A. Krithivas, M. Fujimoro, M. Weidner, D. B. Young, and S. D. Hayward, "Protein interactions targeting the latency-associated nuclear antigen of Kaposi's sarcoma associated herpesvirus to cell chromosomes," *Journal of Virology*, vol. 76, no. 22, pp. 11596–11604, 2002.

[103] S. C. Verma, Q. Cai, E. Kreider, J. Lu, and E. S. Robertson, "Comprehensive analysis of LANA interacting proteins essential for viral genome tethering and persistence," *PLoS ONE*, vol. 8, no. 9, Article ID e74662, 2013.

[104] A. L. Franks and J. E. Slansky, "Multiple associations between a broad spectrum of autoimmune diseases, chronic inflammatory diseases and cancer," *Anticancer Research*, vol. 32, no. 4, pp. 1119–1136, 2012.

[105] R. E. Petty, T. R. Southwood, P. Manners et al., "International League of Associations for Rheumatology classification of juvenile idiopathic arthritis: second revision, Edmonton, 2001," *The Journal of Rheumatology*, vol. 31, no. 2, pp. 390–392, 2004.

[106] M. Wahren-Herlenius and T. Dörner, "Immunopathogenic mechanisms of systemic autoimmune disease," *The Lancet*, vol. 382, no. 9894, pp. 819–831, 2013.

[107] S. Ringkowski, P. S. Thomas, and C. Herbert, "Interleukin-12 family cytokines and sarcoidosis," *Frontiers in Pharmacology*, vol. 5, article 233, 2014.

[108] K. J. Murray, W. Szer, A. A. Grom et al., "Antibodies to the 45 kDa DEK nuclear antigen in pauciarticular onset juvenile rheumatoid arthritis and iridocyclitis: selective association with MHC gene," *The Journal of Rheumatology*, vol. 24, no. 3, pp. 560–567, 1997.

[109] H. Sierakowska, K. R. Williams, I. S. Szer, and W. Szer, "The putative oncoprotein DEK, part of a chimera protein associated with acute myeloid leukaemia, is an autoantigen in juvenile rheumatoid arthritis," *Clinical and Experimental Immunology*, vol. 94, no. 3, pp. 435–439, 1993.

[110] L. Forero, N. W. Zwirner, C. W. Fink, M. A. Fernández-Viña, and P. Stastny, "Juvenile arthritis, HLA-A2 and binding of DEK oncogene-peptides," *Human Immunology*, vol. 59, no. 7, pp. 443–450, 1998.

[111] N. Mor-Vaknin, F. Kappes, A. E. Dick et al., "DEK in the synovium of patients with juvenile idiopathic arthritis: characterization of DEK antibodies and posttranslational modification of the DEK autoantigen," *Arthritis and Rheumatism*, vol. 63, no. 2, pp. 556–567, 2011.

[112] W. Brintnell, E. Zeggini, A. Barton et al., "Evidence for a novel rheumatoid arthritis susceptibility locus on chromosome 6p," *Arthritis & Rheumatism*, vol. 50, no. 12, pp. 3823–3830, 2004.

[113] I. Wichmann, J. R. Garcia-Lozano, N. Respaldiza, M. F. Gonzalez-Escribano, and A. Nuñez-Roldan, "Autoantibodies to transcriptional regulation proteins DEK and ALY in a patient with systemic lupus erythematosus," *Human Immunology*, vol. 60, no. 1, pp. 57–62, 1999.

[114] X. Dong, M. A. Michelis, J. Wang, R. Bose, T. DeLange, and W. H. Reeves, "Autoantibodies to DEK oncoprotein in a patient with systemic lupus erythematosus and sarcoidosis," *Arthritis & Rheumatism*, vol. 41, no. 8, pp. 1505–1510, 1998.

[115] I. Wichmann, N. Respaldiza, J. R. Garcia-Lozano, M. Montes, J. Sanchez-Roman, and A. Nuñez-Roldan, "Autoantibodies to DEK oncoprotein in systemic lupus erythematosus (SLE)," *Clinical and Experimental Immunology*, vol. 119, no. 3, pp. 530–532, 2000.

[116] B. S. Adams, H. C. Cha, J. Cleary et al., "DEK binding to class II MHC Y-box sequences is gene- and allele-specific," *Arthritis Research & Therapy*, vol. 5, no. 4, pp. R226–R233, 2003.

[117] J. Zheng, M. E. Kohler, Q. Chen et al., "Serum from mice immunized in the context of Treg inhibition identifies DEK as a neuroblastoma tumor antigen," *BMC Immunology*, vol. 8, article 4, 2007.

[118] M. Makita, T. Azuma, H. Hamaguchi et al., "Leukemia-associated fusion proteins, dek-can and bcr-abl, represent immunogenic HLA-DR-restricted epitopes recognized by fusion peptide-specific CD4+ T lymphocytes," *Leukemia*, vol. 16, no. 12, pp. 2400–2407, 2002.

[119] Z. G. Fridlender and S. M. Albelda, "Tumor-associated neutrophils: friend or foe?" *Carcinogenesis*, vol. 33, no. 5, pp. 949–955, 2012.

[120] I. Langers, V. M. Renoux, M. Thiry, P. Delvenne, and N. Jacobs, "Natural killer cells: role in local tumor growth and metastasis," *Biologics: Targets and Therapy*, vol. 6, pp. 73–82, 2012.

[121] R. Noy and J. W. Pollard, "Tumor-associated macrophages: from mechanisms to therapy," *Immunity*, vol. 41, pp. 49–61, 2014.

[122] S. Choi, S.-Y. Park, J. Jeong et al., "Identification of toxicological biomarkers of di(2-ethylhexyl) phthalate in proteins secreted by HepG2 cells using proteomic analysis," *Proteomics*, vol. 10, no. 9, pp. 1831–1846, 2010.

[123] S. Choi, S.-Y. Park, D. Kwak et al., "Proteomic analysis of proteins secreted by HepG2 cells treated with butyl benzyl phthalate," *Journal of Toxicology and Environmental Health Part A: Current Issues*, vol. 73, no. 21-22, pp. 1570–1585, 2010.

[124] K. Liu, T. Feng, J. Liu, M. Zhong, and S. Zhang, "Silencing of the DEK gene induces apoptosis and senescence in CaSki cervical carcinoma cells via the up-regulation of NF-κB p65," *Bioscience Reports*, vol. 32, no. 3, pp. 323–332, 2012.

[125] M. Sammons, S. W. Shan, N. L. Vogel, E. J. Mientjes, G. Grosveld, and B. P. Ashburner, "Negative regulation of the RelA/p65 transactivation function by the product of the DEK proto-oncogene," *The Journal of Biological Chemistry*, vol. 281, no. 37, pp. 26802–26812, 2006.

[126] C. Sandén, M. Ageberg, J. Petersson, A. Lennartsson, and U. Gullberg, "Forced expression of the DEK-NUP214 fusion protein promotes proliferation dependent on upregulation of mTOR," *BMC Cancer*, vol. 13, article 440, 2013.

[127] J. Wang, L. Sun, M. Yang et al., "DEK depletion negatively regulates Rho/ROCK/MLC pathway in non-small cell lung cancer," *Journal of Histochemistry and Cytochemistry*, vol. 61, no. 7, pp. 510–521, 2013.

[128] A. Oeckinghaus and S. Ghosh, "The NF-kappaB family of transcription factors and its regulation," *Cold Spring Harbor Perspectives in Biology*, vol. 1, no. 4, Article ID a000034, 2009.

[129] V. F.-S. Shih, R. Tsui, A. Caldwell, and A. Hoffmann, "A single NFκB system for both canonical and non-canonical signaling," *Cell Research*, vol. 21, no. 1, pp. 86–102, 2011.

[130] M. M. Chaturvedi, B. Sung, V. R. Yadav, R. Kannappan, and B. B. Aggarwal, "NF-kappaB addiction and its role in cancer: one size does not fit all," *Oncogene*, vol. 30, no. 14, pp. 1615–1630, 2011.

[131] B. Hoesel and J. A. Schmid, "The complexity of NF-κB signaling in inflammation and cancer," *Molecular Cancer*, vol. 12, no. 1, article 86, 2013.

[132] G. Maeda, T. Chiba, S. Kawashiri, T. Satoh, and K. Imai, "Epigenetic inactivation of IκB kinase-A in oral carcinomas and tumor progression," *Clinical Cancer Research*, vol. 13, no. 17, pp. 5041–5047, 2007.

[133] N. D. Perkins, "NF-κB: tumor promoter or suppressor?" *Trends in Cell Biology*, vol. 14, no. 2, pp. 64–69, 2004.

[134] D. J. Wang, N. M. Ratnam, J. C. Byrd, and D. C. Guttridge, "NF-kappaB functions in tumor initiation by suppressing the surveillance of both innate and adaptive immune cells," *Cell Reports*, vol. 9, no. 1, pp. 90–103, 2014.

[135] A. Iannetti, A. C. Ledoux, S. J. Tudhope et al., "Regulation of p53 and Rb links the alternative NF-κB pathway to EZH2 expression and cell senescence," *PLoS Genetics*, vol. 10, no. 9, Article ID e1004642, 2014.

[136] M. Karam, M. Thenoz, V. Capraro et al., "Chromatin redistribution of the DEK oncoprotein represses hTERT transcription in leukemias," *Neoplasia*, vol. 16, no. 1, pp. 21–30, 2014.

[137] M. Campillos, M. A. García, F. Valdivieso, and J. Vázquez, "Transcriptional activation by AP-2α is modulated by the oncogene DEK," *Nucleic Acids Research*, vol. 31, no. 5, pp. 1571–1575, 2003.

[138] R. I. Koleva, S. B. Ficarro, H. S. Radomska et al., "C/EBPα and DEK coordinately regulate myeloid differentiation," *Blood*, vol. 119, no. 21, pp. 4878–4888, 2012.

[139] D. W. Kim, J. I. Y. Kim, S. Choi, S. Rhee, Y. Hahn, and S.-B. Seo, "Transcriptional regulation of 1-cys peroxiredoxin by the proto-oncogene protein DEK," *Molecular Medicine Reports*, vol. 3, no. 5, pp. 877–881, 2010.

[140] K.-S. Lee, D.-W. Kim, J.-Y. Kim, J.-K. Choo, K. Yu, and S.-B. Seo, "Caspase-dependent apoptosis induction by targeted expression of DEK in *Drosophila* involves histone acetylation inhibition," *Journal of Cellular Biochemistry*, vol. 103, no. 4, pp. 1283–1293, 2008.

[141] S. Waidmann, B. Kusenda, J. Mayerhofer, K. Mechtler, and C. Jonak, "A DEK domain-containing protein modulates chromatin structure and function in arabidopsis," *The Plant Cell Online*, vol. 26, no. 11, pp. 4328–4344, 2014.

[142] S. A. Eming, T. Krieg, and J. M. Davidson, "Inflammation in wound repair: molecular and cellular mechanisms," *Journal of Investigative Dermatology*, vol. 127, no. 3, pp. 514–525, 2007.

2

Overexpression of Activation-Induced Cytidine Deaminase in MTX- and Age-Related Epstein-Barr Virus-Associated B-Cell Lymphoproliferative Disorders of the Head and Neck

Kentaro Kikuchi,[1] Toshiyuki Ishige,[2] Fumio Ide,[1] Yumi Ito,[3]
Ichiro Saito,[4] Miyako Hoshino,[5] Harumi Inoue,[1] Yuji Miyazaki,[1]
Tadashige Nozaki,[6] Masaru Kojima,[7] and Kaoru Kusama[1]

[1]*Division of Pathology, Department of Diagnostic and Therapeutic Sciences, Meikai University School of Dentistry,*
 1-1 Keyakidai, Sakado, Saitama 350-0283, Japan
[2]*Department of Pathology, Nihon University School of Medicine, 30-1 Oyaguchi-Kamimachi, Itabashi-ku, Tokyo 173-8610, Japan*
[3]*Division of Diagnostic Pathology, Tsurumi University Dental Hospital, 2-1-3 Tsurumi, Tsurumi-ku, Yokohama 230-8501, Japan*
[4]*Department of Pathology, Tsurumi University School of Dental Medicine, 2-1-3 Tsurumi, Tsurumi-ku, Yokohama 230-8501, Japan*
[5]*Second Division of Oral and Maxillofacial Surgery, Department of Diagnostic and Therapeutic Sciences,*
 Meikai University School of Dentistry, 1-1 Keyakidai, Sakado, Saitama 350-0283, Japan
[6]*Department of Pharmacology, Osaka Dental University, 8-1 Kuzuhahanazono-cho, Hirakata, Osaka 573-1211, Japan*
[7]*Department of Anatomic and Diagnostic Pathology, Dokkyo Medical University School of Medicine, 880 Oaza-kitakobayashi,*
 Mibu-machi, Shimotsuga-gun, Tochigi 321-0293, Japan

Correspondence should be addressed to Kentaro Kikuchi; k-kikuchi@dent.meikai.ac.jp

Academic Editor: James L. Mulshine

Recent research has shown that activation-induced cytidine deaminase (AID) triggers somatic hypermutation and recombination, in turn contributing to lymphomagenesis. Such aberrant AID expression is seen in B-cell leukemia/lymphomas, including Burkitt lymphoma which is associated with *c-myc* translocation. Moreover, Epstein-Barr virus (EBV) latent membrane protein-1 (LMP-1) increases genomic instability through early growth transcription response-1 (Egr-1) mediated upregulation of AID in B-cell lymphoma. However, few clinicopathological studies have focused on AID expression in lymphoproliferative disorders (LPDs). Therefore, we conducted an immunohistochemical study to investigate the relationship between AID and LMP-1 expression in LPDs (MTX-/Age-related EBV-associated), including diffuse large B-cell lymphomas (DLBCLs). More intense AID expression was detected in LPDs (89.5%) than in DLBCLs (20.0%), and the expression of LMP-1 and EBER was more intense in LPDs (68.4% and 94.7%) than in DLBCLs (10.0% and 20.0%). Furthermore, stronger Egr-1 expression was found in MTX/Age-EBV-LPDs (83.3%) than in DLBCLs (30.0%). AID expression was significantly constitutively overexpressed in LPDs as compared with DLBCLs. These results suggest that increased AID expression in LPDs may be one of the processes involved in lymphomagenesis, thereby further increasing the survival of genetically destabilized B-cells. AID expression may be a useful indicator for differentiation between LPDs and DLBCLs.

1. Introduction

Epstein-Barr virus (EBV) is associated with a variety of lymphoproliferative disorders (LPDs) and other malignancies [1–5], including nasopharyngeal carcinoma, Hodgkin disease, and Burkitt lymphoma [6–9]. EBV-driven B-cell LPDs can be age-related or can occur in patients who are immunosuppressed due to primary immune deficiency, HIV infection, organ transplantation, and treatment with methotrexate or tumor necrosis factor-α antagonist for rheumatoid arthritis

TABLE 1: Case mix of patient with MTX-/Age-EBV-LPDs and DLBCLs in the head and neck.

Case number	Diagnosis	Age (y)/sex	Biopsy site	Collagen disease	Treatment of collagen disease	Histological type	ISH and immunohistochemistry			
							EBER-ISH	LMP-1	AID	Egr-1
1	MTX-LPD	32/F	LN (neck/axilla)	RA	MTX	NA	+ (M)	+ (W)	+++ (S)	+++ (S)
2	MTX-LPD	57/M	LN (neck)	RA	MTX	LPL	+++ (M)	+ (M)	+++ (S)	++ (M)
3	MTX-LPD	73/F	Oral mucosa (?)	RA	MTX/PSL	LPL	++ (M)	+ (M)	+ (W)	NA
4	MTX-LPD	52/M	LN (neck)	RA	MTX	HDMC	++ (M)	++ (W)	+++ (S)	+++ (S)
5	MTX-LPD	57/F	LN (left neck and axilla)	RA	MTX/PSL	HDNS	+++ (M)	+ (S)	+++ (S)	+++ (S)
6	MTX-LPD	71/F	Septonasal mucosa	RA	MTX	NA	++ (M)	+ (M)	+++ (S)	+++ (S)
7	MTX-LPD	60/F	LN (neck)	RA	MTX/PSL	LPL	++ (M)	+ (M)	+++ (S)	-/± (W)
8	MTX-LPD	64/M	LN (neck)	RA	MTX/PSL	DLBCL	++ (M)	+ (M)	+++ (S)	+++ (S)
9	MTX-LPD	44/M	Gingiva (right upper)	(Still's disease) RA	MTX/PSL	DLBCL	++ (M)	+ (M)	+++ (S)	++ (S)
10	MTX-LPD	69/F	Gingiva (left upper)	RA	MTX	HD-like	++ (M)	+ (M)	+++ (S)	+++ (S)
11	MTX-LPD	76/F	Gingiva (right upper)	RA	MTX	HD-like	++ (M)	+ (M)	+++ (S)	+++ (S)
12	MTX-LPD	67/M	Hard palate (midline)	RA	MTX	NA	+ (M)	-/±, (W)	-/± (W)	+ (M)
13	MTX-LPD	67/M	LN (neck)	RA	MTX/PSL	Follicular	++ (M)	+ (W)	++ (S)	++ (S)
14	MTX-LPD	56/F	LN (left neck)	RA	MTX/PSL	MALT	+ (M)	+ (W)	+++ (S)	+++ (S)
15	MTX-LPD	64/F	Skin (?)	RA	MTX/PSL	DLBCL	++ (M)	++ (S)	++ (S)	+++ (S)
16	MTX-LPD	59/M	Thyroid gland	RA	MTX/PSL	DLBCL	++ (M)	++ (W)	++ (S)	+++ (S)
17	MTX-LPD	74/F	Parotid gland (left)	RA	MTX/PSL	DLBCL	+ (M)	++ (S)	+++ (S)	++ (S)
18	Age-LPD	71/M	Mandibular bone (intraosseous)	N	NT	Polymorphous	++ (S)	++ (S)	+++ (S)	+++ (S)
19	Age-LPD	76/M	Tongue/floor of mouth (right)	N	NT	Intermediate, DLBCL/CHL	+ (W)	+ (M)	+++ (S)	+++ (S)
20	DLBCL	78/M	Maxillary sinus (right)	N	NT	DLBCL	-/± (W)	++ (M)	-/± (W)	+++ (S)
21	DLBCL	63/M	LN (left submandibular)	N	NT	DLBCL	+ (W)	-/± (N)	-/± (W)	-/± (M)
22	DLBCL	64/M	Gingiva (upper)	N	NT	DLBCL	+ (W)	-/± (N)	-/± (W)	-/± (M)
23	DLBCL	82/F	Gingiva (right lower)	N	NT	DLBCL	-/± (N)	++ (W)	++ (M)	++ (S)
24	DLBCL	69/F	Gingiva (left upper)	N	NT	DLBCL	+ (M)	-/± (W)	-/± (W)	+ (M)
25	DLBCL	56/M	Gingiva (right upper)	N	NT	DLBCL	+ (M)	-/± (W)	+ (M)	+ (S)
26	DLBCL	52/F	Gingiva (upper)	N	NT	DLBCL	-/± (N)	-/± (N)	-/± (W)	+ (W)
27	DLBCL	46/M	Gingiva (left lower)	N	NT	DLBCL	-/± (W)	-/± (N)	-/± (N)	-/± (N)
28	DLBCL	70/F	LN (left neck)	N	NT	DLBCL	-/± (W)	-/± (N)	-/± (W)	+ (M)
29	DLBCL	71/F	Maxillary sinus (left)	N	NT	DLBCL	-/± (N)	-/± (N)	-/± (W)	++ (M)

MTX: methotrexate; LPD: lymphoproliferative disorder; DLBCL: diffuse large B-cell lymphoma; RA: rheumatoid arthritis; LPL: lymphoplasmacytic lymphoma; HDMC: Hodgkin disease, mixed cellularity; HDNS: Hodgkin disease, nodular sclerosis; MALT: mucosa-associated lymphoid tissue; CHL: classical Hodgkin lymphoma; HD-like: Hodgkin disease-like; NA: not available; NT: no treatment; PSL: prednisolone; ?: unknown; LN: lymph node; LMP-1: Epstein-Barr virus- (EBV-) latent infection membrane protein-1; ISH: *in situ* hybridization; EBER: EBV-encoded small RNA; AID: activation-induced cytidine deaminase; Egr-1: early growth response transcription factor-1; diffuse: +++ (≧75%); focal: ++ (<75% to ≧25%); few: −/± (negative/<5% or nonspecific); (S): strongly positive; (M): moderately positive; (W): weakly positive; (N): negative; M: male; F: female.

TABLE 2: Antibodies and dilutions used in this study.

Antigen	Clone	Dilution	Pretreatment	Primary antibody incubation time	Source
AID	—	1 : 50 (rabbit polyclonal)	MW	Overnight (about 15 h, 4°C)	Serotec
LMP-1	CS. 1–4	1 : 100 (mouse monoclonal)	—	Overnight (about 15 h, 4°C)	Dako
Egr-1	—	1 : 100 (rabbit polyclonal)	—	Nonovernight (1 h, RT)	Rockland

AID: activation-induced cytidine deaminase; LMP-1: latent membrane protein-1; Egr-1: early growth response-1; MW: microwave oven (for 1 min at high voltage and then for 10 min at low voltage); —: none; RT: room temperature.

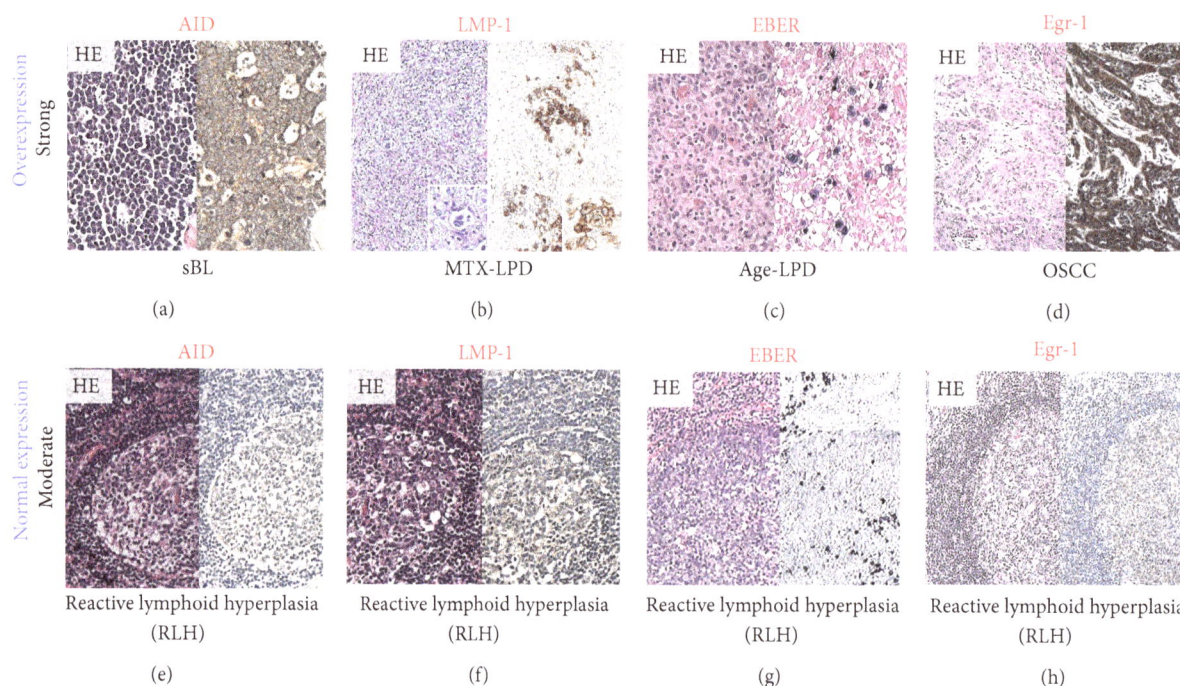

FIGURE 1: Positive control for AID, LMP-1, EBER, and Egr-1 in the overexpression and normal expression. (a) Sporadic Burkitt lymphoma (sBL) [34], (b) MTX-LPD [35], (c) Age-LPD [36], and (d) oral squamous cell carcinoma (OSCC) were used as an aberrant positive control (strong intensity/overexpression) for AID, LMP-1, EBER, and Egr-1 (hematoxylin-eosin staining: HE, left panel; immunohistochemical staining: IHC, right panel) ((a)–(d) original magnification ×100). Reactive lymphoid hyperplasia (RLH) was used as normally positive control (moderate/normal expression) for (e) AID, (f) LMP-1, (g) EBER, and (h) Egr-1 ((e)–(h) original magnification ×100). (g) Germinal center B-cells were moderate/normal positive for EBER, and plasma cells were strongly positive for EBER (right panel).

[10, 11]. The major EBV oncogene, latent membrane protein-1 (LMP-1), activates signaling pathways such as those involving nuclear factor-kappa-light-chain-enhancer of activated B-cells (NF-κB), which enhances B-cell survival and is essential for EBV-induced transformation [12–16]. LMP-1 is a 63 kDa integral membrane protein with three domains and contains two distinct functional regions within its C-terminus, designated C-terminal activating regions 1 and 2 (CTAR1 and CTAR2). The protein also protects cancer cells from apoptosis, by inducing antiapoptotic proteins, including BCL-2, MCL-1, A20, early growth response transcription factor-1 (Egr-1), and SNARK [17–19]. Recent studies have shown that EBV-infected cells undergo hypermutation or switching of recombination in vivo via upregulation of activation-induced cytidine deaminase (AID) [20] and also that EBV-induced

AID is associated with oncogene mutations, which contribute to lymphomagenesis [21]. The relationship between LMP-1 and cancer has been relatively well established, while the molecular mechanisms underlying AID induction remain to be fully clarified.

AID is normally expressed in germinal center (GC) B-cells [22], where it plays a central role in both somatic hypermutation and class switch recombination in humans and mice [23, 24]. AID converts single-stranded genomic cytidine into uracil, with pronounced activity in the immunoglobulin variable and switch regions [25–28]. Aberrant expression of AID and abnormal targeting of AID activation in both B- and non-B-cells cause DNA double-strand breaks (DSBs) and DNA point mutations in both Ig and non-Ig genes, inducing tumorigenesis [29]. AID is required for chromosomal DSBs

MTX-LPD case number 8   Age-LPD case number 19   DLBCL case number 21

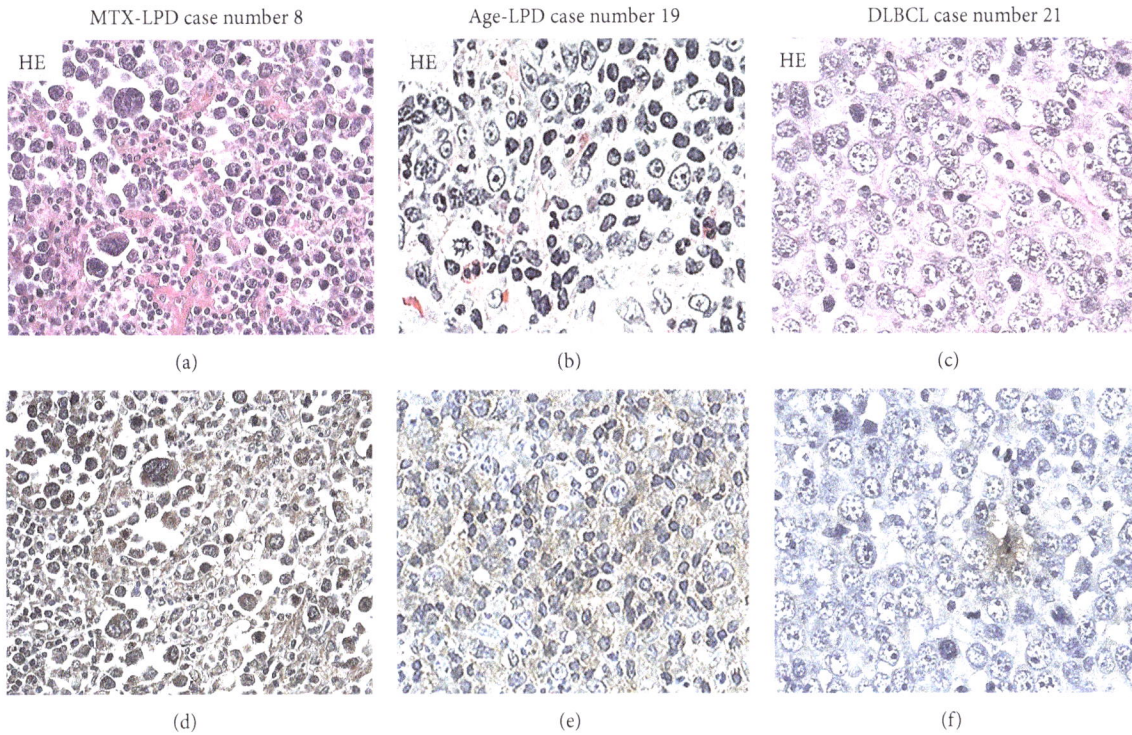

FIGURE 2: Distribution and intensity of AID expression in MTX-/Age-EBV-LPDs and DLBCLs in biopsy specimens. ((a)–(c)) HE stain and ((d)–(f)) AID by IHC (brownish color). AID positive atypical lymphoid cells were diffuse in (d) MTX-LPD and (e) Age-LPD but were few in (f) DLBCL. AID positive cells were of strong intensity in (d) MTX-LPD and (e) Age-LPD and were of (f) weak or moderate intensity in DLBCL ((a)–(f) original magnification, ×200).

MTX-LPD case number 13   Age-LPD case number 18   DLBCL case number 24

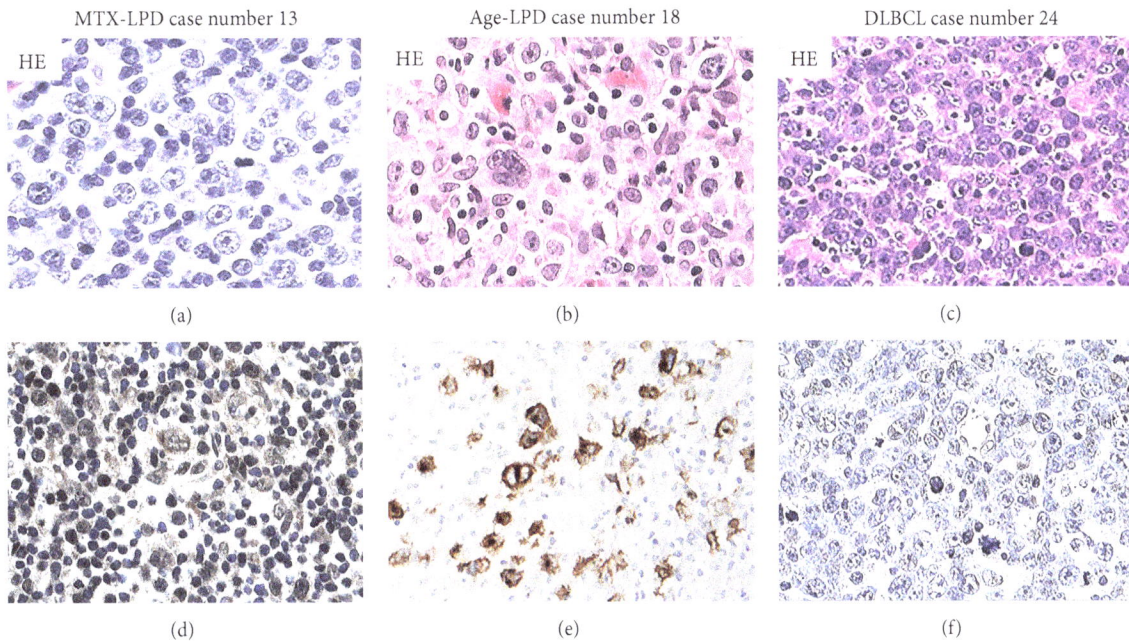

FIGURE 3: Distribution and intensity of LMP-1 expression in MTX-/Age-EBV-LPDs and DLBCLs in biopsy specimens. ((a)–(c)) HE stain and ((d)–(f)) LMP-1 by IHC. LMP-1 positive atypical lymphoid cells (brownish color) were diffuse or sporadic diffuse in (d) MTX-LPD or (e) Age-LPD but were not verifiable in (f) DLBCL. LMP-1 positive cells were of moderate or strong intensity in (d) MTX-LPD and (e) Age-LPD and were of weak or nonspecific intensity in (f) DLBCL ((a)–(f) original magnification, ×200).

MTX-LPD case number 2

Age-LPD case number 18

DLBCL case number 26

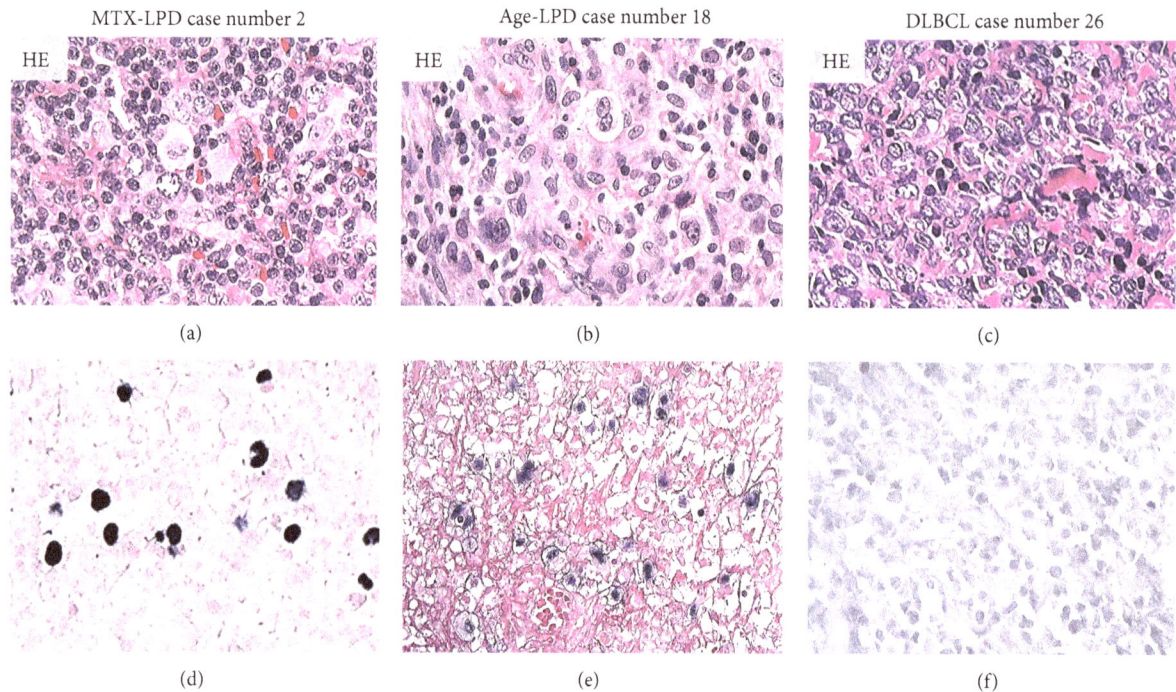

(a)

(b)

(c)

(d)

(e)

(f)

FIGURE 4: Distribution and intensity of EBER expression in MTX-/Age-EBV-LPDs and DLBCLs in biopsy specimens. ((a)–(c)) HE stain and ((d)–(f)) EBER by ISH (blackish color). EBER positive atypical lymphoid cells were sporadic diffuse in (d) MTX-LPD and (e) Age-LPD but were not verifiable in (f) DLBCL. EBER positive cells were of almost strong intensity in (d) MTX-LPD and (e) Age-LPD and were of weak or nonspecific intensity in (f) DLBCL ((a)–(f) original magnification, ×200).

at the *c-myc* and *IgH* loci, which lead to reciprocal *c-myc/IgH* translocations, resulting in the development of B-cell lymphomas, such as Burkitt lymphoma in humans and plasmacytoma in mice [30]. AID protein is localized more in the cytoplasm than in the nucleus in normal and neoplastic B-cells, and cytoplasmic AID protein relocates to the nucleus when pathological change occurs in B-cells [31, 32].

A recent *in vitro* study by Kim et al. [33] has shown that LMP-1 increases genomic instability through Egr-1-mediated upregulation of AID in B-cell lymphoma cell lines. However, to our knowledge, no clinicopathological case study has examined the expression of LMP-1, AID, and Egr-1, including the distribution and density of positive cells, on LPDs. It is therefore important to clarify the expression pathway and distribution of positive cells in lesions of human tissues. We considered that AID positive cells would be more numerous in the EBV-driven LPDs than in DLBCLs showing a monotonous growth pattern. Therefore, we conducted an immunohistochemical study to investigate the relationship between LMP-1, AID, and Egr-1 expression in LPDs (MTX-/Age-related EBV-associated), including DLBCLs.

2. Materials and Methods

2.1. Tissue Samples. A total of 29 biopsy specimens were retrieved from the three hospitals to which the authors have contributed pathological diagnosis and were presented for

investigation. Tissue samples from 17 cases of MTX-EBV-LPD, 2 cases of Age-EBV-LPD, and 10 cases of DLBCL were used (Table 1). Sporadic-Burkitt lymphoma (sBL) [34], MTX-LPD [35], Age-LPD [36], and oral squamous cell carcinoma (OSCC) were used as an overexpressing positive control for AID, LMP-1, EBV-encoded small RNA (EBER), and Egr-1. Ten samples of cervical lymph nodes (LNs) showing reactive lymphoid hyperplasia (RLH) were used as normal positive controls for AID, LMP-1, EBER, and Egr-1. Each section was prepared for immunohistochemical analysis (IHC) and *in situ* hybridization (ISH). The case study protocol was reviewed and approved by the Research Ethics Committee of Meikai University School of Dentistry (A0832, A1321).

2.2. Immunohistochemistry. Deparaffinized sections were immersed for 15 min at room temperature in absolute methanol containing 0.3% H_2O_2 to block endogenous peroxidase activity and then treated with 2% bovine serum albumin for 15 min to block nonspecific reactions. After washing, they were incubated with an appropriately diluted mouse monoclonal antibody against human LMP-1 and rabbit polyclonal antibodies against AID and Egr-1 (Table 2). After washing, the sections were incubated with a prediluted anti-mouse or rabbit IgG antibody conjugated with peroxidase (Nichirei, Tokyo, Japan) for 30 min at room temperature. They were then immersed for 8 min in 0.05% 3,3′-diaminobenzidine tetrahydrochloride (DAB) in 0.05 M Tris-HCl buffer (pH 8.5) containing 0.01% H_2O_2 and counterstained with Mayer's haematoxylin for 90 s.

(a)

(b)

(c)

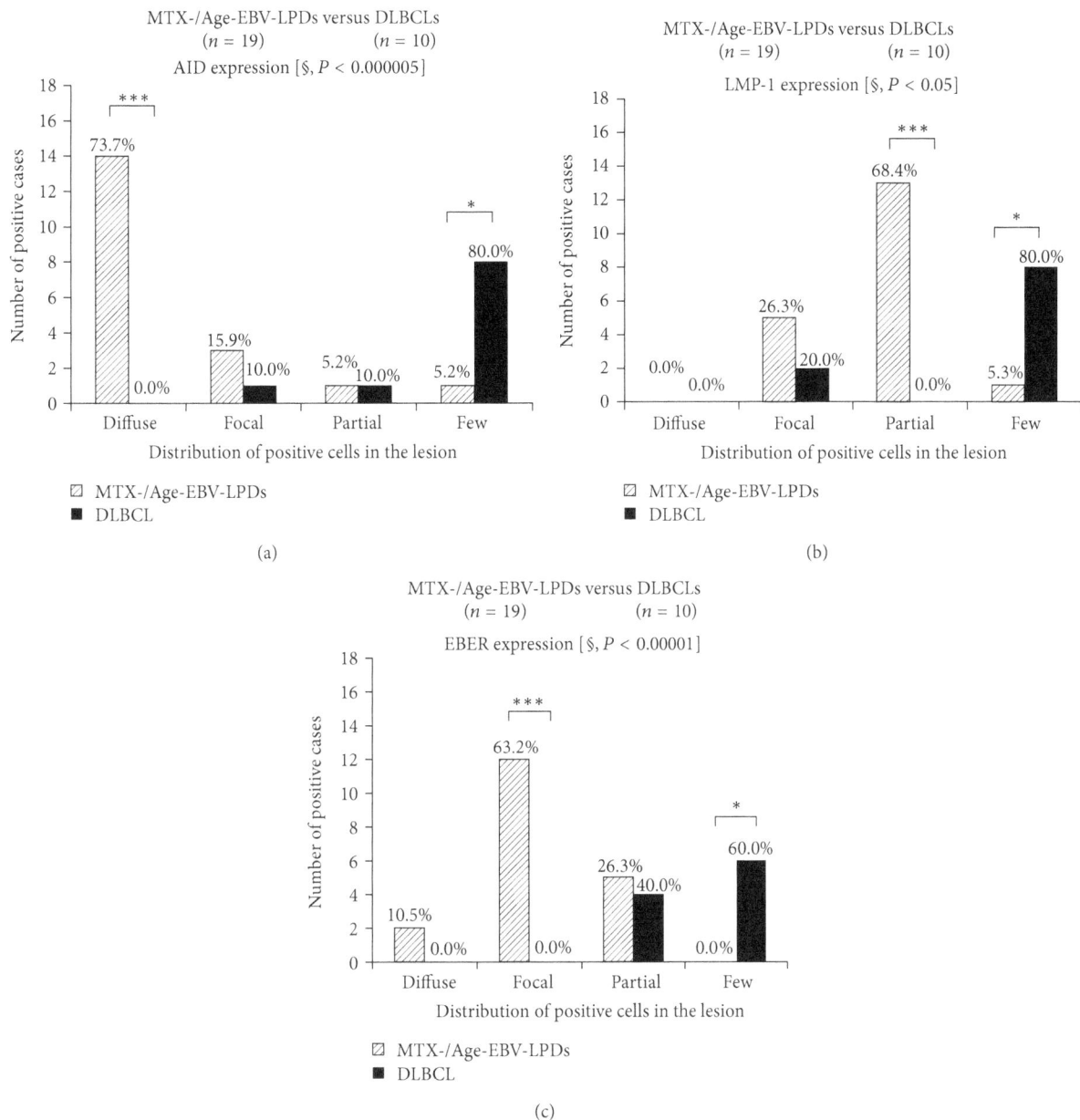

FIGURE 5: Distribution of AID, LMP, and EBER expression in MTX-/Age-EBV-LPDs and DLBCLs. ((a), (b), and (c)) The distribution of positive cells for AID, LMP, and EBER was more extensive in MTX-/Age-EBV-LPDs than in DLBCLs. P values were examined by Mann-Whitney U test [§] or Exact Binominal test (${}^{*}P < 0.05$, ${}^{**}P < 0.01$, and ${}^{***}P < 0.001$).

2.3. In Situ Hybridization. ISH for EBER oligonucleotides was performed to detect the presence of EBV small RNA in formalin-fixed paraffin-embedded sections using a hybridization kit (Dako, A/S, Denmark) in accordance with the manufacturer's instructions. Age-EBV-LPD was used as a positive control for EBER [36].

2.4. Assessment of AID, LMP-1, EBER, and Egr-1 Expression in Biopsy Specimens. Reactivity for each of the antigens and EBER was evaluated semiquantitatively using a light microscope (model BH2, Olympus Corp.). The distribution of the staining was categorized semiquantitatively according

to the ratio of the positive area as follows: diffuse (+++) ≧75%; focal (++) <75% to ≧25%; partial (+) <25% to ≧5%; few (−/±) negative/<5% or nonspecific. The intensity of the staining was categorized semiquantitatively as strong (S), moderate (M), weak (W), or negative (N) relative to each control specimen. AID intensity was compared with that in the sBL case sample used as a positive control [34] and expressed as strong (S) when higher or of the same intensity as that in sBL, moderate (M) when lower than that in sBL or of the same intensity as that in RLH, weak (W) when lower than that in RLH, and negative (N) in case of no staining or nonspecific staining. LMP-1 and EBER intensity were compared with those in

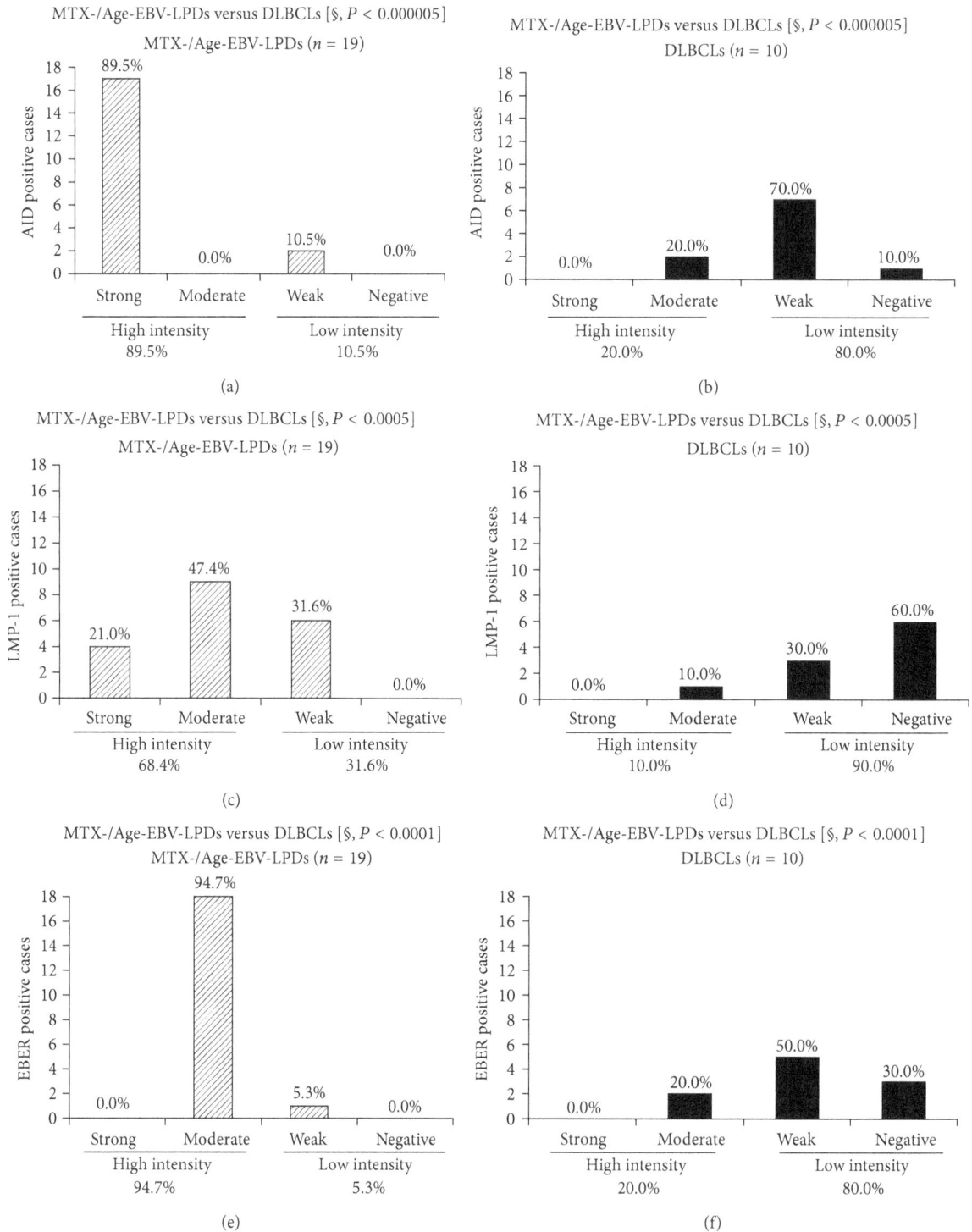

FIGURE 6: Intensity of AID, LMP-1, and EBER expression in MTX-/Age-EBV-LPDs and DLBCLs. High intensity rate of AID was higher in (a) MTX/Age-EBV-LPDs (89.5%) than in (b) DLBCLs (20.0%). Conversely, low intensity rate of AID was higher in (b) DLBCLs (80.0%) than in (a) MTX/Age-EBV-LPDs (10.5%). $P < 0.000005$ by Mann-Whitney U test [§]. High intensity rate of LMP-1 was higher in (c) MTX/Age-EBV-LPDs (68.4%) than in (d) DLBCLs (10.0%). Conversely, low intensity rate of LMP-1 was higher in (d) DLBCLs (90.0%) than in (c) MTX/Age-EBV-LPDs (31.6%). $P < 0.0005$ by Mann-Whitney U test [§]. High intensity rate of EBER was higher in (e) MTX/Age-EBV-LPDs (94.7%) than in (f) DLBCLs (20.0%). Conversely, low intensity rate of EBER was higher in (f) DLBCLs (80.0%) than in (e) MTX/Age-EBV-LPDs (5.3%). $P < 0.0001$ by Mann-Whitney U test [§].

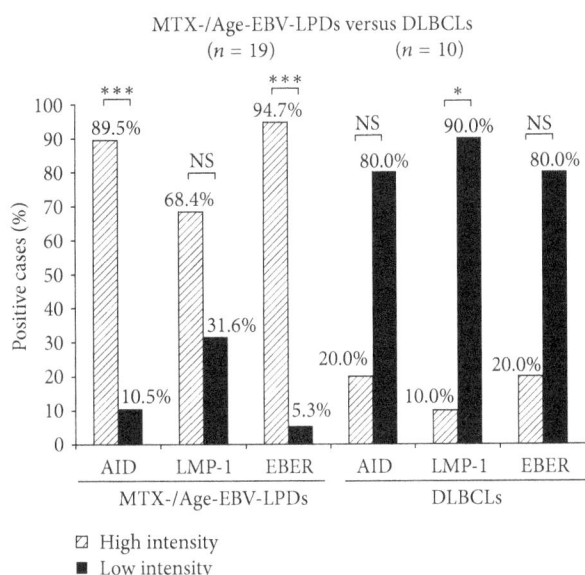

FIGURE 7: Comparison of the intensity of AID, LMP-1, and EBER expression between MTX/Age-EBV-LPDs and DLBCLs. High intensity showed strongly and moderately positive cases, and low intensity showed weakly positive and negative cases. Although a high intensity of expression (AID, LMP-1, and EBER) was greater in MTX-/Age-EBV-LPDs than in DLBCLs, a low intensity of those was smaller in the former than in the latter. P values were examined by Exact Binominal test ($^{*}P < 0.05$, $^{**}P < 0.01$, and $^{***}P < 0.001$). NS: not significant.

MTX-LPD and Age-EBV-LPD used as a positive control [35, 36] and evaluated in the same manner as those for AID. Egr-1 intensity was compared with that in OSCC used as a positive control and evaluated in the same manner as that for AID.

2.5. Statistical Analysis. The significance of differences between the mean values was determined by using the Mann-Whitney U test or Exact Binominal test for comparing two categories. The accepted level of significance was $P < 0.05$.

3. Results

Strong AID, LMP-1, EBER, and Egr-1 reactivity were observed in overexpressing positive control specimens in sBL, MTX-LPD, Age-LPD, and OSCC by IHC and ISH (Figures 1(a)–1(d)). Moderate AID, LMP-1, EBER, and Egr-1 reactivity were observed in normal positive control specimens RLM by IHC and ISH (Figures 1(e)–1(h)). AID expression was diffuse and strongly positive in MTX-/Age-EBV-LPDs (Figures 2(a), 2(b), 2(d), and 2(e)) and was few and moderately positive in DLBCLs (Figures 2(c) and 2(f)). Although LMP-1 expression was diffuse and strongly positive in MTX-/Age-EBV-LPDs (Figures 3(a), 3(b), 3(d), and 3(e)), the expression was few and weakly positive in DLBCLs (Figures 3(c) and 3(f)). EBER expression was sporadic diffuse and strongly positive in MTX-/Age-EBV-LPDs (Figures 4(a), 4(b), 4(d), and 4(e)), while EBER reactivity was negative in DLBCLs (Figures 4(c)

and 4(f)). Expression of AID, LMP-1, and EBER was higher in MTX-/Age-EBV-LPDs than in DLBCLs. Staining patterns, AID, LMP-1, and EBER, were compared between different lesion types (Table 1).

The distribution of AID ($P < 0.000005$), LMP-1 ($P < 0.05$), and EBER ($P < 0.00001$) expression was significantly more extensive in the MTX-/Age-EBV-LPDs than in the DLBCLs (Figures 5(a)–5(c)). In addition, AID expression was significantly more intense in MTX-/Age-EBV-LPDs than in DLBCLs ($P < 0.000005$) (Figures 6(a) and 6(b)), and expression of LMP-1 ($P < 0.0005$) (Figures 6(c) and 6(d)) and EBER ($P < 0.0001$) was more intense in MTX-/Age-EBV-LPDs than in DLBCLs (Figures 6(e) and 6(f)). The high intensity (strong and moderate) of AID, LMP-1, and EBER expression was greater in MTX/Age-EBV-LPDs (89.5%, 68.4%, and 94.7%) than in DLBCLs (20.0%, 10.0%, and 20.0%) (Figures 6 and 7). Conversely, the low intensity (weak and negative) of AID, LMP-1, and EBER expression was greater in DLBCLs (80.0%, 90.0%, and 80.0%) than in MTX/Age-EBV-LPDs (10.5%, 31.6%, and 5.3%) (Figures 6 and 7). In MTX-/Age-EBV-LPDs, the intensity of AID, LMP-1, and EBER expression was stronger than in DLBCLs (Figure 7). Egr-1 expression was diffuse and strongly positive in MTX-/Age-EBV-LPDs (Figures 8(a)–8(c)) and was a positive variety in the DLBCLs (Figures 8(d)–8(f)). Distribution of Egr-1 expression was significantly more extensive in MTX-/Age-EBV-LPDs than in the DLBCLs ($P < 0.001$) (Figure 9(a)). The intensity of Egr-1 was significantly different between MTX-/Age-EBV-LPDs and DLBCLs ($P < 0.01$) (Figures 9(b) and 9(c)). Although the high intensity of Egr-1 expression was comparable rate in both MTX-/Age-EBV-LPDs (94.4%) and DLBCLs (80.0%), strong intensity was higher in MTX-/Age-EBV-LPDs (83.3%) (Figure 9(b)) than in DLBCLs (30.0%) (Figure 9(c)).

4. Discussion

Immunohistochemical analysis in this study revealed that the expression of AID, LMP-1, and Egr-1 had a much more diffuse distribution and was stronger in intensity in LPD than in DLBCL cases. Furthermore, LPD cases showed a more diffuse distribution and stronger intensity of EBER-ISH than DLBCL cases.

EBV is associated with a variety of LPDs and malignant lymphomas [1, 3–5]. EBV-driven B-cell LPDs occur in patients who are immunosuppressed due to primary immune deficiency, HIV infection, or organ transplantation or patients who have received other treatments including methotrexate and tumor necrosis factor-α antagonists [10, 11]. Primary EBV infection is usually asymptomatic and leads to latent infection in memory B-cells, which do not permit viral replication [37]. Although newly infected naive B-cells have the phenotypes of transformed cells, they are controlled by both EBV-specific cytotoxic T lymphocytes and natural killer cells unless immunity is suppressed [37, 38]. In immunocompromised hosts, transformed cells become proliferating blasts that can result in symptomatic disease, such as immunodeficiency-associated LPD [1, 10, 37, 38]. LPD is

MTX-LPD case number 13   MTX-LPD case number 8   Age-LPD case number 18

(a)   (b)   (c)

DLBCL case number 20   DLBCL case number 23   DLBCL case number 27

(d)   (e)   (f)

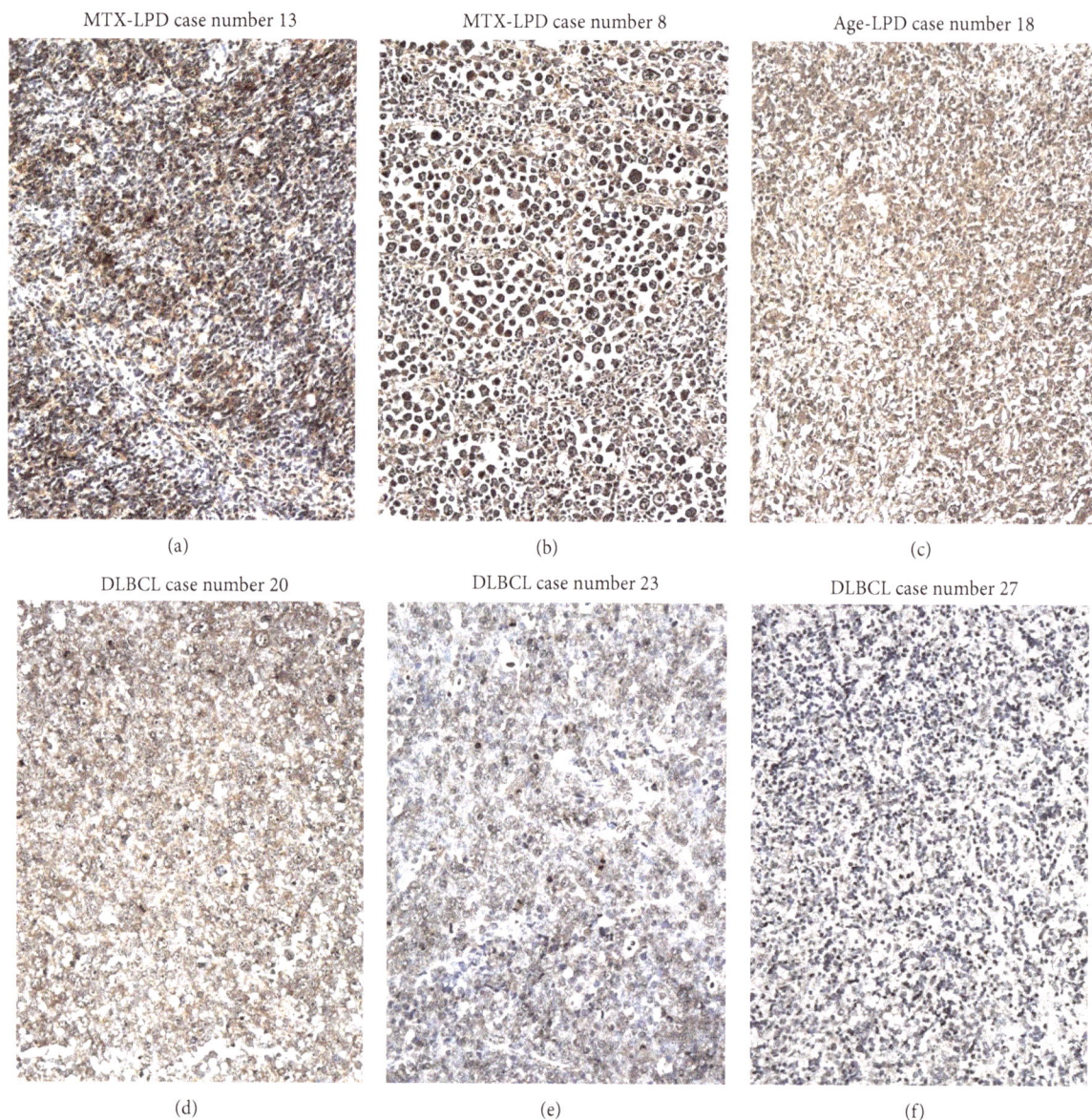

FIGURE 8: Distribution and intensity of Egr-1 expression in MTX-/Age-LPDs and DLBCLs in biopsy specimens. Egr-1 positive cells (brownish color) were diffuse and of strong intensity in ((a), (b)) MTX-LPDs and (c) Age-LPD and were a variety in ((d)–(f)) DLBCLs ((a)–(f) original magnification ×100).

characterized pathologically by focal or diffuse proliferation of atypical large B-cells including Reed-Sternberg-like cells with reactive components, which pose a diagnostic problem for pathologists. The spectrum of EBV-LPD is broad, ranging from benign polyclonal reactivation lesions to monoclonal EBV-DLBCL [39].

The major EBV-encoded LMP-1 is an integral membrane protein, which activates signaling pathways such as that involving NF-κB, which increases B-cell survival and induces transformation [12–16] by inducing antiapoptotic protein [17–19]. An *in vitro* study has reported that EBV-infected cells undergo hypermutation or switching of recombination via AID upregulation [20], and EBV-induced AID is also associated with oncogene mutations, which contribute to lymphomagenesis [21]. In a mouse bone marrow transplantation model, AID overexpression was reported to promote B-cell lymphomagenesis [40]. Although the relationship between LMP-1 and lymphomagenesis has been relatively well established, the molecular mechanisms underlying AID induction remain to be fully clarified. Recently, Kim et al. have reported that LMP-1 increases genomic instability through Egr-1-mediated upregulation of AID in B-cell lymphoma [18]. The Egr-1 gene (also named zif268, NGFI-A, or Krox24) encodes an 80 kDa DNA-binding transcription factor [41]. Egr-1 is an exceptionally multifunctional transcription factor. In response to growth factors and cytokine signaling, Egr-1 regulates cell growth, differentiation, and apoptosis [42]. Egr-1 has been associated with EBV infection, a human gamma herpes virus closely associated with several lymphoid and epithelial malignancies [43]. First, Egr-1 is upregulated when

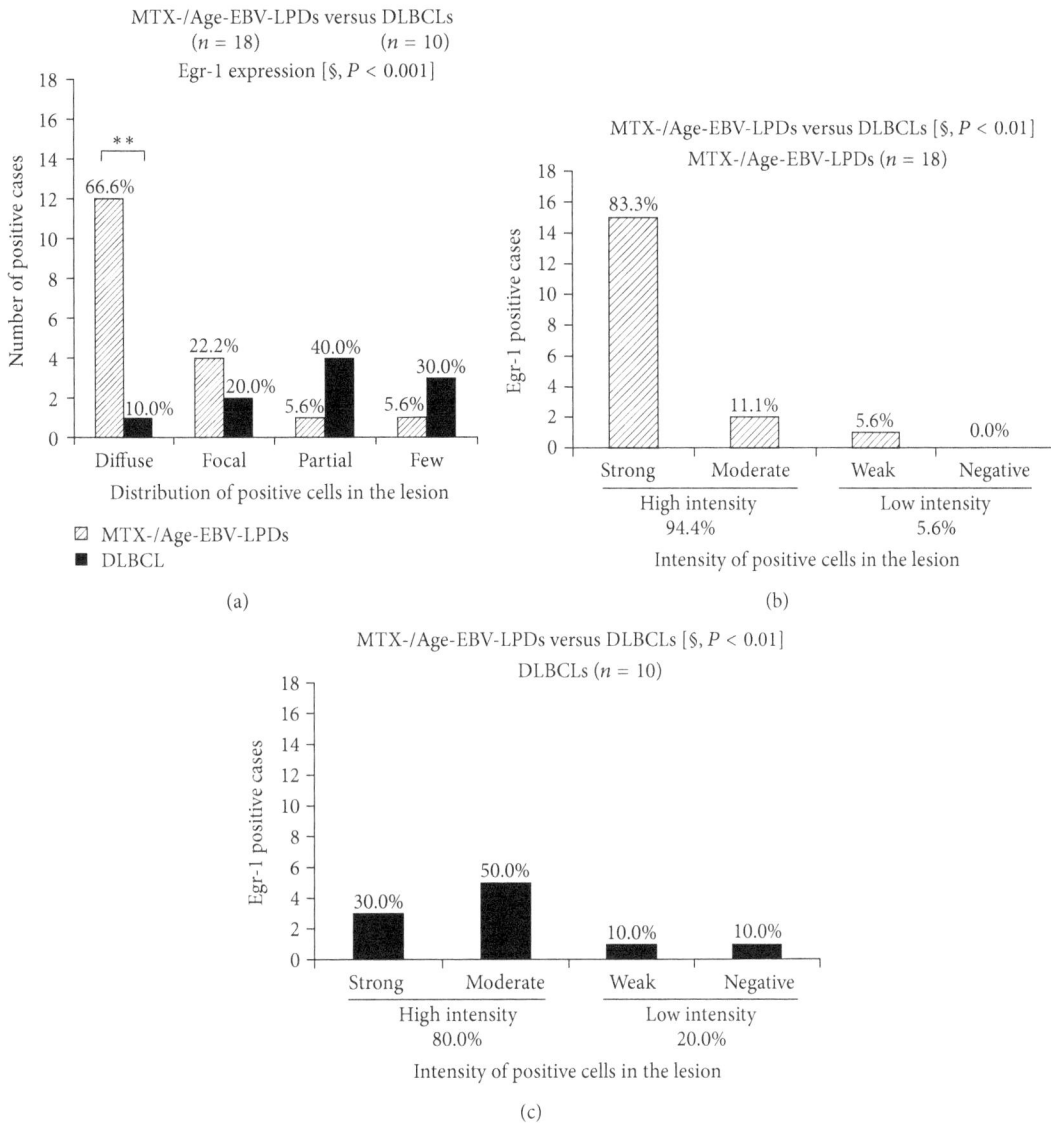

(a)

(b)

(c)

FIGURE 9: Distribution and intensity of Egr-1 expression in MTX-/Age-EBV-LPDs and DLBCLs. (a) Distribution of Egr-1-positive cells was more extensive in MTX-/Age-EBV-LPDs than in DLBCLs ($P < 0.001$). (a) In diffuse category, distribution of Egr-1 was significantly greater in MTX-/Age-EBV-LPDs (66.6%) than in DLBCLs (10.0%). ((b), (c)) Although the intensity of Egr-1 expression was high in both MTX/Age-EBV-LPDs (94.4%) and DLBCLs (80.0%), in the strong category, it was greater in the former (83.3%) than in the latter (30.0%). P values were examined by Mann-Whitney U test [§] or Exact Binominal test ($^*P < 0.05$, $^{**}P < 0.01$, and $^{***}P < 0.001$).

EBV interacts with B lymphocytes at the initial infection stage, and constitutive expression of Egr-1 correlates with certain types of EBV latency in B-lymphoid cell lines [44]. EBV reactivation is associated with upregulation of Egr-1, and Egr-1 can be induced as an EBV lytic transactivator [45]. However, there are no reports of any clinicopathological studies on LMP-1, AID, and Egr-1 in samples of human tissue. Therefore, we examined the density and distribution of AID, LMP-1, EBER, and Egr-1 in 19 cases of LPD and 10 cases of DLBCL.

The distribution of AID, LMP-1, and EBER expression was more extensive in patients with LPD than in patients with DLBCL. The intensity of AID, LMP-1, and EBER expression was higher in LPD (89.5%, 68.4%, and 94.7%) than in DLBCL

(20.0%, 10.0%, and 20.0%) patients (Figure 7). Although a higher intensity of expression was seen in LPD (94.4%) and DLBCL (80%), the intensity of Egr-1 expression was stronger in the former (83.3%) than in the latter (30.0%) (Figures 9(b) and 9(c)). These *in vivo* results partly supported the previous *in vitro* study by Kim et al. [18] and suggest that overexpression of AID in LPDs may be one process in the course of tumorigenic transformation.

The factor responsible for the lack of lymphoid tissue involvement in oral areas in patients with primary lymphoma/LPD is unclear, but there may be some association with bacteria in and around the teeth, together with chronic inflammation such as apical and marginal periodontitis. The copy number of EBV-DNA in subgingival plaque is associated with the presence of some periodontal bacteria [46]. A recent study has shown that periodontal disease could act as a risk factor for HIV reactivation [47] and similarly induce EBV reactivation [48]. Thus, there may be a relationship between AID, LMP-1, and Egr-1 expression in EBV-infected B-cells. Further studies, including the head and neck, will be needed to confirm the causal link between oral bacteria and EBV-positive lymphoma/LPDs of the oral cavity.

These results suggest that increased AID expression in LPDs may be part of the process of lymphomagenesis, thereby further increasing the survival of genetically destabilized B-cells. The reason why AID, LMP-1, and EBER were expressed more in the EBV related LPDs compared to DLBCL could be either the EBV infection or immunosuppression that is predominant in age-related lymphoma or in autoimmune diseases of patients taking methotrexate. The intensity and distribution of AID expression may be an indicator for differentiating EBV-driven LPDs from DLBCLs.

Conflict of Interests

The authors declare that there is no conflict of interests regarding the publication of this paper.

References

[1] B. Borisch, M. Raphael, S. H. Swerdlow et al., "Immunodeficiency associated lymphoproliferative disorders," in *World Health Organization Classification of Tumours: Pathology and Genetics of Tumours of Haematopoietic and Lymphoid Tissues*, E. S. Jaffe, N. L. Harris, H. Stein, and J. W. Vardiman, Eds., pp. 255–271, International Agency for Research on Cancer, Lyon, France, 2001.

[2] S. Nakamura, E. S. Jaffe, and S. H. Swerdlow, "BV-positive diffuse large B-cell lymphoma of the elderly," in *World Health Organization Classification of Tumours of Haematopoietic and Lymphoid Tissues*, S. J. Swerdlow, E. Campo, N. L. Harris et al., Eds., pp. 243–244, IARC, Lyon, France, 2008.

[3] R. F. Ambinder, "Epstein-Barr virus-associated lymphoproliferative disorders," *Reviews in Clinical and Experimental Hematology*, vol. 7, no. 4, pp. 362–374, 2003.

[4] J. Diebold, E. S. Jaffe, M. Raphael, and R. A. Warnke, "Burkitt lymphoma," in *Pathology and Genetics of Tumours of Haematopoietic and Lymphoid Tissues*, E. S. Jaffe, N. L. Harris, H. Stein, and J. W. Vardiman, Eds., World Health Organization Classification of Tumours, pp. 181–185, IARC, Lyon, France, 2001.

[5] J. K. C. Chan, E. S. Jaffe, and E. Ralfkiaer, "Extranodal NK/T-cell lymphoma, nasal type," in *World Health Organization Classification of Tumours. Pathology and Genetics of Tumours of Haematopoietic and Lymphoid Tissues*, E. S. Jaffe, N. L. Harris, H. Stein, and J. W. Vardiman, Eds., pp. 204–207, International Agency for Research on Cancer (IARC), Lyon, France, 2001.

[6] R. Fåhraeus, H. L. Fu, I. Ernberg et al., "Expression of Epstein-Barr virus-encoded proteins in nasopharyngeal carcinoma," *International Journal of Cancer*, vol. 42, no. 3, pp. 329–338, 1988.

[7] L. M. Weiss, L. A. Movahed, R. A. Warnke, and J. Sklar, "Detection of Epstein-Barr viral genomes in Reed-Sternberg cells of Hodgkin's disease," *The New England Journal of Medicine*, vol. 320, no. 8, pp. 502–506, 1989.

[8] D. Shibata and L. M. Weiss, "Epstein-Barr virus-associated gastric adenocarcinoma," *American Journal of Pathology*, vol. 140, no. 4, pp. 769–774, 1992.

[9] J. M. Kwon, Y. H. Park, J. H. Kang et al., "The effect of Epstein-Barr virus status on clinical outcome in Hodgkin's lymphoma," *Annals of Hematology*, vol. 85, no. 7, pp. 463–468, 2006.

[10] E. S. Jaffe, N. L. Harris, S. J. Swerdlow et al., "Immunodeficiency-associated lymphoproliferative disorder," in *World Health Organization Classification of Tumors of Haematopoietic and Lymphoid Tissues*, S. J. Swerdlow, E. Campo, N. L. Harris et al., Eds., pp. 335–351, IARC, Lyon, France, 2008.

[11] T. Oyama, K. Ichimura, R. Suzuki et al., "Senile EBV⁺ B-cell lymphoproliferative disorders: a clinicopathologic study of 22 patients," *The American Journal of Surgical Pathology*, vol. 27, no. 1, pp. 16–26, 2003.

[12] P. G. Murray, L. S. Young, M. Rowe, and J. Crocker, "Immunohistochemical demonstration of the Epstein-Barr virus-encoded latent membrane protein in paraffin sections of Hodgkin's disease," *The Journal of Pathology*, vol. 166, no. 1, pp. 1–5, 1992.

[13] M. Peng and E. Lundgren, "Transient expression of the Epstein-Barr virus LMP1 gene in human primary B cells induces cellular activation and DNA synthesis," *Oncogene*, vol. 7, no. 9, pp. 1775–1782, 1992.

[14] D. S. Huen, S. A. Henderson, D. Croom-Carter, and M. Rowe, "The Epstein-Barr virus latent membrane protein-1 (LMP1) mediates activation of NF-κB and cell surface phenotype via two effector regions in its carboxy-terminal cytoplasmic domain," *Oncogene*, vol. 10, no. 3, pp. 549–560, 1995.

[15] O. Gires, U. Zimber-Strobl, R. Gonnella et al., "Latent membrane protein 1 of Epstein-Barr virus mimics a constitutively active receptor molecule," *The EMBO Journal*, vol. 16, no. 20, pp. 6131–6140, 1997.

[16] E. D. C. McFarland, K. M. Izumi, and G. Mosialos, "Epstein-Barr virus transformation: involvement of latent membrane protein 1-mediated activation of NF-κB," *Oncogene*, vol. 18, no. 49, pp. 6959–6964, 1999.

[17] K. R. N. Baumforth, L. S. Young, K. J. Flavell, C. Constandinou, and P. G. Murray, "The Epstein-Barr virus and its association with human cancers," *Journal of Clinical Pathology—Molecular Pathology*, vol. 52, no. 6, pp. 307–322, 1999.

[18] J. H. Kim, W. S. Kim, J. H. Kang, H.-Y. Lim, Y.-H. Ko, and C. Park, "Egr-1, a new downstream molecule of Epstein-Barr virus latent membrane protein 1," *FEBS Letters*, vol. 581, no. 4, pp. 623–628, 2007.

[19] J. H. Kim, W. S. Kim, and C. Park, "SNARK, a novel downstream molecule of EBV latent membrane protein 1, is associated with resistance to cancer cell death," *Leukemia and Lymphoma*, vol. 49, no. 7, pp. 1392–1398, 2008.

[20] B. He, N. Raab-Traub, P. Casali, and A. Cerutti, "EBV-encoded latent membrane protein 1 cooperates with BAFF/BLyS and APRIL to induce T cell-independent Ig heavy chain class switching," *The Journal of Immunology*, vol. 171, no. 10, pp. 5215–5224, 2003.

[21] M. Epeldegui, Y. P. Hung, A. McQuay, R. F. Ambinder, and O. Martínez-Maza, "Infection of human B cells with Epstein-Barr virus results in the expression of somatic hypermutation-inducing molecules and in the accrual of oncogene mutations," *Molecular Immunology*, vol. 44, no. 5, pp. 934–942, 2007.

[22] M. Muramatsu, V. S. Sankaranand, S. Anant et al., "Specific expression of activation-induced cytidine deaminase (AID),

a novel member of the RNA-editing deaminase family in germinal center B cells," *The Journal of Biological Chemistry*, vol. 274, no. 26, pp. 18470–18476, 1999.

[23] P. Revy, T. Muto, Y. Levy et al., "Activation-induced cytidine deaminase (AID) deficiency causes the autosomal recessive form of the hyper-IgM syndrome (HIGM2)," *Cell*, vol. 102, no. 5, pp. 565–575, 2000.

[24] M. Muramatsu, K. Kinoshita, S. Fagarasan, S. Yamada, Y. Shinkai, and T. Honjo, "Class switch recombination and hypermutation require activation-induced cytidine deaminase (AID), a potential RNA editing enzyme," *Cell*, vol. 102, no. 5, pp. 553–563, 2000.

[25] V. G. De Yábenes and A. R. Romiro, "Activation-induced deaminase: light and dark sides," *Trends in Molecular Medicine*, vol. 12, no. 9, pp. 432–439, 2006.

[26] S. Longerich, U. Basu, F. Alt, and U. Storb, "AID in somatic hypermutation and class switch recombination," *Current Opinion in Immunology*, vol. 18, no. 2, pp. 164–174, 2006.

[27] R. K. Delker, S. D. Fugmann, and F. N. Papavasiliou, "A coming-of-age story: activation-induced cytidine deaminase turns 10," *Nature Immunology*, vol. 10, no. 11, pp. 1147–1153, 2009.

[28] M. Kuraoka, L. McWilliams, and G. Kelsoe, "AID expression during B-cell development: searching for answers," *Immunologic Research*, vol. 49, no. 1–3, pp. 3–13, 2011.

[29] S.-R. Park, "Activation-induced cytidine deaminase in B cell immunity and cancers," *Immune Network*, vol. 12, no. 6, pp. 230–239, 2012.

[30] D. F. Robbiani and M. C. Nussenzweig, "Chromosome translocation, B cell lymphoma, and activation-induced cytidine deaminase," *Annual Review of Pathology: Mechanisms of Disease*, vol. 8, pp. 79–103, 2013.

[31] L. Pasqualucci, R. Guglielmino, J. Houldsworth et al., "Expression of the AID protein in normal and neoplastic B cells," *Blood*, vol. 104, no. 10, pp. 3318–3325, 2004.

[32] G. Cattoretti, M. Büttner, R. Shaknovich, E. Kremmer, B. Alobeid, and G. Niedobitek, "Nuclear and cytoplasmic AID in extrafollicular and germinal center B cells," *Blood*, vol. 107, no. 10, pp. 3967–3975, 2006.

[33] J. H. Kim, W. S. Kim, and C. Park, "Epstein-Barr virus latent membrane protein 1 increases genomic instability through Egr-1-mediated up-regulation of activation-induced cytidine deaminase in B-cell lymphoma," *Leukemia and Lymphoma*, vol. 54, no. 9, pp. 2035–2040, 2013.

[34] K. Kikuchi, H. Inoue, Y. Miyazaki et al., "Adult sporadic burkitt lymphoma of the oral cavity: a case report and literature review," *Journal of Oral and Maxillofacial Surgery*, vol. 70, no. 12, pp. 2936–2943, 2012.

[35] K. Kikuchi, Y. Miyazaki, A. Tanaka et al., "Methotrexate-related Epstein-Barr Virus (EBV)-associated lymphoproliferative disorder–so-called 'Hodgkin-like lesion'—of the oral cavity in a patient with rheumatoid arthritis," *Head and Neck Pathology*, vol. 4, no. 4, pp. 305–311, 2010.

[36] K. Kikuchi, S. Fukunaga, H. Inoue et al., "A case of age-related Epstein-Barr virus (EBV)-associated B cell lymphoproliferative disorder, so-called polymorphous subtype, of the mandible, with a review of the literature," *Head and Neck Pathology*, vol. 7, no. 2, pp. 178–187, 2013.

[37] H. Kimura, Y. Ito, R. Suzuki, and Y. Nishiyama, "Measuring Epstein–Barr virus (EBV) load: the significance and application for each EBV-associated disease," *Reviews in Medical Virology*, vol. 18, no. 5, pp. 305–319, 2008.

[38] J. I. Cohen, "Epstein-Barr virus infection," *The New England Journal of Medicine*, vol. 343, no. 7, pp. 481–492, 2000.

[39] Y. Shimoyama, N. Asano, M. Kojima et al., "Age-related EBV-associated B-cell lymphoproliferative disorders: diagnostic approach to a newly recognized clinicopathological entity," *Pathology International*, vol. 59, no. 12, pp. 835–843, 2009.

[40] Y. Komeno, J. Kitaura, N. Watanabe-Okochi et al., "AID-induced T-lymphoma or B-leukemia/lymphoma in a mouse BMT model," *Leukemia*, vol. 24, no. 5, pp. 1018–1024, 2010.

[41] J. Milbrandt, "A nerve growth factor-induced gene encodes a possible transcriptional regulatory factor," *Science*, vol. 238, no. 4828, pp. 797–799, 1987.

[42] S. Bhattacharyya, F. Fang, W. Tourtellotte, and J. Varga, "Egr-1: new conductor for the tissue repair orchestra directs harmony (regeneration) or cacophony (fibrosis)," *Journal of Pathology*, vol. 229, no. 2, pp. 286–297, 2013.

[43] A. B. Rickinson and E. Kieff, "Epstein-Barr virus," in *Fields Virology*, D. M. Knipe and P. M. Howley, Eds., pp. 2575–2627, Lippincott Williams & Wilkins, Philadelphia, Pa, USA, 4th edition, 2001.

[44] A. Calogero, L. Cuomo, M. D'Onofrio et al., "Expression of Egr-1 correlates with the transformed phenotype and the type of viral latency in EBV genome positive lymphoid cell lines," *Oncogene*, vol. 13, no. 10, pp. 2105–2112, 1996.

[45] Y. Chang, H. H. Lee, Y. T. Chen et al., "Induction of the early growth response 1 gene by Epstein-Barr virus lytic transactivator Zta," *Journal of Virology*, vol. 80, no. 15, pp. 7748–7755, 2006.

[46] D. R. Dawson III, C. Wang, R. J. Danaher et al., "Real-time polymerase chain reaction to determine the prevalence and copy number of epstein-barr virus and cytomegalovirus DNA in subgingival plaque at individual healthy and periodontal disease sites," *Journal of Periodontology*, vol. 80, no. 7, pp. 1133–1140, 2009.

[47] K. Imai, K. Ochiai, and T. Okamoto, "Reactivation of latent HIV-1 infection by the periodontopathic bacterium *Porphyromonas gingivalis* involves histone modification," *The Journal of Immunology*, vol. 182, no. 6, pp. 3688–3695, 2009.

[48] K. Imai, H. Inoue, M. Tamura et al., "The periodontal pathogen Porphyromonas gingivalis induces the Epstein-Barr virus lytic switch transactivator ZEBRA by histone modification," *Biochimie*, vol. 94, no. 3, pp. 839–846, 2012.

3

Right Ventricular Dysfunction in Patients Experiencing Cardiotoxicity during Breast Cancer Therapy

Anna Calleja,[1] **Frédéric Poulin,**[1,2] **Ciril Khorolsky,**[1] **Masoud Shariat,**[3]
Philippe L. Bedard,[4] **Eitan Amir,**[4] **Harry Rakowski,**[1] **Michael McDonald,**[1]
Diego Delgado,[1] **and Paaladinesh Thavendiranathan**[1,3]

[1]*Division of Cardiology, Peter Munk Cardiac Center, Toronto General Hospital, University Health Network, University of Toronto, 200 Elizabeth Street, Toronto, ON, Canada M5G 2C4*
[2]*Division of Cardiology, Hôpital du Sacré-Coeur de Montréal, University of Montreal, 5400 Boulevard Gouin Ouest, Montreal, QC, Canada H4J 1C5*
[3]*Division of Medical Imaging, Peter Munk Cardiac Center, Toronto General Hospital, University Health Network, University of Toronto, 200 Elizabeth Street, Toronto, ON, Canada M5G 2C4*
[4]*Division of Medical Oncology & Hematology, Princess Margaret Cancer Center, University Health Network, University of Toronto, 610 University Avenue, Toronto, ON, Canada M5T 2M9*

Correspondence should be addressed to Paaladinesh Thavendiranathan; dinesh.thavendiranathan@uhn.ca

Academic Editor: Daniel Lenihan

Background. Right ventricular (RV) dysfunction during cancer therapy related cardiotoxicity and its prognostic implications have not been examined. *Aim.* We sought to determine the incidence and prognostic value of RV dysfunction at time of LV defined cardiotoxicity. *Methods.* We retrospectively identified 30 HER2+ female patients with breast cancer treated with trastuzumab (± anthracycline) who developed cardiotoxicity and had a diagnostic quality transthoracic echocardiography. LV ejection fraction (LVEF), RV fractional area change (RV FAC), and peak systolic longitudinal strain (for both LV and RV) were measured on echocardiograms at the time of cardiotoxicity and during follow-up. Thirty age balanced precancer therapy and HER2+ breast cancer patients were used as controls. *Results.* In the 30 patients with cardiotoxicity (mean ± SD age 54 ± 12 years) RV FAC was significantly lower (42 ± 7 versus 47 ± 6%, $P = 0.01$) compared to controls. RV dysfunction defined by global longitudinal strain (GLS < −20.3%) was seen in 40% ($n = 12$). During follow-up in 16 out of 30 patients (23 ± 15 months), there was persistent LV dysfunction (EF < 55%) in 69% ($n = 11$). Concomitant RV dysfunction at the time of LV cardiotoxicity was associated with reduced recovery of LVEF during follow-up although this was not statistically significant. *Conclusion.* RV dysfunction at the time of LV cardiotoxicity is frequent in patients with breast cancer receiving trastuzumab therapy. Despite appropriate management, LV dysfunction persisted in the majority at follow-up. The prognostic value of RV dysfunction at the time of cardiotoxicity warrants further investigation.

1. Introduction

Breast cancer is the leading cause of cancer in women worldwide [1, 2]. Survival from breast cancer has improved significantly over the past 15–20 years primarily due to advances in cancer treatment [3]. However, many anticancer drugs used for the treatment of patients with breast cancer have the potential to cause cardiac toxicity (cardiotoxicity). Anthracycline-based chemotherapy and trastuzumab

(TZM), a monoclonal antibody against the HER2 receptor, are of particular concern due to the high incidence of cardiotoxicity individually and with combined use [4, 5]. Once left ventricular (LV) dysfunction or heart failure (HF) occurs from anthracycline and/or TZM based therapy the prognosis can be poor with lack of LV function recovery in up to 40–58% of the patients and subsequent major adverse cardiac events [6, 7]. Due to the poor prognosis of advanced cardiac dysfunction [6, 8], many argue for efforts to identify early cardiac dysfunction so that appropriate intervention can be initiated to prevent HF [9]. This can include administration of cardiac treatment such as beta-blockers, ACE inhibitors, and dexrazoxane; selection of alternative cancer regimens or dose adjustment; and transient cessation of cancer treatment [9]. In TZM treated patients in particular, early cardiac dysfunction is identified by repeated cardiac imaging performed prior and during cancer therapy. Cardiotoxicity is commonly defined based on a symptomatic fall in LVEF of >5 percentage points or an asymptomatic fall of >10 percentage points to <55% between pre- and during treatment measurements as defined by the cardiac review and evaluation committee criteria (CREC) [10].

To date, there has been very little focus on the toxic effects of cancer therapy on the right ventricle (RV) [11, 12]. Given the thinner structure of the RV with fewer myofibrils, the RV may also be susceptible to damage by cardiotoxic therapy. Several studies have shown that RV wall motion abnormalities [13] or functional abnormalities [12, 14] occur *during cancer therapy*; however, this finding has not been universally observed [11, 15]. The presence of RV dysfunction at the *time of LV cardiotoxicity* and whether it has prognostic implications has not been examined. However, in many other cardiovascular diseases the concomitant RV dysfunction is associated with worse outcomes [16–18]. In this study we sought to determine the incidence of RV dysfunction at the time of cardiotoxicity in women with HER2+ breast cancer receiving treatment with trastuzumab using measurements of fractional area change and myocardial peak systolic longitudinal strain. Secondly as a hypothesis generating objective we examined the prognostic value of RV dysfunction in subsequent LV function recovery during follow-up in a subgroup of patients who had follow-up imaging after completion of cancer therapy.

2. Methods

2.1. Study Population. We retrospectively identified all women >18 years of age with HER2/neu overexpressing (HER2+) breast cancer of any stage treated with TZM with or without anthracyclines at a large cancer referral center (Princess Margaret Cancer Center, Toronto, Canada) between 2006 and 2013 from the hospital pharmacy database. We included patients who (1) developed cardiotoxicity during the treatment course using the CREC criteria [10] and (2) had an echocardiogram with adequate image quality at the time of diagnosis of cardiotoxicity. For each patient the following data were obtained through electronic patient records: patient demographics, cardiac risk factors, previous cardiac history, cardiac medication use, cancer history, cancer therapy with doses used, radiotherapy history, LVEF and RVEF measurements by multigated acquisition (MUGA) pre-cancer therapy and at the time of cardiotoxicity, clinical symptoms of heart failure, and management of cardiotoxicity. The study protocol was approved by the institutional Research Ethics Board.

2.2. Controls. Age and cardiac risk factor balanced women with a diagnosis of HER2+ breast cancer without history of any previous cardiovascular disease and who had an echocardiogram prior to initiation of any cancer therapy were included as controls. This was necessary as currently existing normal values for some of the myocardial function measures used in this study such as RV strain are variable and age- and vendor-specific and have never been studied in patients with cancer. Also during the study period it was routine for patients at our center to be followed by MUGA scans as opposed to echocardiography. Therefore, since baseline echocardiography was not available in our patients with cardiotoxicity this comparison with a control group was essential.

2.3. Transthoracic Echocardiogram: Conventional Parameters and Myocardial Strain. Echocardiography studies from patients at the time of LV cardiotoxicity and from the control group were read together blinded to the group designation and clinical history. LVEF was calculated using the Biplane Simpson's method and RV FAC (analogous to LVEF) following existing American Society of Echocardiography (ASE) guidelines [19, 20].

Myocardial peak systolic longitudinal strain was measured offline for both the LV and RV based on the ASE recommendations [21] using commercially available software (Vector Velocity Imaging (VVI) 3.0, Siemens Medical Solutions, Mountain View, CA) using the speckle tracking technique. Briefly, apical 4-, 3-, and 2-chamber images of the LV and an apical 4-chamber view of the RV in DICOM format were obtained for each patient and loaded into the VVI software. Endocardial contours were drawn along the LV and RV border separately for measurement of respective longitudinal strain values (Figures 1 and 2). The contours were adjusted as needed to ensure adequate visual tracking of the endocardium. Any segments that were not tracked adequately after 5 attempts at adjustment were excluded from the analysis. LV peak systolic global longitudinal endocardial strain (GLS) was measured by taking the average of the peak endocardial strain curves in the apical 4-, 3-, and 2-chamber views (16-segment model) (Figure 1). As conventionally done, RV peak systolic global longitudinal endocardial strain (RVGLS) was measured from all 6 RV myocardial segments from an apical 4-chamber view (3 segments of the free wall and 3 segments of the interventricular septum) while the RV free wall peak systolic longitudinal strain (RVFWLS) was obtained from the 3 RV free wall segments only (Figure 2). This distinction is made since measurement of RVGLS based on the inclusion of the interventricular septum may partially reflect changes in the left ventricle as the septum is shared by both ventricles. RVFWLS focuses only on the RV free wall and does not include contribution of the septum; however, it does not account for potential changes that may occur in the RV septum.

2.4. Follow-Up. As a hypothesis generating objective, to examine the prognostic value of RV dysfunction on subsequent LV function recovery after completion of all cancer therapy, we identified those who had at least one follow-up echocardiogram ≥3 months after completion of their cancer therapy with adequate image quality. In these patients the last

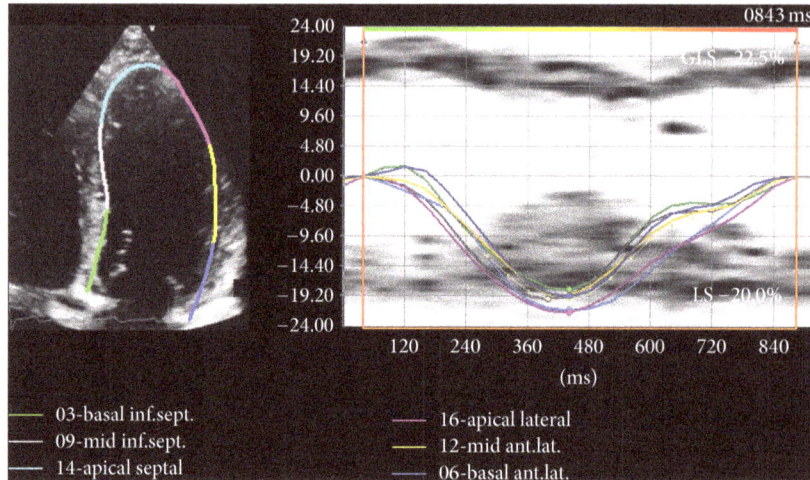

(a)

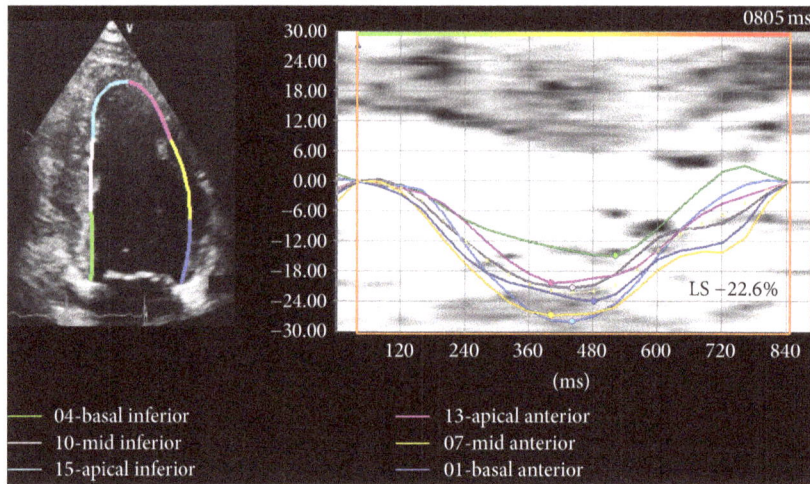

(b)

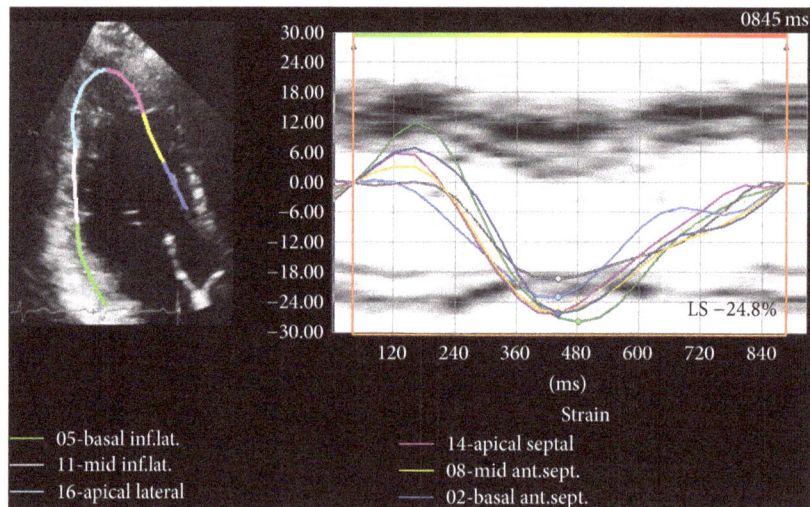

(c)

FIGURE 1: Left ventricular peak systolic longitudinal strain. Representative example of normal left ventricular peak endocardial strain curves: left panel shows B-mode images with endocardial tracings in the (a) 4-chamber, (b) 2-chamber, and (c) 3-chamber views with their corresponding longitudinal strain curves to its right. For each view 5-6 curves are shown representing strain values for each of the myocardial segments. Peak global longitudinal strain (GLS) is an average of the longitudinal strain (LS) values obtained from each view and a total of 16 segments (6 basal, 6 midventricular, and 4 apical segments).

(a)

(b)

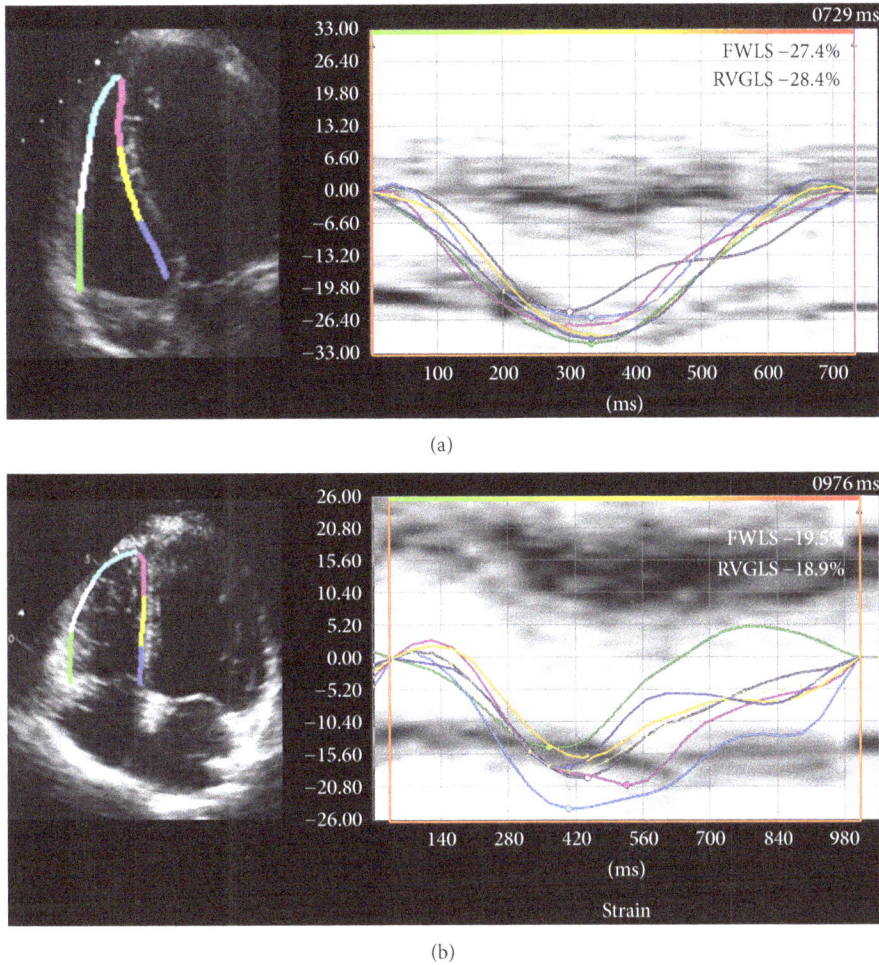

FIGURE 2: Right ventricular systolic longitudinal strain. Right ventricular peak endocardial strain curves. Left panel shows B-mode images of the RV in 4-chamber view with endocardial tracing and to its right is the corresponding strain curve in (a) control and (b) during cardiotoxicity. Right ventricular free wall longitudinal strain (RVFWLS) is composed of 3 segments while right ventricular peak systolic global longitudinal strain (RVGLS) includes all 6 segments (RV free wall and septum).

available echocardiogram was used to measure LVEF, FAC, and strain values. In addition the following clinical history was obtained through EPR: cardiac symptoms, medication use, and new diagnosis of other cardiac conditions.

2.5. Interobserver and Intraobserver Variability. Twenty randomly selected studies were reanalyzed by the same observer (AC) several months after the initial analysis and a second observer (FP) blinded to the original measurements for the assessment of intra- and interobserver variability of RV strain measurements.

2.6. Statistical Analysis. Normality for each variable was tested using a combination of quantile-quantile plots and the Kolmogorov-Smirnov test. Depending on the normality, variables are expressed as mean ± SD or median and interquartile range (IQR). Independent sample t-test or Wilcoxon rank sum test was used to compare continuous data between groups. A paired t-test or a Wilcoxon sign rank test was used to compare patients at the time of cardiotoxicity and

at follow-up. Fisher's exact test was used to compare categorical data between the groups. Intraclass correlation coefficient (ICC) was used to assess interobserver and intraobserver variability. A P value of <0.05 was considered statistically significant. All statistical analyses were performed using MedCalc software (ver 11.4.2 Belgium).

3. Results

3.1. Patients and Cancer Treatment. A total of 598 female patients with breast cancer received trastuzumab treatment between 2006 and 2013 at the Princess Margaret Cancer Center. Amongst these patients 30 (5%) were identified as having experienced cardiotoxicity, had a diagnostic quality echocardiogram at the time of cardiotoxicity, and met our inclusion criteria. The remaining 568 patients were either not identified as having cardiotoxicity by the treating oncologist, had an echocardiography study with poor image quality at the time of cardiotoxicity, or were only followed by MUGA studies. Amongst the 30 included patients, 26 (87%) had early stage breast cancer (≤ stage III) and 4 patients had

TABLE 1: Patient and control demographics.

	Control $n = 30$	Cohort $n = 30$
Age	51 ± 8	54 ± 12
Stages (I–III)	30 (100%)	26 (87%)
NYHA II-III	—	16 (53%)
Cardiac risk factor		
Coronary artery disease	—	—
Hypertension	5 (17%)	6 (20%)
Diabetes mellitus	1 (3%)	3 (10%)
Dyslipidemia	—	3 (10%)
Smoker	3 (10%)	1 (3%)
Chemotherapeutic regimen		
AC-TH		13 (43%)
Epirubicin mg/m^2	—	*302.4 ± 10
FEC + DH		9 (30%)
Doxorubicin mg/m^2	—	*231.2 ± 18.7
TCH		3 (10%)
TH		5 (17%)
Radiation		23 (77%)
Mastectomy		21 (70%)
Previous cancer[†]		6 (20%)
Ventricular systolic function by MUGA (%)		
LVEF		
Prechemo	—	62 ± 5
At time of cardiotoxicity		48 ± 4
RVEF		
Prechemo		45 ± 4
At time of cardiotoxicity		43 ± 6

[*] Mean cumulative dose, [†] 4 were previously diagnosed with breast tumor and at the time of the study were being treated for recurrence, and 2 had previous history of Ewing's Sarcoma and Hodgkin's lymphoma. AC-TH: doxorubicin and cyclophosphamide followed by either paclitaxel or docetaxel and trastuzumab; FEC-DH: 5-fluorouracil, epirubicin, and cyclophosphamide followed by docetaxel and trastuzumab; TCH: docetaxel, carboplatin or cyclophosphamide, and trastuzumab; TH: trastuzumab and docetaxel or paclitaxel.

metastatic disease. In patients with early stage disease, 13 received doxorubicin and cyclophosphamide followed by either paclitaxel or docetaxel and TZM (AC-TH) while 9 received 5-fluorouracil, epirubicin, and cyclophosphamide followed by docetaxel and TZM (FEC-DH), and 3 patients received docetaxel, carboplatin or cyclophosphamide, and TZM (TCH). One patient with early stage disease with history of prior early breast cancer treated with FEC twelve years before her new breast cancer diagnosis received only TZM and docetaxel. The 4 patients with metastatic disease received a combination of a taxane (either paclitaxel or docetaxel) and TZM. In patients who received anthracyclines, the mean cumulative dose of epirubicin administered was 302 ± 10 mg/m^2 while in those who received doxorubicin the mean dose was 231 ± 19 mg/m^2 (Table 1).

TABLE 2: Conventional and strain parameters measured by echocardiography in patients with cardiotoxicity and the control group.

	Control $n = 30$	Cardiotoxicity $n = 30$	P
Left ventricle			
EF Biplane (%)	59 ± 2	46 ± 6	<0.0001
GLS	−21.1 ± 1.2	−15.5 ± 2.4	<0.0001
Right ventricle			
RVSP mmHg	24 ± 6.4	29 ± 7.5	0.01
FAC (%)	47 ± 6	42 ± 7	0.01
RVFWLS	−28.8 ± 3.6	−25.0 ± 4.3	0.0005
RVGLS	−25.7 ± 2.7	−21.0 ± 3.1	<0.0001

GLS: global longitudinal strain, FAC: fractional area change, RVFWLS: right ventricular free wall longitudinal strain (3 segments), and RVGLS: right ventricular global longitudinal strain (includes all 6 segments).

3.2. Timing and Management of Cardiotoxicity.

All patients with cardiotoxicity had normal pre-chemotherapy LV and RV function by MUGA with a mean LVEF of 62 ± 5% and mean RVEF of 45 ± 5%. In patients who received anthracycline followed by trastuzumab ($n = 22$), cardiotoxicity occurred immediately after anthracycline therapy in one and during trastuzumab treatment in the rest with a median (IQR) time to occurrence of 5.0 (5.0) months. In the 8 patients who received trastuzumab without anthracyclines, the median (IQR) time to cardiotoxicity was 7.5 months (5.7). At the time of cardiotoxicity, 17 (57%) patients reported symptoms consistent with NYHA 2-3, while the rest were NYHA 1. Management of cardiotoxicity included withholding TZM treatment only in 10 patients, adding ACE inhibitors and/or beta-blockers along with withholding TZM in 9 patients, and starting ACE inhibitors and/or beta blockers while continuing TZM in 4. In 7 patients, TZM was continued with close monitoring. The latter reflects the variability in clinical practice.

3.3. Ventricular Function at Time of Cardiotoxicity.

LV function by MUGA was significantly reduced to 48 ± 4% compared to pretreatment values of 62 ± 5% ($P < 0.0001$). LVEF by MUGA and echo at the time of cardiotoxicity were not significantly different (48 ± 4% versus 46 ± 6%, $P = 0.13$). When compared to controls, the LVEF by echocardiography in patients with cardiotoxicity was significantly lower as expected (59 ± 2% versus 46 ± 6, $P < 0.0001$). Similarly LV peak systolic global longitudinal strain (GLS −21.1 ± 1.2% versus −15.5 ± 2.4%, $P < 0.0001$) was significantly lower in patients with cardiotoxicity compared to controls (Table 2). This value is also significantly lower than the published lower limit of normal for LV GLS of −18.9% ($P < 0.001$) [9, 22].

Precancer treatment RV function by MUGA was 45 ± 4% (normal) [23] while at the time of cardiotoxicity it was 43 ± 6 ($P = 0.19$). None of the patients had abnormal RV function pretherapy. By echocardiography at the time of cardiotoxicity the mean RV function by FAC was significantly lower than the controls although still in the normal range (42 ± 7% versus 47 ± 6% $P = 0.01$) with 3 (10%) patients having

TABLE 3: Ventricular function at the time of cardiotoxicity by chemotherapy agent received.

	(+) Anthracycline $n = 22$	(−) Anthracycline $n = 8$
Time to toxicity in months*	5 (5)	7.5 (5.7)
Left ventricle		
Baseline EF by MUGA (%)	62 ± 6	60 ± 3
Cardiotoxicity EF by MUGA (%)	48 ± 4	47 ± 4
Cardiotoxicity EF by ECHO (%)	46 ± 6	44 ± 5
Cardiotoxicity GLS	−15.5 ± 2.5	−15.7 ± 2.5
Right ventricle		
Baseline EF by MUGA (%)	46 ± 4	43 ± 3
Cardiotoxicity EF by MUGA (%)	44 ± 6	40 ± 5
Cardiotoxicity FAC by ECHO (%)	42 ± 8	43 ± 5
Cardiotoxicity RVFWLS	−24.1 ± 3.9	−27.4 ± 4.6
Cardiotoxicity RVGLS	−20.4 ± 2.8	−22.8 ± 3.2

*Median (IQR) onset of cardiotoxicity which occurred after initiation of TZM therapy in 21 patients; in 1 patient toxicity occurred after 3 months from the start of chemotherapy. Abbreviations as per Table 2.

TABLE 4: Ventricular function at time of cardiotoxicity and at follow-up ($n = 16$) in patients with only left ventricular dysfunction at the time of cardiotoxicity and in those with biventricular dysfunction.

	Cardiotoxicity	Posttreatment
Left ventricular dysfunction $n = 10$		
EF Biplane (%)	44 ± 7	51 ± 9
GLS	−15.7 ± 2.4	−17.6 ± 3.1
FAC (%)	44 ± 5	46 ± 9
RVGLS	−22.2 ± 1.4	−23.2 ± −5.5
RVFWLS	−27.0 ± 3.2	−26.1 ± 6.6
Biventricular dysfunction based on RVGLS $n = 6$		
EF biplane (%)	47 ± 3	52 ± 3
LV GLS	−14.4 ± 1.7	−16.4 ± 1.6
FAC	39 ± 11	48 ± 6
RVGLS	−17.8 ± 1.2	−22.3 ± 2.9
RVFWLS	−21.6 ± 2.8	−26.3 ± 5.0
Biventricular dysfunction based on RVFWLS $n = 3$		
EF biplane (%)	49 ± 5	52 ± 2.5
LV GLS	−15.6 ± 0.8	−16.1 ± 1.1
FAC	33 ± 11	48 ± 3
RVGLS	−14.6 ± 0.7	−21.8 ± 2.1
RVFWLS	−19.5 ± 1.1	−23.5 ± 2.4

Abbreviations as per Table 2.

an abnormal FAC (<35%). The RV strain was significantly decreased (*i.e., less negative*) in patients with cardiotoxicity compared to controls for both RVGLS (−21.0 ± 3.1% versus −25.7 ± 2.7%, $P < 0.0001$) and RVFWLS (−25.0 ± 4.3% versus −28.8 ± 3.6%, $P = 0.005$) (Table 2). Using a cut-off value of −20.3% for RVGLS and −21.6% for RVFWLS (2SD below mean value for the controls), 12 (40%) and 5 patients (17%), respectively, had reduced RV function by strain analysis. The RVSP (a marker of pulmonary systolic pressures) was also slightly higher in patients with cardiotoxicity compared to controls (Table 2) although still within the normal range. The changes in LV and RV parameters at the time of cardiotoxicity in patients who received anthracycline versus those who did not are summarized in Table 3.

3.4. Ventricular Function at Follow-Up. Follow-up echocardiograms at least *3 months after completion of cancer therapy* were available in 16 of the 30 patients. Mean time from completion of therapy to follow-up echocardiogram was 23 ± 15 months. At follow-up, compared to the time of cardiotoxicity, there was significant improvement in LVEF (from 45 ± 6% to 52 ± 7%, $P = 0.0001$) and LV GLS (−15.2 ± 2.2 to −17.2 ± 2.6%, $P = 0.004$). However, only 5 patients at follow-up had a Biplane LVEF in the normal range (i.e., ≥55%). The mean RV function measured by FAC did not change significantly between the time of

cardiotoxicity and follow-up (43 ± 8% to 46 ± 8%, $P = 0.13$). Likewise there was no significant improvement in RVGLS (−20.5 ± 2.6% to −22.9 ± 5% $P = 0.09$) or RVFWLS (−25.0 ± 3.9% to −26.2 ± 5.9% $P = 0.48$) at follow-up. The changes in LV and RV parameters between time of cardiotoxicity and follow-up in patients with LV dysfunction only versus those with coexisting LV and RV dysfunction at the time of cardiotoxicity is summarized in Table 4. Also ventricular function parameters at baseline, at the time of cardiotoxicity, and at follow-up are provided separately for patients with and without LVEF recovery in Table 5.

We also examined the association between RV strain abnormalities at the time of cardiotoxicity and subsequent recovery of LVEF at follow-up. LVEF recovery was seen in only 1 out of 6 patients (17%) with abnormal RVGLS at the time of cardiotoxicity while it was seen in 4 out of 10 patients (40%) with normal RVGLS ($P = 0.59$). Similarly, recovery in LVEF did not occur in any of the 3 patients (0%) with abnormal RVFWLS at the time of cardiotoxicity while it occurred 5 out of 13 patients (38%) with normal RVFWLS ($P = 0.51$). When patients with and without LV function recovery were compared, none of the patients with ventricular function recovery had any cardiac risk factors (diabetes, hypertension, or hypercholesterolemia) while 64% of the patients without recovery had at least 1 cardiac risk factors. There was no difference in mean age (57 ± 24 years

TABLE 5: Ventricular function parameters at the time of cardiotoxicity and at follow-up ($n = 16$) in patients with and without left ventricular ejection fraction recovery to ≥55%.

	(+) LV recovery $n = 5$	(−) LV recovery $n = 11$
Left ventricle		
Baseline EF by MUGA (%)	62 ± 8	61 ± 4
Cardiotoxicity EF by MUGA (%)	49 ± 3	45 ± 3
Cardiotoxicity EF by ECHO (%)	49 ± 6	44 ± 6
Post-treatment EF by ECHO (%)	59 ± 2	48 ± 6
Cardiotoxicity GLS	−15.6 ± 2.8	−15.0 ± 1.9
Post-treatment GLS	−19.8 ± 2.3	−16.0 ± 1.8
Right ventricle		
Baseline EF by MUGA (%)	48 ± 3	48 ± 4
Cardiotoxicity EF by MUGA (%)	41 ± 5	42 ± 4
Cardiotoxicity FAC by ECHO (%)	45 ± 3	42 ± 9
Post-treatment FAC by ECHO (%)	54 ± 4	43 ± 8
Cardiotoxicity RVFWLS	−25.3 ± 2.2	−24.8 ± 4.6
Post-treatment RVFWLS	−32.1 ± 5.3	−23.4 ± 3.8
Cardiotoxicity RVGLS	−21.1 ± 1.8	−20.2 ± 2.8
Post-treatment RVGLS	−24.6 ± 3.7	−22.1 ± 4.9

Abbreviations as per Table 2; recovery is defined as an LVEF ≥55% at last follow-up.

versus 56 ± 9 years, $P = 0.87$), mean duration of follow-up (26 ± 14 versus 22 ± 15 $P = 0.58$), the proportion that received anthracyclines (80% versus 73%, $P = 0.99$), and the lowest mean LVEF during cardiotoxicity (49 ± 6% versus 44 ± 6%, $P = 0.14$), between patients with and without recovery, respectively. In the 5 patients with LVEF recovery, 2 were treated with cardiac medications at 1.5 and 4 months from the diagnosis of cardiotoxicity, while in 11 patients without recovery 8 received cardiac medications, with 6 treated at mean of 1.7 ± 1.4 months from diagnosis of cardiotoxicity and 2 patients were treated after 3.5 months due to fluctuating LVEF.

In the remaining 14 out of 30 patients not described above; repeat imaging was done in 11 during the course of cancer treatment but not afterwards, 2 patients had echocardiograms early after treatment completion but were technically inadequate for strain analysis, and one patient was lost to follow up. When these 14 patients were compared to the 16 patients above, there was no statistically significant

difference in age (51 ± 14 versus 58 ± 11, $P = 0.10$) or echocardiographic parameters at the time of cardiotoxicity: LVEF (46 ± 6% versus 45 ± 6% $P = 0.97$), GLS (−15.9 ± 2.7% versus −15.2 ± 2.2%, $P = 0.27$), RV FAC (42 ± 6% versus 43 ± 8%, $P = 0.57$), RVFWLS (−25.1 ± 4.8% versus −25.0 ± 3.9%, $P = 0.68$), and RVGLS (−21.6 ± 3.6% versus −20.5 ± 2.6%, $P = 0.62$). In the 13 patients, LVEF at interim follow-up was significantly higher compared to the time of cardiotoxicity (45 ± 6 versus 53 ± 12, $P = 0.02$); however only 7 patients had LVEF >55% at the last available study.

3.5. Intraobserver and Interobserver Variability. For the measurement of RVFWLS and RVGLS the intraobserver ICC were 0.97 and 0.97, respectively, while the interobserver ICC were 0.80 and 0.90, respectively.

4. Discussion

Our study demonstrates that in women with HER2+ breast cancer that experienced LV cardiotoxicity during treatment with trastuzumab (with or without anthracycline therapy), RV function at the time of cardiotoxicity is lower than controls as measured using FAC (a measure analogous to ejection fraction for the LV) and strain. RV dysfunction was seen in 10% of the patients by FAC and in up to 40% of the patients based on strain analysis by speckle tracking echocardiography. The proportion of patients with abnormal strain was larger than those with abnormal FAC demonstrating the sensitivity of strain measures to identify subtle ventricular dysfunction. In a subgroup of patients with a mean follow-up of 23 months after completion of cancer therapy, LV dysfunction persisted despite appropriate management. Finally, recovery of LV function was lower in patients who had concomitant RV dysfunction at the time of cardiotoxicity compared to those who did not (17% versus 40%); however, this did not reach statistical significance, likely reflecting our small sample size.

4.1. Right Ventricular Dysfunction and Cardiotoxicity. In women with HER2+ breast cancer receiving trastuzumab therapy alone or in combination with anthracyclines the incidence of cardiotoxicity (defined by fall in LVEF) in clinical trials has been reported to be as high as 14% [24]. However, in retrospective population based studies the rates are much higher ranging from 15.5 to 41.9% especially in older women and over long term follow-up [25, 26]. The identification of cardiotoxicity has been primarily based on development of LV systolic dysfunction and eventual HF. Currently, RV dysfunction is not considered in the diagnosis of cardiotoxicity and its incidence and prognostic value in patients receiving cancer therapy is unknown. The limited literature on the impact of cancer therapy on the RV may reflect the absence of robust techniques for the assessment of RV function. However, given the thinner structure of the RV with fewer myofibrils, the RV may also be susceptible to damage by cardiotoxic cancer therapy as we have shown in this study. In fact the recent ASE expert consensus statement on the multimodality imaging of adult patients receiving cancer therapy recommends monitoring RV function during cancer therapy [9].

The effect of cancer therapy on the RV was first demonstrated in an older study of 41 doxorubicin treated patients with various cancers where RV wall motion abnormalities were more common than LV abnormalities on radionuclide ventriculography [13]. More recently, a cardiac MRI study of 46 women with breast cancer receiving anthracyclines with or without trastuzumab illustrated RV dysfunction in 34% of the patients by 12 months, while LV dysfunction was seen in 26% [12]. Interestingly RV dysfunction was present as early as 4 months into therapy and was felt to represent an early sign of myocardial injury. Another echocardiography study identified mild reduction in RV FAC and tricuspid annular plane systolic excursion (TAPSE) even as early as the 3rd cycle of doxorubicin therapy in 37 anthracycline treated patients with breast cancer [14]. Two other studies of 19 and 56 survivors of pediatric cancers have shown a reduction in RV free wall strain values (a marker of subclinical ventricular dysfunction) at cumulative anthracycline (various) doses <300 mg/m^2 [27, 28]. In more recent study of patients with advanced HF receiving LV mechanical circulatory support, patients with chemotherapy induced cardiomyopathy were significantly more likely to also require RV mechanical support [29]. However, these findings have not been consistent amongst studies. Two small studies of patients treated with similar doxorubicin equivalent doses as above studies did not demonstrate RV dysfunction by radionuclide angiography and echocardiography when comparing pre- to posttherapy time points [11, 15]. Also, the incidence of concomitant RV dysfunction *at the time of cardiotoxicity* has not been previously studied.

Our work builds on the existing literature by demonstrating that, in women with HER2+ breast cancer receiving trastuzumab therapy, RV dysfunction is seen *at the time of cardiotoxicity*. When compared to controls, the mean FAC, RVGLS, and RVFWLS were significantly reduced in patients experiencing cardiotoxicity. In addition 10% of the patients had abnormal RV function by FAC. Similarly using a threshold for abnormal strain generated based on the control group; up to 40% of patients had abnormal RVGLS or RVFWS. The higher incidence of RV dysfunction based on strain abnormality reflects the higher sensitivity of this measure for myocardial dysfunction. Ventricular strain is a marker of myocardial deformation and has been used widely for the detection of subclinical cardiotoxicity in many diseases including patients receiving cancer therapy [30]. We demonstrate the use of these measures for the first time for the assessment of RV dysfunction *at the time cardiotoxicity* in patients treated with trastuzumab.

4.2. Recovery of Ventricular Function. Generally in trastuzumab treated patients with breast cancer, LV dysfunction that occurs at the time of cardiotoxicity is thought to recover with cessation of trastuzumab [31]. However, this finding has not been universal with some studies demonstrating lack of recovery in LV function in as many as 40% of the patients despite receiving appropriate cardiac therapy [7]. Our study demonstrates that 69% of the patients had persistently abnormal LVEF (<55%) at follow-up, and 3 (19%) remained symptomatic (NYHA $\geq$ 2). Although the incidence likely exaggerated due to incomplete follow-up, our data suggest that LV dysfunction persists in a significant proportion of patients who experience cardiotoxicity during trastuzumab therapy despite appropriate management. A recent study demonstrated that persistent LV dysfunction in follow-up in patients treated for cancer was associated with higher mortality [32]. Mortality data was not available in our study. Also, interestingly our study demonstrates that a significant proportion of patients with abnormal RV function measured by strain at the time of cardiotoxicity did not have subsequent recovery in LV function at follow-up. This suggests that concomitant RV dysfunction may be a marker of more significant cardiac injury and a potential risk factor for persistent LV dysfunction during follow-up. However, given our small sample size this difference did not reach statistical significance. These findings are hypothesis generating and will need to be confirmed in larger studies.

4.3. Limitations. This was a retrospective study from a single center with a relative small sample size. However, the low rates of cardiotoxicity at our center and the fact that cardiac function is generally followed by MUGA as opposed to echocardiography explain our small sample size. Also we did not have baseline echocardiography in our patients with cardiotoxicity to ensure that their LV and RV function were normal pre-cancer therapy and to compare strain and EF values at baseline to the time of cardiotoxicity. However, by MUGA, all of the patients had normal pre-cancer therapy LV and RV function. Furthermore, we used an age and cardiac risk factor balanced control group of HER2+ breast cancer patients who had echocardiography prior to any cancer treatment to account for this limitation. Post-cancer therapy follow-up data was only present in 53% of the patients. This reflects the retrospective nature of the study, and the fact that many patients are not routinely followed with cardiac imaging at our tertiary care center once cancer therapy is completed. Therefore our estimates of ventricular function recovery must be considered in the context of this limitation and is likely higher than expected in clinical practice. We have however shown that the 14 patients without postcancer treatment follow-up were similar to the 16 patients with follow-up with respect to clinical and echocardiographic parameters. We did not include these latter 14 in the follow-up cohort as any conclusion about ventricular function recovery is hampered by ongoing cancer treatment. We also had patients with variability in the cancer treatment. However, all patients received trastuzumab therapy with a majority (73%) also having received anthracyclines. We also did not report measures of TAPSE and systolic annular velocities as additional measures of RV function as this was not consistently available in all the patients. However, we did measure RVGLS in our patients and this has been shown to be a good marker of RV function when compared to the gold-standard of cardiac MRI [33]. Cardiac MRI is considered the reference standard for RV function assessment, but we did not have cardiac MRI data in our patients as this was not standard of care. Finally we did not do a logistic regression analysis of predictors of LV recovery as the number of events was small to meaningfully adjust for confounders.

4.4. Clinical Implication. The finding of RV dysfunction during the diagnosis of cardiotoxicity in our study demonstrates the need to assess both ventricles during cancer therapy in patients with breast cancer receiving trastuzumab therapy. This is consistent with recent guidelines from the American Society of Echocardiography, which encourages routine follow-up of both LV and RV functions during cancer treatment [9]. Also, our findings of persistent LV dysfunction during follow-up have implications for cardiac therapy in patients experiencing cardiotoxicity. The appropriate length of treatment with cardiac medications such as beta-blockers and ACE inhibitors in patients experiencing cardiotoxicity during cancer therapy is unknown. Based on our findings of persistently reduced LVEF it may be necessary to continue cardiac treatment for a prolonged period of time. In addition, these patients may need close cardiology follow-up.

5. Conclusion

In patients with HER2+ breast cancer treated with trastuzumab with or without anthracyclines who experienced cardiotoxicity (based on reduction in LVEF), concomitant RV dysfunction was seen in up to 40% of the patients based on RV strain measurements. During follow-up after completion of cancer therapy, LV dysfunction (LVEF < 55%) persisted in 69%. Patients with concomitant LV and RV dysfunction at the time of cardiotoxicity had a lower propensity for subsequent ventricular function recovery although this did not reach statistical significance. The prognostic value of RV dysfunction and its persistence during follow-up needs to be assessed in larger studies.

Conflict of Interests

None of the authors have any conflict of interests.

Acknowledgments

This work was partially funded by the Heart and Stroke Foundation, University of Toronto, Polo Chair in Cardiology Grant and the Canadian Institute of Health Research Grant to Dr. Paaladinesh Thavendiranathan. Dr. Philippe L. Bedard received research funding from Roche and Genentech.

References

[1] American Cancer Society, *Cancer Facts & Figures*, American Cancer Society, Washington, DC, USA, 2014.

[2] Canadian Cancer Society's Advisory Committee on Cancer Statistics, *Canadian Cancer Statistics 2014*, 2014.

[3] M. P. Coleman, D. Forman, H. Bryant et al., "Cancer survival in Australia, Canada, Denmark, Norway, Sweden, and the UK, 1995–2007 (the international cancer benchmarking partnership): an analysis of population-based cancer registry data," *The Lancet*, vol. 377, no. 9760, pp. 127–138, 2011.

[4] M. Y. Su, L. Y. Lin, and Y. H. Tseng, "CMR-verified diffuse myocardial fibrosis is associated with diastolic dysfunction in HFpEF," *JACC: Cardiovascular Imaging*, vol. 7, no. 10, pp. 991–997, 2014.

[5] J. M. Isner, V. J. Ferrans, S. R. Cohen et al., "Clinical and morphologic cardiac findings after anthracycline chemotherapy. Analysis of 64 patients studied at necropsy," *The American Journal of Cardiology*, vol. 51, no. 7, pp. 1167–1174, 1983.

[6] D. Cardinale, A. Colombo, G. Lamantia et al., "Anthracycline-induced cardiomyopathy: clinical relevance and response to pharmacologic therapy," *Journal of the American College of Cardiology*, vol. 55, no. 3, pp. 213–220, 2010.

[7] D. Cardinale, A. Colombo, R. Torrisi et al., "Trastuzumab-induced cardiotoxicity: clinical and prognostic implications of troponin I evaluation," *Journal of Clinical Oncology*, vol. 28, no. 25, pp. 3910–3916, 2010.

[8] G. M. Felker, R. E. Thompson, J. M. Hare et al., "Underlying causes and long-term survival in patients with initially unexplained cardiomyopathy," *The New England Journal of Medicine*, vol. 342, no. 15, pp. 1077–1084, 2000.

[9] J. C. Plana, M. Galderisi, A. Barac et al., "Expert consensus for multimodality imaging evaluation of adult patients during and after cancer therapy: a report from the American Society of Echocardiography and the European Association of Cardiovascular Imaging," *Journal of the American Society of Echocardiography*, vol. 27, no. 9, pp. 911–939, 2014.

[10] A. Seidman, C. Hudis, M. K. Pierri et al., "Cardiac dysfunction in the trastuzumab clinical trials experience," *Journal of Clinical Oncology*, vol. 20, no. 5, pp. 1215–1221, 2002.

[11] Y. Cottin, C. Touzery, B. Coudert et al., "Diastolic or systolic left and right ventricular impairment at moderate doses of anthracycline? A 1-year follow-up study of women," *European Journal of Nuclear Medicine*, vol. 23, no. 5, pp. 511–516, 1996.

[12] S. Grover, D. P. Leong, A. Chakrabarty et al., "Left and right ventricular effects of anthracycline and trastuzumab chemotherapy: a prospective study using novel cardiac imaging and biochemical markers," *International Journal of Cardiology*, vol. 168, no. 6, pp. 5465–5467, 2013.

[13] E. C. Barendswaard, H. Prpic, E. E. van der Wall, J. A. J. Camps, H. J. Keizer, and E. K. J. Pauwels, "Right ventricle wall motion abnormalities in patients treated with chemotherapy," *Clinical Nuclear Medicine*, vol. 16, no. 7, pp. 513–516, 1991.

[14] A. Tanindi, U. Demirci, G. Tacoy et al., "Assessment of right ventricular functions during cancer chemotherapy," *European Journal of Echocardiography*, vol. 12, no. 11, pp. 834–840, 2011.

[15] S. S. Ayhan, K. Özdemir, M. Kayrak et al., "The evaluation of doxorubicin-induced cardiotoxicity: comparison of Doppler and tissue Doppler-derived myocardial performance index," *Cardiology Journal*, vol. 19, no. 4, pp. 363–368, 2012.

[16] C. Chrysohoou, C.-K. Antoniou, I. Kotrogiannis et al., "Role of right ventricular systolic function on long-term outcome in patients with newly diagnosed systolic heart failure," *Circulation Journal*, vol. 75, no. 9, pp. 2176–2181, 2011.

[17] S. Guendouz, S. Rappeneau, J. Nahum et al., "Prognostic significance and normal values of 2D strain to assess right ventricular systolic function in chronic heart failure," *Circulation Journal*, vol. 76, no. 1, pp. 127–136, 2012.

[18] F. Haddad, R. Doyle, D. J. Murphy, and S. A. Hunt, "Right ventricular function in cardiovascular disease, part II: pathophysiology, clinical importance, and management of right ventricular failure," *Circulation*, vol. 117, no. 13, pp. 1717–1731, 2008.

[19] R. M. Lang, M. Bierig, R. B. Devereux et al., "Recommendations for chamber quantification: a report from the American Society of Echocardiography's guidelines and standards committee and the Chamber Quantification Writing Group, developed in conjunction with the European Association of Echocardiography, a branch of the European Society of Cardiology," *Journal of the American Society of Echocardiography*, vol. 18, no. 12, pp. 1440–1463, 2005.

[20] S. F. Nagueh, C. P. Appleton, T. C. Gillebert et al., "Recommendations for the evaluation of left ventricular diastolic function by echocardiography," *Journal of the American Society of Echocardiography*, vol. 22, no. 2, pp. 107–133, 2009.

[21] V. Mor-Avi, R. M. Lang, L. P. Badano et al., "Current and evolving echocardiographic techniques for the quantitative evaluation of cardiac mechanics: ASE/EAE consensus statement on methodology and indications endorsed by the Japanese Society of Echocardiography," *Journal of the American Society of Echocardiography*, vol. 24, no. 3, pp. 277–313, 2011.

[22] T. Yingchoncharoen, S. Agarwal, Z. B. Popović, and T. H. Marwick, "Normal ranges of left ventricular strain: a meta-analysis," *Journal of the American Society of Echocardiography*, vol. 26, no. 2, pp. 185–191, 2013.

[23] M. E. Pfisterer, A. Battler, and B. L. Zaret, "Range of normal values for left and right ventricular ejection fraction at rest and during exercise assessed by radionuclide angiocardiography," *European Heart Journal*, vol. 6, no. 8, pp. 647–655, 1985.

[24] E. Tan-Chiu, G. Yothers, E. Romond et al., "Assessment of cardiac dysfunction in a randomized trial comparing doxorubicin and cyclophosphamide followed by paclitaxel, with or without trastuzumab as adjuvant therapy in node-positive, human epidermal growth factor receptor 2-overexpressing breast cancer: NSABP B-31," *Journal of Clinical Oncology*, vol. 23, no. 31, pp. 7811–7819, 2005.

[25] J. Chen, J. B. Long, A. Hurria, C. Owusu, R. M. Steingart, and C. P. Gross, "Incidence of heart failure or cardiomyopathy after adjuvant trastuzumab therapy for breast cancer," *Journal of the American College of Cardiology*, vol. 60, no. 24, pp. 2504–2512, 2012.

[26] X. L. Du, R. Xia, K. Burau, and C.-C. Liu, "Cardiac risk associated with the receipt of anthracycline and trastuzumab in a large nationwide cohort of older women with breast cancer, 1998–2005," *Medical Oncology*, vol. 28, no. 1, supplement, pp. S80–S90, 2011.

[27] J. Ganame, P. Claus, A. Uyttebroeck et al., "Myocardial dysfunction late after low-dose anthracycline treatment in asymptomatic pediatric patients," *Journal of the American Society of Echocardiography*, vol. 20, no. 12, pp. 1351–1358, 2007.

[28] B. Yağci-Küpeli, A. Varan, H. Yorgun, B. Kaya, and M. Büyükpamukçu, "Tissue Doppler and myocardial deformation imaging to detect myocardial dysfunction in pediatric cancer patients treated with high doses of anthracyclines," *Asia-Pacific Journal of Clinical Oncology*, vol. 8, no. 4, pp. 368–374, 2012.

[29] G. H. Oliveira, M. Dupont, D. Naftel et al., "Increased need for right ventricular support in patients with chemotherapy-induced cardiomyopathy undergoing mechanical circulatory support: outcomes from the intermacs registry (interagency registry for mechanically assisted circulatory support)," *Journal of the American College of Cardiology*, vol. 63, no. 3, pp. 240–248, 2014.

[30] P. Thavendiranathan, F. Poulin, K. D. Lim, J. C. Plana, A. Woo, and T. H. Marwick, "Use of myocardial strain imaging by echocardiography for the early detection of cardiotoxicity in patients during and after cancer chemotherapy: a systematic review," *Journal of the American College of Cardiology*, vol. 63, no. 25PA, pp. 2751–2768, 2014.

[31] E. H. Romond, J.-H. Jeong, P. Rastogi et al., "Seven-year follow-up assessment of cardiac function in NSABP B-31, a randomized trial comparing doxorubicin and cyclophosphamide followed by paclitaxel (ACP) with ACP plus trastuzumab as adjuvant therapy for patients with node-positive, human epidermal growth factor receptor 2-positive breast cancer," *Journal of Clinical Oncology*, vol. 30, no. 31, pp. 3792–3799, 2012.

[32] G. H. Oliveira, S. Mukerji, A. V. Hernandez et al., "Incidence, predictors, and impact on survival of left ventricular systolic dysfunction and recovery in advanced cancer patients," *The American Journal of Cardiology*, vol. 113, no. 11, pp. 1893–1898, 2014.

[33] B. H. Freed, W. Tsang, N. M. Bhave et al., "Right ventricular strain in pulmonary arterial hypertension: a 2D echocardiography and cardiac magnetic resonance study," *Echocardiography*, 2014.

4

Tumor Suppressor Inactivation in the Pathogenesis of Adult T-Cell Leukemia

Christophe Nicot

Department of Pathology and Laboratory Medicine, Center for Viral Oncology, University of Kansas Medical Center, 3901 Rainbow Boulevard, Kansas City, KS 66160, USA

Correspondence should be addressed to Christophe Nicot; cnicot@kumc.edu

Academic Editor: Michiel W. M. van den Brekel

Tumor suppressor functions are essential to control cellular proliferation, to activate the apoptosis or senescence pathway to eliminate unwanted cells, to link DNA damage signals to cell cycle arrest checkpoints, to activate appropriate DNA repair pathways, and to prevent the loss of adhesion to inhibit initiation of metastases. Therefore, tumor suppressor genes are indispensable to maintaining genetic and genomic integrity. Consequently, inactivation of tumor suppressors by somatic mutations or epigenetic mechanisms is frequently associated with tumor initiation and development. In contrast, reactivation of tumor suppressor functions can effectively reverse the transformed phenotype and lead to cell cycle arrest or death of cancerous cells and be used as a therapeutic strategy. Adult T-cell leukemia/lymphoma (ATLL) is an aggressive lymphoproliferative disease associated with infection of CD4 T cells by the Human T-cell Leukemia Virus Type 1 (HTLV-I). HTLV-I-associated T-cell transformation is the result of a multistep oncogenic process in which the virus initially induces chronic T-cell proliferation and alters cellular pathways resulting in the accumulation of genetic defects and the deregulated growth of virally infected cells. This review will focus on the current knowledge of the genetic and epigenetic mechanisms regulating the inactivation of tumor suppressors in the pathogenesis of HTLV-I.

1. Introduction

The first description of HTLV-I came after the discovery of the human T-cell growth factor (interleukin-2; IL-2), allowing long-term *in vitro* culture of T cells and the establishment of T-cell lines from a patient with a cutaneous T-cell lymphoma [1–3]. Afterward, this virus was identified as the etiological agent of ATLL and the terminology HTLV-I was adopted. HTLV-I is transmitted through sexual contacts and contaminated blood and from mother to child by breast-feeding [4]. HTLV-I is mainly found in endemic areas such as Japan, Africa, South America, the Caribbean basin, southern parts of North America, and Eastern Europe [5]. The diversity in clinical presentation and prognosis of patients with ATLL has led to its classification into distinct subtypes referred to as smoldering, chronic, and acute or lymphoma type [6, 7]. In patients circulating atypical multinucleated lymphocytes termed "flower cells" are considered pathognomonic of ATLL. Tumor ATLL cells are of clonal origin and usually carry a single copy of integrated virus [8, 9]. The fact that

the different clinical forms of ATLL have distinct genomic alterations and variable clinical progression is consistent with the fact that these diseases necessitate different treatments [10]. However, most of the current treatments for ATLL fail to induce long-term remission and do not offer the prospect of a cure. Even the clinically less aggressive forms of ATLL eventually progress to the acute form. The 4-year survival rate for acute, lymphoma, chronic, and smoldering type ATLL is 5.0, 5.7, 26.9, and 62.8%, respectively [11, 12]. The poor prognosis of ATLL patients is associated with the resistance of neoplastic cells to the conventional combination of high-dose chemotherapy and radiotherapy. While most HTLV-I-infected individuals remain asymptomatic carriers, 1 to 5% of infected individuals will develop ATLL in their lifetime. The disease usually develops after a long latency of several decades, although faster disease progression has been reported in individuals coinfected with parasites. The low incidence and long latency of HTLV-I-associated ATLL suggest that, in addition to viral infection, accumulations of genetic alterations are required for cellular transformation *in vivo.* These observations are consistent with the fact that HTLV-I does not transduce an oncogene and that the viral oncoprotein Tax has a low transforming activity in human T cells [13, 14]. Although HTLV-I integrates into open transcriptionally active chromatin [15], the provirus does not integrate at specific sites within the human genome and therefore HTLV-I is not associated with insertional mutagenesis by either disruption of tumor suppressor or activation of oncogene. The mechanism by which HTLV-I induces T-cell transformation is still unclear but recent studies suggest that the virus may reprogram infected cells to a mutator phenotype. HTLV-I viral proteins can inflict DNA breaks and simultaneously prevent proper repair through the homologous recombination DNA repair pathway, resulting in the accumulation of mutations and small deletions. If the longevity of infected cells is extended through reactivation of hTERT, then the cumulative risk of acquiring a sufficient number of oncogenic events for transformation is significantly increased. This review will describe how common tumor suppressors frequently inactivated in human cancers are affected in ATLL tumor cells and the significance of these alterations in terms of disease progression and therapeutic opportunities.

2. Review

2.1. Inactivation of Cell Cycle Checkpoints Leads to Uncontrolled Proliferation of ATLL Cells

2.1.1. p53 and p73. In contrast to oncogenic events, inactivation of tumor suppressor functions requires the loss of both alleles. Consistent with this notion, monoallelic loss of the 17p13.1 region, where the p53 gene is located [16, 17], is consistently associated with mutations of the residual p53 allele to inactivate the remaining p53 function [18, 19]. While p53 mutations are relatively uncommon in non-HTLV-I-associated T-cell neoplasms and found in less than 3% of patients [20], it has been reported in approximately 30% of ATLL patients [21–24]. In addition, functional inactivation of p53 in the absence of genetic mutations has been reported in a majority of ATLL patients [25–27]. Further studies demonstrated that the viral Tax protein plays an active part in this process and inactivates p53 transcriptional functions [28–32]. Since significant Tax mRNA expression is detected in approximately 50% of fresh ATLL patient samples analyzed [33, 34], it is unclear if and how p53 is inactivated in ATLL cells in which Tax is not expressed and in the absence of mutations. MdmX is upregulated in HTLV-I-transformed cells *in vitro* and *in vivo* and may play an important role in the inactivation of p53 in the absence of Tax expression. In addition, while p53 mutations in ALL are very rare, hypermethylation of the p53 promoter can be detected in 30% of ALL patients [35]. Such a mechanism could also take part in ATLL and this warrants additional studies. Interestingly, microRNA miR-150 has been shown to target p53 and to play an important role in NSCLC tumorigenesis [36]. Along these lines, miR-150 expression has been found to be upregulated in ATLL patient samples, suggesting that it may be involved in inhibition of p53 in ATLL cells [37].

Similarly, studies have demonstrated that p53 inactivation involves activation of the canonical NF-kB pathway [38] and activation of NF-kB in the absence of Tax can be achieved in ATLL cells through upregulated expression of miR-31 [39], suggesting that miR-31 may play a role in p53 inactivation. Although p53 is transcriptionally inactive in a majority of ATLL patients, several studies have demonstrated that inactivation mechanisms are reversible and that reactivation of p53 functions can activate the senescence or apoptosis pathway and efficiently eliminate HTLV-I-transformed cells [40, 41]. Coexistence of tumor clones with wild type p53 and p53 mutated has been reported in previously untreated ATLL patients. In this patient treatment leading to the eradication of the p53 wild type tumor clone resulted in disease relapse, the emergence of the p53 mutated tumor clone, and aggressive disease progression [41].

The p53-related gene, p73, is located in a chromosome region (1p36) which is a locus that is frequently deleted in human tumors but infrequently mutated [42, 43]. Existence of p73 as a tumor suppressor is debated. Hypermethylation-associated loss of p73 gene expression in various types of leukemia has been reported [44] and, similarly, p73 is inactivated by methylation in 30% of smoldering ATLL but surprisingly at a much lower rate in chronic and acute types of ATLL, with an overall methylation rate of 10% in ATLL [45]. In addition to epigenetic inactivation, the viral Tax protein has been shown to inhibit p73 functions [46, 47].

2.1.2. CDKN2 Genes. The CDKN2A locus located at chromosome 9p21.3 encodes p14ARF and p16INK4a while the CDKN2B locus encodes p15INK4b, a functional homolog of p16INK4a. The p14ARF and p16INK4a genes have been implicated as tumor suppressor genes and are frequently mutated, deleted, or inactivated through promoter hypermethylation in human cancers [48]. P16INK4a is a cyclin-dependent kinase inhibitor (CDKI) that complexes with CDK4 or CDK6 and prevents the activation of CDK-cyclin D and cell cycle progression from G1 to S phase.

While mutations of p16INK4a have been frequently reported in pancreatic adenocarcinoma and melanoma [49–51], genetic mutations have not been reported in ATLL patients. In contrast, homozygous deletion or promoter hypermethylation of the CDKN2A genes has been described in at least 20% of acute ATLL patients and loss of CDKN2A was infrequent in chronic or smoldering ATLL [52–54]. Consistent with its role as a tumor suppressor, azacitidine-mediated demethylation of the p16INK4a locus significantly increased expression of p16INK4a and inhibited the growth of ATLL cells [55]. Remarkably, most of the patients with CDKN2 gene alterations had the acute and most aggressive form of ATLL, which is consistent with the fact that p16INK4A expression is a biomarker associated with a more favorable prognosis as measured by cancer-specific survival (CSS) and recurrence-free survival (RFS) in many human cancers. In pediatric cases of ATLL (2–18 years old), frequency of deletion of the CDKN2A locus or mutation of p53 was found in five of the eight patients, suggesting that alteration in these genes is associated with a more rapid progression of ATLL [56]. Additional epigenetic control of

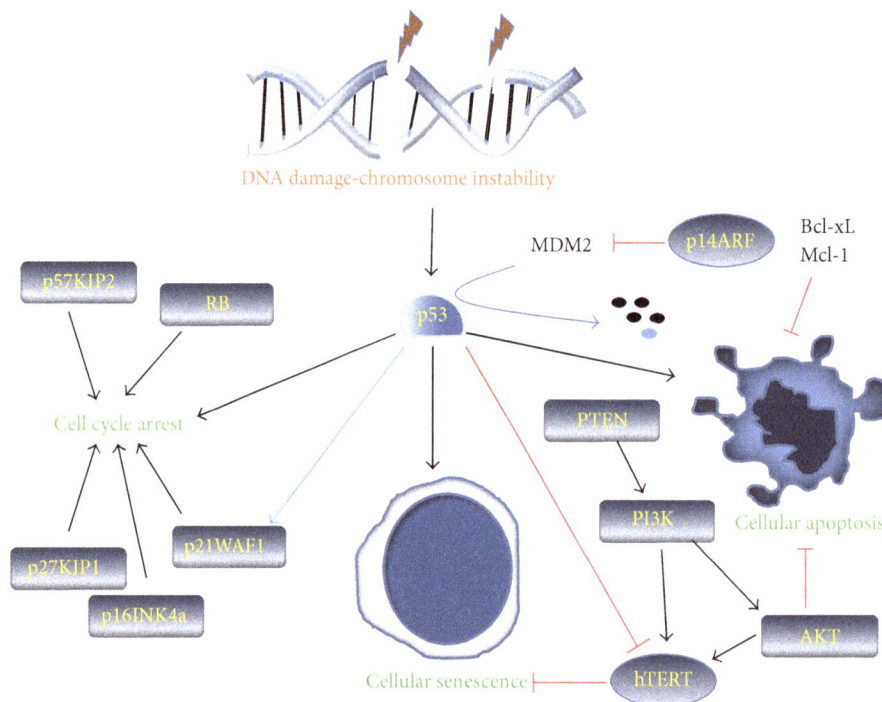

FIGURE 1: Schematic representation of DNA damage-induced p53 pathway and how other tumor suppressors are connected to activate cell cycle arrest, senescence, or apoptosis to prevent cellular transformation.

P16INK4a, P19INK4d, and p14ARF expression by microRNAs miR-31 and miR-24 has previously been observed [57, 58]. However, loss of miR-31 expression has been detected in ATLL cells [59] and expression of miR-24 has not been reported. In addition to genetic or epigenetic control of p16INK4A, several studies have shown that the viral Tax protein directly interacts with p16INK4A and prevents its inhibitory activity towards CDK4 [60, 61]. Tax was also shown to bind to p15INK4b similarly to p16INK4a, but not to p18INK4c and p19INK4d. However, expression of p18INK4c was suppressed by Tax at the transcriptional level through the E-box element present in the p18INK4c promoter [60].

P14ARF is encoded from an alternative reading frame of the CDKN2A locus. P14ARF interacts with and sequesters MDM2, thereby preventing the ubiquitination and degradation of p53 (Figure 1). Although P16INK4a and P14ARF act on distinct targets, they share functional similarity by preventing cell cycle progression through inactivation of RB and p53, respectively. However, P14ARF can also inhibit proliferation in cells lacking expression of p53 or p53 and Mdm2 [62]. Like p16INK4A, P14ARF is silenced by promoter hypermethylation or deletion. Although mutations that impair p14ARF functions have been reported in melanoma, colon, pancreatic, and lung cancer [63–65], no data is available for ATLL.

2.1.3. CIP/KIP Family. The CIP/KIP members act as CDKI and have a wider specificity for CDKs than the INK4 members. At low levels p21CIP1/WAF1 and p27KIP1 stimulate the assembly of the CDK4-cyclin D complex, whereas at higher levels p21CIP1/WAF1 and p27KIP1 inhibit the activity of the CDK-cyclin heterodimers [66, 67]. Similarly, at low concentrations p57KIP2 is able to form an active complex with CDK2-cyclin A, whereas at higher levels p57KIP2 prevents the kinase activity of CDK2 [68].

CDKN1A (p21CIP1/WAF1) located at chromosome 6p21.2 is transcriptionally activated in a p53-dependent and independent manner [69], inhibits the activity of cyclin-CDK2, cyclin-CDK1, and cyclin-CDK4/6 complexes, and negatively regulates cell cycle progression from G1 to S [70]. Although expression of p21CIP1/WAF1 has been reported to be increased in HTLV-I-transformed cells *in vitro* [71], additional studies revealed that p21CIP1/WAF1 expression was frequently downregulated through promoter hypermethylation in acute ATLL cells, complete methylation was found in 25% of patients, and partial methylation was found in 70% of ATLL patients [72]. The fact that an increased level of p21WAF1/CIP1 is not associated with cell cycle arrest in HTLV-I-transformed cells *in vitro* may be explained by p21CIP1/WAF1 phosphorylation at Threonine 145 by the PI3K/AKT pathway resulting in cytoplasmic retention and inactive p21CIP1/WAF1 [72]. Additional regulation of p21CIP1/WAF1 by microRNA miR-93 has been described [73]. Since miR-93 is upregulated in ATLL cells it may play a role in tumor cell proliferation by reducing the p21CIP1/WAF1 level [74].

CDKN1B (p27KIP1) is located at chromosome 12p13.1 and its loss has been proposed to play an essential role in T-cell transformation following HTLV-I infection [75]. P27KIP1 is rarely mutated or deleted in ATLL. Homozygous deletions of p27KIP1 and expression of a truncated nonfunctional p27KIP1 protein (amino acid 76*) have been reported in two cases of lymphoma ATLL [76]. In contrast, P27KIP1 expression was downregulated at the posttranscriptional level in HTLV-I-transformed cells *in vitro* [75]. In addition, in cells with physiological levels of p27KIP1, AKT-mediated phosphorylation of p27KIP1 at amino acid residue Threonine 157 resulted in its cytoplasmic localization and inactivity in ATLL cells [72].

CDKN1C (p57, KIP2) is located in the telomeric end of chromosome 11 at the 11p15 locus, which contains several imprinted genes. In addition to its role in the G1-to-S transition, p57KIP2 also contributes to the M-to-G1 transition through activation by p73 [77]. Mutations of CDKN1C are associated with sporadic cancers and with Beckwith-Wiedemann syndrome, a disease characterized by an increased risk of tumor formation in childhood [78, 79]. Loss of heterozygosity (LOH) of p57KIP2 is frequently observed in human cancers [80]. Expression of p57KIP2 is transcriptionally regulated through distinct epigenetic mechanisms. Histone methyltransferase EZH2 has also been shown to suppress p57KIP2 expression through histone H3 lysine 27 trimethylation (H3K27me3) [81] and p57KIP2 is methylated in nearly 50% of newly diagnosed ALL patients [82]. In addition, several microRNAs have also been shown to downregulate p57KIP2 expression, including miR-221 and miR-222 [73, 83, 84], miR-25 [73], and miR-92b [85]. However, there is currently no information about the relative expression of these microRNAs in ATLL patient samples and expression of p57KIP2 in ATLL has not been reported.

2.1.4. Retinoblastoma (RB). The RB locus is located at chromosome 13q14.1. In resting cells inhibition of the cyclin D-CDK4/6 complexes maintains RB and its related proteins (p107 and RB2/p130) in a hypophosphorylated state and sequesters the E2F transcription factor [86]. Following activation of the cyclin D-CDK4/6 complexes, RB becomes hyperphosphorylated and dissociates from E2F, allowing the latter to stimulate expression of the genes involved in the progression to S phase of the cell cycle. RB is progressively dephosphorylated during the M-to-G1 transition [87]. Genetic mutation in the RB gene has been reported in various human cancers [88].

Homozygous loss of RB exon 1 has been reported in one of 21 acute ATLL, one of 15 chronic ATLL, and none of four lymphoma ATLL samples. In that study no point mutations were found in the entire RB gene coding sequence [89]. Hence, the overall rate of RB alteration in ATLL is approximately 5%. Interestingly, the authors observed that none of the samples with an altered RB gene had any defect in CDKI genes and vice versa, suggesting that these tumor suppressor genes likely operate in a common pathway and alteration of either can provide these cells with a growth advantage [89]. These results are consistent with another study suggesting that RB is infrequently mutated or deleted in ATLL tumor cells [22]. In addition, mutations of the RB2/p130 gene have been found in approximately 2.5% of ATLL patients [90, 91]. Despite a low level of genetic alterations in the RB gene in ATLL, almost 50% of patients demonstrate very low levels of expression of an RB protein, which has led to the hypothesis that RB is posttranscriptionally downregulated in ATLL cells [91]. This

observation is clinically relevant since lower pRB levels in ATLL patients have been correlated with poor prognosis and shorter survival [92]. Epigenetic control by microRNA may in part explain lower levels of RB protein in the absence of decreased RNA levels. Along these lines, several studies have shown that RB is targeted by several microRNAs, including miR-155 [93], and since miR-155 is highly expressed in ATLL cells [37], this may explain the partial loss of RB. Finally, as indicated above for other tumor suppressors, the viral Tax protein is also able to inactivate RB. Direct binding of Tax to RB targeted the latter for proteasomal degradation and stimulation of cell cycle progression [94].

3. Phosphatase and Tensin Homolog (PTEN)/Src Homology 2 Domain Containing Inositol

3.1. Polyphosphate Phosphatase (SHP1/PTPN6). PTEN is located at chromosome 10q23.3 [95] and is among the most frequent tumor suppressors lost in human cancers [96]. PTEN acts as a phosphatase to deactivate phosphatidylinositol (3,4,5)-trisphosphate (PIP3) and inhibit the activation of the PI3K/AKT prosurvival pathway [97]. Germline PTEN mutations and sporadic mutations have been reported in various human cancers [98] but to date no study has investigated the presence of mutations or methylation of the PTEN promoter in ATLL cells. Although PTEN is downregulated at the protein level, in a majority of IL-2-independent HTLV-I-transformed cells *in vitro*, PTEN protein expression is not altered in ATLL tumor cells [99].

SHP1 is located on chromosome 12p13, a region commonly involved in leukemia-associated chromosomal abnormalities. Like PTEN, SHP1 is also implicated in the degradation of PIP3 and inhibition of the PI3K/AKT pathway [100, 101]. In addition, loss of SHP1 enhances JAK3/STAT3 signaling and decreases proteasome degradation of JAK3. Hypermethylation of the SHP1 promoter is associated with loss of SHP1 expression [102, 103], which coincides with the IL-2-independent transformation of T cells by HTLV-I *in vitro* [104, 105]. Consistent with these observations, SHP1 is one of the most frequently altered genes in ATLL patients, with an overall hypermethylation rate of 90% [45]. Interestingly, methylation inactivation of the SHP1 promoter was more frequently seen in the acute (60%) and the lymphoma (80%) form of ATLL, which have the worst prognosis and lowest survival rate [45]. Additional epigenetic control of PTEN and SHP1 has been reported, such as miR-221, miR-222 [106], miR-21 [107], and miR-155 [108]. Among these microRNAs, miR-155 is the only one that has been shown to be upregulated in HTLV-I-transformed T cells *in vitro* as well as in ATLL cells [37].

3.2. Secreted Frizzled-Related Protein 1 (SFRP1). SFRP1 is located at chromosome 8 p12, a region frequently deleted in human cancers [109, 110]. SFRP1 functions as a tumor suppressor and its expression is lost in many patient tumors because of promoter hypermethylation [109, 111, 112]. Point mutation is not a frequent method of inactivation of the

SFRP1 gene in cancer [109]. Inactivation of SFRP1 is associated with constitutive Wnt signaling and an increased proliferation in tumor cells [113]. Although potential alterations in SFRP1 have not yet been investigated in HTLV-I-transformed cells, it has been found that the noncanonical Wnt pathway is activated and Wnt5a overexpressed in ATLL cells.

3.3. Additional Tumor Suppressor Pathways. In addition to tumor suppressors involved in cell cycle control and proliferation, cancer is frequently associated with inactivation of tumor suppressors involved in other cellular pathways. Among those, activation of senescence or apoptosis limits survival and prevents the growth of pretumoral cells. Other tumor suppressors are responsible for activation of DNA damage responses and DNA repair pathways, and their inactivation increases the cumulative risk of oncogenic genetic and genomic alterations. Finally, some tumor suppressor genes are involved in the control of adhesion molecules and their loss leads to increased metastasis.

3.4. Senescence and Apoptosis. In nontumoral cells the progressive shortening of the telomeres after each cell division limits the proliferative potential by activating the senescence program and permanent cell cycle arrest. Consequently, senescence impedes the accumulation of mutations and genomic defects that are needed for initiation and progression of cellular transformation. In cancer cells, preservation of sufficient telomere ends is ensured by reactivation of human telomerase endogenous reverse transcriptase (hTERT). Initiation of senescence is regulated by the p16INK4a/RB-dependent pathway and a p53-dependent DNA damage response (DDR) pathway. As discussed above, most cancer cells avoid senescence by disruption of tumor suppressor genes p53 and p16INK4a and reactivation of hTERT. Like most other human cancers, reactivation of hTERT expression and activity is found in HTLV-I-associated leukemia and required for long-term proliferation of tumor cells [114]. Some studies reported a correlation between telomerase activity and the progression of ATLL [115, 116]. Apoptosis is a tumor suppressor mechanism that is used to eliminate precancerous cells. HTLV-I-transformed cells and ATLL cells are highly resistant to multiple proapoptotic stimuli, including death receptor-mediated and DNA damage-induced agents compared to normal cells. One major player of ATLL cell resistance to apoptosis is the activation of the NF-kB pathway which controls transcription of numerous antiapoptotic proteins such as Bcl-xL and Mcl-1 or inhibitor of apoptosis (IAP) overexpressed in ATLL cells [117–120]. Additional epigenetic alterations have been reported in ATLL. For instance, hypermethylation of the death-associated protein kinase (DAPK) promoter was identified as one of the contributing factors for the progression of the asymptomatic carrier or smoldering type of ATLL to the acute or lymphoma type ATLL and was altered in 55% of patients [45]. MicroRNAs miR-132 and miR-125a are downregulated in ATLL cells [37]. These microRNAs are downregulated through promoter-mediated methylation in various cancers [121, 122]. miR-132 has been shown to target prosurvival proteins in solid tumors while loss of miR-125 protects myeloid leukemia cells from apoptosis [121, 122]. Overall, alteration in the ability of tumor cells to activate the senescence or apoptosis pathway increases resistance to therapies and is associated with a poor prognosis.

4. DNA Repair Pathways and Genome Instability

Genome instability is a hallmark of tumor cells and is involved in the transformation process. ATLL has numerous structural and numerical genomic alterations. Although there is not a specific chromosome alteration typifying ATLL, some genomic defects such as translocations involving 14q32 (28%) or 14q11 (14%) and deletion of 6q (23%) occur more frequently and may play a role in disease progression [123, 124]. Alterations of the DDR and the DNA repair pathways are intimately linked to genome and chromosome integrity. HTLV-I Tax protein inhibits DDR and predisposes to accumulation of genomic mutations [125–127]. Although aneuploidy is frequently observed in HTLV-I-transformed and ATLL cells, it is not linked to defects in the mitotic spindle checkpoint, which is fully functional in these cells [128]. In contrast, centrosome amplification-associated aneuploidy has been reported in ATLL cells and may be involved in chromosome instability and tumor progression [129]. Alternatively, defects in the homologous recombination (HR) pathway observed in Tax-expressing cells [130, 131] may also be responsible for chromosome instability and increased aneuploidy [132].

4.1. Single-Strand DNA Damage Repair Pathways. Microsatellite instability (MSI) has been linked to a defect of the DNA mismatch repair (MMR) pathway and has been implicated in a wide array of human cancers. The incidence of MSI in ATLL is significantly higher than in other hematological diseases, suggesting that MSI is a feature of ATLL and may be involved in the progression of the disease [133, 134]. In fact, the hMSH2 gene that contributes to DNA mismatch repair demonstrated two types of polymorphisms (CTT to TTT resulting in Leu changing to Phe at codon 390 in exon 7 and CAG to AAG resulting in Gin changing to Arg at codon 419 in exon 7) in ATLL cells [135]. Additional studies demonstrated loss of MMR-related genes in ATLL cells [136]. HTLV-I viral protein Tax-mediated increased expression of proliferating cell nuclear antigen (PCNA) has been shown to inhibit the activity of the nucleotide excision repair (NER) pathway [137, 138]. Similarly, Tax was also shown to inhibit the base excision repair (BER) pathway [139].

4.2. Double-Strand DNA Damage Repair Pathway. Tax has been shown to associate with the minichromosome maintenance MCM2-7 helicase and stimulate premature S phase progression leading to genomic lesions [140]. Follow-up studies confirmed these results and demonstrated that Tax acts as an inducer of genomic DNA double-strand breaks (DDSB) during DNA replication by blocking progression of the replication fork [130, 131]. Importantly, Tax-mediated NF-kB activation prevented DDSB repair by homologous recombination (HR) and increased usage of the error-prone nonhomologous end joining (NHEJ) repair pathway [130, 131].

In addition, reduced expression of human translesion synthesis (TLS) DNA polymerases Pol-H and Pol-K in HTLV-I-transformed T cells and ATLL cells was associated with an increase in DNA breaks at particular genomic regions, such as the c-Myc and the Bcl-2 major breakpoints [130].

5. Loss of Adhesion Molecules Stimulates Metastasis of ATLL Cells

Studies have reported that the tumor suppressor in lung cancer 1 (TSLC1/IgSF4/CADM1) is overexpressed in the acute type of ATLL [141]. In addition, others had shown that expression of TSLC1 plays an important role in the organ infiltration of ATLL cells [142]. High levels of intracellular and serum levels of MMP-9 have been reported in ATLL patients and correlated with organ involvement, suggesting that overexpression of MMP-9 in ATLL cells may be in part responsible for their invasiveness potential [143]. Likewise, analyses of histopathological tissue sections from ATLL patients with skin infiltrations revealed increased expression of MMP-2 in fibroblasts surrounding infiltrating ATLL cells, but not in fibroblast biopsies from nondiseased areas. Emmprin was found to be overexpressed and it facilitates MMP-2 production via interactions with fibroblasts, thereby facilitating stromal invasion by tumor cells [144]. Additional studies found that the CADM1 protein is overexpressed in ATLL cells. CADM1 interacted with T-lymphoma invasion and metastasis 1 (Tiam1) leading to Rac activation and stimulated infiltration of tumor cells into various organs [145].

Disclaimer

The content is solely the responsibility of the author and does not necessarily represent the official views of the National Institutes of Health.

Conflict of Interests

The author declares that there is no conflict of interests regarding the publication of this paper.

Acknowledgments

The author would like to thank Brandi Miller for editorial assistance. This work was supported by NIH Grant CA106258 to Christophe Nicot.

References

[1] B. J. Poiesz, F. W. Ruscetti, A. F. Gazdar, P. A. Bunn, J. D. Minna, and R. C. Gallo, "Detection and isolation of type C retrovirus particles from fresh and cultured lymphocytes of a patient with cutaneous T-cell lymphoma," *Proceedings of the National Academy of Sciences of the United States of America*, vol. 77, no. 12, pp. 7415–7419, 1980.

[2] M. Yoshida, I. Miyoshi, and Y. Hinuma, "Isolation and characterization of retrovirus from cell lines of human adult T-cell leukemia and its implication in the disease," *Proceedings of the National Academy of Sciences of the United States of America*, vol. 79, no. 6, pp. 2031–2035, 1982.

[3] M. Yoshida, I. Miyoshi, and Y. Hinuma, "A retrovirus from human leukemia cell lines: its isolation, characterization, and implication in human adult T-cell leukemia (ATL)," *Princess Takamatsu Symposia*, vol. 12, pp. 285–294, 1982.

[4] A. Gessain and O. Cassar, "Epidemiological aspects and world distribution of HTLV-1 infection," *Frontiers in Microbiology*, vol. 3, article 388, Article ID Article 388, 2012.

[5] M. Iwanaga, T. Watanabe, and K. Yamaguchi, "Adultt-cell leukemia: a review of epidemiological evidence," *Frontiers in Microbiology*, vol. 3, article 322, 2012.

[6] K. Takatsuki, K. Yamaguchi, F. Kawano et al., "Clinical diversity in adult T-cell leukemia-lymphoma," *Cancer Research*, vol. 45, pp. 4644s–4645s, 1985.

[7] K. Tsukasaki, O. Hermine, A. Bazarbachi et al., "Definition, prognostic factors, treatment, and response criteria of adult T-cell leukemia-lymphoma: a proposal from an international consensus meeting," *Journal of Clinical Oncology*, vol. 27, no. 3, pp. 453–459, 2009.

[8] F. Wong-Staal, B. Hahn, V. Manzari et al., "A survey of human leukaemias for sequences of a human retrovirus," *Nature*, vol. 302, no. 5909, pp. 626–628, 1983.

[9] M. Yoshida, M. Seiki, K. Yamaguchi, and K. Takatsuki, "Monoclonal integration of human T-cell leukemia provirus in all primary tumors of adult T-cell leukemia suggests causative role of human T-cell leukemia virus in the disease," *Proceedings of the National Academy of Sciences of the United States of America*, vol. 81, no. 8, pp. 2534–2537, 1984.

[10] A. Bazarbachi, F. Suarez, P. Fields, and O. Hermine, "How I treat adult T-cell leukemia/lymphoma," *Blood*, vol. 118, no. 7, pp. 1736–1745, 2011.

[11] M. Shimoyama, "Diagnostic criteria and classification of clinical subtypes of adult T-cell leukaemia-lymphoma. A report from the lymphoma study group (1984–87)," *British Journal of Haematology*, vol. 79, no. 3, pp. 428–437, 1991.

[12] A. Bazarbachi, Y. Plumelle, J. C. Ramos et al., "Meta-analysis on the use of zidovudine and interferon-alfa in adult T-cell leukemia/lymphoma showing improved survival in the leukemic subtypes," *Journal of Clinical Oncology*, vol. 28, no. 27, pp. 4177–4183, 2010.

[13] Y. Kfoury, R. Nasr, C. Journo, R. Mahieux, C. Pique, and A. Bazarbachi, "The multifaceted oncoprotein Tax. subcellular localization, posttranslational modifications, and NF-κB activation," *Advances in Cancer Research*, vol. 113, pp. 85–120, 2012.

[14] M. Bellon, H. H. Baydoun, Y. Yao, and C. Nicot, "HTLV-I tax-dependent and -independent events associated with immortalization of human primary T lymphocytes," *Blood*, vol. 115, no. 12, pp. 2441–2448, 2010.

[15] N. A. Gillet, N. Malani, A. Melamed et al., "The host genomic environment of the provirus determines the abundance of HTLV-1-infected T-cell clones," *Blood*, vol. 117, no. 11, pp. 3113–3122, 2011.

[16] C. Miller, T. Mohandas, D. Wolf, M. Prokocimer, V. Rotter, and H. P. Koeffler, "Human p53 gene localized to short arm of chromosome 17," *Nature*, vol. 319, no. 6056, pp. 783–784, 1986.

[17] O. W. McBride, D. Merry, and D. Givol, "The gene for human p53 cellular tumor antigen is located on chromosome 17 short arm (17p13)," *Proceedings of the National Academy of Sciences of the United States of America*, vol. 83, no. 1, pp. 130–134, 1986.

[18] S. J. Baker, E. R. Fearon, J. M. Nigro et al., "Chromosome 17 deletions and p53 gene mutations in colorectal carcinomas," *Science*, vol. 244, no. 4901, pp. 217–221, 1989.

[19] J. M. Nigro, S. J. Baker, A. C. Preisinger et al., "Mutations in the p53 gene occur in diverse human tumour types," *Nature*, vol. 342, no. 6250, pp. 705–708, 1989.

[20] G. Gaidano, P. Ballerini, J. Z. Gong et al., "p53 mutations in human lymphoid malignancies: association with Burkitt lymphoma and chronic lymphocytic leukemia," *Proceedings of the National Academy of Sciences of the United States of America*, vol. 88, no. 12, pp. 5413–5417, 1991.

[21] A. Sakashita, T. Hattori, C. W. Miller et al., "Mutations of the p53 gene in adult T-cell leukemia," *Blood*, vol. 79, no. 2, pp. 477–480, 1992.

[22] E. Cesarman, A. Chadburn, G. Inghirami, G. Gaidano, and D. M. Knowles, "Structural and functional analysis of oncogenes and tumor suppressor genes in adult T-cell leukemia/lymphoma shows frequent p53 mutations," *Blood*, vol. 80, no. 12, pp. 3205–3216, 1992.

[23] H. Nagai, T. Kinoshita, J. Imamura et al., "Genetic alteration of p53 in some patients with adult T-cell leukemia," *Japanese Journal of Cancer Research*, vol. 82, no. 12, pp. 1421–1427, 1991.

[24] M. Tawara, S. J. Hogerzeil, Y. Yamada et al., "Impact of p53 aberration on the progression of Adult T-cell leukemia/lymphoma," *Cancer Letters*, vol. 234, no. 2, pp. 249–255, 2006.

[25] K. Yamato, T. Oka, M. Hiroi et al., "Aberrant expression of the p53 tumor suppressor gene in adult T-cell leukemia and HTLV-I-infected cells," *Japanese Journal of Cancer Research*, vol. 84, no. 1, pp. 4–8, 1993.

[26] R. L. Reid, P. F. Lindholm, A. Mireskandari, J. Dittmer, and J. N. Brady, "Stabilization of wild-type p53 in human T-lymphocytes transformed by HTLV-I," *Oncogene*, vol. 8, no. 11, pp. 3029–3036, 1993.

[27] S. Takemoto, R. Trovato, A. Cereseto et al., "p53 Stabilization and functional impairment in the absence of genetic mutation or the alteration of the p14(APF)-MDM2 loop in ex vivo and cultured adult T-cell leukemia/lymphoma cells," *Blood*, vol. 95, no. 12, pp. 3939–3944, 2000.

[28] T. Akagi, H. Ono, N. Tsuchida, and K. Shimotohno, "Aberrant expression and function of p53 in T cells immortalized by HTLV-I Tax1," *FEBS Letters*, vol. 406, no. 3, pp. 263–266, 1997.

[29] C. A. Pise-Masison, K.-S. Choi, M. Radonovich, J. Dittmer, S.-J. Kim, and J. N. Brady, "Inhibition of p53 transactivation function by the human T-cell lymphotropic virus type 1 Tax protein," *Journal of Virology*, vol. 72, no. 2, pp. 1165–1170, 1998.

[30] C. A. Pise-Masison, R. Mahieux, H. Jiang et al., "Inactivation of p53 by human T-cell lymphotropic virus type 1 tax requires activation of the NF-κB pathway and is dependent on p53 phosphorylation," *Molecular and Cellular Biology*, vol. 20, no. 10, pp. 3377–3386, 2000.

[31] J. C. Mulloy, T. Kislyakova, A. Cereseto et al., "Human T-cell lymphotropic/leukemia virus type 1 tax abrogates p53-induced cell cycle arrest and apoptosis through its CREB/ATF functional domain," *Journal of Virology*, vol. 72, no. 11, pp. 8852–8860, 1998.

[32] C. A. Pise-Masison, R. Mahieux, M. Radonovich, H. Jiang, and J. N. Brady, "Human T-lymphotropic virus type I Tax protein utilizes distinct pathways for p53 inhibition that are cell type-dependent," *The Journal of Biological Chemistry*, vol. 276, no. 1, pp. 200–205, 2001.

[33] N. L. Ko, J. M. Taylor, M. Bellon et al., "PA28γ is a novel corepressor of HTLV-1 replication and controls viral latency," *Blood*, vol. 121, no. 5, pp. 791–800, 2013.

[34] Y. Satou, J. I. Yasunaga, M. Yoshida, and M. Matsuoka, "HTLV-I basic leucine zipper factor gene mRNA supports proliferation of adult T cell leukemia cells," *Proceedings of the National Academy of Sciences of the United States of America*, vol. 103, no. 3, pp. 720–725, 2006.

[35] X. Agirre, F. J. Novo, M. J. Calasanz et al., "TP53 is frequently altered by methylation, mutation, and/or deletion in acute lymphoblastic leukaemia," *Molecular Carcinogenesis*, vol. 38, no. 4, pp. 201–208, 2003.

[36] D.-T. Wang, Z.-L. Ma, Y.-L. Li et al., "miR-150, p53 protein and relevant miRNAs consist of a regulatory network in NSCLC tumorigenesis," *Oncology Reports*, vol. 30, no. 1, pp. 492–498, 2013.

[37] M. Bellon, Y. Lepelletier, O. Hermine, and C. Nicot, "Deregulation of microRNA involved in hematopoiesis and the immune response in HTLV-I adult T-cell leukemia," *Blood*, vol. 113, no. 20, pp. 4914–4917, 2009.

[38] S.-J. Jeong, M. Radonovich, J. N. Brady, and C. A. Pise-Masison, "HTLV-I Tax induces a novel interaction between p65/RelA and p53 that results in inhibition of p53 transcriptional activity," *Blood*, vol. 104, no. 5, pp. 1490–1497, 2004.

[39] M. Yamagishi, K. Nakano, A. Miyake et al., "Polycomb-mediated loss of miR-31 activates nik-dependent NF-κB pathway in adult T cell leukemia and other cancers," *Cancer Cell*, vol. 21, no. 1, pp. 121–135, 2012.

[40] K.-J. Jung, A. Dasgupta, K. Huang et al., "Small-molecule inhibitor which reactivates p53 in human T-cell leukemia virus type 1-transformed cells," *Journal of Virology*, vol. 82, no. 17, pp. 8537–8547, 2008.

[41] A. Datta, M. Bellon, U. Sinha-Datta et al., "Persistent inhibition of telomerase reprograms adult T-cell leukemia to p53-dependent senescence," *Blood*, vol. 108, no. 3, pp. 1021–1029, 2006.

[42] S. Ichimiya, Y. Nimura, H. Kageyama et al., "p73 at chromosome 1p36.3 is lost in advanced stage neuroblastoma but its mutation is infrequent," *Oncogene*, vol. 18, no. 4, pp. 1061–1066, 1999.

[43] M. Kaghad, H. Bonnet, A. Yang et al., "Monoallelically expressed gene related to p53 at 1p36, a region frequently deleted in neuroblastoma and other human cancers," *Cell*, vol. 90, no. 4, pp. 809–819, 1997.

[44] S. Kawano, C. W. Miller, A. Gombart et al., "Loss of p73 gene expression in leukemias/lymphomas due to hypermethylation," *Blood*, vol. 94, no. 3, pp. 1113–1120, 1999.

[45] H. Sato, T. Oka, Y. Shinnou et al., "Multi-step aberrant CpG island hyper-methylation is associated with the progression of adult T-cell leukemia/lymphoma," *The American Journal of Pathology*, vol. 176, no. 1, pp. 402–415, 2010.

[46] I. Lemasson and J. K. Nyborg, "Human T-cell leukemia virus type I tax repression of p73β is mediated through competition for the C/H1 domain of CBP," *The Journal of Biological Chemistry*, vol. 276, no. 19, pp. 15720–15727, 2001.

[47] A. Kaida, Y. Ariumi, Y. Ueda et al., "Functional impairment of p73 and p51, the p53-related proteins, by the human T-cell leukemia virus type 1 Tax oncoprotein," *Oncogene*, vol. 19, no. 6, pp. 827–830, 2000.

[48] R. T. Williams and C. J. Sherr, "The INK4-ARF (CDKN2A/B) locus in hematopoiesis and BCR-ABL-induced leukemias," *Cold Spring Harbor Symposia on Quantitative Biology*, vol. 73, pp. 461–467, 2008.

[49] C. Caldas, S. A. Hahn, L. T. da Costa et al., "Frequent somatic mutations and homozygous deletions of the p16 (*MTS1*) gene in

pancreatic adenocarcinoma," *Nature Genetics*, vol. 8, no. 1, pp. 27–32, 1994.

[50] D. Bartsch, D. W. Shevlin, W. S. Tung, O. Kisker, S. A. Wells Jr., and P. J. Goodfellow, "Frequent mutations of CDKN2 in primary pancreatic adenocarcinomas," *Genes Chromosomes and Cancer*, vol. 14, no. 3, pp. 189–195, 1995.

[51] L. Liu, N. J. Lassam, J. M. Slingerland et al., "Germline p16INK4A mutation and protein dysfunction in a family with inherited melanoma," *Oncogene*, vol. 11, no. 2, pp. 404–412, 1995.

[52] R. Trovato, A. Cereseto, S. Takemoto et al., "Deletion of the p16^{INK4A} gene in *ex vivo* acute adult T cell lymphoma/leukemia cells and methylation of the p16^{INK4A} promoter in HTLV type I-infected T cell lines," *AIDS Research and Human Retroviruses*, vol. 16, no. 8, pp. 709–713, 2000.

[53] T. Uchida, T. Kinoshita, T. Murate, H. Saito, and T. Hotta, "CDKN2 (MTS1/p16^{INK4A}) gene alterations in adult T-cell leukemia/lymphoma," *Leukemia & Lymphoma*, vol. 29, no. 1-2, pp. 27–35, 1998.

[54] Y. Hatta, T. Hirama, C. W. Miller, Y. Yamada, M. Tomonaga, and H. P. Koeffler, "Homozygous deletions of the p15 (MTS2) and p16 (CDKN2/MTS1) genes in adult T-cell leukemia," *Blood*, vol. 85, no. 10, pp. 2699–2704, 1995.

[55] K. Uenogawa, Y. Hatta, N. Arima et al., "Azacitidine induces demethylation of p16INK4a and inhibits growth in adult T-cell leukemia/lymphoma," *International Journal of Molecular Medicine*, vol. 28, no. 5, pp. 835–839, 2011.

[56] M. S. Pombo-de-Oliveira, J. A. Dobbin, P. Loureiro et al., "Genetic mutation and early onset of T-cell leukemia in pediatric patients infected at birth with HTLV-I," *Leukemia Research*, vol. 26, no. 2, pp. 155–161, 2002.

[57] M. J. Bueno and M. Malumbres, "MicroRNAs and the cell cycle," *Biochimica et Biophysica Acta*, vol. 1812, no. 5, pp. 592–601, 2011.

[58] M. J. Bueno, I. P. de Castro, and M. Malumbres, "Control of cell proliferation pathways by microRNAs," *Cell Cycle*, vol. 7, no. 20, pp. 3143–3148, 2008.

[59] M. Yamagishi, K. Nakano, A. Miyake et al., "Polycomb-mediated loss of miR-31 activates nik-dependent NF-κB pathway in adult T cell leukemia and other cancers," *Cancer Cell*, vol. 21, no. 1, pp. 121–135, 2012.

[60] T. Suzuki, T. Narita, M. Uchida-Toita, and M. Yoshida, "Downregulation of the INK4 family of cyclin-dependent kinase inhibitors by tax protein of HTLV-1 through two distinct mechanisms," *Virology*, vol. 259, no. 2, pp. 384–391, 1999.

[61] T. Suzuki, S. Kitao, H. Matsushime, and M. Yoshida, "HTLV-1 tax protein interacts with cyclin-dependent kinase inhibitor p16INK4A and counteracts its inhibitory activity towards CDK4," *The EMBO Journal*, vol. 15, no. 7, pp. 1607–1614, 1996.

[62] D. Bertwistle, M. Sugimoto, and C. J. Sherr, "Physical and functional interactions of the Arf tumor suppressor protein with nucleophosmin/B23," *Molecular and Cellular Biology*, vol. 24, no. 3, pp. 985–996, 2004.

[63] H. Rizos, A. P. Darmanian, E. A. Holland, G. J. Mann, and R. F. Kefford, "Mutations in the INK4a/ARF melanoma susceptibility locus functionally impair p14ARF," *The Journal of Biological Chemistry*, vol. 276, no. 44, pp. 41424–41434, 2001.

[64] N. Burri, P. Shaw, H. Bouzourene et al., "Methylation silencing and mutations of the p14ARF and p16INK4a genes in colon cancer," *Laboratory Investigation*, vol. 81, no. 2, pp. 217–229, 2001.

[65] D. K. Bartsch, M. Sina-Frey, S. Lang et al., "CDKN2A germline mutations in familial pancreatic cancer," *Annals of Surgery*, vol. 236, no. 6, pp. 730–737, 2002.

[66] S. W. Blain, E. Montalvo, and J. Massagué, "Differential interaction of the cyclin-dependent kinase (CDK) inhibitor p27^{Kip1} with cyclin A-Cdk2 and cyclin D2-Cdk4," *The Journal of Biological Chemistry*, vol. 272, no. 41, pp. 25863–25872, 1997.

[67] J. Labaer, M. D. Garrett, L. F. Stevenson et al., "New functional activities for the p21 family of CDK inhibitors," *Genes and Development*, vol. 11, no. 7, pp. 847–862, 1997.

[68] Y. Hashimoto, K. Kohri, Y. Kaneko et al., "Critical role for the 3_{10} helix region of p57^{Kip2} in cyclin-dependent kinase 2 inhibition and growth suppression," *The Journal of Biological Chemistry*, vol. 273, no. 26, pp. 16544–16550, 1998.

[69] W. S. El-Deiry, T. Tokino, V. E. Velculescu et al., "WAF1, a potential mediator of p53 tumor suppression," *Cell*, vol. 75, no. 4, pp. 817–825, 1993.

[70] A. L. Gartel and S. K. Radhakrishnan, "Lost in transcription: p21 repression, mechanisms, and consequences," *Cancer Research*, vol. 65, no. 10, pp. 3980–3985, 2005.

[71] C. de la Fuente, F. Santiago, L. Deng et al., "Overexpression of p21(waf1) in human T-cell lymphotropic virus type 1-infected cells and its association with cyclin A/cdk2," *Journal of Virology*, vol. 74, no. 16, pp. 7270–7283, 2000.

[72] M. Watanabe, S. Nakahata, M. Hamasaki et al., "Downregulation of CDKN1A in adult T-cell leukemia/lymphoma despite overexpression of CDKN1A in human T-lymphotropic virus 1-infected cell lines," *Journal of Virology*, vol. 84, no. 14, pp. 6966–6977, 2010.

[73] Y.-K. Kim, J. Yu, T. S. Han et al., "Functional links between clustered microRNAs: suppression of cell-cycle inhibitors by microRNA clusters in gastric cancer," *Nucleic Acids Research*, vol. 37, no. 5, pp. 1672–1681, 2009.

[74] G. C. Sampey, R. Van Duyne, R. Currer, R. Das, A. Narayanan, and F. Kashanchi, "Complex role of microRNAs in HTLV-1 infections," *Frontiers in Genetics*, vol. 3, article 295, 2012.

[75] A. Cereseto, R. W. Parks, E. Rivadeneira, and G. Franchini, "Limiting amounts of p27^{Kip1} correlates with constitutive activation of cyclin E-CDK2 complex in HTLV-I-transformed T cells," *Oncogene*, vol. 18, no. 15, pp. 2441–2450, 1999.

[76] R. Morosetti, N. Kawamata, A. F. Gombart et al., "Alterations of the p27KIP1 Gene in Non-Hodgkin's Lymphomas and Adult T-Cell Leukemia/Lymphoma," *Blood*, vol. 86, no. 5, pp. 1924–1930, 1995.

[77] W. Roeb, A. Boyer, W. K. Cavenee, and K. C. Arden, "PAX3-FOXO1 controls expression of the p57Kip2 cell-cycle regulator through degradation of EGR1," *Proceedings of the National Academy of Sciences of the United States of America*, vol. 104, no. 46, pp. 18085–18090, 2007.

[78] S. Matsuoka, M. C. Edwards, C. Bai et al., "P57KIP2, a structurally distinct member of the p21CIP1 Cdk inhibitor family, is a candidate tumor suppressor gene," *Genes and Development*, vol. 9, no. 6, pp. 650–662, 1995.

[79] I. Hatada, A. Nabetani, H. Morisaki et al., "New p57^{KIP2} mutations in Beckwith-Wiedemann syndrome," *Human Genetics*, vol. 100, no. 5-6, pp. 681–683, 1997.

[80] I. S. Pateras, K. Apostolopoulou, K. Niforou, A. Kotsinas, and V. G. Gorgoulis, "p57KIP2: 'kip'ing the cell under control," *Molecular Cancer Research*, vol. 7, no. 12, pp. 1902–1919, 2009.

[81] X. Yang, R. K. M. Karuturi, F. Sun et al., "*CDKN1C* (p57^{KIP2}) is a direct target of EZH2 and suppressed by multiple epigenetic mechanisms in breast cancer cells," *PLoS ONE*, vol. 4, Article ID e5011, 2009.

[82] L. Shen, M. Toyota, Y. Kondo et al., "Aberrant DNA methylation of p57KIP2 identifies a cell-cycle regulatory pathway with prognostic impact in adult acute lymphocytic leukemia," *Blood*, vol. 101, no. 10, pp. 4131–4136, 2003.

[83] F. Fornari, L. Gramantieri, M. Ferracin et al., "MiR-221 controls CDKN1C/p57 and CDKN1B/p27 expression in human hepatocellular carcinoma," *Oncogene*, vol. 27, no. 43, pp. 5651–5661, 2008.

[84] R. Medina, S. K. Zaidi, C.-G. Liu et al., "MicroRNAs 221 and 222 bypass quiescence and compromise cell survival," *Cancer Research*, vol. 68, no. 8, pp. 2773–2780, 2008.

[85] S. Sengupta, J. Nie, R. J. Wagner, C. Yang, R. Stewart, and J. A. Thomson, "MicroRNA 92b controls the G1/S checkpoint gene p57 in human embryonic stem cells," *Stem Cells*, vol. 27, no. 7, pp. 1524–1528, 2009.

[86] D. G. Johnson and R. Schneider-Broussard, "Role of E2F in cell cycle control and cancer," *Frontiers in Bioscience*, vol. 3, pp. d447–d448, 1998.

[87] S. A. Henley and F. A. Dick, "The retinoblastoma family of proteins and their regulatory functions in the mammalian cell division cycle," *Cell Division*, vol. 7, article 10, 2012.

[88] P. Indovina, E. Marcelli, N. Casini, V. Rizzo, and A. Giordano, "Emerging roles of RB family: new defense mechanisms against tumor progression," *Journal of Cellular Physiology*, vol. 228, no. 3, pp. 525–535, 2013.

[89] Y. Hatta, Y. Yamada, M. Tomonaga, and H. P. Koeffler, "Extensive analysis of the retinoblastoma gene in adult T cell leukemia/lymphoma (ATL)," *Leukemia*, vol. 11, no. 7, pp. 984–989, 1997.

[90] S. Takeuchi, N. Takeuchi, K. Tsukasaki et al., "Mutations in the retinoblastoma-related gene RB2/p130 in adult T-cell leukaemia/lymphoma," *Leukemia and Lymphoma*, vol. 44, no. 4, pp. 699–701, 2003.

[91] A. Hangaishi, S. Ogawa, N. Imamura et al., "Inactivation of multiple tumor-suppressor genes involved in negative regulation of the cell cycle, MTS1/p16INK4A/CDKN2, MTS2/p15INK4B, p53, and Rb genes in primary lymphoid malignancies," *Blood*, vol. 87, no. 12, pp. 4949–4958, 1996.

[92] K. Nakayama, Y. Yamada, T. Koji, T. Hayashi, M. Tomonaga, and S. Kamihira, "Expression and phosphorylation status of retinoblastoma protein in adult T-cell leukemia/lymphoma," *Leukemia Research*, vol. 24, no. 4, pp. 299–305, 2000.

[93] D. Jiang and R. C. T. Aguiar, "MicroRNA-155 controls RB phosphorylation in normal and malignant B lymphocytes via the noncanonical TGF-β1/SMAD5 signaling module," *Blood*, vol. 123, no. 1, pp. 86–93, 2014.

[94] K. Kehn, C. de la Fuente, K. Strouss et al., "The HTLV-I Tax oncoprotein targets the retinoblastoma protein for proteasomal degradation," *Oncogene*, vol. 24, no. 4, pp. 525–540, 2005.

[95] P. A. Steck, M. A. Pershouse, S. A. Jasser et al., "Identification of a candidate tumour suppressor gene, MMAC1, at chromosome 10q23.3 that is mutated in multiple advanced cancers," *Nature Genetics*, vol. 15, no. 4, pp. 356–362, 1997.

[96] Y. Yin and W. H. Shen, "PTEN: a new guardian of the genome," *Oncogene*, vol. 27, no. 41, pp. 5443–5453, 2008.

[97] E. C. Chu and A. S. Tarnawski, "PTEN regulatory functions in tumor suppression and cell biology," *Medical Science Monitor*, vol. 10, no. 10, pp. RA235–RA241, 2004.

[98] M. C. Hollander, G. M. Blumenthal, and P. A. Dennis, "PTEN loss in the continuum of common cancers, rare syndromes and mouse models," *Nature Reviews Cancer*, vol. 11, no. 4, pp. 289–301, 2011.

[99] J. Pancewicza, J. M. Taylora, A. Dattaa et al., "Notch signaling contributes to proliferation and tumor formation of human T-cell leukemia virus type 1-associated adult T-cell leukemia," *Proceedings of the National Academy of Sciences of the United States of America*, vol. 107, no. 38, pp. 16619–16624, 2010.

[100] J. E. Damen, L. Liu, P. Rosten et al., "The 145-kDa protein induced to associate with Shc by multiple cytokines is an inositol tetraphosphate and phosphatidylinositol 3,4,5-trisphosphate 5-phosphatase," *Proceedings of the National Academy of Sciences of the United States of America*, vol. 93, no. 4, pp. 1689–1693, 1996.

[101] G. Krystal, J. E. Damen, C. D. Helgason et al., "SHIPs ahoy," *International Journal of Biochemistry and Cell Biology*, vol. 31, no. 10, pp. 1007–1010, 1999.

[102] K. Nakase, J. Cheng, Q. Zhu, and W. A. Marasco, "Mechanisms of SHP-1 P2 promoter regulation in hematopoietic cells and its silencing in HTLV-1-transformed T cells," *Journal of Leukocyte Biology*, vol. 85, no. 1, pp. 165–174, 2009.

[103] Q. Zhang, P. N. Raghunath, E. Vonderheid, N. Odum, and M. A. Wasik, "Lack of phosphotyrosine phosphatase SHP-1 expression in malignant T-cell lymphoma cells results from methylation of the SHP-1 promoter," *American Journal of Pathology*, vol. 157, no. 4, pp. 1137–1146, 2000.

[104] J. Cheng, D. Zhang, C. Zhou, and W. A. Marasco, "Downregulation of SHP1 and up-regulation of negative regulators of JAK/STAT signaling in HTLV-1 transformed cell lines and freshly transformed human peripheral blood CD4+ T cells," *Leukemia Research*, vol. 28, no. 1, pp. 71–82, 2004.

[105] T.-S. Migone, N. A. Cacalano, N. Taylor, T. Yi, T. A. Waldmann, and J. A. Johnston, "Recruitment of SH2-containing protein tyrosine phosphatase SHP-1 to the interleukin 2 receptor; loss of SHP-1 expression in human T-lymphotropic virus type I-transformed T cells," *Proceedings of the National Academy of Sciences of the United States of America*, vol. 95, no. 7, pp. 3845–3850, 1998.

[106] M. Garofalo, G. Di Leva, G. Romano et al., "miR-221&222 regulate TRAIL resistance and enhance tumorigenicity through PTEN and TIMP3 downregulation," *Cancer Cell*, vol. 16, no. 6, pp. 498–509, 2009.

[107] Y.-N. Bai, Z.-Y. Yu, L.-X. Luo, J. Yi, Q.-J. Xia, and Y. Zeng, "MicroRNA-21 accelerates hepatocyte proliferation *in vitro* via PI3K/Akt signaling by targeting PTEN," *Biochemical and Biophysical Research Communications*, vol. 443, no. 3, pp. 802–807, 2014.

[108] R. M. O'Connell, A. A. Chaudhuri, D. S. Rao, and D. Baltimore, "Inositol phosphatase SHIP1 is a primary target of miR-155," *Proceedings of the National Academy of Sciences of the United States of America*, vol. 106, no. 17, pp. 7113–7118, 2009.

[109] G. M. Caldwell, C. Jones, K. Gensberg et al., "The Wnt antagonist sFRP1 in colorectal tumorigenesis," *Cancer Research*, vol. 64, no. 3, pp. 883–888, 2004.

[110] R. Stoehr, C. Wissmann, H. Suzuki et al., "Deletions of chromosome 8p and loss of sFRP1 expression are progression markers of papillary bladder cancer," *Laboratory Investigation*, vol. 84, no. 4, pp. 465–478, 2004.

[111] M. L. Gumz, H. Zou, P. A. Kreinest et al., "Secreted frizzled-related protein 1 loss contributes to tumor phenotype of clear cell renal cell carcinoma," *Clinical Cancer Research*, vol. 13, no. 16, pp. 4740–4749, 2007.

[112] T. Fukui, M. Kondo, G. Ito et al., "Transcriptional silencing of secreted frizzled related protein 1 (SFRP1) by promoter

hypermethylation in non-small-cell lung cancer," *Oncogene*, vol. 24, no. 41, pp. 6323–6327, 2005.

[113] E. Dahl, J. Veeck, H. An et al., "Epigenetic inactivation of the WNT antagonist SFRP1 in breast cancer," *Verhandlungen der Deutschen Gesellschaft für Pathologie*, vol. 89, pp. 169–177, 2005.

[114] U. Sinha-Datta, I. Horikawa, E. Michishita et al., "Transcriptional activation of hTERT through the NF-kappaB pathway in HTLV-I-transformed cells," *Blood*, vol. 104, no. 8, pp. 2523–2531, 2004.

[115] N. Uchida, T. Otsuka, F. Arima et al., "Correlation of telomerase activity with development and progression of adult T-cell leukemia," *Leukemia Research*, vol. 23, no. 3, pp. 311–316, 1999.

[116] Y. Kubuki, M. Suzuki, H. Sasaki et al., "Telomerase activity and telomere length as prognostic factors of adult T-cell leukemia," *Leukemia and Lymphoma*, vol. 46, no. 3, pp. 393–399, 2005.

[117] C. Nicot, R. Mahieux, S. Takemoto, and G. Franchini, "Bcl-X(L) is up-regulated by HTLV-I and HTLV-II in vitro and in ex vivo ATLL samples," *Blood*, vol. 96, no. 1, pp. 275–281, 2000.

[118] Y. B. Choi, E. W. Harhaj, and S. R. Ross, "HTLV-1 tax stabilizes MCL-1 via TRAF6-dependent K63-linked polyubiquitination to promote cell survival and transformation," *PLoS Pathogens*, vol. 10, no. 10, 2014.

[119] A. Kawakami, T. Nakashima, H. Sakai et al., "Inhibition of caspase cascade by HTLV-I tax through induction of NF-κB nuclear translocation," *Blood*, vol. 94, no. 11, pp. 3847–3854, 1999.

[120] H. Macaire, A. Riquet, V. Moncollin et al., "Tax protein-induced expression of antiapoptotic Bfl-1 protein contributes to survival of human T-cell leukemia virus type 1 (HTLV-1)-infected T cells," *The Journal of Biological Chemistry*, vol. 287, no. 25, pp. 21357–21370, 2012.

[121] A. Formosa, A. M. Lena, E. K. Markert et al., "DNA methylation silences miR-132 in prostate cancer," *Oncogene*, vol. 32, no. 1, pp. 127–134, 2013.

[122] M. L. Ufkin, S. Peterson, X. Yang, H. Driscoll, C. Duarte, and P. Sathyanarayana, "miR-125a regulates cell cycle, proliferation, and apoptosis by targeting the ErbB pathway in acute myeloid leukemia," *Leukemia Research*, vol. 38, no. 3, pp. 402–410, 2014.

[123] T. Itoyama, R. S. K. Chaganti, Y. Yamada et al., "Cytogenetic analysis and clinical significance in adult T-cell leukemia/ lymphoma: a study of 50 cases from the human T-cell leukemia virus type-1 endemic area, Nagasaki," *Blood*, vol. 97, no. 11, pp. 3612–3620, 2001.

[124] N. Kamada, M. Sakurai, K. Miyamoto et al., "Chromosome abnormalities in adult T-cell leukemia/lymphoma: a Karyotype Review Committee report," *Cancer Research*, vol. 52, no. 6, pp. 1481–1493, 1992.

[125] T. Dayaram, F. J. Lemoine, L. A. Donehower, and S. J. Marriott, "Activation of WIP1 phosphatase by HTLV-1 Tax mitigates the cellular response to DNA damage," *PLoS ONE*, vol. 8, no. 2, Article ID e55989, 2013.

[126] C. Chandhasin, R. I. Ducu, E. Berkovich, M. B. Kastan, and S. J. Marriott, "Human T-cell leukemia virus type 1 tax attenuates the ATM-mediated cellular DNA damage response," *Journal of Virology*, vol. 82, no. 14, pp. 6952–6961, 2008.

[127] H. U. Park, S.-J. Jeong, J.-H. Jeong, J. H. Chung, and J. N. Brady, "Human T-cell leukemia virus type 1 Tax attenuates γ-irradiation- induced apoptosis through physical interaction with Chk2," *Oncogene*, vol. 25, no. 3, pp. 438–447, 2006.

[128] B. Liu, M.-H. Liang, Y.-L. Kuo et al., "Human T-lymphotropic virus type 1 oncoprotein tax promotes unscheduled degradation

of Pds1p/securin and Clb2p/cyclin B1 and causes chromosomal instability," *Molecular and Cellular Biology*, vol. 23, no. 15, pp. 5269–5281, 2003.

[129] T. Nitta, M. Kanai, E. Sugihara et al., "Centrosome amplification in adult T-cell leukemia and human T-cell leukemia virus type 1 Tax-induced human T cells," *Cancer Science*, vol. 97, no. 9, pp. 836–841, 2006.

[130] H. Chaib-Mezrag, D. Lemaçon, H. Fontaine et al., "Tax impairs DNA replication forks and increases DNA breaks in specific oncogenic genome regions," *Molecular Cancer*, vol. 13, article 205, 2014.

[131] H. H. Baydoun, X. T. Bai, S. Shelton, and C. Nicot, "HTLV-I tax increases genetic instability by inducing DNA double strand breaks during DNA replication and switching repair to NHEJ," *PLoS ONE*, vol. 7, no. 8, Article ID e42226, 2012.

[132] J. German, "Bloom's syndrome. I. Genetical and clinical observations in the first twenty-seven patients.," *The American Journal of Human Genetics*, vol. 21, no. 2, pp. 196–227, 1969.

[133] Y. Hatta, Y. Yamada, M. Tomonaga, I. Miyoshi, J. W. Said, and H. P. Koeffler, "Microsatellite instability in adult T-cell leukaemia," *British Journal of Haematology*, vol. 101, no. 2, pp. 341–344, 1998.

[134] Y. Hayami, H. Komatsu, S. Iida et al., "Microsatellite instability as a potential marker for poor prognosis in adult T cell leukemia/lymphoma," *Leukemia and Lymphoma*, vol. 32, no. 3-4, pp. 345–349, 1999.

[135] Y. Hatta, M. Wada, S. Takeuchi et al., "Mutational analysis of the hMSH2 gene in a wide variety of tumors," *International Journal of Oncology*, vol. 11, no. 3, pp. 465–469, 1997.

[136] H. Morimoto, J. Tsukada, Y. Kominato, and Y. Tanaka, "Reduced expression of human mismatch repair genes in adult T-cell leukemia," *The American Journal of Hematology*, vol. 78, no. 2, pp. 100–107, 2005.

[137] F. J. Lemoine, S.-Y. Kao, and S. J. Marriott, "Suppression of DNA repair by HTLV type 1 Tax correlates with Tax transactivation of proliferating cell nuclear antigen gene expression," *AIDS Research and Human Retroviruses*, vol. 16, no. 16, pp. 1623–1627, 2000.

[138] S.-Y. Kao and S. J. Marriott, "Disruption of nucleotide excision repair by the human T-cell leukemia virus type 1 Tax protein," *Journal of Virology*, vol. 73, no. 5, pp. 4299–4304, 1999.

[139] S. M. Philpott and G. C. Buehring, "Defective DNA repair in cells with human T-cell leukemia/bovine leukemia viruses: role of tax gene," *Journal of the National Cancer Institute*, vol. 91, no. 11, pp. 933–942, 1999.

[140] M. Boxus, J.-C. Twizere, S. Legros, R. Kettmann, and L. Willems, "Interaction of HTLV-1 Tax with minichromosome maintenance proteins accelerates the replication timing program," *Blood*, vol. 119, no. 1, pp. 151–160, 2012.

[141] H. Sasaki, I. Nishikata, T. Shiraga et al., "Overexpression of a cell adhesion molecule, TSLC1, as a possible molecular marker for acute-type adult T-cell leukemia," *Blood*, vol. 105, no. 3, pp. 1204–1213, 2005.

[142] M. Z. Dewan, N. Takamatsu, T. Hidaka et al., "Critical role for TSLC1 expression in the growth and organ infiltration of adult T-cell leukemia cells in vivo," *Journal of Virology*, vol. 82, no. 23, pp. 11958–11963, 2008.

[143] N. Mori, H. Sato, T. Hayashibara et al., "Human T-cell leukemia virus type I Tax transactivates the matrix metalloproteinase-9 gene: potential role in mediating adult T-cell leukemia invasiveness," *Blood*, vol. 99, no. 4, pp. 1341–1349, 2002.

[144] K. Nabeshima, J. Suzumiya, M. Nagano et al., "Emmprin, a cell surface inducer of matrix metalloproteinases (MMPs), is expressed in T-cell lymphomas," *The Journal of Pathology*, vol. 202, no. 3, pp. 341–351, 2004.

[145] M. Masuda, T. Maruyama, T. Ohta et al., "CADM1 interacts with Tiam1 and promotes invasive phenotype of human T-cell leukemia virus type I-transformed cells and adult T-cell leukemia cells," *The Journal of Biological Chemistry*, vol. 285, no. 20, pp. 15511–15522, 2010.

Pulmonary Venous Obstruction in Cancer Patients

Chuang-Chi Liaw,[1] Hung Chang,[1] Tsai-Sheng Yang,[1] and Ming-Sheng Wen[2]

[1]*Division of Hemato-Oncology, Department of Internal Medicine,*
  Chang-Gung Memorial Hospital and Chang-Gung University College of Medicine, Taoyuan 33305, Taiwan
[2]*Division of Cardiology, Department of Internal Medicine,*
  Chang-Gung Memorial Hospital and Chang-Gung University College of Medicine, Taoyuan 33305, Taiwan

Correspondence should be addressed to Chuang-Chi Liaw; e102309@adm.cgmh.org.tw

Academic Editor: Sandra Cascio

Background. We study the clinical significance and management of pulmonary venous obstruction in cancer patients. *Methods*. We conducted a prospective cohort study to characterize the syndrome that we term "pulmonary vein obstruction syndrome" (PVOS) between January 2005 and March 2014. The criteria for inclusion were (1) episodes of shortness of breath; (2) chest X-ray showing abnormal pulmonary hilum shadow with or without presence of pulmonary edema and/or pleural effusion; (3) CT scan demonstrating pulmonary vein thrombosis/tumor with or without tumor around the vein. *Results*. Two hundred and twenty-two patients developed PVOS. Shortness of breath was the main symptom, which was aggravated by chemotherapy in 28 (13%), and medical/surgical procedures in 21 (9%) and showed diurnal change in intensity in 32 (14%). Chest X-rays all revealed abnormal pulmonary hilum shadows and presence of pulmonary edema in 194 (87%) and pleural effusion in 192 (86%). CT scans all showed pulmonary vein thrombosis/tumor (100%) and surrounding the pulmonary veins by tumor lesions in 140 patients (63%). PVOS was treated with low molecular weight heparin in combination with dexamethasone, and 66% of patients got clinical/image improvement. *Conclusion*. Physicians should be alert to PVOS when shortness of breath occurs and chest X-ray reveals abnormal pulmonary hilum shadows.

1. Introduction

Cancer cells can pass through a lung capillary and/or direct extension into pulmonary vein [1]. Tumor that extends into pulmonary veins may cause the pulmonary vein flow stasis, and/or vascular injury results in thrombosis generation [2–5]. Pulmonary veins infiltration by tumors or compression by affected lymph nodes result in venous stasis is also a potential reason to develop thrombosis [2–5]. Multiple pulmonary venous thrombosis/tumor is a potentially fatal condition. Impedance of blood flow from the pulmonary vein to the left atrium may cause pulmonary edema or pleural effusion.

In the present prospective case series study, we investigate the clinical significance of pulmonary vein obstruction in cancer patients and better characterize the syndrome that we term "pulmonary vein obstruction syndrome" (PVOS). The management of PVOS is also studied.

2. Materials and Methods

2.1. Patients. Between January 2005 and March 2014, we conduct a prospective case series study. Data collected from 1117 patients hospitalized in oncology wards of the Chang-Gung Memorial Hospital. Our data source mainly came from a single physician. The urological cancer was our area of expertise; most of these patients had urothelial carcinomas.

2.2. Diagnostic Criteria of PVOS. The criteria for PVOS diagnosis inclusion/diagnosis are listed as symptoms, chest X-ray findings, and CT findings, and that all 3 were required. The criteria for inclusion were (1) episodes of shortness of breath; (2) chest X-ray showing unilateral or bilateral abnormal pulmonary hilum shadow with or without presence of pulmonary edema and/or pleural effusion; (3) CT (computed tomography) scan demonstrating pulmonary vein thrombosis/tumor with or without lesions sticking to the outer vein surface. When dyspnea occurred and chest X-ray shows abnormal hilum shadow, CT scan was traced to detect pulmonary vein thrombosis/tumor. The majority of patients did a CT scan before the onset of symptom. But CT scans were not sensitive enough to separate thrombosis from tumor embolism. No patients had prior congestive heart failure history. The study was approved by the hospital ethics committee.

2.3. Clinical Investigation. The characteristics of PVOS included the presence of acute respiratory distress, combined with other thromboembolic complications and with other paraneoplastic syndromes. Acute respiratory distress was described as aggravated by chemotherapy, aggravated by medical/surgical procedures, and subject to diurnal fluctuation in intensity. Common thromboembolism-associated complications included consciousness loss/mental change [6, 7], paraneoplastic pain, and iliofemoral venous thrombosis symptoms. Paraneoplastic pain was defined as breakthrough pain occurring in the absence of an identifiable precipitating cause [8]. Cerebral thromboembolic complication and/or paraneoplastic pain in most patients were clinically suspected because of difficulty in definite diagnosis. Paraneoplastic syndromes included neoplastic fever (tumor-related fever with good response to naproxen test) [9], cachexia syndrome (simultaneous presence of weight loss > 5% within 6 months, reduced food intake, and muscle wasting) [10].

2.4. Laboratory Study. The D-dimer test, complete blood counts, liver function test, renal function test as checked in all patients with PVOS, APTT (active partial thromboplastin time) and PT (prothrombin time), calcium, C-reactive protein, blood gas, and pleural effusion study were checked in selected patients when diagnosing PVOS. The cutoff D-dimer value was 500 ng/mL. Paraneoplastic syndromes included hypercalcemia (serum calcium level more than 11 mg/dL), leukemoid reaction (peripheral count to more than $20,000/\mu L$ without evidence of infection or leukemia), and prerenal azotemia was defined as BUN-to-creatinine ratio greater than 20.

2.5. Image Study. Chest plain film findings included the location of abnormal pulmonary hilum shadows, presence of pulmonary edema, and presence of pleural effusion. CT scan findings included pulmonary vein obstruction sites, presence of pulmonary embolism, and presence of pleural effusion. Echocardiography and lung ventilation/perfusion scan were performed in selected patients when diagnosing PVOS.

2.6. Therapy. Treatment included subcutaneous injection of low molecular weight heparin (LMWH) either Fraxiparin (GlaxoSmithKline) or Enoxaparin (Sanofi-Aventis), intravenous dexamethasone, and intravenous fluids with or without furosemide when PVOS with acute respiratory distress occurred. Further use of chemotherapy or targeted therapy or hormone therapy depended on the patient's condition. CT scans were obtained from the hospital picture archiving and communication system (PACS).

2.7. Statistical Methods. Continuous data (presented as mean ± standard deviation) were used for D-dimer, C-reactive protein, BUN, creatinine, and BUN-to-creatinine ratio analysis. Survival was calculated from the time of the diagnosis of PVOS to death. Survival curves were determined using Kaplan-Meier methods. The significance of difference between survival curves was measured by log-rank test.

3. Results

3.1. Patient Characteristics. Of 1117 patients, 222 patients (20%) were documented to have PVOS. The data for 222 consecutive cancer patients (139 men and 83 women; 27–93 years old; median age, 69) was collected for evaluation of PVOS. The patients' characteristics and important laboratory and imaging findings of PVOS were shown in Table 1. PVOS occurred in patients with various metastatic tumors. One hundred and sixty-seven patients (75%) had an Eastern Cooperative Oncology Group (ECOG) performance status of 2 or greater. Common association with thromboembolic complications occurred in 146 patients (66%): consciousness disturbance ($n = 103$), paraneoplastic pain ($n = 53$), and iliofemoral venous thrombosis symptom ($n = 16$). Of them, 62 associated with multiple thromboembolic presentations. Of 103 patients with consciousness disturbance, 16 had CT scan- or magnetic resonance imaging- (MRI-) evidence of cerebral infarction and/or their angiographic proven. Common association with paraneoplastic syndromes occurred in 101 patients (45%): cachexia syndrome ($n = 79$), neoplastic fever ($n = 23$), leukemic-like reactions ($n = 18$), hypercalcemia ($n = 4$), and lactic acidosis ($n = 3$). Of them, 15 had multiple syndromes.

3.2. Clinical Outcome. Shortness of breath was the main symptom. Acute respiratory distress ($n = 222$) was aggravated by chemotherapy ($n = 28; 13\%$) and medical/surgical procedures ($n = 21; 9\%$) and fluctuated diurnally in intensity ($n = 32, 14\%$). Blood gas tests in 126 patients found acidity (pH less than 7.3) in 24 (19%), $PaCO_2 > 50$ mmHg in 23 (18%), $PaO_2 < 60$ mmHg in 36 (29%), $HCO_3- < 18$ mEq/L in 35 (28%), and $SaO_2 < 90\%$ in 35 (28%). Pleural effusion tests in 32 patients found exudate in 28 (88%), erythrocyte count < 500 in 14 (44%), leukocyte count < 500 in 22 (69%), and lymphocytes predominant in 25 (78%).

D-dimer and complete blood counts were checked in all patients. Mean D-dimer value was 3354 ± 2187 ng/mL (265 to greater than 10,000 ng/mL). D-dimer values 1001–3000 ng/mL in 35% of patients was the most common. There were 132 patients (59%) with hemoglobin levels below 10 g/dL, 95 patients (43%) with elevated white blood counts (>$10,000/\mu L$), and 21 patients (9%) with decreased platelet counts (<$100,000/\mu L$). APTT (active partial thromboplastin time) was checked in 100 patients and PT (prothrombin time) was checked in 109 patients; of these, 34 (34%) had APTT values above 36 seconds and 29 (27%) had PT values above 15 seconds. Albumin values were below 3.0 g/dL in 78 (41%) of the 189 patients. C-reactive protein was monitored in 111 patients. Mean C-reactive protein value was 114 ± 96 mg/L (0.7 to 384 mg/L). Of these 105 patients (95%) with

TABLE 1: Characteristics and important laboratory and imaging findings of 222 cancer patients with pulmonary vein obstruction syndrome (PVOS).

Characteristics	Number of patients (%)
Age (years)	
Median (range)	69 (27–93)
Sex	
Male/female	139/83
Primary sites: number/total hospitalized number (%)	
All patients	222/1117 (20)
Urinary tract	80/395 (20)
Lung	31/115 (27)
Colorectum	15/67 (22)
Breast	18/58 (31)
Pancreas	8/46 (17)
Stomach	7/38 (18)
Prostate	7/29 (24)
Others	56/369 (13)
Performance status: number/total number (%)	
0-1	55/222 (25)
≥2	167/222 (75)
Associated with other thromboembolic complications: number/total number (%)	
Yes	146/222 (66)
No	76/222 (34)
Associated with other paraneoplastic syndromes: *number/total number* (%)	
Yes	101/222 (45)
No	121/222 (55)
Acute respiratory distress: number/total number	
Aggravated by chemotherapy	28/222 (13)
Aggravated by medical/surgical procedure	21/222 (9)
Showed diurnal rhythm	32/222 (14)
D-dimer (ng/mL): number/total number (%)	
≤1000	25/222 (11)
1001–3000	78/222 (35)
3001–5000	51/222 (23)
>5000	68/222 (31)
C-reactive protein (mg/L): number/total number	
≤10	6/111 (5)
>11	105/111 (95)
Chest plain film: number/total number	
Abnormal hilum shadow	222/222 (100)
By side	
Bilateral lung	175/222 (79)
Unilateral lung	47/222 (21)
By location	
Upper lung + lower lung	186/222 (84)
Upper lung only	19/222 (9)
Lower lung only	17/222 (8)
Pulmonary edema	194/222 (87)
Pleural effusion	192/222 (86)

TABLE 1: Continued.

Characteristics	Number of patients (%)
CT scan: number/total number	
Pulmonary veins thrombosis/tumor	222/222 (100)
Surrounding pulmonary veins by tumor/atelectasis/consolidation	140/222 (63)
By side	
Bilateral lung	204/222 (92)
Unilateral lung	18/222 (8)
By location	
Both superior and inferior pulmonary vein	203/222 (91)
Superior pulmonary vein only	11/222 (5)
Inferior pulmonary vein only	8/222 (4)
Pulmonary artery emboli	70/222 (32)
Pleural effusion	155/222 (70)

elevation. Renal insufficiency was detected in 30 patients (16%). Of them mean BUN value, creatinine value, and BUN-to-creatinine ratio were 79.3±41.6 mg/dL (36.3 to 163 mg/dL), 3.7 ± 2.7 mg/dL (0.65 to 12.3 mg/dL), and 21.4 ± 15.5 (6.9 to 60.5), respectively.

Chest plain X-rays of 222 patients before and at the onset of PVOS were shown in Figures 1(a), 1(b), 2(a), 2(b), 3(a), 3(b), 4(a), and 4(b). All revealed an increase pulmonary hilum shadows when PVOS developed. Abnormal hilum shadows were bilateral in 175 (79%) and unilateral in 47 (21%) and present in both lobes in 186 (84%), upper lobes in 19 (9%), and lower lobes in 17 (8%). Chest plain X-rays showed pulmonary edema in 194 patients (87%) and pleural effusion in 192 patients (86%) (Figures 1(b), 2(b), 3(b), and 4(b)).

CT scans that revealed tumor/thrombosis located in pulmonary veins were shown in Figures 1(c), 1(d), 2(c), 2(d), 3(c), 3(d), 4(c), and 4(d). The separate time between doing CT scan and detecting abnormal hilum shadows by chest films due to PVOS was 149 patients (67%) within 1 month, 46 (21%) in 1-2 months, 20 (9%) in 2-3 months, and 7 (3%) more than 3 months. All demonstrated pulmonary vein thrombosis or tumor. Tumor or atelectic lesions surrounding the pulmonary vein (Figures 4(c) and 4(d)) were seen in 140 (63%). Pulmonary vein obstructions were present bilaterally in 204 (92%) and unilaterally in 18 (8%), in both the superior and inferior pulmonary vein in 203 (91%), in the superior pulmonary vein only in 11 (5%), and inferior pulmonary vein only in 8 (4%). Chest CT scan detected pleural effusion in 155 patients (70%), pulmonary artery embolism in 70 patients (32%), peripheral tumor/thrombi lesions (Figures 2(c) and 2(d)) in 72 patients (32%), and cardiac tumor/thrombi lesions (Figures 3(c) and 3(d)) in 7 patients (3%), and lung ventilation-perfusion scan in 5 patients found two (40%) with a pulmonary embolism and echocardiography in 29 patients found 14 (48%) with left atrium enlargement (≥38 mm).

3.3. Treatment Outcome and Survival Data. LMWH therapy was given to 170 patients with PVOS, including 113 on Fraxiparin (3800 IU or 5700 IU daily) and 57 on Enoxaparin

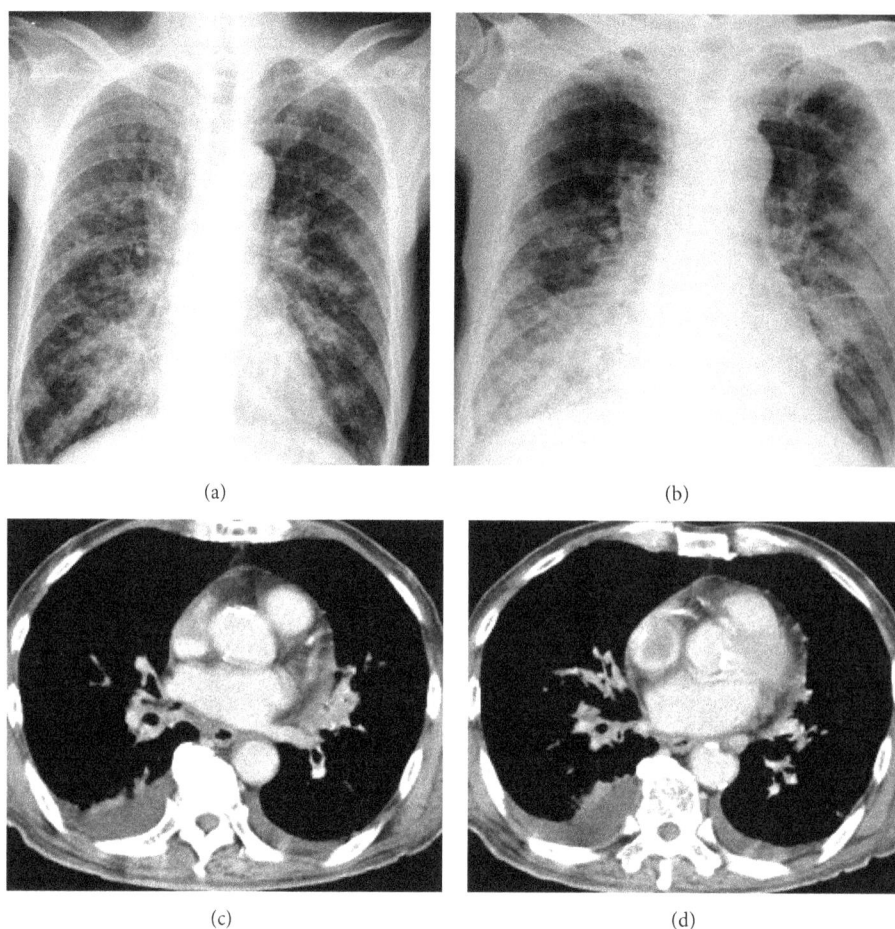

FIGURE 1: Pulmonary vein obstructive syndrome (PVOS). A 78-year-old man with rectal cancer. Chest X-ray (a) before and (b) at the onset of PVOS showed right low lung and pulmonary hilum increase haziness. CT scan ((c) and (d)) revealed tumor/thrombosis located in the bilateral superior and inferior pulmonary veins.

(6000 IU daily). And intravenous dexamethasone was also used in 133 patients. Symptoms and/or image improvement in 113 (66%) including 99 of those treated with dexamethasone. Of them, 37 patients continued their LMWH for secondary prevention.

Of 69 patients who received therapy, including chemotherapy in 59, targeted therapy in 9, and hormone therapy in one, 46 (68%) had disease control. PVOS developed again after disease progression in 32 patients (74%), including 20 with their LMWH for secondary prevention.

Follow-up periods ranged from 1 day to 267 weeks. Besides the fact that 12 patients were lost to follow-up, 210 patients could be followed until death or up to the present. Four patients were still alive. Median overall survival time by Kaplan-Meier methods was 5 weeks. Three-month, 6-month, 1-year, and 2-year-survival probabilities were 30%, 13%, 9%, and 1%, respectively. For 52 patients not receiving LMWH therapy patients, median overall survival time was 4 weeks. For 170 patients receiving LMWH ± dexamethasone therapy showed clinical/image improvement in 114 patients. The composite survival rate for those with clinical/image improvement was superior to those without clinical/image

improvement. The median survival rate was 11 weeks versus 2 weeks by log-rank test ($P = 0.001$). Flow chart of 222 patients with PVOS was shown in Figure 5.

The predeath status could be identified in 198 patients as respiratory failure ($n = 90$; 45%) and consciousness loss ($n = 108$; 55%). Sixty-three patients (32%) died of septicemia and/or febrile neutropenia, including 34 with respiratory failure and 28 with consciousness loss.

4. Discussion

PVOS occurred in 20% of our hospitalized patients with various malignancies.

PVOS is frequently associated with other thromboembolic complications and is a Trousseau's syndrome. Trousseau's syndromein is characterixed by spontaneous, multiple, recurrent, and migratory venous thrombosis, and arterial emboli [11–13]. A few patients also exhibit other paraneoplastic syndromes related to cytokine production [8–10].

Virchow describes the three elements, including venous stasis, endothelial injury, and hypercoagulability that are thought to contribute to venous thromboembolism (VTE)

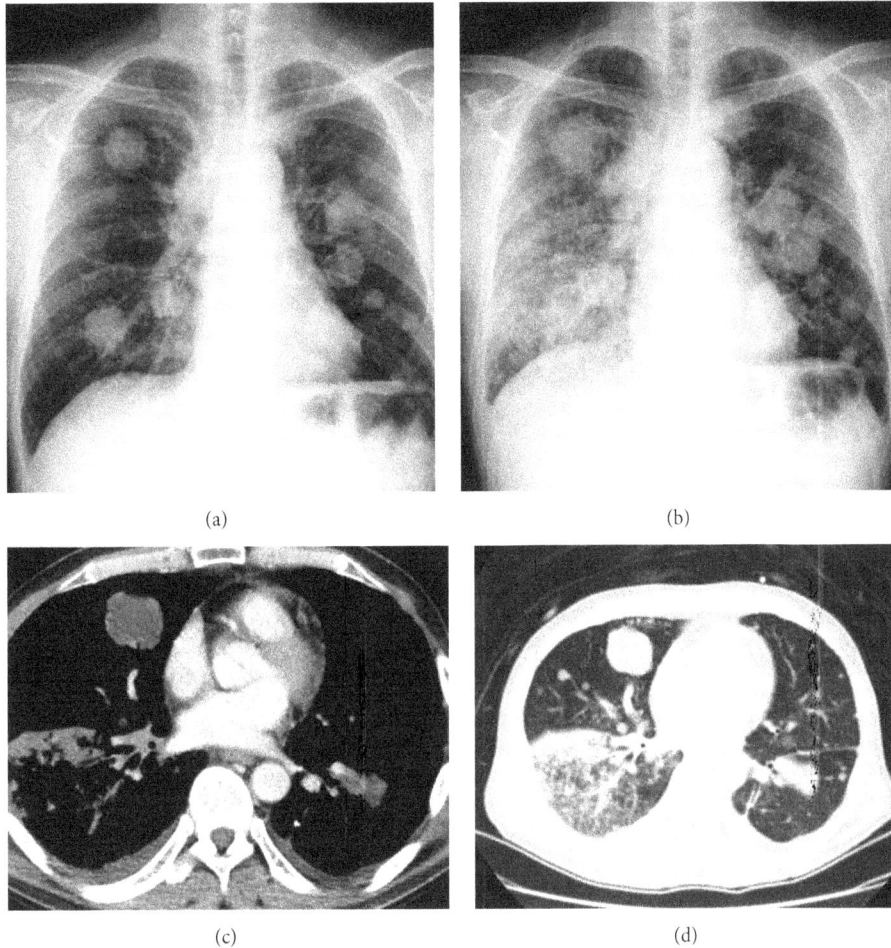

FIGURE 2: Pulmonary vein obstructive syndrome (PVOS). A 54-year-old man with bladder cancer. Chest X-ray (a) before and (b) at the onset of PVOS showed right low lung and hilum increase haziness. CT scan ((c) and (d)) revealed tumor/thrombosis located in right inferior pulmonary veins with peripheral extension.

[14, 15]. The mechanism of prothrombotic state is particularly complex in cancer patients. Cancer cells can activate the hemostatic system through the expression of adhesion molecules, release of inflammatory cytokines, and production of hemostatic factors [16–20]. Activation of blood coagulation results in thrombin generation and intravascular fibrin formation [16–20]. Thrombin-activated tumor cell adhesion to host cells also enhances tumor cell growth, tumor cell seeding, and spontaneous metastasis and stimulates tumor angiogenesis [16–19]. Once cancer cells enter into and/or approach to the pulmonary vein, they result in blood flow stasis and vascular injury. Cancer patients can be in a hypercoagulable status. But the cytokine production is the primary culprit to the development of PVOS. The increase cytokine production among cancer patients have been well recognized in sepsis, surgery/medical procedures and chemotherapy [20–22].

Three lines of evidence are presented in the study to indicate that PVOS is a real model of the thromboembolic complication [16, 17]. First, CT scans demonstrated pulmonary vein thrombosis/tumor. Tumor surrounding the pulmonary vein was noted in 63% of patients. Tumor cells result in pulmonary vein injury and/or stasis is essential. Second, acute respiratory distress is aggravated by chemotherapy and medical/surgical procedures and fluctuates diurnally in intensity. Cancer itself, its treatments, and its complications can activate cytokine signaling pathways including those of nuclear factor kappa B (NFκB) and p38 mitogen-activated protein kinase (MAPK) [23]. Circadian rhythms of cytokine release have been demonstrated in people with advanced neoplasms [24]. Third, D-dimer and CRP levels were elevated in 89% and 95%, respectively, of our patients, as occurs in cases of VTE and PE [25, 26]. Elevated D-dimer or CRP has been associated with increased risk of VTE [27].

A rise in hydrostatic pressure occurs due to blood flow through the pulmonary vein to the left atrium stasis. Symptoms such as pulmonary edema and pleural effusion develop. A few patients already had an oncological emergency (i.e., respiratory failure with hypoxemia, hypercapnia, decreased pH, or low SaO_2). A complex cause of pleural effusion

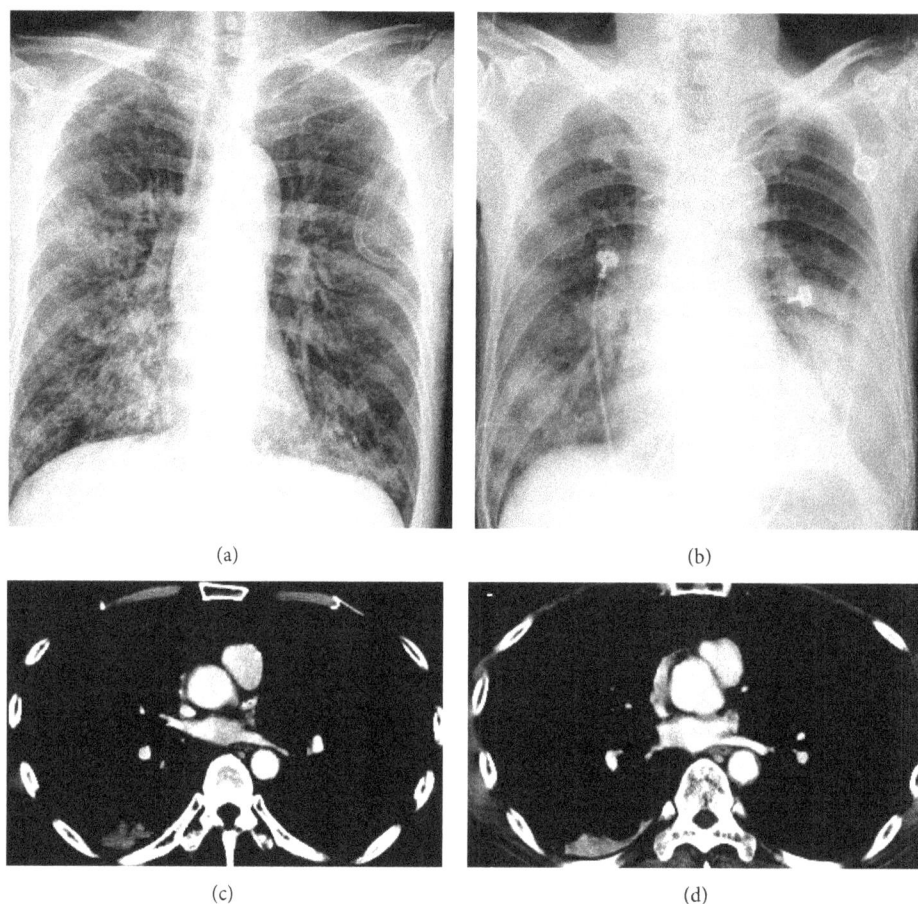

FIGURE 3: Pulmonary vein obstructive syndrome (PVOS). A 51-year-old man with oral cancer. Chest X-ray (a) before and (b) at the onset of PVOS showed a left low lung and hilum increase haziness. CT scan ((c) and (d)) revealed tumor/thrombosis located in superior and inferior pulmonary veins with left atrium extension.

noted in PVOS patients, and 69% had leukocyte count less than 500 on the pleural fluids. The reason in part for the low leukocyte count is that, in PVOS (like heart failure), hydrostatic pressure is also increased.

Cancer can induce pulmonary embolism (PE) formation and thrombotic formation and can invade large veins [28–30]. Extensive tumor-associated thromboemboli in the pulmonary microvasculature have been reported in a cancer patient with dyspnea [28–30]. However, microscopic tumor embolism is rarely recognized before death. The diagnosis was often identified from postmortem examination [28–30]. PVOS can combined with pulmonary artery embolism; tumor/thrombi from pulmonary veins can extend peripherally [28, 29] or enter left atrium [31]. Pulmonary artery embolism, peripheral pulmonary tumor/thrombi lesion, and cardiac tumor/thrombi lesions were 32%, 32%, and 3% of our patients, respectively.

The appearance of abnormal pulmonary hilum shadows on chest plain X-ray films (which are due to pulmonary hypertension) is essential for raising suspicion of PVOS [32]. Pulmonary edema and/or pleural effusion on chest plain films indicate severe blockade of pulmonary veins. CT scans

are vital for the diagnosis of PVOS and can show pulmonary vein thrombosis, tumor, and pulmonary vein stricture especially from their abnormal pulmonary hilum shadows [33]. Pulmonary edema and/or pleural effusion may be unilateral or bilateral and may arise from the superior pulmonary vein, inferior pulmonary vein, or both. Bilateral lung and pulmonary veins involvement are seen in most of our patients. In the present study, pleural effusion was detected in 86% of our cases on plain chest X-ray films but in only 70% on CT scans. The discrepancy may be due to the timing of the CT scan, which was usually performed before the PVOS attack. Echocardiography found left atrium enlargement (thought to be due to stenosis of the pulmonary vein distal to the left atrium) in approximately 48% of our cases. In cancer patients, it is important to recognize that early appearance on chest X-ray of abnormal pulmonary shadows can result in a misdiagnosis of lung infection and acute respiratory distress syndrome.

The principle of treatment is based on procoagulant mechanisms. LMWH is used to improve the hemostatic condition [34]. Cytokine and NFκB inhibitors, such as dexamethasone, are used to suppress cytokine formation in acute

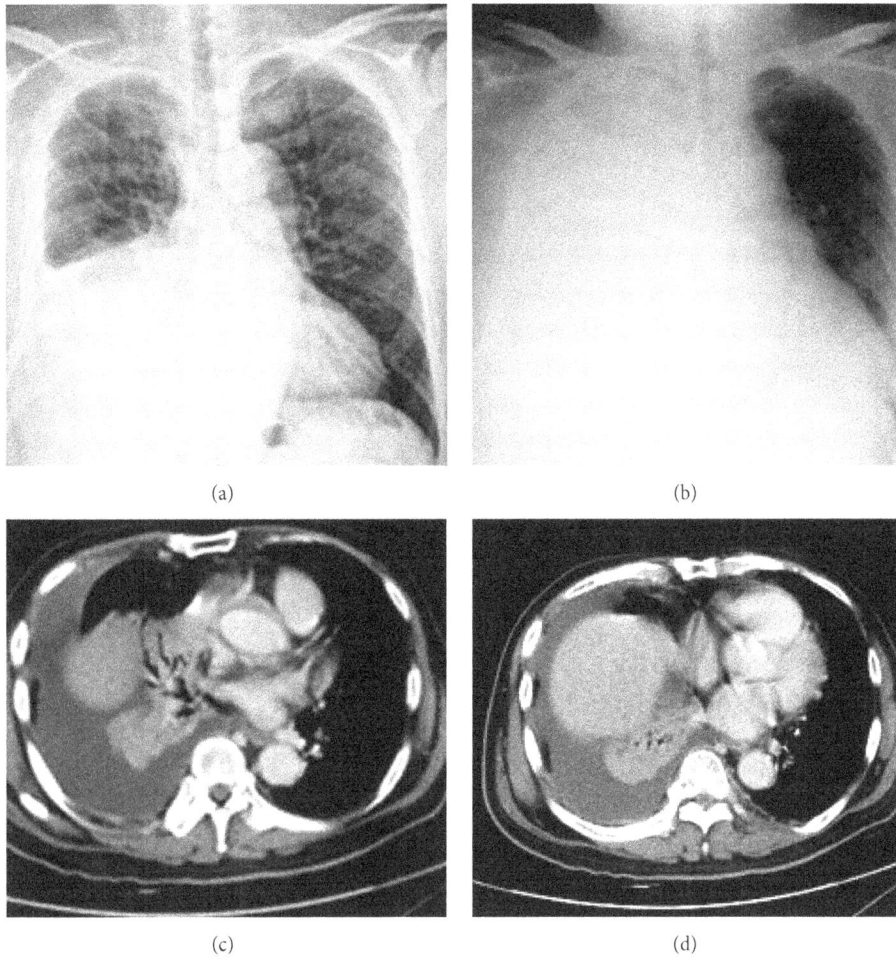

FIGURE 4: Pulmonary vein obstructive syndrome (PVOS). A 61-year-old man with lung cancer. Chest X-ray (a) before and (b) at the onset of PVOS showed right low lung increase haziness to total opacity. CT scan ((c) and (d)) revealed lung tumor and atelectatic lesions surrounding the superior and inferior pulmonary veins with right pleural effusion.

stage [35]. Stress related to cytokines can influence the course of neoplastic diseases [36]. Preventing unnecessary procedures and calming the patients can reduce cytokine overproduction. Knowing aggravated factors can cause PVOS. When an infection occurs, antibiotics is given immediately. Adequate fluids supplement is necessary for maintaining good perfusion of vital organ (brain, coronary artery, and kidney) [6, 7, 37, 38]. The importance of cancer-associated hyper-coagulation is an etiology of acute ischemic stroke [6, 7] and probably a leading death in our patients. Renal insufficiency had been linked to increased mortality from the literature [38] and prerenal azotemia pattern in our 16% patients. Furosemide for preload reduction can provide immediate symptom relief when acute respiratory distress with pulmonary edema occurs. Blood gas analysis can help the assessment of disease condition. Maintenance of LMWH is suggested for secondary prevention [39, 40] and probably a survival benefit [41–43]. Underlying disease therapy can be treated if feasible. Clinical/image improved in 66% of our patients after LMWH with or without combination with dexamethasone. Disease control was achieved in 68% of these

patients after further anticancer therapy. The survival rate for those with clinical/image improvement was superior to those without clinical/image improvement.

The outcome of PVOS was dismal (median survival time, 6 weeks). The cause of death was either respiratory failure or consciousness disturbance and related to thromboembolic complications. Two-thirds patients died of septicemia and/or febrile neutropenia. In the pathogenesis of sepsis, inflammation and coagulation play a pivotal literature [19]. Sepsis increases cytokine production and is considered to be an aggravating factor of thromboembolic complications.

Our study has several important limitations. First, the data was collected from prospective case cohort study in a single center mainly from a single physician. Secondary, image study included chest plain film and CT scan was probably not done simultaneously. Third, pulmonary vein thrombosis, tumor, or mixed type was difficult judge from CT scan. Fourth, consciousness/mental change related to thromboembolic complication seldom proven by image study. Fifth, the absence of tissue confirmation was either by biopsy or autopsy. Sixth, no cytokine study was demonstrated.

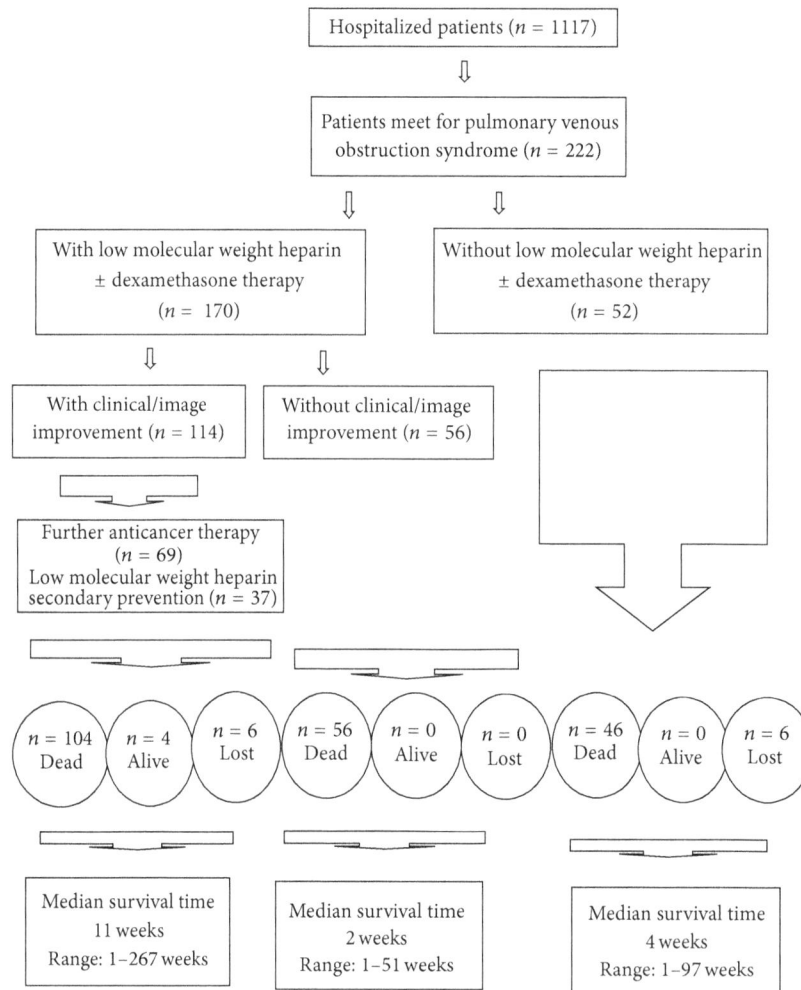

FIGURE 5: Flowchart of 222 cancer patients with pulmonary vein obstruction syndrome (PVOS).

5. Conclusion

PVOS is a common but neglected thromboembolic complication. Physicians should be alert to PVOS when shortness of breath occurs and chest X-ray reveals abnormal pulmonary hilum shadows. Medical/surgical procedures, therapy, and infection can aggravate PVOS. Symptoms can be relieved by the administration of LMWH, dexamethasone, prevent unnecessary procedures, calm the patients, adequate fluids, furosemide given when there is acute respiratory distress, and antibiotics given immediately when there is an infection.

Conflict of Interests

The authors declare that they have no conflict of interests regarding the publication of this paper.

Acknowledgment

The authors thank our oncology nurse staff for providing the best supportive care to these patients.

References

[1] R. W. Dudek and T. M. Louis, *High-Yield Gross Anatomy*, Lippincott Williams & Wilkins, London, UK, 5th edition, 2014.

[2] M. Takahashi, Y. Murakami, N. Nitta et al., "Pulmonary infarction associated with bronchogenic carcinoma," *Radiation Medicine*, vol. 26, no. 2, pp. 76–80, 2008.

[3] I. B. Wilson and W. I. Onuigbo, "Direct extension of cancer between pulmonary veins and the left atrium," *Chest*, vol. 62, no. 4, pp. 4044–4046, 1972.

[4] J. M. Stinson and R. A. Goodwin Jr., "Pulmonary vein obstruction by bronchogenic carcinoma," *Southern Medical Journal*, vol. 69, no. 1, pp. 1482–1483, 1976.

[5] N. B. N. Ibrahim, H. Burnley, K. A. Gaber et al., "Segmental pulmonary veno-occlusive disease secondary to lung cancer," *Journal of Clinical Pathology*, vol. 58, no. 4, pp. 434–436, 2005.

[6] C. J. Schwarzbach, A. Schaefer, A. Ebert et al., "Stroke and cancer: the importance of cancer-associated hypercoagulation as a possible stroke etiology," *Stroke*, vol. 43, no. 11, pp. 3029–3034, 2012.

[7] F. J. Álvarez-Pérez, I. Verde, M. Usón-Martín, A. Figuerola-Roig, J. Ballabriga-Planas, and A. Espino-Ibañez, "Frequency

and mechanism of ischemic stroke associated with malignancy: a retrospective series," *European Neurology*, vol. 68, no. 4, pp. 209–213, 2012.

[8] C. I. Ripamonti, D. Santini, E. Maranzano, M. Berti, and F. Roila, "Management of cancer pain: ESMO clinical practice guidelines," *Annals of Oncology*, vol. 23, supplement 7, pp. vii139–vii154, 2012.

[9] J. C. Chang and H. M. Gross, "Neoplastic fever responds to the treatment of an adequate dose of naproxen," *Journal of Clinical Oncology*, vol. 3, no. 4, pp. 552–558, 1985.

[10] K. C. Fearon, A. C. Voss, and D. S. Hustead, "Definition of cancer cachexia: effect of weight loss, reduced food intake, and systemic inflammation on functional status and prognosis," *The American Journal of Clinical Nutrition*, vol. 83, no. 6, pp. 1345–1350, 2006.

[11] M. B. Donati, "Thrombosis and cancer: trousseau syndrome revisited," *Best Practice & Research: Clinical Haematology*, vol. 22, no. 1, pp. 3–8, 2009.

[12] G. H. Sack Jr., J. Levin, and W. R. Bell, "Trousseau's syndrome and other manifestations of chronic disseminated coagulopathy in patients with neoplasms: clinical, pathophysiologic, and therapeutic features," *Medicine*, vol. 56, no. 1, pp. 1–37, 1977.

[13] A. Varki, "Trousseau's syndrome: multiple definitions and multiple mechanisms," *Blood*, vol. 110, no. 6, pp. 1723–1729, 2007.

[14] C. N. Bagot and R. Arya, "Virchow and his triad: a question of attribution," *British Journal of Haematology*, vol. 143, no. 2, pp. 180–190, 2008.

[15] A. S. Wolberg, M. M. Aleman, K. Leiderman, and K. R. Machlus, "Procoagulant activity in hemostasis and thrombosis: virchow's triad revisited," *Anesthesia and Analgesia*, vol. 114, no. 2, pp. 275–285, 2012.

[16] A. Falanga, M. Marchetti, and A. Vignoli, "Coagulation and cancer: biological and clinical aspects," *Journal of Thrombosis and Haemostasis*, vol. 11, no. 2, pp. 223–233, 2013.

[17] E. A. Beleva and J. Grudeva-Popova, "From Virchow's triad to metastasis: circulating hemostatic factors as predictors of risk for metastasis in solid tumors," *Journal of Balkan Union of Oncology*, vol. 18, no. 1, pp. 25–33, 2013.

[18] S. Margetic, "Inflammation and haemostasis," *Biochemia Medica*, vol. 22, no. 1, pp. 49–62, 2012.

[19] M. Levi and T. van der Poll, "Inflammation and coagulation," *Critical Care Medicine*, vol. 38, no. 62, pp. S26–S34, 2010.

[20] H. C. Kwaan and B. McMahon, "The role of plasminogen-plasmin system in cancer," *Cancer Treatment and Research*, vol. 148, pp. 43–66, 2009.

[21] G. H. Lyman, L. Eckert, Y. Wang, H. Wang, and A. Cohen, "Venous thromboembolism risk in patients with cancer receiving chemotherapy: a real-world analysis," *The Oncologist*, vol. 18, no. 12, pp. 1321–1329, 2013.

[22] G. H. Lyman, "Thromboprophylaxis with low-molecular-weight heparin in medical patients with cancer," *Cancer*, vol. 115, no. 24, pp. 5637–5650, 2009.

[23] A. H. Miller, S. Ancoli-Israel, J. E. Bower, L. Capuron, and M. R. Irwin, "Neuroendocrine-immune mechanisms of behavioral comorbidities in patients with cancer," *Journal of Clinical Oncology*, vol. 26, no. 6, pp. 971–982, 2008.

[24] B. Zubelewicz-Szkodzinska, M. Muc-Wierzgon, J. Wierzgon, and A. Brodziak, "Dynamics of circardian fluctuations in serum concentration of cortisol and TNF-α soluble receptors in gastrointestinal cancer patients," *Oncology Reports*, vol. 8, no. 1, pp. 207–212, 2001.

[25] F. Parent, S. Maître, G. Meyer et al., "Diagnostic value of D-dimer in patients with suspected pulmonary embolism: results from a multicentre outcome study," *Thrombosis Research*, vol. 120, no. 2, pp. 195–200, 2007.

[26] K. L. Dunn, J. P. Wolf, D. M. Dorfman, P. Fitzpatrick, J. L. Baker, and S. Z. Goldhaber, "Normal D-dimer levels in emergency department patients suspected of acute pulmonary embolism," *Journal of the American College of Cardiology*, vol. 40, no. 8, pp. 1475–1478, 2002.

[27] R. Kanz, T. Vukovich, R. Vormittag et al., "Thrombosis risk and survival in cancer patients with elevated C-reactive protein," *Journal of Thrombosis and Haemostasis*, vol. 9, no. 1, pp. 57–63, 2011.

[28] M. Sakuma, S. Fukui, M. Nakamura et al., "Cancer and pulmonary embolism—thrombotic embolism, tumor embolism, and tumor invasion into a large vein," *Circulation Journal*, vol. 70, no. 6, pp. 744–749, 2006.

[29] S. Mehrishi, A. Awan, A. Mehrishi, and A. Fein, "Pulmonary tumor microembolism," *Hospital Physicians*, vol. 40, no. 6, pp. 23–30, 2004.

[30] K. E. Roberts, D. Hamele-Bena, A. Saqi, C. A. Stein, and R. P. Cole, "Pulmonary tumor embolism: a review of the literature," *The American Journal of Medicine*, vol. 115, no. 3, pp. 228–232, 2003.

[31] M.-T. Lin, S.-C. Ku, M.-Z. Wu, and C.-J. Yu, "Intracardiac extension of lung cancer via the pulmonary vein," *Thorax*, vol. 63, no. 12, article 1122, 2008.

[32] W. R. Webb, "The pulmonary hila," in *Thoracic Imaging: Pulmonary and Cardiovascular Radiology*, pp. 148–174, Lippincott Williams & Wilkins, Philadelphia, Pa, USA, 1st edition, 2004.

[33] D. H. Choe, J. H. Lee, B. H. Lee et al., "Obliteration of the pulmonary vein in lung cancer: significance in assessing local extent with CT," *Journal of Computer Assisted Tomography*, vol. 22, no. 4, pp. 587–591, 1998.

[34] A. Y. Y. Lee, "Treatment of venous thromboembolism in cancer patients," *Best Practice & Research: Clinical Haematology*, vol. 22, no. 1, pp. 93–101, 2009.

[35] Y. Yamamoto and R. B. Gaynor, "Therapeutic potential of inhibition of the NF-κB pathway in the treatment of inflammation and cancer," *Journal of Clinical Investigation*, vol. 107, no. 2, pp. 135–142, 2001.

[36] I. J. Elenkov and G. P. Chrousos, "Stress, cytokine patterns and susceptibility to disease," *Baillière's Best Practice & Research in Clinical Endocrinology & Metabolism*, vol. 13, no. 4, pp. 583–595, 1999.

[37] A. A. Khorana, C. W. Francis, E. Culakova, N. M. Kuderer, and G. H. Lyman, "Thromboembolism is a leading cause of death in cancer patients receiving outpatient chemotherapy," *Journal of Thrombosis and Haemostasis*, vol. 5, no. 3, pp. 632–634, 2007.

[38] F. Scotté, J. B. Rey, and V. Launay-Vacher, "Thrombosis, cancer and renal insufficiency: low molecular weight heparin at the crossroads," *Supportive Care in Cancer*, vol. 20, no. 12, pp. 3033–3042, 2012.

[39] R. L. Bick, "Cancer-associated thrombosis: focus on extended therapy with dalteparin," *Journal of Supportive Oncology*, vol. 4, no. 3, pp. 115–120, 2006.

[40] M. Carrier and A. Y. Y. Lee, "Thromboprophylaxis in cancer patients," *Seminars in Thrombosis and Hemostasis*, vol. 40, no. 3, pp. 395–400, 2014.

[41] A. K. Kakkar, M. N. Levine, Z. Kadziola et al., "Low molecular weight heparin, therapy with dalteparin, and survival in

advanced cancer: the fragmin advanced malignancy outcome study (FAMOUS)," *Journal of Clinical Oncology*, vol. 22, no. 10, pp. 1944–1948, 2004.

[42] A. Falanga, A. Vignoli, E. Diani, and M. Marchetti, "Comparative assessment of low-molecular-weight heparins in cancer from the perspective of patient outcomes and survival," *Patient Related Outcome Measures*, vol. 2, pp. 175–188, 2011.

[43] D. H. Che, J. Y. Cao, L. H. Shang, Y. C. Man, and Y. Yu, "The efficacy and safety of low-molecular-weight heparin use for cancer treatment: a meta-analysis," *The European Journal of Internal Medicine*, vol. 24, no. 5, pp. 433–439, 2013.

6

Stereotactic Radiosurgery for Renal Cancer Brain Metastasis: Prognostic Factors and the Role of Whole-Brain Radiation and Surgical Resection

Franziska M. Ippen,[1] **Anand Mahadevan,**[2] **Eric T. Wong,**[3] **Erik J. Uhlmann,**[3]
Soma Sengupta,[3] **and Ekkehard M. Kasper**[1]

[1]*Department of Neurosurgery, Beth Israel Deaconess Medical Center, Harvard Medical School, Boston, MA 02445, USA*
[2]*Department of Radiation Oncology, Beth Israel Deaconess Medical Center, Harvard Medical School, Boston, MA 02445, USA*
[3]*Department of Neuro-Oncology, Beth Israel Deaconess Medical Center, Harvard Medical School, Boston, MA 02445, USA*

Correspondence should be addressed to Anand Mahadevan; amahadev@bidmc.harvard.edu

Academic Editor: Akira Hara

Background. Renal cell carcinoma is a frequent source of brain metastasis. We present our consecutive series of patients treated with Stereotactic Radiosurgery (SRS) and analyse prognostic factors and the interplay of WBRT and surgical resection. *Methods.* This is a retrospective study of 66 patients with 207 lesions treated with the Cyberknife radiosurgery system in our institution. The patients were followed up with imaging and clinical examination 1 month and 2-3 months thereafter for the brain metastasis. Patient, treatment, and outcomes characteristics were analysed. *Results.* 51 male (77.3%) and 15 female (22.7%) patients, with a mean age of 58.9 years (range of 31–85 years) and a median Karnofsky Performance Status (KPS) of 90 (range of 60–100), were included in the study. The overall survival was 13.9 months, 21.9 months, and 5.9 months for the patients treated with SRS only, additional surgery, and WBRT, respectively. The actuarial 1-year Local Control rates were 84%, 94%, and 88% for SRS only, for surgery and SRS, and for WBRT and additional SRS, respectively. *Conclusions.* Stereotactic radiosurgery is a safe and effective treatment option in patients with brain metastases from RCC. In case of a limited number of brain metastases, surgery and SRS might be appropriate.

1. Background

Renal cell carcinoma (RCC) accounts for about 2% of all cancer cases worldwide and represents the sixth leading cause of all cancer deaths [1, 2]. One-third of patients present at advanced stages of disease, and up to 40% of patients who underwent local surgical resection will have disease recurrence [3, 4].

Despite its relatively low incidence, RCC presents itself as one of the most common sources of brain metastases along with lung and breast cancer, melanoma, and colorectal carcinoma [5]. Approximately 1,200 to 1,500 cases of brain metastases from RCC are diagnosed annually [6], and 4% to 17% of all patients with RCC will develop brain metastases during their clinical course of disease [7].

The median survival of patients with untreated brain metastases from primary RCC is reported to be approximately 1 to 2 months [7], whereas the median survival time after radiotherapy and corticosteroid treatment for patients with this type of malignancy was reported to be 2 to 8 months [8]. Since surgical resection is not always possible, WBRT has played an important role in the treatment of patients with RCC brain metastasis but has yielded unsatisfactory results in terms of overall survival and local tumor control in these patients due to the relative radioresistant nature of RCC to conventional radiation therapy [9]. Due to the potential neurotoxic effects of WBRT as well as the radioresistant features of this primary, WBRT may not be the treatment of choice in these patients, particularly with oligometastatic disease [10].

Stereotactic radiosurgery (SRS) is a minimally invasive radiation technique that delivers a highly conformal, high dose of radiation to a prescribed target volume [11, 12]. This procedure can be completed in one up to five treatment sessions and offers the possibility to treat multiple tumor sites during one treatment session [12]. Stereotactic radiosurgery is increasingly used for the treatment of brain metastases with or without prior microsurgical resection [13, 14], as tumors traditionally considered to be radioresistant such as renal cell carcinoma have shown favorable response rates in various studies [7, 15–20]. However, the optimal treatment of these patients still remains controversial.

In this study, our aim was to analyze the outcomes after SRS for the treatment of brain metastases from RCC. Furthermore, we examined potential prognostic factors that correlate with improved survival and local tumor control in these patients.

2. Methods

2.1. Study Design.
This is a retrospective evaluation of all patients treated with SRS for brain metastases from primary RCC at our institution. Patients' medical records were reviewed to obtain patient, tumor, and treatment characteristics and follow-up data. Neuroimaging studies for each individually treated lesion were reviewed prior to radiosurgical treatment and at regular intervals (1, 3, 6, 9, 12, and 24 months) after completion of SRS. Data were collected by personnel not directly involved in either direct patient care or any related treatment decision-making process. The design and analysis of this study were approved by the Institutional Review Board (IRB) of Dana Farber/Harvard Cancer Center (DF/HCC) (IRB#09-451).

2.2. Patient Selection.
The study cohort consists of 76 patients with RCC brain metastases treated with SRS at BIDMC between August 2005 and December 2013. For 10 (13.2%) patients, no follow-up was available because they transferred their care to other facilities. These patients were excluded from any further analysis. Evaluation of overall survival, local and distant brain tumor control were performed for the remaining 66 patients with a total of 207 lesions, for which all follow-up data sets were available and analysis was completed.

In 65/66 patients (98.5%), brain metastases from RCC were diagnosed by magnetic resonance imaging (MRI). In one patient (1.5%), the diagnosis was based on computed tomography (CT) alone, since the patient harbored a contraindication to undergo MRI scanning. Each patient's performance status was assessed at each visit using the Karnofsky Performance Status (KPS) and was further classified by prognosticators for assessment of their outcomes.

2.3. SRS Planning and Treatment.
All patients were treated in the Cyberknife (Accuray Inc., Sunnyvale, California) robotic frameless stereotactic radiosurgery system. Diagnostic thin slice (1 mm) gadolinium enhanced axial MRI images were fused with CT scan obtained in an immobilization mask at planning. Image fusion and nonisocentric treatment planning were performed with the multiplan treatment planning software.

2.4. Follow-Up.
Patients were followed up from the time of SRS with clinical examination and neuroimaging with contrast enhanced MRI 1 month after treatment and every 2-3 months thereafter until the last follow-up appointment or until the date of death.

2.5. Outcome Measures.
Overall survival, local control, distant brain control, local progression-free survival, and distant brain progression-free survival were assessed after SRS. Overall survival was calculated as the time in months from SRS until the date of death. In case of censored data, the patients' last date of clinical follow-up visit was used to determine overall survival.

A determination of the cause of death was attempted for all patients who died during the observation period. Patients were considered to have died due to neurologic causes if they had either absent or stable systemic disease and progressive neurologic dysfunction. If patients had developed fatal organ failure, infection, or hemorrhage, in the setting of a stable neurological examination at the last clinic visit, they were considered to have died from progression of systemic disease or intercurrent disease (e.g., pulmonary embolus) and not due to neurological causes.

Treatment response was evaluated according to the updated Response Evaluation Criteria in Solid Tumors (RECIST). Local control (LC) was defined as no further tumor growth after treatment, subdivided into complete response (CR), partial response (PR), or stable disease (SD) on follow-up CT and/or MRI scans. In lesions which underwent resection prior to SRS, LC was defined as the absence of new nodular contrast enhancement adjacent to the resection cavity on MRI. Local failure (LF) was defined as tumor recurrence at the site of the targeted lesion and was further classified as progressive disease (PD). Distant brain control (DC) was defined as the absence of new intracranial lesions after treatment, whereas distant brain failure (DF) was defined by the appearance of new brain metastases or leptomeningeal disease outside the lesions previously treated with SRS. Actuarial local progression-free survival (LPFS) and distant brain progression-free survival (DPFS) were calculated in months from the date of SRS to the date of CT/MR-imaging showing local or distant brain failure. Otherwise, patients were censored at the time of their last MRI scan. For patients receiving WBRT for salvage, control rates were censored at the time of WBRT.

2.6. Statistical Analysis.
Descriptive statistics were obtained for a variety of patient and treatment characteristics in this study. Actuarial OS, LC, and DF rates were calculated using the Kaplan-Meier method. Univariate analysis was performed using the log-rank test for categorical data. Multivariate analysis was performed using Cox proportional hazards regression for continuous variables and in order to identify prognostic factors for OS and LPFS. For both

univariate and multivariate analyses, statistical significance was defined as a level of $\alpha = 0.05$ value.

Kaplan-Meier curves for OS, LPFS, and DPFS and univariate analysis were conducted using Graph Pad Prism version 6.00 software for Mac (Graph Pad Software, San Diego, CA; Windows; Microsoft, Seattle, WA). Descriptive statistics and multivariate analyses were performed using the STATA 13 software package (STATA Corp., College Station, TX, USA).

3. Results

In a total of 66 patients with 207 brain metastases, the median follow-up after SRS was 10 months (mean, 15.8 months; range, 6–84 months).

3.1. Patient Characteristics. Of the analyzed 66 patients, 51 were male (77.3%) and 15 were female (22.7%). The patients ranged in age from 31 to 85 years (mean age of 58.9 years) at the time of their initial brain metastasis diagnosis. The median Karnofsky Performance Status (KPS) was 90 (range of 60–100). Thirty-nine patients (59.1%) presented with a single brain metastasis; 27 patients (40.9%) had two or more brain metastases at time of diagnosis. At the time of SRS treatments, 56 patients (84.8%) were found to have uncontrolled systemic disease and 10 patients (15.2%) were found to have controlled systemic disease. According to the Recursive Partitioning Analysis (RPA) by the Radiation Therapy Oncology Group (RTOG), 3 patients (4.5%) were classified as RPA class I, 59 patients (89.4%) as RPA class II, and 4 patients (6.1%) as RPA class III. Patients were also classified into subgroups according to the Score Index for Radiosurgery (SIR) and the Basic Score for Brain Metastases (BSBM) to allow a prognostic determination of patients with brain metastasis who underwent SRS and to make this data set comparable to other available literature. According to the SIR, 35 patients (53%) were found to have a score less than 6, and 31 patients (47%) were found to have a score equal to and more than 6. According to the BSBM, 12 patients (18.2%) had a score of 0, whereas 44 patients (66.7%) had a score of 1 and 8 patients (12.1%) were found to have a score of 2. Two patients (3%) had a score of 3. According to the Disease-Specific Graded Prognostic Assessment (Ds-GPA), 27 patients (40.9%) were classified as Ds-GPA 4, 18 (27.3%) as Ds-GPA 3, 14 (21.2%) as Ds-GPA 2, 6 (9.1%) as Ds-GPA 1, and 1 (1.5%) as Ds-GPA 0.

In 51 patients (77.3%), the histologic subtype was defined as clear cell carcinoma, but also two cases of papillary RCC (4.5%) and one case of chromophobe RCC (1.5%) were observed. In 12 patients (18.2%) with brain metastases from RCC, the histologic subtype remained unclassified.

At the time of diagnosis of the first brain metastasis, 63 patients (95.5%) also had extra cranial metastases. Patient and disease characteristics are shown in Table 1.

3.2. Treatment Characteristics. Stereotactic radiosurgery with the Cyberknife (Accuray, Sunnyvale, CA) technique was used to treat all patients in this cohort with brain metastases from RCC. A total of 207 lesions were treated in

179 separate sessions via a total of 132 treatment plans. An average of 1.2 lesions was irradiated in each treatment session and an average of 1.6 lesions was irradiated in each treatment plan (range, 1–6).

The median prescription dose was 22 Gy, the median conformality index was 1.3 (range of 1.03–6.96), and the median homogeneity index was 1.32 (range, 1.12–1.72). The median prescribed isodose line was 76% (range of 58–89%) and the median coverage of each individual lesion was 96.39% (range, 84.2%–100%). All patients received prophylactic corticosteroids (dexamethasone) and anticonvulsants (levetiracetam) during and after the SRS treatment.

56 patients (84.8%) received additional systemic therapy during their course of disease. Of those, 25 patients (44.6%) received standard systemic therapy (e.g., high dose IL2; sunitinib and pazopanib), 5 patients (9%) were treated with IRB-approved experimental study therapy regimens (e.g. bevacizumab + interferon α; bevacizumab versus erlotinib; and pazopanib versus sunitinib, or tivozanib), and 26 patients (46.4%) were treated with a combination of both. 10 patients (15.2%) had received no systemic therapy at all at the time of SRS treatment.

As an initial treatment, 24 patients (36.4%) underwent surgical resection before SRS, 36 patients (54.5%) were treated with SRS only, and 6 patients (9.1%) had received prior WBRT (median dose, 30 Gy; range, 20–30 Gy). Six patients (9.1%) were treated with WBRT for salvage after SRS and 2 patients (3%) had resection due to progression after treatment with SRS. In patients initially treated with surgical resection prior to SRS, gross total resection could be achieved in 22 patients (91.7%). Treatment characteristics are shown in Table 2.

3.3. Overall Survival. At the time of analysis (6 months after the last SRS treatment), 48 patients were dead (72.7%) and 18 were alive (27.3%). Most of the deceased patients (24; 50%) died from documented progression of systemic disease (nonneurological death), whereas in 21 patients (43.75%), the specific cause of death was unknown in the setting of a stable neurological examination at last visit and 3 patients (6.25%) died from progression of intracranial disease (neurological death). The median overall survival was 72.2 months (95% CI 45.2–95.5 months) from the diagnosis of the primary tumor, 17.5 months (95% CI 11.5–22.5 months) from the diagnosis of the first brain metastasis, and 13.9 months (95% CI 9.7–21.3 months) from the time of SRS for the analyzed study population. Actuarial survival rates for the analyzed patient cohort calculated from the time of SRS were 98.5% ($n = 65$) at 1 month, 87.4% ($n = 55$) at 3 months, 77.8% ($n = 49$) at 6 months, 68% ($n = 41$) at 9 months, 54.8% ($n = 33$) at 12 months, and 34.1% ($n = 18$) at 24 months (Figure 1). The median overall survival from the time of SRS for the 39 patients with a single brain metastasis was 20.3 months (95% CI 13.6–29.2 months) compared to 5.4 months (95% CI 1.3–10.2 months) in 8 patients with multiple (>3) brain metastases ($p = 0.0022$) (Figure 2). No statistically significant difference in median overall survival was found when comparing patients with a single brain metastasis to patients with two (11.2 months) or three brain metastases (9.7 months) at initial

TABLE 1: Patient and disease characteristics by treatment group.

Characteristics	SRS	Surgery + SRS	WBRT + SRS	p value
Number of patients	36	24	6	
Age (years)				
Median age	60.5	58	59	
Mean age	58.6	58.1	62.8	0.5622
Range	31–79	40–85	54–81	
Sex				
Male	37 (75%)	19 (79.2%)	1 (16.7%)	0.909
Female	9 (25%)	5 (20.8%)	5 (83.3%)	
Systemic disease status at the time of SRS				
Controlled	3 (8.3%)	6 (25%)	1 (16.7%)	0.169
Uncontrolled	33 (91.7%)	18 (75%)	5 (83.3%)	
Intracranial disease status at the time of SRS				
Controlled	0 (0%)	12 (50%)	1 (16.7%)	<0.0001
Uncontrolled	36 (100%)	12 (50%)	5 (83.3%)	
RPA				
I	0 (0%)	3 (12.5%)	0 (0%)	
II	34 (94.4%)	20 (83.3%)	5 (83.3%)	0.1379
III	2 (5.6%)	1 (4.2%)	1 (16.7%)	
KPS				
≥70	34 (94.4%)	23 (95.8%)	5 (83.3%)	0.521
<70	2 (5.6%)	1 (4.2%)	1 (16.7%)	
SIR				
≥6	20 (55.6%)	11 (45.8%)	0 (0%)	0.041
<6	16 (44.4%)	13 (54.2%)	6 (100%)	
Ds-GPA				
4	18 (50%)	9 (37.5%)	0 (0%)	
3	8 (22.2%)	9 (37.5%)	1 (16.7%)	
2	8 (22.2%)	4 (16.7%)	2 (33.3%)	0.0073
1	2 (5.6%)	2 (8.3%)	2 (33.3%)	
0	0 (0%)	0 (0%)	1 (16.7%)	
BSBM				
3	0 (0%)	2 (8.3%)	0 (0%)	
2	3 (8.3%)	4 (16.7%)	1 (16.7%)	0.6526
1	28 (77.8%)	13 (64.2%)	3 (50%)	
0	5 (13.9%)	5 (20.8%)	2 (33.3%)	
Number of brain metastases				
≤3	33 (91.7%)	23 (95.8%)	2 (33.3%)	0.002
>3	3 (8.7%)	1 (4.2%)	4 (66.7%)	
Initial tumor volume (cm^3)				
Median initial tumor volume	1.151	11.746	1.945	
Mean initial tumor volume	3.3770	11.411	9.295	0.0001
Range	0.241–27.73	2.178–26.51	0.192–33.57	

Fisher and Kruskal-Wallis test.

presentation ($p = 0.1853$). The median OS was significantly different for the three different RPA classes ($p = 0.0001$). In patients stratified into RPA class I, median OS was not reached because all 3 patients were still alive at the time of analysis. Patients in RPA class II and III only had a median survival of 14.1 months and 4.1 months respectively (Figure 3).

Stratifying the patients cohort by their initial treatment modality (surgery prior to SRS, SRS, and WBRT prior to SRS) resulted in a median survival for patients initially treated with SRS only ($n = 36$) of 13.6 months (95% CI 6.9–23.5 months) and a median survival of 21.9 months (95% CI 10.5–70.4 months) for patients who underwent surgical resection

TABLE 2: Treatment characteristics.

Characteristics	n (%)
Stereotactic radiosurgery	
Median tumor volume (cm^3)	0.688
Range tumor volume (cm^3)	0.056–33.57
Median number of beams	202
Median number of monitor units	14741.26
Median dose per fraction (Gy)	22
Range dose per fraction (Gy)	5–22
Median total dose (Gy)	22
Range total dose (Gy)	12–30
Median number of fractions	1
Range number of fractions	1–5
Median coverage (%)	96.39
Median isodose line (%)	76
Range isodose line (%)	58–89
Median conformality index	1.3
Median homogeneity index	1.32
Median minimum dose (Gy)	2037.18
Median maximum dose (Gy)	2822.02
Surgical resection	
N (patients)	24
Gross total resection	22 (91.7)
Subtotal resection	2 (8.3)
Whole-brain radiation therapy (WBRT)	
N total	12 (18.2)
N WBRT prior to SRS	6 (9.1)
N WBRT after SRS	6 (9.1)
Median total dose (Gy)	30
Dose range (Gy)	20–37.5
Median dose for WBRT prior to SRS (Gy)	30
Dose range for WBRT prior to SRS (Gy)	20–30
Systemic therapy	
N (patients)	56 (84.8)
Standard	25 (44.6)
Experimental	5 (9)
Both	26 (46.4)

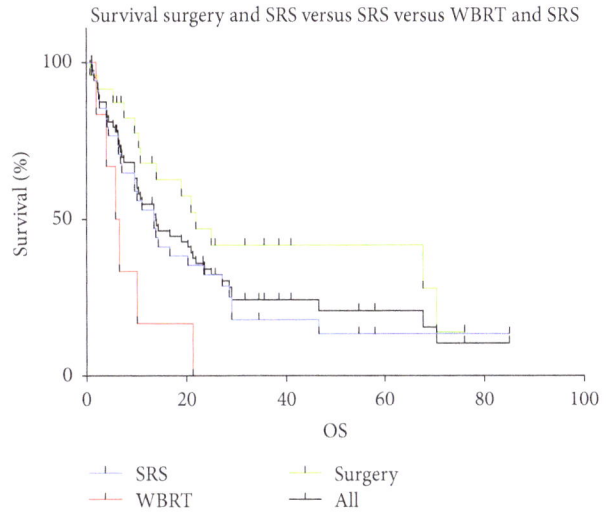

FIGURE 1: Overall survival by treatment modality.

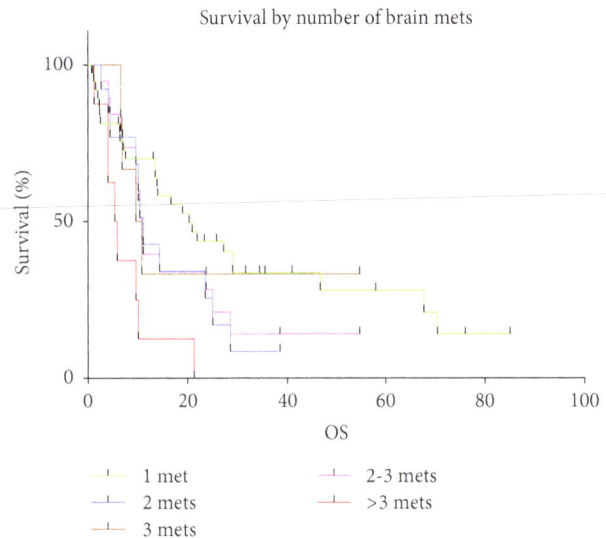

FIGURE 2: Overall survival by number of brain metastases.

(n = 24) as an initial treatment. Patients who underwent WBRT (n = 6) before treatment with SRS had a median survival of 5.9 months after SRS (Figure 1). The actuarial one-year overall survival rates for patients treated with those different approaches were 55.9% for patients who underwent SRS as a sole treatment, 67.8% for patients who underwent surgical resection prior to SRS, and 16.7% for patients treated with WBRT prior to SRS (p = 0.011). No significant difference in overall survival was detected between patients treated with SRS only and patients treated with surgery + SRS (p = 0.1141).

In univariate analysis of the entire cohort age (p = 0.0000), prior surgery (p = 0.0486), RPA class (p = 0.0000), KPS ($\geq$70 versus <70, p = 0.0000), SIR ($\geq$6 versus <6, p = 0.0093), BSBM (p = 0.0027), number of brain metastases (>3 versus $\leq$3, p = 0.0009), initial tumor volume (p = 0.0000),

and Ds-GPA (p = 0.0002) were associated with significantly better overall survival. Prior WBRT (p = 0.0097) was found to be significantly associated with poor overall survival.

Sex, systemic and intracranial disease status at the time of SRS, and whether the patients had received systemic treatment during their course of systemic disease were not found to be significantly associated with a difference in overall survival.

In multivariate Cox analysis, factors associated with a significantly better overall survival were age (p = 0.038), RPA class (p = 0.000), KPS ($\geq$70 versus <70, p = 0.000), and the initial number of brain metastases (>3 versus $\leq$3, p = 0.002). Again, prior WBRT was significantly associated with poorer overall survival (p = 0.014). Prior surgery (p = 0.053) was only found to be borderline significant in multivariate Cox regression.

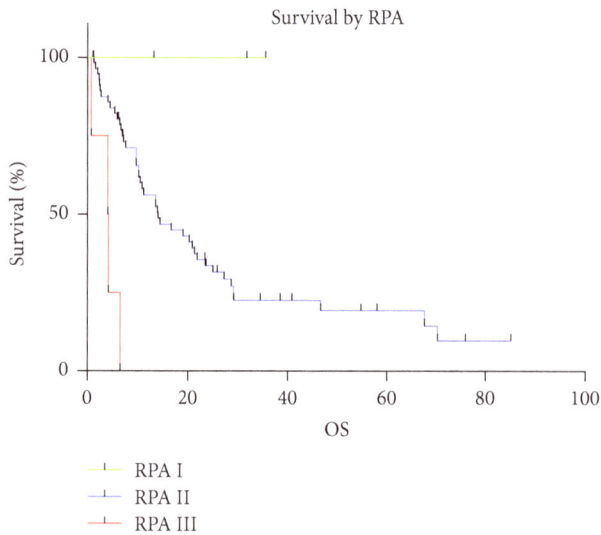

FIGURE 3: Overall survival by RPA (Recursive Partitioning Analysis) class.

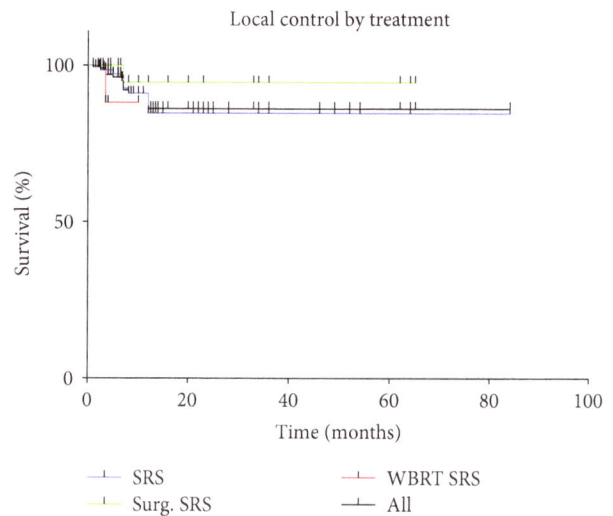

FIGURE 4: Local control by treatment modality.

Factors not found to be significantly associated with better overall survival were sex, systemic and intracranial disease status at the time of SRS, whether the patients had received systemic treatment during their course of systemic disease, and initial tumor volume (Table 3).

In univariate analysis of the two subgroups initially treated with SRS and surgical resection followed by SRS, age ($p = 0.0000$), RPA class ($p = 0.0001$), KPS ($\geq$70 versus <70, $p = 0.0001$), SIR ($\geq$6 versus <6, $p = 0.0385$), BSBM ($p = 0.0147$), Ds-GPA ($p = 0.0001$), initial tumor volume ($p = 0.0000$), and the initial number of brain metastases (>3 versus $\leq$3, $p = 0.0002$) were found to have a significant impact on overall survival. In multivariate Cox analysis of these two subgroups, again RPA class ($p = 0.000$), KPS ($\geq$70 versus <70, $p = 0.001$), SIR ($\geq$6 versus <6, $p = 0.043$), Ds-GPA ($p = 0.003$), BSBM ($p = 0.008$), and the initial number of brain metastases (>3 versus $\leq$3, $p = 0.001$) were found to be prognostic for better overall survival. In multivariate analysis, the initial tumor volume was not found to be a prognostic factor for overall survival.

3.4. Local Control. Over the course of the entire follow-up period, local control was achieved in 193 (93.2%) of 207 treated lesions. Of the 138 lesions treated with SRS only in a total of 51 patients, local failure was noted in 10 lesions (7.2%) of 8 patients (15.7%) during the entire follow-up period. In a total of 25 lesions treated with surgery and SRS as an adjunct in 24 patients, local failure was noted in 1 lesion (4%) in 1 patient (4.2%). Of the 44 lesions treated with WBRT prior to SRS in a total of 6 patients, local failure was observed in 3 lesions (6.8%) in 1 patient (16.7%). Actuarial 1-year local control rates for lesions treated with SRS as a sole treatment, surgical resection + SRS, and WBRT + SRS were 84%, 94%, and 88%, respectively (Figure 4).

In univariate analysis, no significant difference in local control was found between lesions treated with the three different approaches ($p = 0.445$). Furthermore, no statistically significant difference in local control could be detected comparing SRS with surgical resection + SRS ($p = 0.3422$), SRS with WBRT + SRS ($p = 0.445$), and WBRT+ SRS with surgical resection + SRS ($p = 0.333$).

Tumor volume was found to be the only significant variable in univariate log-rank analysis ($p = 0.0000$); however, in multivariate Cox analysis, neither tumor volume nor surgical resection or the number of brain metastases was found to be prognostic for local progression-free survival.

3.5. Distant Brain Progression-Free Survival. Distant brain failure was observed in 34 (51.5%) patients. The median time until distant brain failure was 7 months after SRS (95% CI 6–15 months). Actuarial freedom from distant brain failure was 90.9% at 1 month, 76.3% at 3 months, 48.9% at 6 months, 41.7% at 9 months, 35.2% at 12 months, and 23.8% at 24 months after SRS. The distant brain progression-free survival for all patients is shown in Figure 5. Median distant brain progression-free survival for patients who initially received SRS alone, surgery + SRS, and WBRT + SRS was 19, 7, and 3.5 months, respectively.

In univariate as well as in multivariate analysis, prior WBRT was significantly associated with better distant tumor control ($p = 0.007$ in univariate analysis and $p = 0.014$ in multivariate analysis).

3.6. Complications after Treatment. 14 (21.2%) patients developed some form of toxicity related to SRS. Of the 24 patients initially treated with surgical resection, 7 had side effects: among this group, 6 patients developed fatigue, one patient additionally experienced worsening of his left-sided weakness after SRS (1/24 acute grade 3 toxicity). Among 36 patients who received SRS only as an initial treatment, 7 patients had side effects. 5 patients developed fatigue, and among those, one patient had seizures due to expanding vasogenic edema after treatment. Of the remaining two patients, one patient experienced worsening edema causing mass effect

TABLE 3: Prognostic factors.

Variable	Log-rank	Multivariate Cox regression		
	p value	p value	Coefficient (Coeff.)	95% Confidence interval (CI)
Survival				
Age	0.0000	0.038	0.0338118	0.0018982–0.0657254
Prior surgery	0.0486	0.053	0.6203678	−1.24931–0.0085739
Prior WBRT	0.0097	0.014	1.104396	0.2219025–1.986891
RPA	0.0000	0.000	2.153972	1.108619–3.199326
KPS (≥70 versus <70)	0.0000	0.000	2.072708	0.9231157–3.222301
SIR (≥6 versus <6)	0.0093	0.011	2.155395	0.1726184–1.36333
BSBM	0.0027	0.003	−0.8503598	−1.402409–−0.2983109
Number of brain metastases (>3 versus ≤3)	0.0009	0.002	1.260513	0.462241–2.058785
Ds-GPA	0.0002	0.000	0.5929137	−0.7985645–−0.2468485
Initial tumor volume	0.0000	0.651	0.008675	−0.0289586–0.0463086
Local control				
Tumor volume	0.0000	0.668	−0.0242895	−0.1353437–0.0867646
Distant brain progression-free survival				
Prior WBRT	0.0072	0.014	1.252507	0.2539636–2.25105

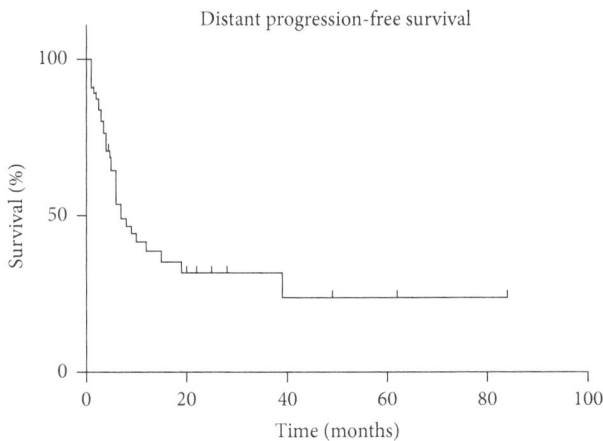

FIGURE 5: Distant brain progression-free survival.

and midline shift (2/24 Acute Grade 3 Toxicity); the other presented with symptomatic radiation necrosis causing left hemiplegia. In the group of patients who received upfront WBRT, one patient developed nausea after treatment with WBRT, before undergoing SRS. Overall, there were 4/66 (4.5%) acute grade ≥ 3 toxicity and 1/66 (1.5%) ≥ grade 3 long term toxicity. The mean volume in patients experiencing toxicity was 12.6 and the median dose was 20 Gy.

4. Discussion

Brain metastases from RCC are reported with a frequency of approximately 4 to 17% of patients during their course of disease [7]. As newer therapies for the management of RCC emerge and standard treatments are further refined, these patients will live longer and, as a consequence, are more likely to develop brain metastases during their course

of disease [21]. In addition, brain metastases from RCC are known for their high propensity of intratumoral hemorrhage and their extensive surrounding edema which is profound when compared to other metastatic brain lesions from other primaries [9]. Surgery may often not be feasible due to location of the lesion and studies on WBRT as a sole treatment in the treatment process of these patients have shown disappointing results regarding overall survival [22–27]. SRS is proving to be a useful modality in the treatment of brain metastasis from RCC.

In this retrospective cohort analysis, we evaluated the effectiveness, safety, and potential prognostic factors of SRS for the treatment of brain metastases from RCC on survival and local and distant tumor control at our institution.

4.1. Stereotactic Radiosurgery and Overall Survival. Stereotactic radiosurgery for brain metastases from RCC has been suggested to prolong overall survival when compared to patients treated with modalities such as WBRT only [15, 20, 28] with median survival rates of 5.1 to 17.8 months. In our study, the median survival of the entire cohort was 13.9 months. The groups treated with SRS only, surgical resection plus subsequent SRS, and WBRT plus SRS achieved a median overall survival of 13.6, 21.9, and 5.9 months, respectively. The results for survival among the three groups were found to be statistically significant. A significant difference in median overall survival was furthermore observed when stratifying the patients into the three different RPA classes. This result confirms findings from previously published series evaluating the role of SRS for patients with brain metastases from this primary [21, 29, 30]. The majority of patients in our series were graded into RPA class II due to the presence of active extracranial disease or advanced age.

4.2. Stereotactic Radiosurgery and Local Tumor Control. Multiple studies have reported the effectiveness of SRS for brain metastases from RCC have reported local control rates ranging from 60.9 to 100% (Table 4) [7, 8, 14–16, 18–21, 24, 28–42]. The majority of patients in these studies were treated with LINAC-based or Gamma Knife-based devices, but comparable data on treatment outcomes for these patients undergoing Cyberknife SRS is lacking. To date, our retrospective study is the largest study conducted so far to evaluate the outcome of patients and potential prognostic factors in the treatment of Cyberknife radiosurgery for brain metastases from RCC.

In our study, actuarial 1-year local control rates for lesions treated with the three different initial treatment approaches were 84% for patients treated with SRS as a sole treatment, 94% for patients who underwent surgical resection plus subsequent SRS, and 88% for patients initially treated with WBRT followed by SRS which is comparable to that in literature. Except for a single report [48], SRS as a sole treatment or in combination with WBRT has shown favorable results comparable to those of surgery plus subsequent WBRT in patients with a single brain metastasis in the current literature [49–51].

Several important factors such as tumor size, location, number of brain metastases, presence of symptomatic peritumoral edema, and mass effect have to be taken into consideration when it comes to the decision whether a patient should undergo surgical resection or SRS. In regard to the tumor size, the RTOG protocol 90-05 established SRS dose-volume prescription criteria, recommending a maximum dose of 24, 18, and 15 Gy in a single fraction for tumors ranging up to 2 cm, between 2 and 3 cm, and greater than 3 cm in diameter, respectively [6, 10]. Other reported optimal doses range from 15 up to 22 Gy, with a median dose of 20 Gy [6].

The treatment of patients with brain metastases from RCC has several advantages: stereotactic radiosurgery is a minimally invasive procedure, usually performed in the outpatient setting, with the potential to treat multiple lesions during one treatment session, and can be performed repeatedly in case of local or distant brain tumor recurrence [12, 52]. However, despite the noted improvements in local tumor control, some questions still remain to be investigated in the field of this treatment modality, such as an appropriate selection of patients for SRS versus surgery, the development of validated prognostic factors after treatment with SRS, and the role of adjuvant WBRT [10]. The role of adjuvant treatment options such as WBRT and targeted systemic treatments especially needs to be further investigated in brain metastases from RCC.

4.3. Stereotactic Radiosurgery Related Toxicities.

During the course of treatment, a total of 4 (6%) patients of the analyzed cohort presented with ≥ grade 3 side effects related to SRS. Especially among the patients with severe complications such as symptomatic radiation necrosis, worsening symptoms, and seizures related to the treated lesion, there was trend towards larger initial tumor volume. The more severe side effects were more common among the patients with larger lesions treated with SRS only than in the surgical group.

4.4. Surgery.

In patients with a single brain metastasis, with good performance status, and limited to controlled systemic disease, surgical resection of brain metastasis has shown survival benefit in randomized data [53], but, however, there is currently no class I evidence available for the optimal surgical treatment of patients with 2 or more brain metastases [54]. Since local failure rates as high as 60% after surgical resection have been reported, adjuvant SRS or WBRT is recommended [54, 55]. Two randomized trials [53, 56] have furthermore shown that the addition of WBRT to either surgery or SRS results in significantly improved local and distant brain tumor control, although improved overall survival has only been reported for surgery plus subsequent WBRT [53].

In addition, Bindal and colleagues [57] reported equivalent survival time of patients with up to three brain metastases and good performance status who had all lesions removed to that of similar patients undergoing surgery for a single brain lesion.

To date, randomized trials reporting significantly improved survival, local and distant brain control after treatment with surgery, and/or SRS have only been including patients with brain metastases from different primary tumors, but no such trials have been conducted on the surgical treatment for patients with brain metastases from renal cell carcinoma [43].

In our study, the group of patients initially treated with surgical resection followed by SRS had a median survival of 21.9 months and the highest 1-year local tumor control rate (94%), although these results failed to show statistically significant difference compared to the outcome of patients initially treated with SRS only, which may be due to the relatively low number of patients in our cohort. This observation should hence be reexamined in a larger sample which can be achieved by pooling data or when patients are accrued in a multicenter trial.

Based on the available data in the current literature, the first-line treatment for accessible brain metastases from RCC has been surgical resection followed by WBRT. To date, six studies have been conducted to evaluate the outcome and prognostic factors of patients who underwent surgical resection for brain metastases from RCC [58–63].

In aggregate, the results of these investigations including our findings support the role of surgery for brain metastases from RCC in selected patients with good prognostic factors, limited or controlled systemic disease, and a single brain metastasis in a surgically accessible location, as surgery usually results in immediate relief of symptoms and can contribute to achieving excellent local tumor control. However, in terms of quality of life, even patients with poor prognostic factors may also benefit from surgical intervention if a lesion causing significant mass effect can be removed [64]. The question whether surgical resection only or a combined approach is more favorable still remains unclear as prospective randomized trials for patients with brain metastases from RCC are lacking.

4.5. WBRT.

Historically, whole-brain radiation therapy (WBRT) has been the mainstay of treatment in the management of patients with brain metastases, although this treatment modality is potentially associated with neurocognitive dysfunction and with suboptimal control rates, especially

TABLE 4: Summary of literature on SRS for renal cell brain metastasis.

Study	Year	Number of patients	Number of lesions	Median tumor volume (cm³)	Dose range (Gy)	Radiosurgery device	Median overall survival (months)	One-year local control (%)	One-year distant progression-free survival (%)
Present study	2014	66	207	0.688	12–30	Cyberknife	13.9	84% (SRS only) 94% (Surgery + SRS) 88% (WBRT + SRS)	35.2
Seastone et al. [31]	2014	166	487	1.96	12–35	Gamma knife	ND	90[a]	ND
Lwu et al. [32]	2013	16	41	0.4[f]	15–25	Gamma knife	ND	91	ND
Kim et al. [9, 14]	2012	46	99	3.0[b]	12–25	Gamma knife	10	84.7[a]	ND
Kano et al. [29]	2011	158	531	2.8	10–22	Gamma knife	8.2	86	45
Nieder et al. [43]	2011	35	ND	ND	ND	ND	10.1	ND	ND
Lo et al. [33]	2011	14	22	4[b,f]	15–22[f]	Gamma knife	6.5[f]	95.5[a]	40.2[f]
Fokas et al. [24]	2010	51	ND	ND	15–22	LINAC	12	81	ND
Marko et al. [34]	2010	19	59	1.72[b]	21.3[b]	Gamma knife	12.58	95[a]	ND
Hara et al. [44]	2009	18	145[f]	1.47[f]	14–24[f]	Cyberknife	14.2	87[f]	38[f]
Shuch et al. [45]	2008	138	ND	1.7	ND	ND	10.7[j]	ND	ND
Powell et al. [35]	2008	23	303[g]	ND	8–30[g]	Gamma knife	5.1[g]	93.6	37.3[g]
Jensen et al. [21]	2008	28	59	0.9	15–22	LINAC	7.03[f]	60.9[a]	ND
Samlowski et al. [36]	2008	32	71	0.03–26.9[d]	15–24	LINAC	6.7	86	ND
Shuto et al. [30]	2006	69	314	1.5[b]	8–30	Gamma knife	9.5	82.6[a]	ND
Manon et al. [46]	2005	14	ND	ND	15–24[g]	ND	8.3[g]	67.8[g,h]	67.8[g,h]
Chang et al. [16]	2005	77	99	1.5	15–24	LINAC	9.1	64.3	60
Muacevic et al. [37]	2004	85	376	1.2	15–35	Gamma knife	11.1	94[a]	ND
Noel et al. [19]	2004	28	65	1.28	10.9–22.3	LINAC	11	93	70
Sheehan et al. [7]	2003	69	146	2.8	12.5–32	Gamma knife	6	96[a]	ND
Petrovich et al. [47]	2002	29	70	ND	20[c]	Gamma knife	12	ND	ND
Hernandez et al. [17]	2002	29	92	4.7	13–30	Gamma knife	7	ND	ND
Siebels et al. [38]	2002	58	277	3.4	15–35	Gamma knife	9.9	95[a]	ND
Wowra et al. [39]	2002	75	350	1.6	15–35	Gamma knife	11	95[i]	ND
Hoshi et al. [18]	2002	42	110	1.5[c,e]	20–30	Gamma knife	12.5	93[a]	ND
Gerosa et al. [40]	2002	74	102	ND	22[b]	Gamma knife	14.6	86[a]	ND
Brown et al. [15]	2002	16	ND	ND	12–25	Gamma knife	17.8	85[a]	ND
Amendola et al. [20]	2000	22	ND	3.9[b]	15–22	Gamma knife	8	98.5[a]	ND
Payne et al. [41]	2000	21	37	4.4	10.5–40	Gamma knife	8	100[a]	ND

TABLE 4: Continued.

Study	Year	Number of patients	Number of lesions	Median tumor volume (cm^3)	Dose range (Gy)	Radiosurgery device	Median overall survival (months)	One-year local control (%)	One-year distant progression-free survival (%)
Goyal et al. [42]	2000	29	66	1.135	7–24	LINAC and Gamma knife	6.7	91[a]	ND
Schöggl et al. [8]	1998	23	44	ND	8–30	Gamma knife	11	96[a]	ND
Mori et al. [28]	1998	35	52	2.4[b]	13–20	Gamma knife	11	90[a]	ND

ND: not defined, LINAC: linear accelerator.
[a]Crude.
[b]Mean.
[c]Median.
[d]Range.
[e]mm tumor diameter.
[f]For melanoma and RCC.
[g]For melanoma, RCC, and sarcoma.
[h]At 6 months.
[i]At 1.5 years.
[j]From the time of diagnosis of the first brain metastasis.

for larger tumors [10, 52]. Outcomes after WBRT appear especially poor for patients with metastatic RCC, as this tumor has traditionally been considered to be relatively radioresistant compared to brain metastases from other primaries, such as lung or breast [9, 10].

In our study, patients treated with WBRT prior to SRS had the second highest local control rate. Furthermore, upfront WBRT was significantly associated with improved distant brain tumor control in univariate and multivariate analysis, although this treatment combination revealed a median survival of 5.9 months in these patients, a significantly worse result compared to the overall survival of patients initially treated with SRS only and patients treated with surgery and SRS as an adjunct. This could be attributed to selection bias.

In three retrospective studies, the outcomes of patients with brain metastasis from RCC treated with WBRT were evaluated: the first study conducted by Wroński et al. [27] revealed a median survival of 3.3 months calculated from the last day of WBRT, with death from neurologic causes in 76% of patients. One year later, another study to further investigate the question whether WBRT is a suitable treatment for patients with metastatic brain lesions from RCC was published by Culine et al. [23]. The median survival of patients who received radiotherapy alone was 7 months, compared to a median survival of 1 month of patients who did not undergo any specific treatment and 10 months of patients who underwent surgery. In 2004, Cannady and colleagues [22] published another study with comparable survival rates to those of Wroński et al., with a median survival after WBRT of 3.3 months in a total of 46 patients who received WBRT as their initial treatment for brain metastasis. Furthermore, the median survival rates for the different RPA classes were evaluated: the median survival for RPA classes I, II, and III was 8.5, 3, and 0.6 months, respectively, but no statistically significant difference was observed among the three classes [22].

In addition, some studies also revealed the potential benefit of dose escalation [22, 65–67]. The most recent study was conducted by Rades et al. [66], in which higher doses of radiation (40 Gy in 20 fractions or 45 Gy in 15 fractions) compared to standard treatment regimens resulted in improved local control and overall survival rates. Patients who were treated with higher doses had a median overall survival of 12 months and 6 months' local control rates of 57%, compared to patients treated with lower doses, who had a median overall survival of 4 months and 6 months' local control rates of 21% [66].

These rather unsatisfactory results of treatment or RCC metastasis with WBRT only led to the implementation of more aggressive treatment approaches for brain metastasis from RCC, such as surgical resection and SRS [10].

In 1987, Gay et al. [25] analyzed the median survival rates of 25 patients who received radiation therapy only (13 weeks) and 7 patients who underwent surgical resection and postoperative radiation (66 weeks). However, interpreting the results of this study, it has to be kept in mind that the patients who underwent surgery were preselected because of stable systemic disease, an accessible single metastatic lesion, and the belief that the tumor burden could be completely resected.

Ikushima et al. [26] extended the available data with their retrospective analysis of the effect of adjuvant fractionated stereotactic radiotherapy (FSRT) after surgery compared to surgical resection with adjuvant WBRT and WBRT alone. The different treatment groups achieved median survival times of 25.6, 18.7, and 4 months, respectively. The results in this study, however, are confounded by the fact that the patients included had a relatively good performance status compared to the patients of other studies conducted on this topic before and FRST was only indicated in patients with a good performance status and a tumor diameter of ≤3 cm and if patients presented with less or equal to 3 lesions [9].

A recent study published by Fokas and colleagues [24] evaluated the role of the treatment with SRS and WBRT in brain metastasis from RCC in a total of 88 patients. Fifty-one patients were treated with SRS, and 17 were treated with

SRS plus adjuvant WBRT, whereas the remaining 20 patients were treated with WBRT only. The median overall survival for these different treatment groups was 12, 16, and 2 months, respectively. Statistically significant difference was found in overall survival rates of patients treated with SRS only as well as patients treated with a combination of SRS and WBRT compared to patients treated with WBRT only [24].

Taking everything into account, the results of these studies, including our retrospective analysis, suggest improved local and distant brain tumor control for brain metastases from RCC when WBRT is administered. Although RCC is considered to be a radioresistant tumor, these results suggest that there might be an effect of WBRT on microscopic metastases from RCC within the brain or a potential delay in the appearance of new brain metastases. However, no significant survival benefit could be demonstrated in these patients. This result might be partially explained by selection bias, because WBRT was more commonly used in patients with a larger number of brain metastases.

Our results suggest that more aggressive treatment options like surgical resection and SRS, possibly in combination with WBRT, might be beneficial for patients with favorable performance status and a limited number of brain lesions. However, WBRT and supportive care continue to be the treatment of choice in patients with multiple brain metastases, poor performance status, uncontrolled systemic disease, and a short life expectancy [52, 68]. As more aggressive treatment options may be associated with an increased risk in these patients, it is important to take into account the prognosis of each patient in order to individualize the treatment approach [69] and to offer the best possible treatment modality for an improved outcome of these patients.

4.6. Limitations of This Study. The present study has inherent limitations based on its retrospective nature, and the obtained results may be somewhat influenced by clinical selection bias. In light of varying treatment regimen during the course of disease of the analyzed patients, reliable prognostic factors remain difficult to assess. Furthermore, complete follow-up was only available for 86.8% of all patients. The other patients were transferred to other facilities for further follow-up and could not be analyzed in this study. Therefore, despite the fact that this cohort is the largest reported series to date, the analyzed cohort is a rather heterogeneous group of patients with a variety of different systemic treatment regimens, prior WBRT, and prior surgery, or patients treated with SRS only. Due to this fact, it is difficult to analyze the exact impact of the different treatment options as well as potential prognostic factors on the outcome of this patient cohort. Randomized controlled trials are needed to further evaluate the impact of SRS and possible combination approaches with surgery or WBRT as well as reliable prognostic factors on survival and tumor control in the future.

5. Conclusion

Stereotactic radiosurgery is a safe and effective treatment option in patients with brain metastases from RCC and results in excellent local control rates. In case of a limited number of brain metastases, surgery or SRS might be appropriate, depending on the individual characteristics of the patients and the number, size, and location of brain metastases. Further investigations such as randomized controlled trials are necessary for a reliable evaluation of prognostic factors and for a comparison of the outcome of patients treated with SRS alone versus combined treatment approaches.

Disclosure

Franziska Ippen and Anand Mahadevan are co-primary authors.

Conflict of Interests

All authors report no conflict of interests.

Authors' Contribution

Franziska Ippen, Anand Mahadevan, and Ekkehard Kasper designed the study, analyzed the patients, performed the statistical analysis, and drafted the paper. Eric T. Wong, Erik Uhlmann, and Soma Sengupta contributed to patient treatment and follow-up data and critically reviewed the paper.

References

[1] P. A. Godley and K. I. Ataga, "Renal cell carcinoma," *Current Opinion in Oncology*, vol. 12, no. 3, pp. 260–264, 2000.

[2] K. Gupta, J. D. Miller, J. Z. Li, M. W. Russell, and C. Charbonneau, "Epidemiologic and socioeconomic burden of metastatic renal cell carcinoma (mRCC): a literature review," *Cancer Treatment Reviews*, vol. 34, no. 3, pp. 193–205, 2008.

[3] N. K. Janzen, H. L. Kim, R. A. Figlin, and A. S. Belldegrun, "Surveillance after radical or partial nephrectomy for localized renal cell carcinoma and management of recurrent disease," *The Urologic Clinics of North America*, vol. 30, no. 4, pp. 843–852, 2003.

[4] Y. G. Najjar and B. I. Rini, "Novel agents in renal carcinoma: a reality check," *Therapeutic Advances in Medical Oncology*, vol. 4, no. 4, pp. 183–194, 2012.

[5] J. Remon, P. Lianes, and S. Martínez, "Brain metastases from renal cell carcinoma. Should we change the current standard?" *Cancer Treatment Reviews*, vol. 38, no. 4, pp. 249–257, 2012.

[6] P. W. Hanson, A. L. Elaimy, W. T. Lamoreaux et al., "A concise review of the efficacy of stereotactic radiosurgery in the management of melanoma and renal cell carcinoma brain metastases," *World Journal of Surgical Oncology*, vol. 10, article 176, 2012.

[7] J. P. Sheehan, M.-H. Sun, D. Kondziolka, J. Flickinger, and L. D. Lunsford, "Radiosurgery in patients with renal cell carcinoma metastasis to the brain: long-term outcomes and prognostic factors influencing survival and local tumor control," *Journal of Neurosurgery*, vol. 98, no. 2, pp. 342–349, 2003.

[8] A. Schöggl, K. Kitz, A. Ertl, K. Dieckmann, W. Saringer, and W. T. Koos, "Gamma-knife radiosurgery for brain metastases of renal cell carcinoma: results in 23 patients," *Acta Neurochirurgica*, vol. 140, no. 6, pp. 549–555, 1998.

[9] Y. H. Kim, J. W. Kim, H.-T. Chung, S. H. Paek, D. G. Kim, and H.-W. Jung, "Brain metastasis from renal cell carcinoma," *Progress in Neurological Surgery*, vol. 25, pp. 163–175, 2012.

[10] A. I. Blanco, B. S. Teh, and R. J. Amato, "Role of radiation therapy in the management of renal cell cancer," *Cancers*, vol. 3, no. 4, pp. 4010–4023, 2011.

[11] A. W. Chan, R. M. Cardinale, and J. S. Loeffler, "Stereotactic irradiation," in *Principles and Practice of Radiation Oncology*, A. P. Carlos, L. W. Brady, E. C. Halperin, and R. K. Schmidt-Ullrich, Eds., pp. 410–427, Lippincott Williams & Wilkins, Philadelphia, Pa, USA, 4th edition, 2004.

[12] J. Loeffler, H. Shih, and M. Khandekar, "Application of current radiation delivery systems and radiobiology," in *Principles of Neurological Surgery*, R. G. Ellenbogen, S. I. Abdulrauf, and L. N. Sekhar, Eds., Elsevier Sauders, Philadelphia, Pa, USA, 3rd edition, 2012.

[13] A. L. Asher, S. H. Burri, and A. Chahlavi, "The management of brain metastases," in *Principles of Neuro-Oncology*, D. Schiff and B. P. O'Neill, Eds., pp. 553–579, McGraw-Hill Medical, New York, NY, USA, 2005.

[14] W. H. Kim, D. G. Kim, J. H. Han et al., "Early significant tumor volume reduction after radiosurgery in brain metastases from renal cell carcinoma results in long-term survival," *International Journal of Radiation Oncology Biology Physics*, vol. 82, no. 5, pp. 1749–1755, 2012.

[15] P. D. Brown, C. A. Brown, B. E. Pollock et al., "Stereotactic radiosurgery for patients with 'radioresistant' brain metastases," *Neurosurgery*, vol. 51, no. 3, pp. 656–667, 2002.

[16] E. L. Chang, U. Selek, S. J. Hassenbusch III et al., "Outcome variation among 'radioresistant' brain metastases treated with stereotactic radiosurgery," *Neurosurgery*, vol. 56, no. 5, pp. 936–945, 2005.

[17] L. Hernandez, L. Zamorano, A. Sloan et al., "Gamma knife radiosurgery for renal cell carcinoma brain metastases," *Journal of Neurosurgery*, vol. 97, no. 5, supplement, pp. 489–493, 2002.

[18] S. Hoshi, H. Jokura, H. Nakamura et al., "Gamma-knife radiosurgery for brain metastasis of renal cell carcinoma: results in 42 patients," *International Journal of Urology*, vol. 9, no. 11, pp. 618–625, 2002.

[19] G. Noel, C.-A. Valery, G. Boisserie et al., "LINAC radiosurgery for brain metastasis of renal cell carcinoma," *Urologic Oncology*, vol. 22, no. 1, pp. 25–31, 2004.

[20] B. E. Amendola, A. L. Wolf, S. R. Coy, M. Amendola, and L. Bloch, "Brain metastases in renal cell carcinoma: management with gamma knife radiosurgery," *Cancer Journal*, vol. 6, no. 6, pp. 372–376, 2000.

[21] R. L. Jensen, A. F. Shrieve, W. Samlowski, and D. C. Shrieve, "Outcomes of patients with brain metastases from melanoma and renal cell carcinoma after primary stereotactic radiosurgery," *Clinical neurosurgery*, vol. 55, pp. 150–159, 2008.

[22] S. B. Cannady, K. A. Cavanaugh, S.-Y. Lee et al., "Results of whole brain radiotherapy and recursive partitioning analysis in patients with brain metastases from renal cell carcinoma: a retrospective study," *International Journal of Radiation Oncology, Biology, Physics*, vol. 58, no. 1, pp. 253–258, 2004.

[23] S. Culine, M. Bekradda, A. Kramar, A. Rey, B. Escudier, and J.-P. Droz, "Prognostic factors for survival in patients with brain metastases from renal cell carcinoma," *Cancer*, vol. 83, no. 12, pp. 2548–2553, 1998.

[24] E. Fokas, M. Henzel, K. Hamm, G. Surber, G. Kleinert, and R. Engenhart-Cabillic, "Radiotherapy for brain metastases from renal cell cancer: should whole-brain radiotherapy be added to stereotactic radiosurgery?: analysis of 88 patients," *Strahlentherapie und Onkologie*, vol. 186, no. 4, pp. 210–217, 2010.

[25] P. C. Gay, W. J. Litchy, and T. L. Cascino, "Brain metastasis in hypernephroma," *Journal of Neuro-Oncology*, vol. 5, no. 1, pp. 51–56, 1987.

[26] H. Ikushima, K. Tokuuye, M. Sumi et al., "Fractionated stereotactic radiotherapy of brain metastases from renal cell carcinoma," *International Journal of Radiation Oncology Biology Physics*, vol. 48, no. 5, pp. 1389–1393, 2000.

[27] M. Wroński, M. H. Maor, B. J. Davis, R. Sawaya, and V. A. Levin, "External radiation of brain metastases from renal carcinoma: a retrospective study of 119 patients from the M.D. Anderson Cancer Center," *International Journal of Radiation Oncology Biology Physics*, vol. 37, no. 4, pp. 753–759, 1997.

[28] Y. Mori, D. Kondziolka, J. C. Flickinger, T. Logan, and L. D. Lunsford, "Stereotactic radiosurgery for brain metastasis from renal cell carcinoma," *Cancer*, vol. 83, no. 2, pp. 344–353, 1998.

[29] H. Kano, A. Iyer, D. Kondziolka, A. Niranjan, J. C. Flickinger, and L. D. Lunsford, "Outcome predictors of gamma knife radiosurgery for renal cell carcinoma metastases," *Neurosurgery*, vol. 69, no. 6, pp. 1232–1239, 2011.

[30] T. Shuto, S. Inomori, H. Fujino, and H. Nagano, "Gamma knife surgery for metastatic brain tumors from renal cell carcinoma," *Journal of Neurosurgery*, vol. 105, no. 4, pp. 555–560, 2006.

[31] D. J. Seastone, P. Elson, J. A. Garcia et al., "Clinical outcome of stereotactic radiosurgery for central nervous system metastases from renal cell carcinoma," *Clinical Genitourinary Cancer*, vol. 12, no. 2, pp. 111–116, 2014.

[32] S. Lwu, P. Goetz, E. Monsalves et al., "Stereotactic radiosurgery for the treatment of melanoma and renal cell carcinoma brain metastases," *Oncology Reports*, vol. 29, no. 2, pp. 407–412, 2013.

[33] S. S. Lo, J. W. Clarke, J. C. Grecula et al., "Stereotactic radiosurgery alone for patients with 1-4 radioresistant brain metastases," *Medical Oncology*, vol. 28, no. 1, pp. S439–S444, 2011.

[34] N. F. Marko, L. Angelov, S. A. Toms et al., "Stereotactic radiosurgery as single-modality treatment of incidentally identified renal cell carcinoma brain metastases," *World Neurosurgery*, vol. 73, no. 3, pp. 186–193, 2010.

[35] J. W. Powell, C. T. Chung, H. R. Shah et al., "Gamma Knife surgery in the management of radioresistant brain metastases in high-risk patients with melanoma, renal cell carcinoma, and sarcoma," *Journal of Neurosurgery*, vol. 109, supplement, pp. 122–128, 2008.

[36] W. E. Samlowski, M. Majer, K. M. Boucher et al., "Multidisciplinary treatment of brain metastases derived from clear cell renal cancer incorporating stereotactic radiosurgery," *Cancer*, vol. 113, no. 9, pp. 2539–2548, 2008.

[37] A. Muacevic, F. W. Kreth, A. Mack, J.-C. Tonn, and B. Wowra, "Stereotactic radiosurgery without radiation therapy providing high local tumor control of multiple brain metastases from renal cell carcinoma," *Minimally Invasive Neurosurgery*, vol. 47, no. 4, pp. 203–208, 2004.

[38] M. Siebels, R. Oberneder, A. Buchner et al., "Ambulatory radiosurgery in cerebral metastatic renal cell carcinoma. 5-year outcome in 58 patients," *Der Urologe A*, vol. 41, no. 5, pp. 482–488, 2002.

[39] B. Wowra, M. Siebels, A. Muacevic, F. W. Kreth, A. Mack, and A. Hofstetter, "Repeated gamma knife surgery for multiple brain metastases from renal cell carcinoma," *Journal of Neurosurgery*, vol. 97, no. 4, pp. 785–793, 2002.

[40] M. Gerosa, A. Nicolato, R. Foroni et al., "Gamma knife radiosurgery for brain metastases: a primary therapeutic option," *Journal of Neurosurgery*, vol. 97, no. 5, supplement, pp. 515–524, 2002.

[41] B. R. Payne, D. Prasad, G. Szeifert, M. Steiner, and L. Steiner, "Gamma surgery for intracranial metastases from renal cell carcinoma," *Journal of Neurosurgery*, vol. 92, no. 5, pp. 760–765, 2000.

[42] L. K. Goyal, J. H. Suh, C. A. Reddy, and G. H. Barnett, "The role of whole brain radiotherapy and stereotactic radiosurgery on brain metastases from renal cell carcinoma," *International Journal of Radiation Oncology Biology Physics*, vol. 47, no. 4, pp. 1007–1012, 2000.

[43] C. Nieder, O. Spanne, T. Nordøy, and A. Dalhaug, "Treatment of brain metastases from renal cell cancer," *Urologic Oncology*, vol. 29, no. 4, pp. 405–410, 2011.

[44] W. Hara, P. Tran, G. Li et al., "CyberKnife for brain metastases of malignant melanoma and renal cell carcinoma," *Neurosurgery*, vol. 64, supplement 2, pp. A26–A32, 2009.

[45] B. Shuch, J. C. La Rochelle, T. Klatte et al., "Brain metastasis from renal cell carcinoma: presentation, recurrence, and survival," *Cancer*, vol. 113, no. 7, pp. 1641–1648, 2008.

[46] R. Manon, A. O'Neill, J. Knisely et al., "Phase II trial of radiosurgery for one to three newly diagnosed brain metastases from renal cell carcinoma, melanoma, and sarcoma: an Eastern Cooperative Oncology Group study (E 6397)," *Journal of Clinical Oncology*, vol. 23, no. 34, pp. 8870–8876, 2005.

[47] Z. Petrovich, C. Yu, S. L. Giannotta, S. O'Day, and M. L. J. Apuzzo, "Survival and pattern of failure in brain metastasis treated with stereotactic gamma knife radiosurgery," *Journal of Neurosurgery*, vol. 97, no. 5, supplement, pp. 499–506, 2002.

[48] A. K. Bindal, R. K. Bindal, K. R. Hess et al., "Surgery versus radiosurgery in the treatment of brain metastasis," *Journal of Neurosurgery*, vol. 84, no. 5, pp. 748–754, 1996.

[49] R. M. Auchter, J. P. Lamond, E. Alexander III et al., "A multiinstitutional outcome and prognostic factor analysis of radiosurgery for resectable single brain metastasis," *International Journal of Radiation Oncology Biology Physics*, vol. 35, no. 1, pp. 27–35, 1996.

[50] B. G. Fuller, I. D. Kaplan, J. Adler, R. S. Cox, and M. A. Bagshaw, "Stereotaxic radiosurgery for brain metastases: the importance of adjuvant whole brain irradiation," *International Journal of Radiation Oncology, Biology, Physics*, vol. 23, no. 2, pp. 413–418, 1992.

[51] M. H. Maor, A. E. Frias, and M. J. Oswald, "Palliative radiotherapy for brain metastases in renal carcinoma," *Cancer*, vol. 62, no. 9, pp. 1912–1917, 1988.

[52] A. Muacevic, M. Siebels, J.-C. Tonn, and B. Wowra, "Treatment of brain metastases in renal cell carcinoma: radiotherapy, radiosurgery, or surgery?" *World Journal of Urology*, vol. 23, no. 3, pp. 180–184, 2005.

[53] R. A. Patchell, P. A. Tibbs, J. W. Walsh et al., "A randomized trial of surgery in the treatment of single metastases to the brain," *The New England Journal of Medicine*, vol. 322, no. 8, pp. 494–500, 1990.

[54] P. K. Brastianos, W. T. Curry, and K. S. Oh, "Clinical discussion and review of the management of brain metastases," *Journal of the National Comprehensive Cancer Network*, vol. 11, no. 9, pp. 1153–1164, 2013.

[55] M. Kocher, R. Soffietti, U. Abacioglu et al., "Adjuvant whole-brain radiotherapy versus observation after radiosurgery or surgical resection of one to three cerebral metastases: results of the EORTC 22952-26001 study," *Journal of Clinical Oncology*, vol. 29, no. 2, pp. 134–141, 2011.

[56] H. Aoyama, H. Shirato, M. Tago et al., "Stereotactic radiosurgery plus whole-brain radiation therapy vs stereotactic radiosurgery alone for treatment of brain metastases: a randomized controlled trial," *The Journal of the American Medical Association*, vol. 295, no. 21, pp. 2483–2491, 2006.

[57] R. K. Bindal, R. Sawaya, M. E. Leavens, and J. J. Lee, "Surgical treatment of multiple brain metastases," *Journal of Neurosurgery*, vol. 79, no. 2, pp. 210–216, 1993.

[58] M. J. O'Dea, H. Zincke, D. C. Utz, and P. E. Bernatz, "The treatment of renal cell carcinoma with solitary metastasis," *The Journal of Urology*, vol. 120, no. 5, pp. 540–542, 1978.

[59] D. A. Decker, V. L. Decker, A. Herskovic, and G. D. Cummings, "Brain metastases in patients with renal cell carcinoma: prognosis and treatment," *Journal of Clinical Oncology*, vol. 2, no. 3, pp. 169–173, 1984.

[60] R. A. Badalament, E. Kreutzer, R. W. Cluck et al., "Surgical treatment of brain metastases from renal cell carcinoma," *Urology*, vol. 36, no. 2, pp. 112–117, 1990.

[61] M. Salvati, M. Scarpinati, E. R. Orlando, P. Celli, and F. M. Gagliardi, "Single brain metastases from kidney tumors. Clinico-pathologic considerations on a series of 29 cases," *Tumori*, vol. 78, no. 6, pp. 392–394, 1992.

[62] M. Wroński, E. Arbit, P. Russo, and J. H. Galicich, "Surgical resection of brain metastases from renal cell carcinoma in 50 patients," *Urology*, vol. 47, no. 2, pp. 187–193, 1996.

[63] Y. Harada, N. Nonomura, M. Kondo et al., "Clinical study of brain metastasis of renal cell carcinoma," *European Urology*, vol. 36, no. 3, pp. 230–235, 1999.

[64] E. C. A. Kaal, C. G. J. H. Niël, and C. J. Vecht, "Therapeutic management of brain metastasis," *The Lancet Neurology*, vol. 4, no. 5, pp. 289–298, 2005.

[65] S. J. DiBiase, R. K. Valicenti, D. Schultz, Y. Xie, L. G. Gomella, and B. W. Corn, "Palliative irradiation for focally symptomatic metastatic renal cell carcinoma: support for dose escalation based on a biological model," *The Journal of Urology*, vol. 158, no. 3, part 1, pp. 746–749, 1997.

[66] D. Rades, C. Heisterkamp, and S. E. Schild, "Do patients receiving whole-brain radiotherapy for brain metastases from renal cell carcinoma benefit from escalation of the radiation dose?" *International Journal of Radiation Oncology Biology Physics*, vol. 78, no. 2, pp. 398–403, 2010.

[67] D. Wilson, L. Hiller, L. Gray, M. Grainger, A. Stirling, and N. James, "The effect of biological effective dose on time to symptom progression in metastatic renal cell carcinoma," *Clinical Oncology*, vol. 15, no. 7, pp. 400–407, 2003.

[68] L. S. Doh, R. J. Amato, A. C. Paulino, and B. S. Teh, "Radiation therapy in the management of brain metastases from renal cell carcinoma," *Oncology*, vol. 20, no. 6, pp. 603–613, 2006.

[69] T. Meyners, C. Heisterkamp, J. D. Kueter et al., "Prognostic factors for outcomes after whole-brain irradiation of brain metastases from relatively radioresistant tumors: a retrospective analysis," *BMC Cancer*, vol. 10, article 582, 2010.

7

Fractal Dimensions of *In Vitro* Tumor Cell Proliferation

George I. Lambrou[1] and Apostolos Zaravinos[2]

[1]*1st Department of Pediatrics, University of Athens, Choremeio Research Laboratory, Thivon & Levadeias, 11527 Athens, Greece*
[2]*Division of Clinical Immunology and Transfusion Medicine, Department of Laboratory Medicine,*
 Karolinska Institute, 171 77 Stockholm, Sweden

Correspondence should be addressed to George I. Lambrou; glamprou@med.uoa.gr

Academic Editor: Vassileios Zoumpourlis

Biological systems are characterized by their potential for dynamic adaptation. One of the challenges for systems biology approaches is their contribution towards the understanding of the dynamics of a growing cell population. Conceptualizing these dynamics in tumor models could help us understand the steps leading to the initiation of the disease and its progression. *In vitro* models are useful in answering this question by providing information over the spatiotemporal nature of such dynamics. In the present work, we used physical quantities such as growth rate, velocity, and acceleration for the cellular proliferation and identified the fractal structures in tumor cell proliferation dynamics. We provide evidence that the rate of cellular proliferation is of nonlinear nature and exhibits oscillatory behavior. We also calculated the fractal dimensions of our cellular system. Our results show that the temporal transitions from one state to the other also follow nonlinear dynamics. Furthermore, we calculated self-similarity in cellular proliferation, providing the basis for further investigation in this topic. Such systems biology approaches are very useful in understanding the nature of cellular proliferation and growth. From a clinical point of view, our results may be applicable not only to primary tumors but also to tumor metastases.

1. Introduction

Population dynamics and population genetics provide a well-developed mathematical theory of evolution [1, 2] and many of these models and techniques have been applied to cancer. Cells growing under normal conditions can manifest proliferation dynamics of nonlinear nature [3, 4]. This nonlinear behavior has also been demonstrated in cells being under the influence of drugs or other environmental factors [5]. Any further knowledge regarding the mechanisms underlying cellular proliferation is of major importance and even the smallest indication towards a certain direction could enable us to discover novel differences in the mechanisms that distinguish healthy from diseased cells.

Genes manifest several patterns of differential expression in cancer [6, 7]. Gene expression is highly correlated to the chromosome level and gene expression data can be simulated using polynomial functions [8–10]. Gene expression has also been suggested to take place discretely and not continuously (i.e., in quanta) [11, 12]. It has also been reported to follow oscillatory patterns, thus complicating things even more regarding the rate of cellular proliferation, be it either growth acceleration or deceleration [13, 14]. In terms of growth rate, this means that cells cannot simply transit from one state to the other. If the hypothesis of oscillatory modulation of gene expression is correct, a much more complicated regulatory pattern should be required by a cell in order to be able to change its state, as a result of environmental stimuli. Biological systems are dynamic systems and it is critical to know how to determine a cell's present state from its previous one. This knowledge can have a vast number of applications, from cancer to insect population control. However, discovering the laws that underlie biological systems is a tedious work. On the one hand it is not easy to model such systems due to their high complexity and, on the other hand, biological dynamical systems possess significant capabilities of adaptation. We tested this hypothesis, adding specific modifications to our previously published experimental setup [15]. Although several studies have dealt with the complex dynamic behavior of animal populations [16–19], little is

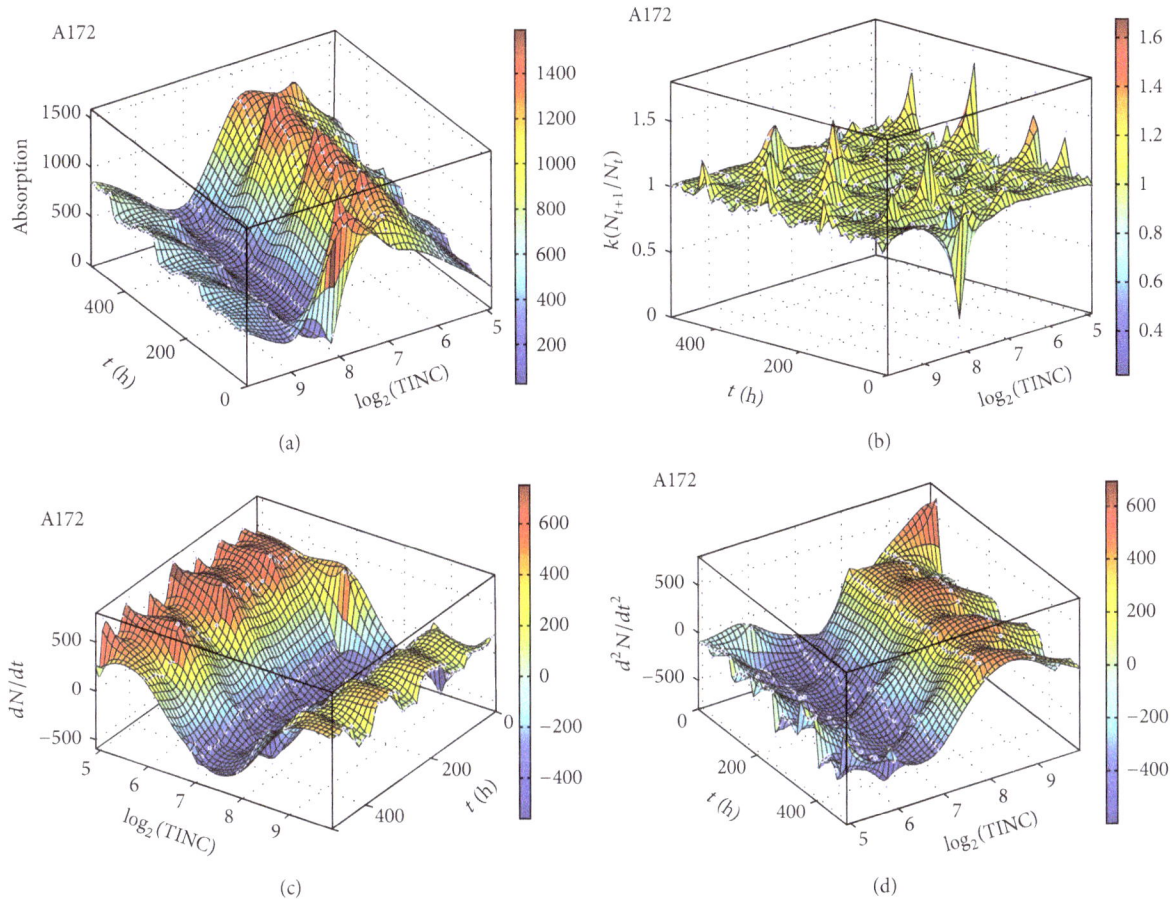

FIGURE 1: Graphical representation of time-series experiments for the A172 (glioblastoma) cells. Factors presented include cell proliferation (a), rate of growth (N_{t+1}/N_t) (b), the speed of growth (dN/dt) (c), and the acceleration of proliferation (d^2N/dt^2) (d). TINC: total initial number of cells.

known regarding the dynamics of tumor cell proliferation [3] and even less is known regarding the state of proliferation dynamics until cells reach an adequate number for the tumor to be diagnosed.

Data regarding the dynamic nature of a tumor can only be collected after it has been diagnosed. Usually, this is too late for the patient, since all the critical steps for the progression of the tumor have already taken place. Therefore, *in vitro* systems provide an excellent opportunity to study effects that are impossible to be measured *in vivo*. Most importantly, *in vitro* systems can be studied in the long term. This is required in order to reach conclusions regarding nonlinearity and chaotic behavior of a cellular system. Since primary cell cultures are short-lived when untransformed (15–20 days), the only way to apply such measurements is to use already established cell lines. For this reason, we developed a modeling approach in order to simulate the *in vivo* conditions, as best as possible. The nature of proliferation dynamics can give insight into the way that not only cells proliferate, but they also differentiate.

In the present study we used systems biology approaches and focused on the dynamics of *in vitro* cellular systems,

using three central nervous system (CNS) tumor and a T-cell acute lymphoblastic leukemia (T-ALL) cell lines. These cells provide an excellent substrate for modeling proliferation dynamics, as previously shown [15]. The questions that we posed were as follows. If certain physical measures, including cellular proliferation, are observed at the phenotypical level of the cells, how can they be translated at the molecular or genomic level? If the proliferation rate of a cellular population increases, does this mean that there are genes being transcribed faster than others and/or at a faster rate than usual? We aimed to test the hypothesis that cell proliferation is of nonlinear nature and manifests self-similarity patterns with its subsequent applications. Our results highlight the fact that tumor cells manifest self-similarities in their proliferation potential. This implies that the trajectory of a cellular population can be predicted and it could be a factor determining metastasis.

2. Materials and Methods

2.1. Cell Cultures. The TE671 (cerebellar rhabdomyosarcoma) [20–23], A172 (glioblastoma) [24], 1321N1 (astrocytoma)

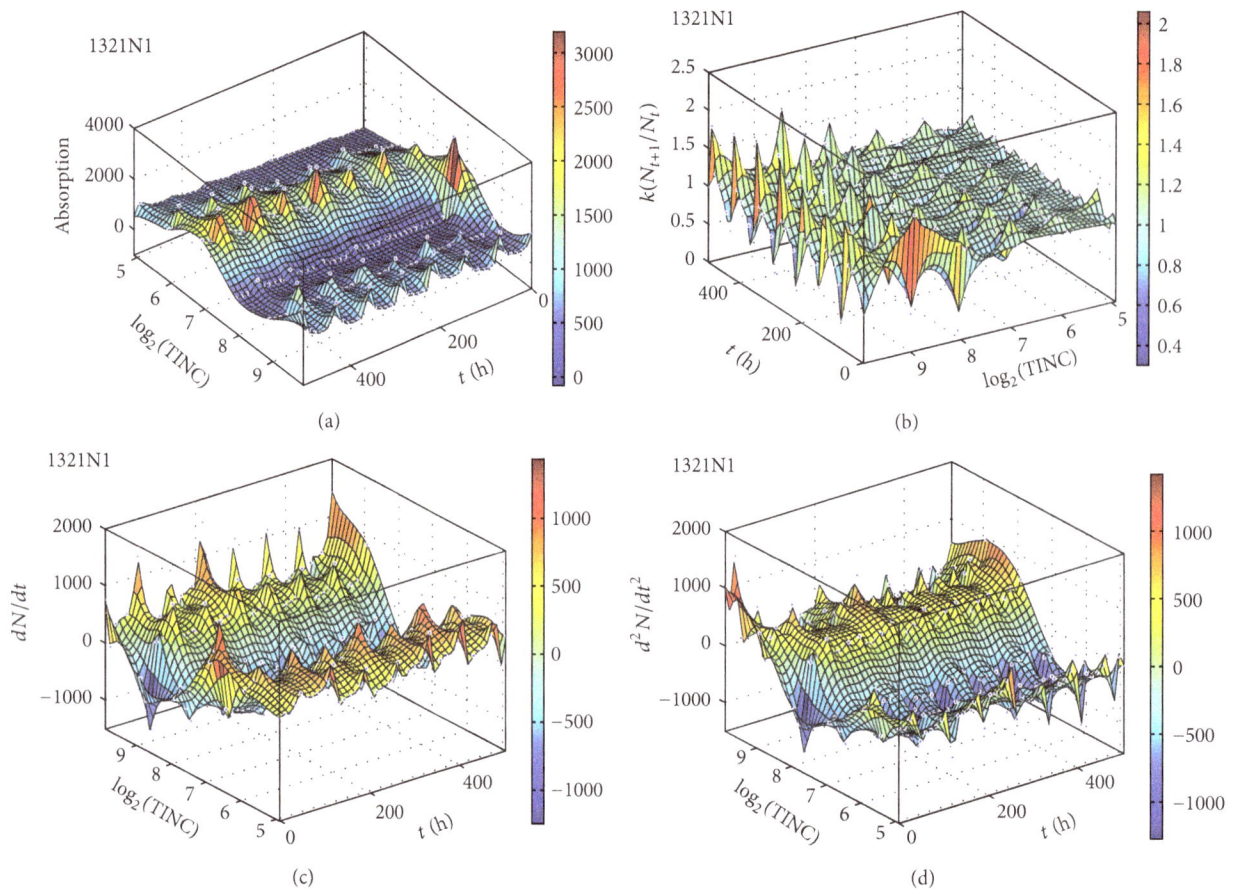

FIGURE 2: Graphical representation of time-series experiments for the 1321N1 (astrocytoma) cells. Factors presented include cell proliferation (a), rate of growth (N_{t+1}/N_t) (b), the speed of growth (dN/dt) (c), and the acceleration of proliferation (d^2N/dt^2) (d). TINC: total initial number of cells.

[25, 26], and CCRF-CEM (T-ALL) [27–31] cell lines were used as the model, obtained from the European Collection of Cell Cultures (ECACC, UK).

2.2. Cell Cultures Conditions. Cells were grown in DMEM and RPMI-1640 medium, 15% FBS, and 0.1x streptomycin/penicillin at 37°C, 5% CO_2, and ~100% humidity. Cells were cultured in 12-well plates and $75 \, cm^2$ flasks in total medium volume of 2 mL and 25 mL, respectively. Cells were seeded at initial concentrations of 20 cells/μL~200 cells/μL for the CCRFCEM cells and 30, 60, 120, 240, 480, and 960 total cells populations were fed at regular intervals thereafter. Medium changes took place by centrifugation at 1000 rpm for 10 min, the supernatant was discarded, and the remaining cells were re-diluted in 25 mL media and were allowed to grow. Measurements were taken every 12 hours for a total of >500 hours. Cells were passaged at regular intervals by removing old media and adding fresh. Cells were not trypsinized and were allowed to grow up to the point of reaching confluence of 80–90%. This practically removed the dead cells from the system and the remaining cells were allowed to grow again in fresh medium. This allowed modelling of the growth of a tumor (CNS tumors or leukemia)

in a space with finite capacity. Removal of cells modelled the circulation that removes dead cells from a particular position in the organism.

2.3. Measurements, Experimental Setup, and Model. The CCRF-CEM cells grow in suspension and can therefore provide an excellent model of avascular growth. In addition, the following assumptions were considered for cellular proliferation: (a) extracellular signal transduction takes place autocrinaly; (b) the cellular distribution at the time of seeding and thereafter is considered to be uniform; and (c) nutrient supply was considered to be stable since cells were fed at regular time intervals. All measurements were performed in triplicate. Wolfrom et al. counted the cell population at the end of a time period varying from 5 to 7 days [3]. At the end of this period, cells were trypsinized, measured, and then seeded at an initial concentration of 10^5 cells per flask. In our study, prior to every measurement, flasks were gently shaken in order to assure that the sample taken consisted of a representative, equally distributed population size. For the cellular growth dynamics study, cells were assayed at least every 48 h and the media renewed every 3–5 days. For the measurements, 200 μL from each flask was measured on an automatic

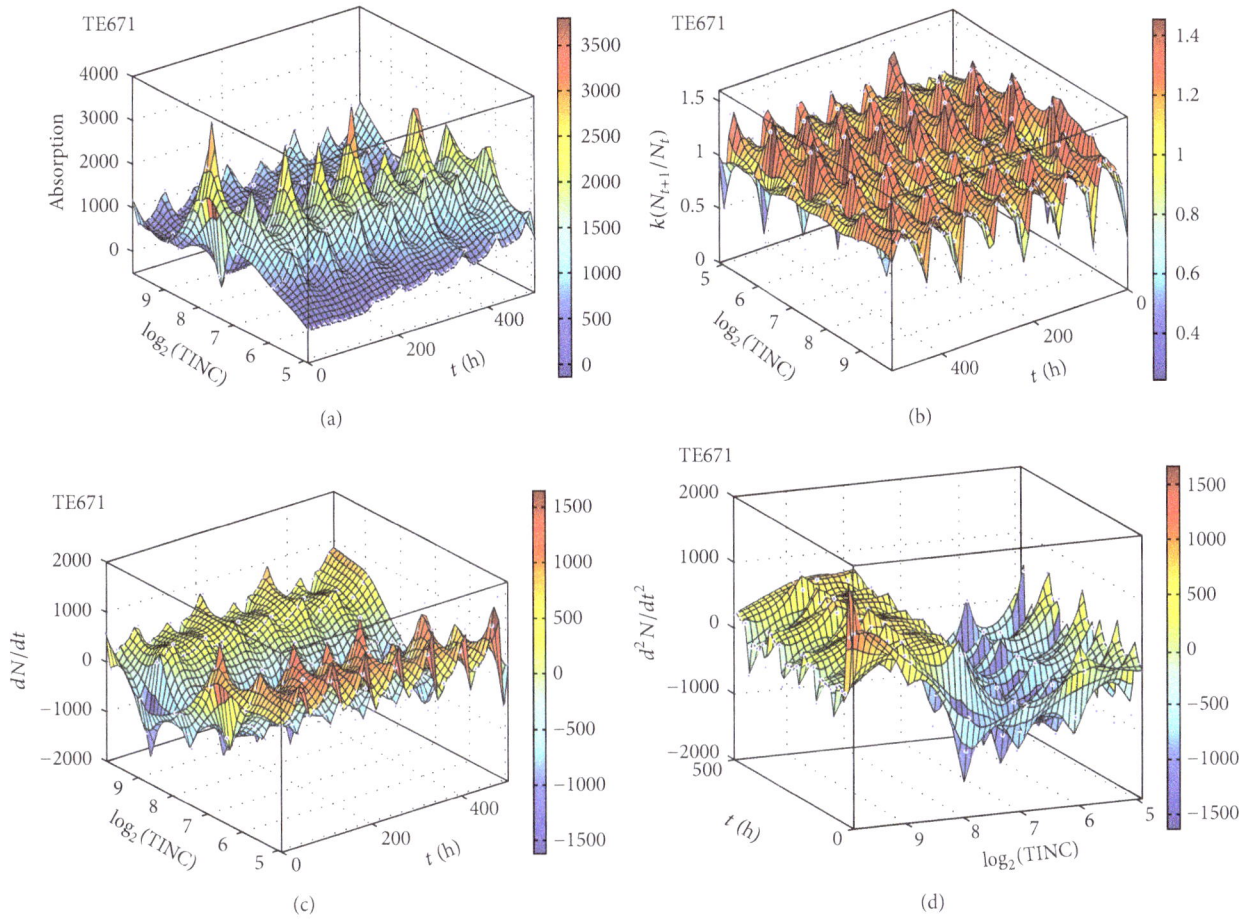

FIGURE 3: Graphical representation of time-series experiments for the TE671 (cerebellar rhabdomyosarcoma) cells. Factors presented include cell proliferation (a), rate of growth (N_{t+1}/N_t) (b), the speed of growth (dN/dt) (c), and the acceleration of proliferation (d^2N/dt^2) (d). TINC: total initial number of cells.

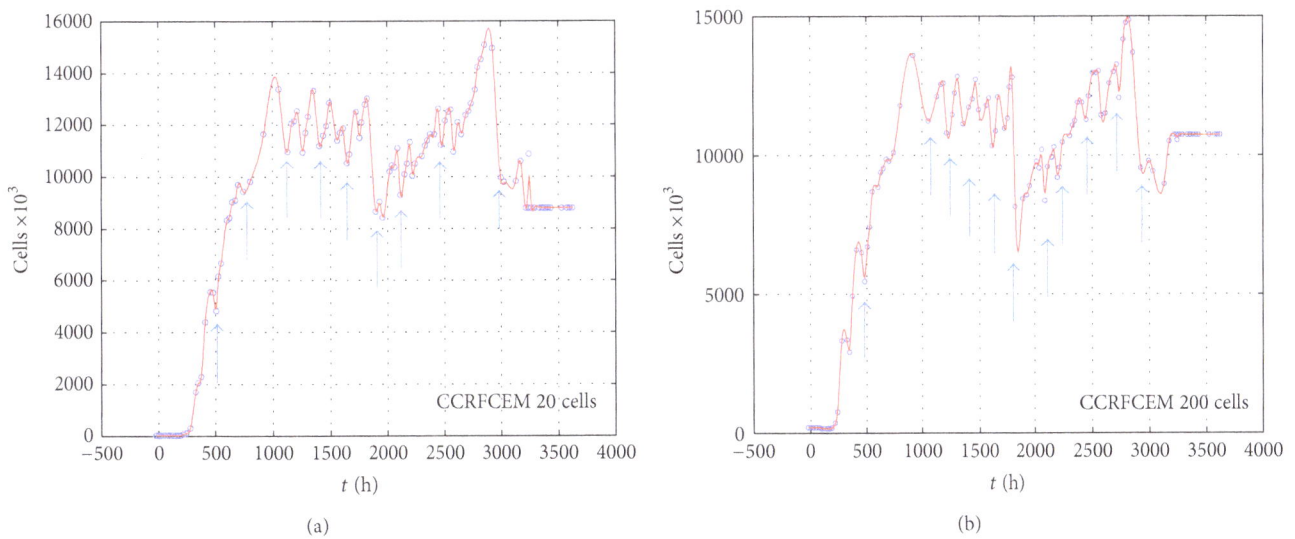

FIGURE 4: Graphical representation of time-series experiments for the CCRCEM (T-cell acute lymphoblastic leukemia) cells. Factors presented include cell proliferation for 20 cells initial population (a) and 200 cells initial population (b).

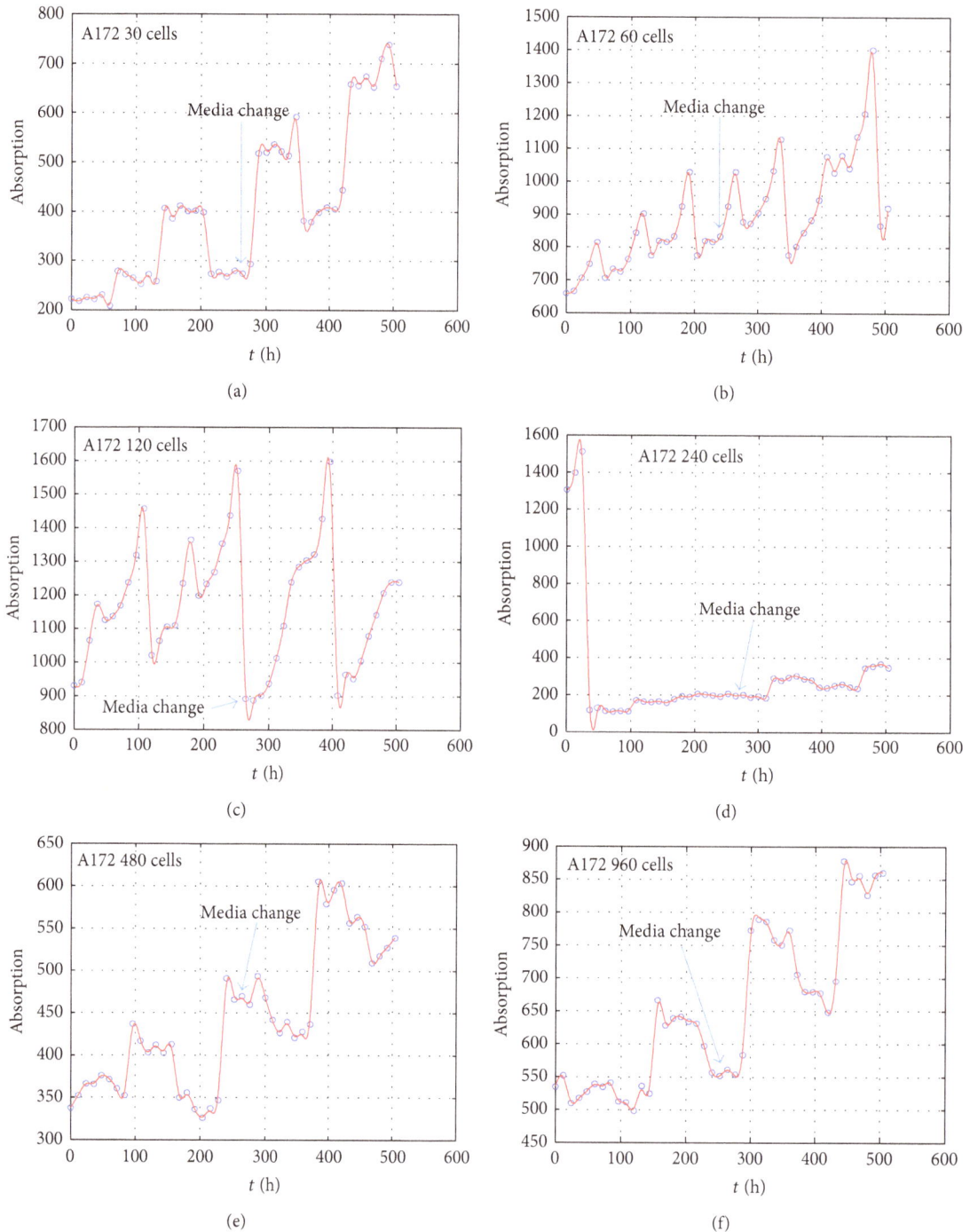

FIGURE 5: Graphical representation of time-series experiments for the A172 (glioblastoma) cells. Factors presented include the cell proliferation measurements as photometric absorption for different initial cells populations: 30 cells (a), 60 cells (b), 120 cells (c), 240 cells (d), 480 cells (e), and 960 cells (f).

hematology analyzer (CellTaq-α, Nihon Kohden). In addition, for the adherent cells, each plate was supplemented with 10% alamarBlue, a nontoxic dye that turns from blue to red due to its oxidation in the mitochondria.

2.4. Mathematical Computations. We used a one-dimensional representation based on the assumption that the pre-

sent state of our system is dependent upon the previous one. So, our system is better described by the logistic equation, as

$$f\left(x_{n+1}\right) = kx_n\left(1 - x_n\right) \qquad (1)$$

and with respect to time

$$\dot{x}_n = kx_n\left(1 - x_n\right) \qquad (2)$$

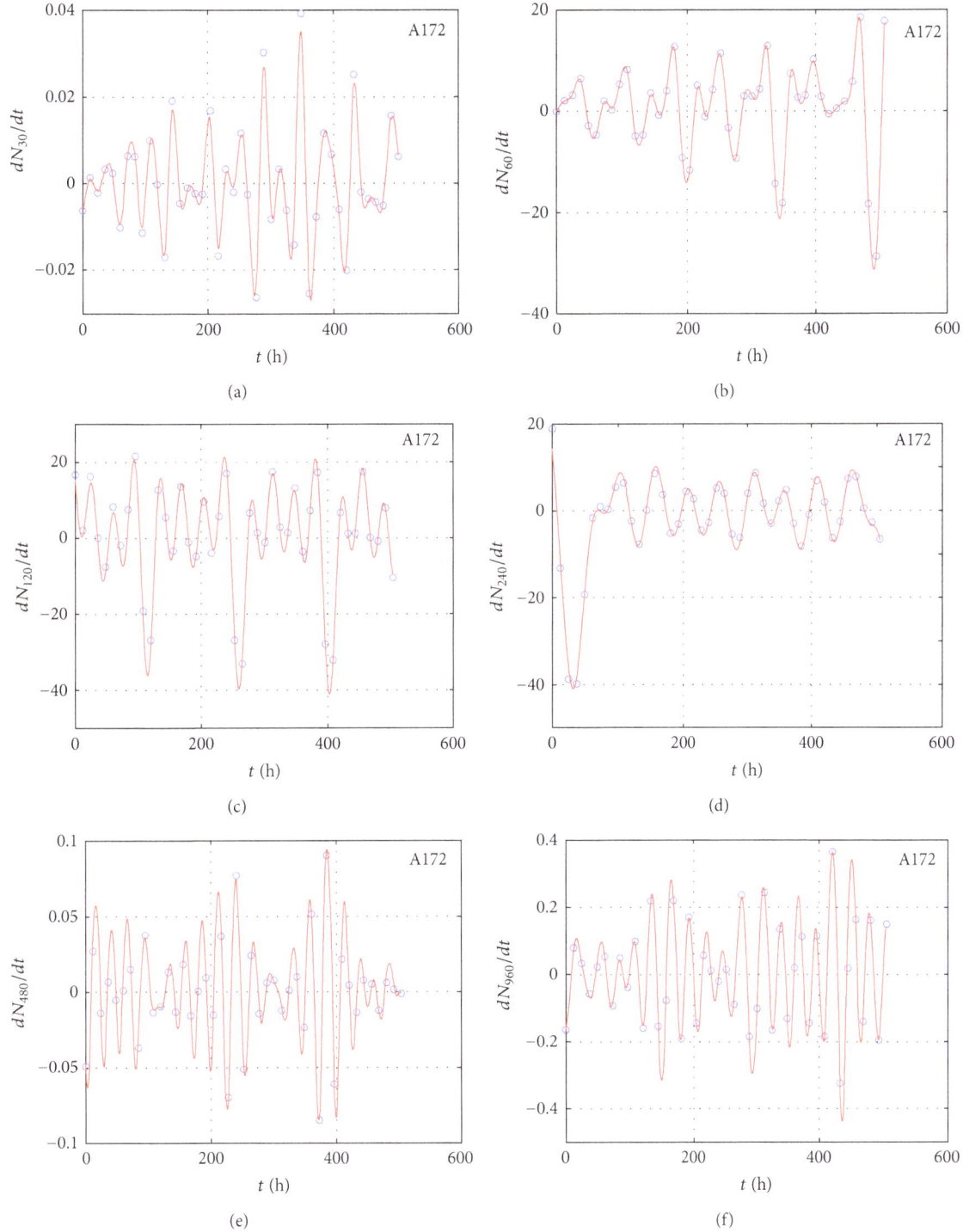

FIGURE 6: Graphical representation of time-series experiments for the A172 (glioblastoma) cells. Factors presented include the dN/dt for different initial cells populations: 30 cells (a), 60 cells (b), 120 cells (c), 240 cells (d), 480 cells (e), and 960 cells (f).

(the *logistic differential equation*). Both equations belong to the family of logistic equations of the form

$$f(x) = kx(1-x), \qquad (3)$$

where k is the proliferation constant. For the analysis of the data we utilized phase-space and return maps and used the geometrical representation, as previously proposed [3]. To

find the fractal dimensions of the measured variables, we calculated two fractal variables: N and R. N represents the number of "squares" needed for a fractal shape to be completed and their respective "square size" R. By definition, if the first derivative of $d \ln N / d \ln R$ remains constant for a space of R, this is the fractal dimension of the shape, in the present case of the cell proliferation trajectory. All mathematical

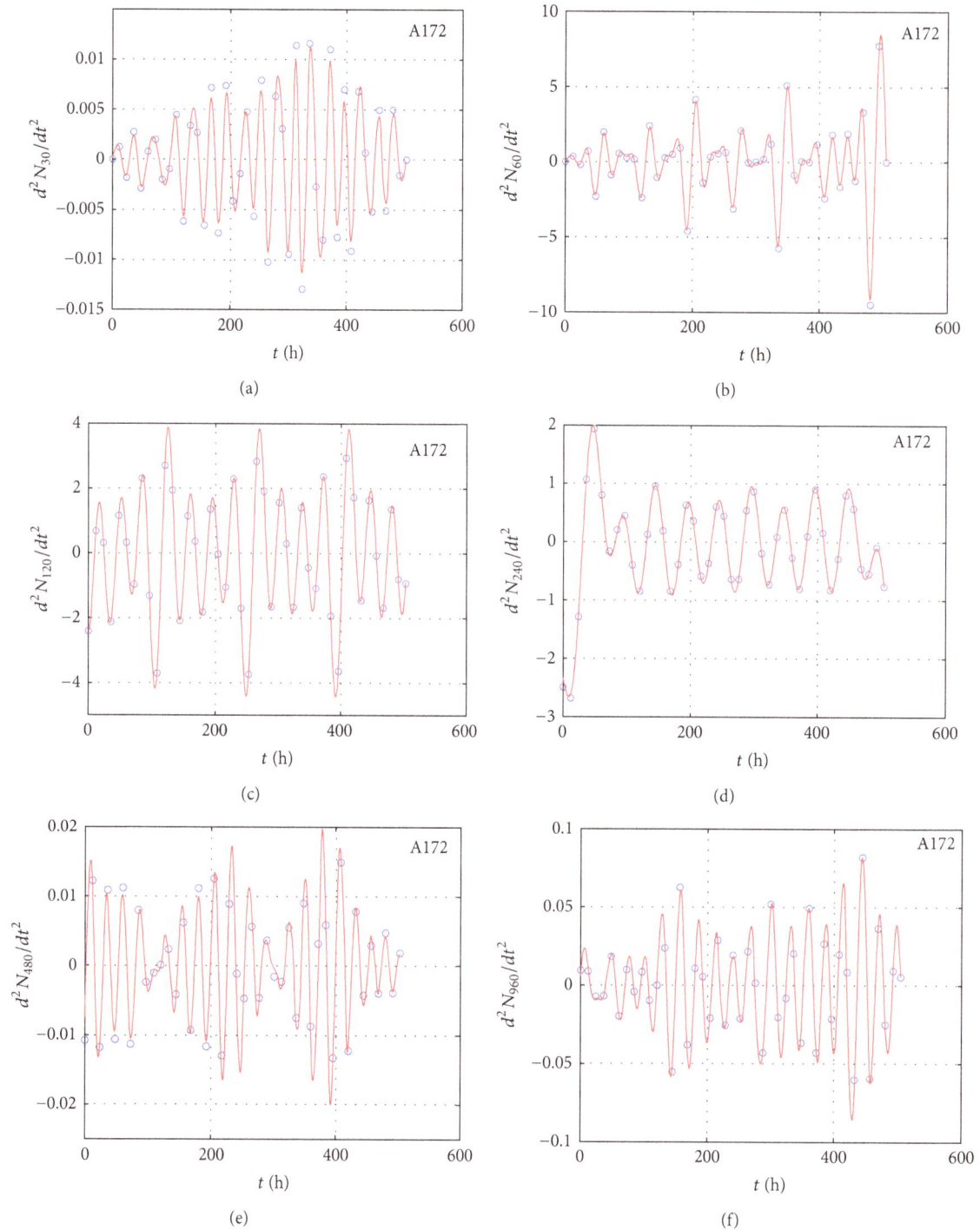

FIGURE 7: Graphical representation of time-series experiments for the A172 (glioblastoma) cells. Factors presented include the d^2N/dt^2 for different initial cells populations: 30 cells (a), 60 cells (b), 120 cells (c), 240 cells (d), 480 cells (e), and 960 cells (f).

computations were performed in the MATLAB computing environment.

3. Results

We measured the proliferation of the three CNS tumor cells and the CCRF-CEM cells *in vitro*. Due to the large amount

of data, the proliferation results are presented in three-dimensional graphs. The time-series proliferation results in the A172, 1321N1, and TE671 cells revealed that proliferation follows an oscillatory pattern (Figures 1–3). The rate of growth $[N(t+1)/Nt]$ appeared to manifest the most stable oscillatory pattern, among all measurements that we performed (Figures 1(b), 2(b), and 3(b)). In order to resolve more the patterns of

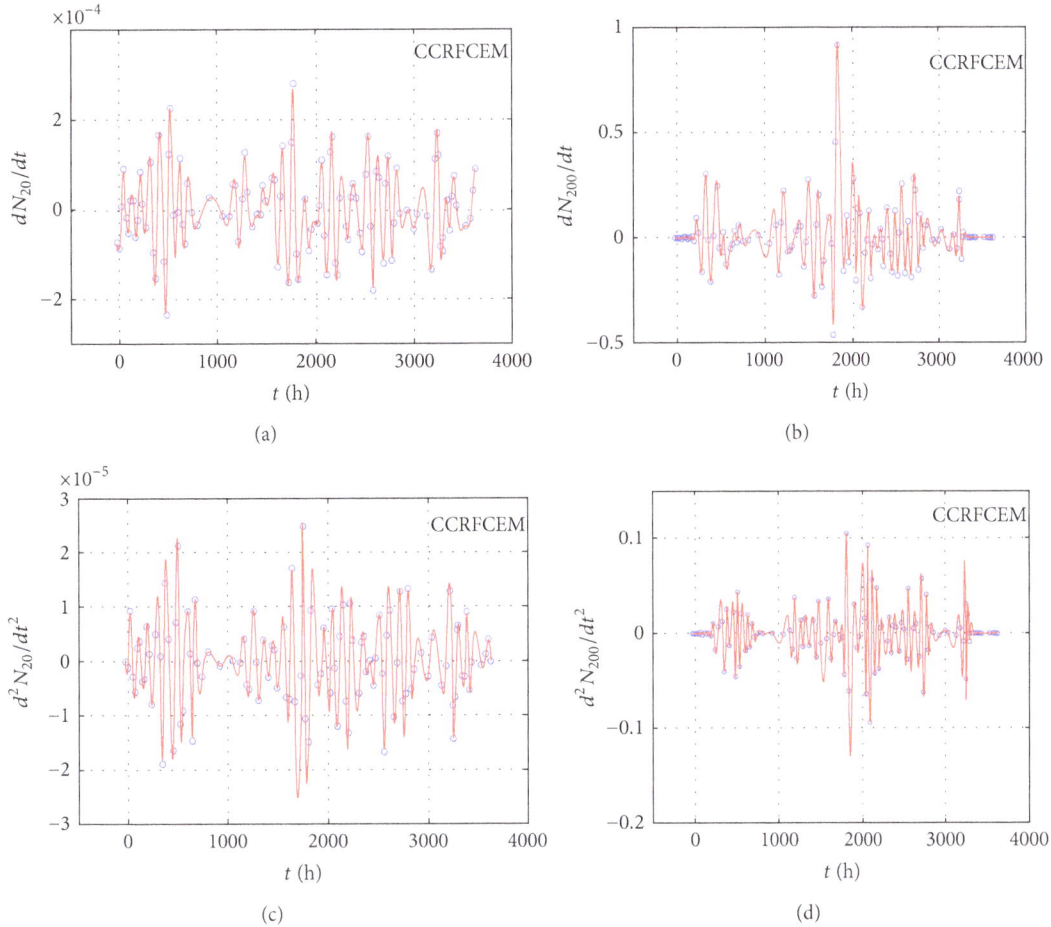

FIGURE 8: Graphical representation of time-series experiments for the CCRFCEM (T-cell acute lymphoblastic leukemia) cells. Factors presented include the dN/dt for different initial cells populations: 20 cells (a), 200 cells (b), the d^2N/dt^2 for the same populations 20 cells (c), and 200 cells (d).

oscillation, we present the proliferative pattern for the CCRF-CEM cells, which resembles that of adherent cells (Figure 4). As a representative resolution, the proliferation dynamics of the A172 cells (Figure 5), characteristic for all adherent cell lines, clearly revealed an oscillatory pattern in cellular growth velocity (Figure 6) and acceleration (Figure 7), respectively. It appears that cells do not proliferate in a linear pattern; rather they oscillate while adapting to the environmental conditions. Apart from testing this in adherent cells, we also applied our question to cells growing in suspension. Of major interest, these cells also exhibited similar dynamics (Figure 8). Therefore, our results support that different cell types manifest similar proliferation patterns, suggesting that a similar self-similarity pattern exists among different cellular types. In order to investigate self-similarity, it was necessary to show that cell proliferation factors follow some form of repetition. In systems biology, when the first derivative $d \ln N / d \ln R$ remains constant in a space R, it is a hint of self-similarity. Interestingly, the rate of proliferation was equal to 1 for all cell types, while for the growth velocity and acceleration for the A172 cells it was equal to 0.80888 (Figure 9). In order to conceive the meaning of those numbers, two shapes with the

same self-similarity measures are mentioned: the *Cantor sets* ($d \ln N / d \ln R = 1$) and the *Apollonian Gasket* (self-similarity value = 0.8). Our results confirmed two interesting points: (1) cell growth factors follow oscillatory dynamics (of nonlinear nature) and (2) different cell types followed similar dynamics of growth, irrespective of whether they grow as adherent or suspension cells, hinting towards a common mechanism of cellular proliferation.

4. Discussion

In the present work we identified nonlinear factors of cellular proliferation, in three CNS tumor cell lines and one leukemic cell line. Since our results show that cell growth is of nonlinear nature, we propose an initial theoretical framework for the analysis of such phenomena and for future considerations. This knowledge could be useful in treating tumors, since by understanding the mechanisms of cellular proliferation we could interpret the factors that determine the progression of the disease and/or metastasis. Biological systems are extremely complicated and manifest non-linear/chaotic phenomena. Among others [15, 32], we strongly support that

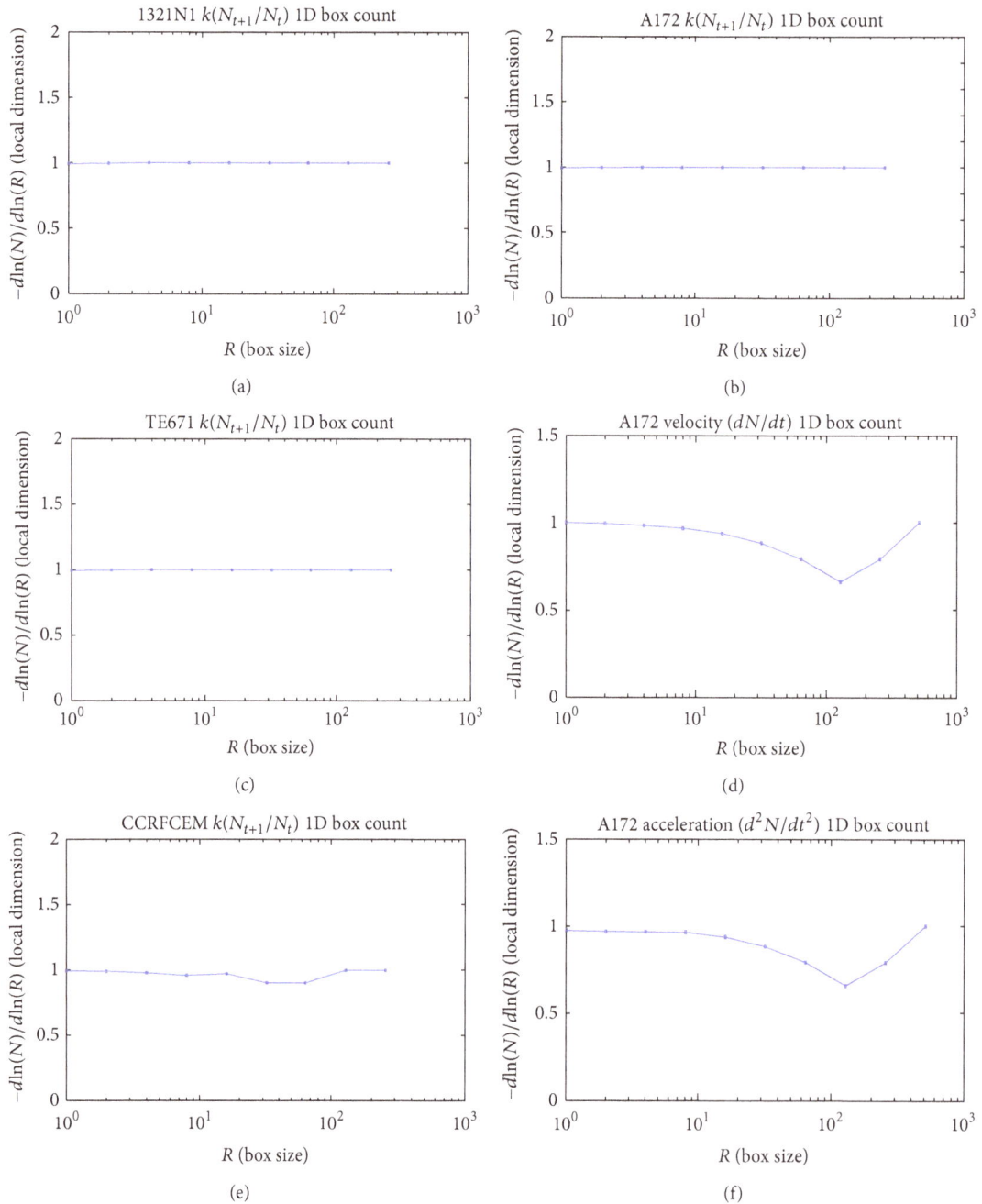

FIGURE 9: Graphical representation of self-similarity calculations for the 1321N1 cells with respect to rate of proliferation (a), for the A172 cells with respect to rate of proliferation (b), for the TE671 cells with respect to the rate of proliferation (c), for the A172 cells with respect to the velocity of cell growth (d), for the CCRFCEM cells with respect to the rate of proliferation (e), and for the A172 cells with respect to the acceleration of cell growth.

the maturity of biological sciences can be achieved through their integration with other disciplines, such as those of mathematics and physics. This integration will enable the research community to give generalized models for phenomena such as the non-linear nature of cellular growth.

We have previously described the chaotic patterns of the leukemic cell line that we used [15]. These patterns were shown by the orbits/trajectories of proliferation and the

Lyapunov exponents (one of the criteria of chaos existence). Such an example is the understanding of cellular proliferation in which we attempted to contribute with our hints. Here, we show that that different cell types follow similar dynamics with respect to proliferation, however their dynamics follow different trajectories. This difference arises from the probable reason that it is possible that all trajectories can be described by the same function, yet with different constants. Another question arising is that when cellular populations are measured with respect to time, they would give natural numbers corresponding to the exact or approximate number of cells present in the system. At the same time, all other physical variables calculated return oscillations. The question posed, concerns the role of gene expression in controlling cellular proliferation. A possible explanation is that cells follow oscillatory dynamics exactly the same way gene expression does [11].

Another issue in tumor proliferation dynamics that remains unanswered is the conditions at the time of the disease onset. The only knowledge we have thus far, concerning tumors, originates from the time of clinical presentation, at diagnosis. Practically, we have complete lack of knowledge from the time of tumor initiation to the time of tumor presentation. In that sense, the understanding of the proliferation dynamics of tumor cells is critical since it could provide insight into the understanding of tumor initiation. Supposing we could describe the dynamics of cellular proliferation in a formal, mathematical form, we would be able not only to predict the time zero (the starting point) but also to understand the mechanics of this progression. Additionally, if we suppose that such a formal description could be applied to several tumor types, we could conclude to a general rule of tumor proliferation. To the best of our knowledge, there are no previous works dealing with this subject and posing these questions.

The implications of the understanding of proliferation dynamics are immense. To date, we do not have a sufficient theory that could allow us understand and predict cellular growth. This is easy to prove if we ask a simple question: given the population of cells today can we predict the population after 24 hours? The answer is no, since the only way we can do it is by approximation and this can be done only statistically. In other words, if we could predict the future cellular population based on the past population, this could lead us to the starting point of cellular proliferation, information that would be of extreme importance in cancer biology.

Concluding, in the present work we aimed to set a framework for the detection of global patterns in cellular proliferation. Considering the fact that our knowledge in tumor biology comes only from the clinical presentation of the disease, the discovery of global models of tumor progression and proliferation could provide more insight in tumor biology and be used for therapeutic or prognostic purposes. Future work should focus on the investigation of the rates of cellular death in the same proliferation models and, most importantly, expand this model to gene expression for the same proliferation models, thus moving from phenotype to the genotype.

Conflict of Interests

The authors declare that there is no conflict of interests regarding the publication of this paper.

References

[1] W. J. Ewens, *Mathematical Population Genetics*, Interdisciplinary Applied Mathematics, Springer, New York, NY, USA, 2nd edition, 2004.

[2] R. Durrett, J. Foo, K. Leder, J. Mayberry, and F. Michor, "Evolutionary dynamics of tumor progression with random fitness values," *Theoretical Population Biology*, vol. 78, no. 1, pp. 54–66, 2010.

[3] C. Wolfrom, N. P. Chau, J. Maigné et al., "Evidence for deterministic chaos in aperiodic oscillations of proliferative activity in long-term cultured Fao hepatoma cells," *Journal of Cell Science*, vol. 113, no. 6, pp. 1069–1074, 2000.

[4] M. Laurent, J. Deschatrette, and C. M. Wolfrom, "Unmasking chaotic attributes in time series of living cell populations," *PLoS ONE*, vol. 5, no. 2, Article ID e9346, 2010.

[5] S. Guerroui, J. Deschatrette, and C. Wolfrom, "Prolonged perturbation of the oscillations of hepatoma Fao cell proliferation by a single small dose of methotrexate," *Pathologie Biologie*, vol. 53, no. 5, pp. 290–294, 2005.

[6] A. Zaravinos, G. I. Lambrou, I. Boulalas, D. Delakas, and D. A. Spandidos, "Identification of common differentially expressed genes in urinary bladder cancer," *PLoS ONE*, vol. 6, no. 4, Article ID e18135, 2011.

[7] A. Zaravinos, G. I. Lambrou, D. Volanis, D. Delakas, and D. A. Spandidos, "Spotlight on differentially expressed genes in urinary bladder cancer," *PLoS ONE*, vol. 6, no. 4, Article ID e18255, 2011.

[8] G. I. Lambrou, M. Adamaki, D. Delakas, D. A. Spandidos, P. Vlahopoulos, and A. Zaravinos, "Gene expression is highly correlated on the chromosome level in urinary bladder cancer," *Cell Cycle*, vol. 12, no. 10, pp. 1544–1559, 2013.

[9] A. Zaravinos, G. Lambrou, I. Boulalas, D. Volanis, D. Delakas, and D. Spandidos, "UP-01.018 linear correlations in chromosomal-based gene expression in urinary bladder cancer," *Urology*, vol. 78, supplement 3, p. S190, 2011.

[10] B. A. Cohen, R. D. Mitra, J. D. Hughes, and G. M. Church, "A computational analysis of whole-genome expression data reveals chromosomal domains of gene expression," *Nature Genetics*, vol. 26, no. 2, pp. 183–186, 2000.

[11] J. C. Mar and J. Quackenbush, "Decomposition of gene expression state space trajectories," *PLoS Computational Biology*, vol. 5, no. 12, Article ID e1000626, 10 pages, 2009.

[12] J. C. Mar, R. Rubio, and J. Quackenbush, "Inferring steady state single-cell gene expression distributions from analysis of mesoscopic samples," *Genome Biology*, vol. 7, article R119, 2006.

[13] J. R. Chabot, J. M. Pedraza, P. Luitel, and A. van Oudenaarden, "Stochastic gene expression out-of-steady-state in the cyanobacterial circadian clock," *Nature*, vol. 450, no. 7173, pp. 1249–1252, 2007.

[14] T. Degenhardt, K. N. Rybakova, A. Tomaszewska et al., "Population-level transcription cycles derive from stochastic timing of single-cell transcription," *Cell*, vol. 138, no. 3, pp. 489–501, 2009.

[15] G. I. Lambrou, A. Zaravinos, M. Adamaki, D. A. Spandidos, F. Tzortzatou-Stathopoulou, and S. Vlachopoulos, "Pathway simulations in common oncogenic drivers of leukemic and rhabdomyosarcoma cells: a systems biology approach," *International Journal of Oncology*, vol. 40, no. 5, pp. 1365–1390, 2012.

[16] R. M. May, "Simple mathematical models with very complicated dynamics," *Nature*, vol. 261, no. 5560, pp. 459–467, 1976.

[17] R. M. May, "Biological populations with nonoverlapping generations: stable points, stable cycles, and chaos," *Science*, vol. 186, no. 4164, pp. 645–647, 1974.

[18] M. C. Mackey and L. Glass, "Oscillation and chaos in physiological control systems," *Science*, vol. 197, no. 4300, pp. 287–289, 1977.

[19] P.-C. Romond, M. Rustici, D. Gonze, and A. Goldbeter, "Alternating oscillations and chaos in a model of two coupled biochemical oscillators driving successive phases of the cell cycle," *Annals of the New York Academy of Sciences*, vol. 879, pp. 180–193, 1999.

[20] R. M. McAllister, H. Isaacs, R. Rongey et al., "Establishment of a human medulloblastoma cell line," *International Journal of Cancer*, vol. 20, no. 2, pp. 206–212, 1977.

[21] M. R. Stratton, J. Darling, G. J. Pilkington, P. L. Lantos, B. R. Reeves, and C. S. Cooper, "Characterization of the human cell line TE671," *Carcinogenesis*, vol. 10, no. 5, pp. 899–905, 1989.

[22] T. R. Chen, C. Dorotinsky, M. Macy, and R. Hay, "Cell identity resolved," *Nature*, vol. 340, no. 6229, p. 106, 1989.

[23] P. J. Syapin, P. M. Salvaterra, and J. K. Engelhardt, "Neuronal-like features of TE671 cells: presence of a functional nicotinic cholinergic receptor," *Brain Research*, vol. 231, no. 2, pp. 365–377, 1982.

[24] O. I. Olopade, R. B. Jenkins, D. T. Ransom et al., "Molecular analysis of deletions of the short arm of chromosome 9 in human gliomas," *Cancer Research*, vol. 52, no. 9, pp. 2523–2529, 1992.

[25] L. C. Showe, M. Ballantine, K. Nishikura, J. Erikson, H. Kaji, and C. M. Croce, "Cloning and sequencing of a c-myc oncogene in a Burkitt's lymphoma cell line that is translocated to a germ line alpha switch region," *Molecular and Cellular Biology*, vol. 5, no. 3, pp. 501–509, 1985.

[26] K. Bhatia, W. Goldschmidts, M. Gutierrez, G. Gaidano, R. Dalla-Favera, and I. Magrath, "Hemi- or homozygosity: a requirement for some but not other p53 mutant proteins to accumulate and exert a pathogenetic effect," *FASEB Journal*, vol. 7, no. 10, pp. 951–956, 1993.

[27] L. Miranda, J. Wolf, S. Pichuantes, R. Duke, and A. Pranzusoff, "Isolation of the human PC6 gene encoding the putative host protease for HIV-1 gp160 processing in CD4+ T lymphocytes," *Proceedings of the National Academy of Sciences of the United States of America*, vol. 93, no. 15, pp. 7695–7700, 1996.

[28] C. Naujokat, O. Sezer, H. Zinke, A. Leclere, S. Hauptmann, and K. Possinger, "Proteasome inhibitors induce caspase-dependent apoptosis and accumulation of p21(WAF1/Cip1) in human immature leukemic cells," *European Journal of Haematology*, vol. 65, no. 4, pp. 221–236, 2000.

[29] G. E. Foley, H. Lazarus, S. Farber, B. G. Uzman, B. A. Boone, and R. E. McCarthy, "Continuous culture of human lymphoblasts from peripheral blood of a child with acute leukemia," *Cancer*, vol. 18, pp. 522–529, 1965.

[30] B. G. Uzman, G. E. Foley, S. Farber, and H. Lazarus, "Morphologic variations in human leukemic lymphoblasts (CCRF-CEM cells) after long-term culture and exposure to chemotherapeutic agents. A study with the electron microscope," *Cancer*, vol. 19, no. 11, pp. 1725–1742, 1966.

[31] P. A. Sandstrom and T. M. Buttke, "Autocrine production of extracellular catalase prevents apoptosis of the human CEM T-cell line in serum-free medium," *Proceedings of the National Academy of Sciences of the United States of America*, vol. 90, no. 10, pp. 4708–4712, 1993.

[32] G. I. Lambrou, A. Chatziioannou, S. Vlahopoulos, M. Moschovi, and G. P. Chrousos, "Evidence for deterministic chaos in aperiodic oscillations of acute lymphoblastic leukemia cells in long-term culture," *Journal of Chaotic Modelling and Simulation*, vol. 1, no. 1, pp. 119–126, 2011.

8

Multimodality Imaging in Cardiooncology

Fausto Pizzino,[1] Giampiero Vizzari,[1] Rubina Qamar,[2] Charles Bomzer,[2] Scipione Carerj,[1] Concetta Zito,[1] and Bijoy K. Khandheria[3]

[1] *Cardiology Unit, Department of Clinical and Experimental Medicine, University of Messina, Azienda Ospedaliera Universitaria "Policlinico G. Martino" and Universita' degli Studi di Messina, Via Consolare Valeria No. 12, 98100 Messina, Italy*
[2] *Aurora Advanced Healthcare, St. Luke's Medical Centers, 2801 W. Kinnickinnic River Parkway, No. 840, Milwaukee, WI 53215, USA*
[3] *Aurora Cardiovascular Services, Aurora Sinai/Aurora St. Luke's Medical Centers, University of Wisconsin School of Medicine and Public Health, 2801 W. Kinnickinnic River Parkway, No. 840, Milwaukee, WI 53215, USA*

Correspondence should be addressed to Bijoy K. Khandheria; publishing22@aurora.org

Academic Editor: Daniel Lenihan

Cardiotoxicity represents a rising problem influencing prognosis and quality of life of chemotherapy-treated patients. Anthracyclines and trastuzumab are the drugs most commonly associated with development of a cardiotoxic effect. Heart failure, myocardial ischemia, hypertension, myocarditis, and thrombosis are typical manifestation of cardiotoxicity by chemotherapeutic agents. Diagnosis and monitoring of cardiac side-effects of cancer treatment is of paramount importance. Echocardiography and nuclear medicine methods are widely used in clinical practice and left ventricular ejection fraction is the most important parameter to asses myocardial damage secondary to chemotherapy. However, left ventricular ejection decrease is a delayed phenomenon, occurring after a long stage of silent myocardial damage that classic imaging methods are not able to detect. New imaging techniques including three-dimensional echocardiography, speckle tracking echocardiography, and cardiac magnetic resonance have demonstrated high sensitivity in detecting the earliest alteration of left ventricular function associated with future development of chemotherapy-induced cardiomyopathy. Early diagnosis of cardiac involvement in cancer patients can allow for timely and adequate treatment management and the introduction of cardioprotective strategies.

1. Introduction

Chemotherapy is widely used in the treatment of several neoplastic diseases, leading to an improvement in survival and prognosis in a large number of patients. Side effects are the most common cause of restriction to its use. Cardiotoxicity represents a frequent complication secondary to the intake of some classes of chemotherapeutic agents, with significant consequences on patients' outcome [1]. Heart failure (HF) is the most common manifestation of chemotherapy induced cardiotoxicity. Although left ventricular ejection fraction (LVEF) is widely utilized in monitoring the cardiac function in clinical practice, it has not demonstrated high sensitivity in detecting subclinical myocardial dysfunction. New parameters and new imaging techniques have been developed in order to overcome the limitations related to isolate evaluation of LVEF [2, 3]. A diagnostic approach based on the integrative use of different imaging techniques can allow early detection of cardiotoxicity, improving the therapeutic management of the neoplastic disease, quality of life, and mortality rate.

2. Clinical Manifestations of Cardiotoxicity

HF occurs with an incidence range included between 0.5 and 28%, depending on the medication used, and is the most common clinical manifestation of the cardiotoxicity induced by chemotherapy [1]. The onset of dyspnea, chest pain, peripheral edema, and asthenia is usually preceded by a variable stage of subclinical myocardial dysfunction. Traditionally cardiotoxicity induced by chemotherapy has been classified into two groups [4]: Type I chemotherapy-related myocardial dysfunction is typical of anthracyclines and has been related to oxidative stress causing myocardiocytes damage and death; it is an irreversible, dose-dependent process and is characterized by ultrastructural alteration identifiable by myocardial biopsy. Type II chemotherapy-related myocardial dysfunction is induced by trastuzumab and is related to the inhibition of ErbB2 pathway. Usually the dysfunction is reversible and not related to the cumulative dose [5].

Coronary artery disease, presenting with asymptomatic T-wave changes, chest pain, acute coronary syndromes, and myocardial infarction, is mainly related to use of antimetabolites (particularly 5-fluorouracil). De Forni reported an incidence of acute coronary syndromes of about 7.6% in patients treated with 5-fluorouracil while cardiac mortality reached 2.2% [6].

Hypertension is a relatively common side effect of several antiangiogenetic drugs like bevacizumab, sunitinib, and sorafenib. Underlying artery hypertension is the most important risk factor for the development of the secondary disease.

Cancer patients have a high incidence of thromboembolic events depending on cancer-related factors (primitive malignancy localization, immobility, HF, arrhythmias, etc.) [7] and additional effects of some chemotherapeutic agents, particularly, cisplatin and thalidomide [8, 9].

3. Cancer Treatment and Cardiotoxicity: Who Are the Actors?

The majority of studies on cardiotoxicity focus on patients treated with anthracyclines and trastuzumab. Anthracyclines (doxorubicin, daunorubicin, and epirubicin) use has been related to onset of HF within 1 year in about 2% of treated patients [1]. The HF incidence increases to 28% when the patients are exposed to the association of anthracyclines and trastuzumab [1]. Cardiotoxic effect has been described for classes of drugs other than the anthracyclines and trastuzumab such as inhibitors of tyrosine kinases (imatinib, dasatinib, nilotinib, sunitinib, sorafenib, and bevacizumab), antimetabolites (5-fluorouracil), alkylating agents (cisplatin, cyclophosphamide), and taxanes (docetaxel and paclitaxel) [10]. Radiotherapy has become an important instrument in the treatment of several malignances and is more often associated to standard chemotherapy treatment. Irradiation of the mediastinum with a cumulative dose >30 Gy and a daily fractioning >2 Gy appeared to be related to a high risk of developing cardiac dysfunction [11].

4. How to Diagnose Cardiotoxicity? The Need for Multimodality Imaging

Myocardial biopsy is still considered the most accurate and specific method in identifying the myocardial damage induced by chemotherapy, detecting the ultrastructural alteration of cardiomyocytes [12]. Nevertheless its invasiveness limited its use in clinical practice. Imaging methods emerged in the last decades as the landmark in monitoring cardiotoxicity in cancer patients. Left ventricular ejection fraction (LVEF) is widely considered the most important parameter for the diagnosis of cardiotoxicity. The most validated definition of cardiotoxicity has been established by the cardiac

review and evaluation committee [13]. Cardiotoxicity can be defined either by the onset of HF symptoms and signs or by an asymptomatic decrease of LVEF as follows.

Cardiac Review and Evaluation Committee Criteria for Diagnosis of Cardiotoxicity. The diagnosis of cardiotoxicity is established if one or more criteria are present:

> cardiomyopathy characterized by a decrease in cardiac LVEF that was either global or more severe in the septum,
>
> symptoms of congestive heart failure,
>
> associated signs of congestive heart failure, including but not limited to third heart sound (S3) gallop, tachycardia, or both,
>
> decline in LVEF of at least 5% to less than 55% with accompanying signs or symptoms of congestive heart failure,
>
> decline in LVEF of at least 10% to below 55% without accompanying signs or symptoms.

Although the evolution of most recent imaging techniques has allowed accurate and reproducible evaluation of volumes and of alteration of LVEF, recently it has appeared evident that the drop of LVEF represents a late phenomenon in the physiopathology of the chemotherapy-induced cardiotoxicity. This evidence has led the clinicians to look to other imaging methods that evaluate cardiac function independently of cardiac volumes changes, aiming to detect the earliest manifestation of cardiotoxicity and allowing for the appropriate management of the therapy. Some of these methods such as speckle tracking imaging have been already introduced in clinical practice whereas others are under investigation in experimental settings.

5. Methods Based on the Evaluation of LVEF: From Echocardiography to Cardiac Magnetic Resonance

5.1. Two-Dimensional Echocardiography. LVEF evaluated by two-dimensional echocardiography (2DE) is the most used parameter in monitoring the cardiac func-tion in chemotherapy-treated patients (Videos 1 and 2; see Supplementary Material available online at http://dx.doi.org/10.1155/2015/263950). The Simpson biplane method is the most validated technique to obtain the left ventricle volumes, while monodimensional measurements are less accurate. However, LVEF derived by the Simpson formula relies on geometrical assumptions and the manual tracking of the endocardial border can differ when performed by different observers, particularly with poor quality images. Indeed, a recent investigation reported that 2DE is unable to estimate a decrease <10% within the 95% of confidence interval when performed by different investigators [14]; considering that cardiotoxicity has been defined as a drop of LVEF ≥10% or ≥5% in presence of HF symptoms, it is clear that the diagnosis provided by 2DE can be burdened by significant inaccuracy. Nevertheless, LVEF derived by 2DE remains the most used method in clinical practice because of its high availability and feasibility.

5.2. Real-Time Three-Dimensional Echocardiography. Real-time three-dimensional echocardiography can obtain a full-volume scan of the left ventricle, providing a quantification of volumes independently of geometrical assumptions. LVEF provided by RT-3DE (Figure 1) demonstrated elevated correlation with the values derived by cardiac magnetic resonance as shown in a study on 50 patients where Walker reported a correlation ranging from 0.90 to 0.97, while 2DE revealed a weak correlation (from 0.31 to 0.53) [15]. LVEF derived by RT-3DE showed the lower intraobserver and interobserver variability (0.017 and 0.027, resp.) and the best minimal detectable variation (4.8% intraobserver and 7.5% interobserver) [14].

5.3. Contrast Echocardiography. The accuracy in the measurement of volumes and LVEF is affected negatively by the poor quality of the acoustic window, which often limits the adequate visualization of the endocardial border. Use of contrast echocardiography demonstrated an incremental value, reducing the interobserver variability in evaluating the cardiac volumes and wall motion score index [16]. Use of contrast associated with 2DE resulted in a reduction of the interreader variability of LVEF from 14.3% (95% confidence interval, 11.7%–16.8%) to 8% (95% CI, 6.3%–9.7%; $P < 0.001$) [17]. Left ventricle opacization is recommended when two or more segments are not well visualized [18, 19]. The value of contrast administration with RT-3DE is uncertain; Hoffmann demonstrated a reduction of interobserver variability from 14.3% to 7.4% [17], while Thavendiranathan did not report any incremental value in comparison to noncontrast RT-3DE [14].

5.4. Nuclear Medicine Imaging. In the past, MUGA has been the most common alternative to echocardiography in the evaluation of chemotherapy-treated patients [20]. MUGA makes use of 99mTC-erythrocyte labeling enabling the visualization of the cardiac blood pool by γ-camera with electrocardiogram-triggered acquisitions. The final result provides a highly reproducible and precise quantification of LV volumes and dyssynchrony independently of geometrical assumption [21]. LVEF values provided by MUGA demonstrated reproducibility and sensitivity comparable to 3D echocardiography and CMR. Walker reported a correlation between LVEF evaluated by MUGA and CMR ranging from 0.87 to 0.97 [15]. Nevertheless, now MUGA is rarely used in clinical practice mainly because of the increased radiation exposure for patients and the introduction of new noninvasive techniques such as CMR and RT-3DE.

5.5. Cardiac Magnetic Resonance (CMR). In the last years, CMR has emerged as the criterion standard technique in the evaluation of LV mass [22] and volumes. It provides a modeling of the cardiac chambers free from geometric assumptions and independently of acoustic window, providing the most accurate evaluation of global and regional myocardial dysfunction [23]. Armstrong demonstrated a decrease of LVEF

and mass in a population of asymptomatic adult survivors of childhood cancer treated with anthracyclines in which other imaging techniques did not detect alterations [24] and similar findings have been reported by Ylänen [25]. CMR is indicated for the evaluation of patients treated with potentially cardiotoxic medications as an alternative to 2DE, particularly in patients with an echocardiographic cardiotoxicity diagnosis in whom the interruption of treatment could be inadvisable or in patients with poor echocardiographic images [26]. Although it has advantages, CMR usage is limited by its low availability and elevated cost. The method is not indicated in patients with metallic prosthesis, and the results are less accurate in subjects with arrhythmias.

6. New Methods and Strategies to Monitor Cardiac Function Independently of LVEF: Clinical Practice and Future Insights

6.1. 2DE and Tissue Doppler Imaging (TDI). Alteration of diastolic function precedes the systolic dysfunction often representing the first sign of early cardiac dysfunction caused by anticancer agents [27]. 2DE is the best method for the evaluation of diastole. The decrease of the early to late ventricular filling velocities (E/A) ratio, the enlargement of the left atrium, and the increase of isovolumic relaxation time are common findings in chemotherapy-treated patients [28, 29] with impairment of diastolic function as well as reduction of E^1/A^1 ratio [5, 30, 31] and the increase of E/E^1 ratio >10 [28]. Although the diastolic dysfunction is frequent in chemotherapy-treated patients, its value in predicting the late development of cardiotoxicity is affected by many factors, such as aging, hypertension, and load conditions. Some authors reported that E, E^1, E/A, and isovolumic relaxation time did not predict late LVEF <50% within three years after the start of treatment [32]. Analysis of systolic function performed by TDI provided contrasting results: in a study by Fallah-Rad 42 patients demonstrated a significant reduction of lateral S^1 within three months from the start of chemotherapy. The decrease was ≥0.6 cm/s in all 10 patients who later developed LVD [33]. However, the result of the study was limited by several biases: above all, there was a high incidence of cardiotoxicity in a relatively small and young population. In effect, other studies failed in revealing a significant reduction of S' in chemotherapy-treated patients [34, 35]. Myocardial deformation analysis derived from TDI demonstrated early alteration of both systolic and diastolic function after chemotherapy [36, 37]. Nevertheless, TDI measurements suffer from angle dependence, noise, translational movements, aliasing, and reverberation. For these reasons, myocardial deformation analysis derived by TDI has been almost totally replaced by speckle tracking echocardiography.

6.2. Two-Dimensional Speckle Tracking Echocardiography. Two-dimensional speckle tracking echocardiography (2D-STE) analyzes the myocardial deformation on two-dimensional images by tracking natural acoustic reflections and interference patterns, called "speckle." The software is able to provide the percentage of distance variation (deformation)

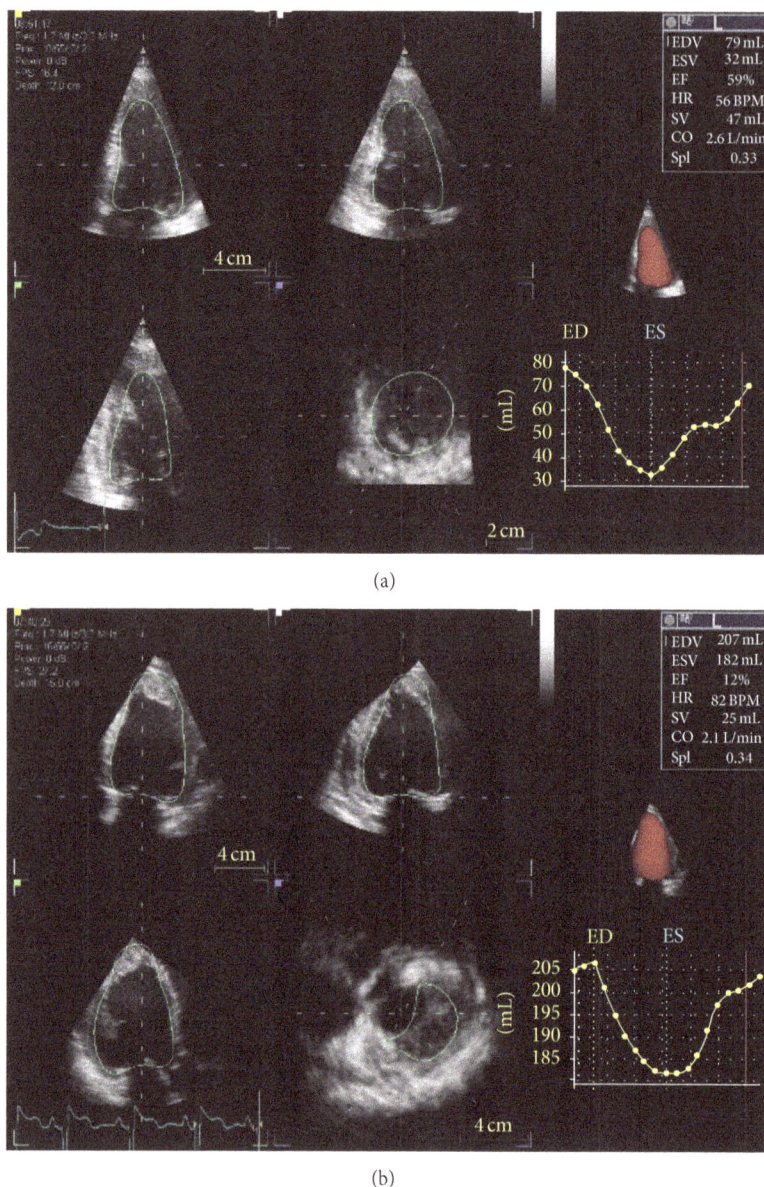

FIGURE 1: Three-dimensional echocardiography: evaluation of left ventricular ejection fraction in a normal patient (a) and in one with impaired function (b).

between speckles within a predefined region of interest, obtaining a value defined as "strain." The velocity of the deformation is defined "strain rate." 2D-STE provides an accurate definition of longitudinal, circumferential, and radial component of the ventricular deformation. Twist, untwist, and torsion are additional parameters that evaluate the torsional deformation of the left ventricle. Strain evaluated by 2D-STE detected early myocardial dysfunction in chemotherapy-treated patients [38, 39] (Figure 2 and Videos 3 and 4). The application of strain and strain rate to cardiotoxicity detection has been evaluated in several relatively small studies. Global longitudinal strain (GLS) appears to be the most sensitive parameter of deformation for the detection of early systolic dysfunction. Negishi demonstrated that, in 81 patients treated for breast cancer, GLS rate and early

diastolic strain rate were significantly decreased at 6 months from treatment, in comparison to baseline value in 30% of patients who developed cardiotoxicity at 12 months. GLS percentage variation was the strongest predictor of cardiotoxicity (area under the curve, 0.84) and a reduction >11% was the optimal cut-off (sensitiveness 65%, specificity 94%) [40]. Similar results have been reported by Plana showing that a decrease of >9% in GLS after the third cycle of epirubicin was the best independent and accurate predictor of cardiotoxicity (sensitiveness 84%, specificity 80%; $P = 0.0001$) in a sample of cancer treated patients [26]. Stoodley showed a correlation between reduction of GLS and cumulative dose of anthracyclines [41]. Thavendiranathan [42] collected the fragmentary data from several studies and reported the results in a comprehensive, systematic review.

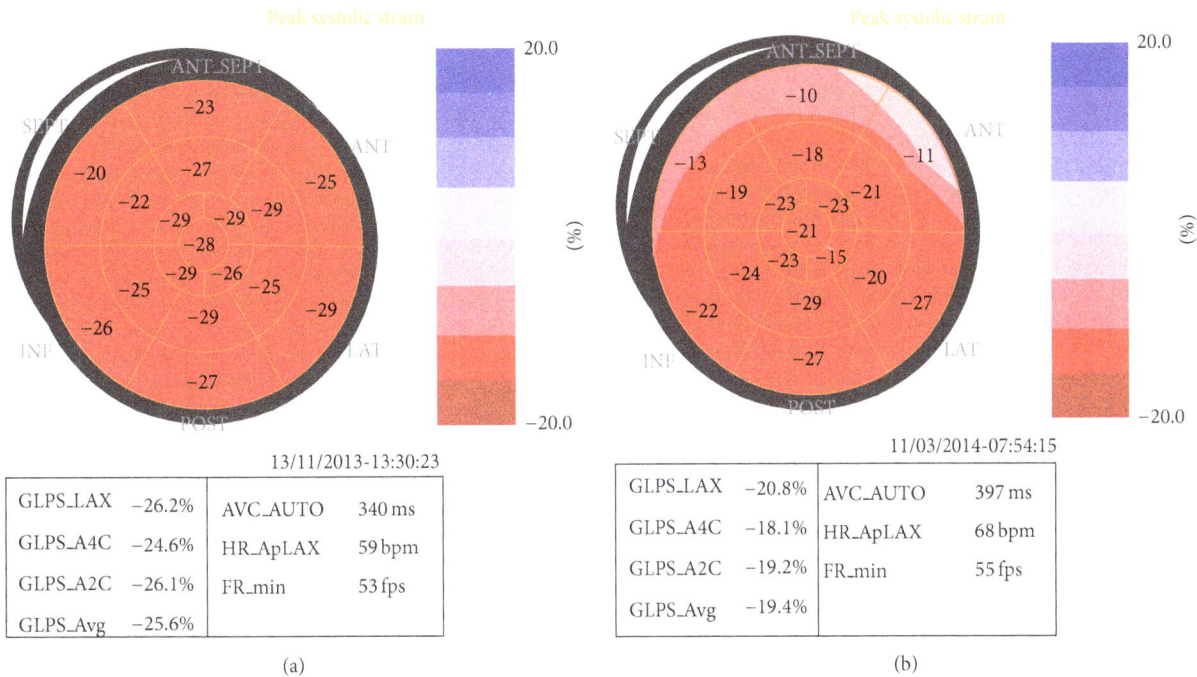

FIGURE 2: Bull's eyes showing a decrease of global and regional strain in a patient before (a) and after (b) treatment with chemotherapy. In the same patient the left ventricular ejection fraction was not significantly altered (see also Supplementary Videos 3 and 4).

The authors established that the percentage of change is a better indicator than a defined cut-off because of the variable baseline values. A variation in GLS ranging from 10% to 15% was the best predictor of future development of cardiotoxicity. Negishi established in 81 women treated with trastuzumab that GLS decrease can predict cardiotoxicity and an 11% reduction was the optimal cut-off (confidence interval 8.3%–14.6%) [40]. According to these findings, the recent consensus document released by the American Society of Echocardiography/European Association of Cardiovascular Imaging (ASE/EACVI) defined that a variation in GLS >15% is strongly predictive of future development of cardiotoxicity, while a variation <8% is not significant [26]. An important limitation associated with the use of STE is represented by differences in the deformation values provided by software from different vendors [43]. Waiting for a full standardization of the measurement, the recommendation is to evaluate the patients with the same software during the follow-up.

6.3. Three-Dimensional Speckle Tracking Echocardiography. Three-dimensional speckle tracking echocardiography (3D-STE) is one of the most advanced techniques in the evaluation of myocardial deformation. The possibility of evaluating the deformation on a full-volume model avoids the errors derived from the use of two-dimensional images. Xu compared 3D-STE to 2D-STE and revealed that GLS evaluation is slightly less feasible in comparison to 2D-STE (84.9% versus 97.2%); however, 3D-STE appeared less time-consuming (50.5 ± 6.4 sec versus 68.0 ± 9.2 sec) and the correlation was good between values obtained by the two methods appearing to be

larger for structural measurements rather than for deformation analysis. Inter- and intraobserver variability ranged from 4.8% to 7.9% [44]. Yu demonstrated that childhood cancer survivors evaluated by 3D-STE had significantly reduced GLS and torsion ($P < 0.001$) and greater systolic dyssynchrony index in comparison to healthy controls [45]. Mornoş found that GLS evaluated by 3D-STE was superior to biomarkers and to LVEF in predicting future development of cardiotoxicity [46]. Although 3D-STE is a promising method, the studies which compared the technique to the other standard methods are few and included a small number of patients. A clear superiority to 2D-STE in predicting development of future cardiotoxicity has not yet been evaluated. Moreover, 3D-STE is not widely available in the echo-labs; thus its use, so far, has to be considered experimental.

6.4. Stress Echocardiography. Stress-echocardiography revealed contrasting results in the evaluation of chemotherapy-treated patients: some studies report a reduction of LVEF during stress in patients treated with chemotherapy in comparison to controls [47], while other studies did not report any incremental value of the technique [48, 49]. The only use of stress echocardiography is the evaluation of inducible ischemia in patients with high or intermediate pretest probability for coronary artery disease treated with drugs associated with ischemia (fluorouracil, bevacizumab, sorafenib, and sunitinib) [50].

6.5. Cardiac Magnetic Resonance. A good incremental value provided by CMR relies on the possibility of the method to perform a tissue characterization, identifying fibrosis and edema. The use of this technique can be used to investigate both early and late myocardial dysfunction in chemotherapy-treated patients.

6.5.1. Detection of Early Cardiotoxicity. Preliminary human studies using T2 weighted sequences showed a significant increase of signal intensity after three days of therapy; this finding is indicative of interstitial edema and was predictive of LVEF reduction at 1 year [51]. A study of 22 patients receiving anthracyclines showed that, after three days of treatment, an increase >5 times of the ratio between signal intensity pre- and postcontrast administration was predictive of reduction of LVEF at 28 days and six months [52]. Delayed enhancement (DE) consists of the acquisition of delayed sequences after administration of gadolinium, which detects tissue with slow contrast washout, usually represented by scar or fibrosis. Fallah-Rad revealed subepicardial linear DE in the lateral wall of LV in all 10 patients with trastuzumab-induced cardiomyopathy even though, in only 40% of cases, DE during therapy was predictive of subsequent decline of LVEF [53]. A contrasting result has been recently presented by Drafts; the authors reported absence of DE during follow-up of anthracycline-treated patients, despite a significant decrease in LVEF [54].

6.5.2. Detection of Late Cardiotoxicity. The improvement of cancer therapy has led to longer survival; accordingly, late cardiotoxic effects of chemotherapy have been observed in many patients. Reduction of LV mass has been evaluated as a marker of late cardiotoxicity. A sample of childhood cancer survivors presented LV mass <2 standard deviation (SD) of the mean value for normal population in 50% of cases [24]. A study carried out by Neilan to evaluate the prognostic value of CMR in adult patients revealed that LV mass index was an independent predictor associated with major adverse cardiovascular events [55].

6.6. Nuclear Medicine Imaging. Nuclear imaging is rapidly evolving, providing new techniques with potential involvement into the evaluation of chemotherapy-treated patients. Functional imaging techniques are able to assess pathophysiologic and neurophysiologic processes at the tissue level. Metaiodobenzylguanidine (MIBG) shares the same metabolic pathway as norepinephrine; when marked with 123I, it is able to represent a scintigraphic image of the efferent sympathetic nervous innervations of the heart. A decrease in myocardial uptake is a strong predictor of mortality and cardiac death [56]. Patients treated with anthracycline in a dose-dependent way showed a quick reduction in 123I MIBG uptake, which was predictive of late cardiotoxicity [57, 58]. A specific anti-myosin antibody marked with 111In has been used to identify cardiomyocyte injury and necrosis in patients treated with anthracyclines, representing a predictor of LVEF decrease [59]. Although these new techniques are very promising for the future, at the moment, their use remains limited to an experimental setting.

7. Conclusions

Use of chemotherapy and radiotherapy is essential for cancer patients and cardiotoxicity represents one of the most frequent causes of treatment interruption with significant implications on the prognosis. Early diagnosis and detection of high risk patients has become a central issue in the management of cancer patients involving both cardiologists and oncologists. Systematic and periodical monitoring of LVEF remains the most used technique to diagnose cardiotoxicity in clinical practice. 2DE is the most used method; however, 3DE has proved to be more accurate and reproducible and is preferable if available. CMR is the criterion standard but its low availability and the high cost limit its use to particular subsets of patients (poor acoustic window or patients in whom treatment interruption is highly hazardous). Nevertheless, the decrease of LVEF occurring only in end-stage has shown that it is not suitable as an early indicator of cardiotoxicity. Among the new techniques that evaluate the cardiac function independently of the analysis of volumes and only GLS derived by 2D-STE has validated supporting evidence in predicting late cardiotoxicity. Baseline and periodical evaluation of GLS is recommended by the recent guidelines by ASE/EACVI [26]. Promising techniques such as 3D-STE and tissue characterization performed by CMR are under investigation and could provide new insights into the future for the evaluation of chemotherapy-treated patients.

Disclosure

Dr. Charles C. Bomzer discloses that he owns publicly held stock in Merck, Inc., and Pfizer, Inc.

Conflict of Interests

There are no conflicts of interest to report for any of the authors relative to this submission.

Acknowledgments

The authors gratefully acknowledge Susan Nord, Jennifer Pfaff, and Katie Klein of Aurora Cardiovascular Services for the editorial preparation of the paper and Brian Miller and Brian Schurrer of Aurora Sinai Medical Center for their help with the figure.

References

[1] E. T. H. Yeh and C. L. Bickford, "Cardiovascular complications of cancer therapy: incidence, pathogenesis, diagnosis, and management," *Journal of the American College of Cardiology*, vol. 53, no. 24, pp. 2231–2247, 2009.

[2] L. Oreto, M. C. Todaro, M. M. Umland et al., "Use of echocardiography to evaluate the cardiac effects of therapies used in cancer treatment: what do we know?" *Journal of the American Society of Echocardiography*, vol. 25, no. 11, pp. 1141–1152, 2012.

[3] L. Oreto, M. C. Todaro, M. M. Umland et al., "Erratum to 'use of echocardiography to evaluate the cardiac effects of therapies used in cancer treatment: what do we know?'," *Journal of the American Society of Echocardiography*, vol. 26, no. 8, p. 845, 2013.

[4] M. S. Ewer and S. M. Lippman, "Type II chemotherapy-related cardiac dysfunction: time to recognize a new entity," *Journal of Clinical Oncology*, vol. 23, no. 13, pp. 2900–2902, 2005.

[5] M. C. Todaro, L. Oreto, R. Qamar, T. E. Paterick, S. Carerj, and B. K. Khandheria, "Cardioncology: state of the heart," *International Journal of Cardiology*, vol. 168, no. 2, pp. 680–687, 2013.

[6] M. de Forni, "Cardiotoxicity of high-dose continuous infusion fluorouracil: a prospective clinical study," *Journal of Clinical Oncology*, vol. 10, no. 11, pp. 1795–1801, 1992.

[7] A. Khorana, N. M. Kuderer, E. Culakova, G. H. Lyman, and C. W. Francis, "Development and validation of a predictive model for chemotherapy-associated thrombosis," *Blood*, vol. 111, no. 10, pp. 4902–4907, 2008.

[8] S. Seng, Z. Liu, S. K. Chiu et al., "Risk of venous thromboembolism in patients with cancer treated with cisplatin: a systematic review and meta-analysis," *Journal of Clinical Oncology*, vol. 30, no. 35, pp. 4416–4426, 2012.

[9] M. Carrier, G. Le Gal, J. Tay, C. Wu, and A. Y. Lee, "Rates of venous thromboembolism in multiple myeloma patients undergoing immunomodulatory therapy with thalidomide or lenalidomide: a systematic review and meta-analysis," *Journal of Thrombosis and Haemostasis*, vol. 9, no. 4, pp. 653–663, 2011.

[10] G. Curigliano, E. L. Mayer, H. J. Burstein, E. P. Winer, and A. Goldhirsch, "Cardiac toxicity from systemic cancer therapy: a comprehensive review," *Progress in Cardiovascular Diseases*, vol. 53, no. 2, pp. 94–104, 2010.

[11] P. Lancellotti, V. T. Nkomo, L. P. Badano et al., "European Society of Cardiology Working Groups on Nuclear Cardiology and Cardiac Computed Tomography and Cardiovascular Magnetic Resonance; American Society of Nuclear Cardiology Society for Cardiovascular Magnetic Resonance, and Society of Cardiovascular Computed Tomography. Expert consensus for multi-modality imaging evaluation of cardiovascular complications of radiotherapy in adults: a report from the European Association of Cardiovascular Imaging and the American Society of Echocardiography," *Journal of the American Society of Echocardiography*, vol. 26, no. 9, pp. 1013–1032, 2013.

[12] J. W. Mason, M. R. Bristow, M. E. Billingham, and J. R. Daniels, "Invasive and noninvasive methods of assessing adriamycin cardiotoxic effects in man: superiority of histopathologic assessment using endomyocardial biopsy," *Cancer Treatment Reports*, vol. 62, no. 6, pp. 857–864, 1978.

[13] A. Seidman, C. Hudis, M. Kathryn Pierri et al., "Cardiac dysfunction in the trastuzumab clinical trials experience," *Journal of Clinical Oncology*, vol. 20, no. 5, pp. 1215–1221, 2002.

[14] P. Thavendiranathan, A. D. Grant, T. Negishi, J. C. Plana, Z. B. Popović, and T. H. Marwick, "Reproducibility of echocardiographic techniques for sequential assessment of left ventricular ejection fraction and volumes: application to patients undergoing cancer chemotherapy," *Journal of the American College of Cardiology*, vol. 61, no. 1, pp. 77–84, 2013.

[15] J. Walker, N. Bhullar, N. Fallah-Rad et al., "Role of three-dimensional echocardiography in breast cancer: comparison with two-dimensional echocardiography, multiple-gated acquisition scans, and cardiac magnetic resonance imaging," *Journal of Clinical Oncology*, vol. 28, no. 21, pp. 3429–3436, 2010.

[16] T. W. Galema, A. R. T. Van De Ven, O. I. I. Soliman et al., "Contrast echocardiography improves interobserver agreement for wall motion score index and correlation with ejection fraction," *Echocardiography*, vol. 28, no. 5, pp. 575–581, 2011.

[17] R. Hoffmann, G. Barletta, S. Von Bardeleben et al., "Analysis of left ventricular volumes and function: a multicenter comparison of cardiac magnetic resonance imaging, cine ventriculography, and unenhanced and contrast-enhanced two-dimensional and three-dimensional echocardiography," *Journal of the American Society of Echocardiography*, vol. 27, no. 3, pp. 292–301, 2014.

[18] R. Olszewski, J. Timperley, S. Cezary et al., "The clinical applications of contrast echocardiography," *European Journal of Echocardiography*, vol. 8, no. 3, pp. S13–S23, 2007.

[19] R. Olszewski, J. Timperley, C. Szmigielski et al., "Erratum in: The clinical applications of contrast echocardiography," *European Journal of Echocardiography*, vol. 8, no. 5, p. 308, 2007, Cezary, Szmigielski [corrected to Szmigielski, Cezary]; Nihoyannopoulis, Petros [corrected to Nihoyannopoulos, Petros].

[20] L.-F. de Geus-Oei, A. M. C. Mavinkurve-Groothuis, L. Bellersen et al., "Scintigraphic techniques for early detection of cancer treatment-induced cardiotoxicity," *Journal of Nuclear Medicine*, vol. 52, no. 4, pp. 560–571, 2011.

[21] S. Takuma, T. Ota, T. Muro et al., "Assessment of left ventricular function by real-time 3-dimensional echocardiography compared with conventional noninvasive methods," *Journal of the American Society of Echocardiography*, vol. 14, no. 4, pp. 275–284, 2001.

[22] A. C. Armstrong, S. Gidding, O. Gjesdal, C. Wu, D. A. Bluemke, and J. A. C. Lima, "LV mass assessed by echocardiography and CMR, cardiovascular outcomes, and medical practice," *Journal of the American College of Cardiology: Cardiovascular Imaging*, vol. 5, no. 8, pp. 837–848, 2012.

[23] G. Pons-Lladó, "Assessment of cardiac function by CMR," *European Radiology, Supplement*, vol. 15, no. 2, pp. B23–B32, 2005.

[24] G. T. Armstrong, J. C. Plana, N. Zhang et al., "Screening adult survivors of childhood cancer for cardiomyopathy: comparison of echocardiography and cardiac magnetic resonance imaging," *Journal of Clinical Oncology*, vol. 30, no. 23, pp. 2876–2884, 2012.

[25] K. Ylänen, T. Poutanen, P. Savikurki-Heikkilä, I. Rinta-Kiikka, A. Eerola, and K. Vettenranta, "Cardiac magnetic resonance imaging in the evaluation of the late effects of anthracyclines among long-term survivors of childhood cancer," *Journal of the American College of Cardiology*, vol. 61, no. 14, pp. 1539–1547, 2013.

[26] J. C. Plana, M. Galderisi, A. Barac et al., "Expert consensus for multimodality imaging evaluation of adult patients during and after cancer therapy: a report from the American Society of Echocardiography and the European Association of Cardiovascular Imaging," *Journal of the American Society Echocardiography*, vol. 27, no. 9, pp. 911–939, 2014.

[27] P. W. Stoodley, D. A. B. Richards, A. Boyd et al., "Altered left ventricular longitudinal diastolic function correlates with reduced systolic function immediately after anthracycline chemotherapy," *European Heart Journal Cardiovascular Imaging*, vol. 14, no. 3, pp. 228–234, 2013.

[28] P. Pellicori, A. Calicchia, F. Lococo, G. Cimino, and C. Torromeo, "Subclinical anthracycline cardiotoxicity in patients with acute promyelocytic leukemia in long-term remission after the AIDA protocol," *Congestive Heart Failure*, vol. 18, no. 4, pp. 217–221, 2012.

[29] F. A. Bu'Lock, M. G. Mott, A. Oakhill, and R. P. Martin, "Left ventricular diastolic function after anthracycline chemotherapy in childhood: relation with systolic function, symptoms, and pathophysiology," *British Heart Journal*, vol. 73, no. 4, pp. 340–350, 1995.

[30] D. Di Lisi, F. Bonura, F. MacAione et al., "Chemotherapy-induced cardiotoxicity: role of the tissue Doppler in the early diagnosis of left ventricular dysfunction," *Anti-Cancer Drugs*, vol. 22, no. 5, pp. 468–472, 2011.

[31] D. di Lisi, F. Bonura, F. Macaione, A. Peritore, M. Meschisi, and F. Cuttitta, "Chemotherapy-induced cardiotoxicity: role of the tissue Doppler in the early diagnosis of left ventricular dysfunction: erratum," *Anti-Cancer Drugs*, vol. 22, no. 8, p. 825, 2011.

[32] S. Tassan-Mangina, D. Codorean, M. Metivier et al., "Tissue Doppler imaging and conventional echocardiography after anthracycline treatment in adults: early and late alterations of left ventricular function during a prospective study," *European Journal of Echocardiography*, vol. 7, no. 2, pp. 141–146, 2006.

[33] N. Fallah-Rad, J. R. Walker, A. Wassef et al., "The utility of cardiac biomarkers, tissue velocity and strain imaging, and cardiac magnetic resonance imaging in predicting early left ventricular dysfunction in patients with human epidermal growth factor receptor iipositive breast cancer treated with adjuvant trastuzumab therapy," *Journal of the American College of Cardiology*, vol. 57, no. 22, pp. 2263–2270, 2011.

[34] M. Lotrionte, E. Cavarretta, A. Abbate et al., "Temporal changes in standard and tissue doppler imaging echocardiographic parameters after anthracycline chemotherapy in women with breast cancer," *The American Journal of Cardiology*, vol. 112, no. 7, pp. 1005–1012, 2013.

[35] J. M. Appel, P. Sogaard, C. E. Mortensen, K. Skagen, and D. L. Nielsen, "Tissue-doppler assessment of cardiac left ventricular function during short-term adjuvant epirubicin therapy for breast cancer," *Journal of the American Society of Echocardiography*, vol. 24, no. 2, pp. 200–206, 2011.

[36] B. Yağci-Küpeli, A. Varan, H. Yorgun, B. Kaya, and M. Büyükpamukçu, "Tissue Doppler and myocardial deformation imaging to detect myocardial dysfunction in pediatric cancer patients treated with high doses of anthracyclines," *Asia-Pacific Journal of Clinical Oncology*, vol. 8, no. 4, pp. 368–374, 2012.

[37] D. S. Jassal, S.-Y. Han, C. Hans et al., "Utility of tissue Doppler and strain rate imaging in the early detection of trastuzumab and anthracycline mediated cardiomyopathy," *Journal of the American Society of Echocardiography*, vol. 22, no. 4, pp. 418–424, 2009.

[38] H. Geyer, G. Caracciolo, H. Abe et al., "Assessment of myocardial mechanics using speckle tracking echocardiography: fundamentals and clinical applications," *Journal of the American Society of Echocardiography*, vol. 23, no. 4, pp. 351–369, 2010.

[39] H. Geyer, G. Caracciolo, H. Abe et al., "Erratum in: Assessment of myocardial mechanics using speckle tracking echocardiography: fundamentals and clinical applications," *Journal of the American Society of Echocardiography*, vol. 23, no. 7, p. 734, 2010.

[40] K. Negishi, T. Negishi, J. L. Hare, B. A. Haluska, J. C. Plana, and T. H. Marwick, "Independent and incremental value of deformation indices for prediction of trastuzumab-induced cardiotoxicity," *Journal of the American Society of Echocardiography*, vol. 26, no. 5, pp. 493–498, 2013.

[41] P. W. Stoodley, D. A. B. Richards, A. Boyd et al., "Left ventricular systolic function in HER2/neu negative breast cancer patients treated with anthracycline chemotherapy: a comparative analysis of left ventricular ejection fraction and myocardial strain imaging over 12 months," *European Journal of Cancer*, vol. 49, no. 16, pp. 3396–3403, 2013.

[42] P. Thavendiranathan, F. Poulin, K. D. Lim, J. C. Plana, A. Woo, and T. H. Marwick, "Use of myocardial strain imaging by echocardiography for the early detection of cardiotoxicity in patients during and after cancer chemotherapy: a systematic review," *Journal of the American College of Cardiology*, vol. 63, no. 25PA, pp. 2751–2768, 2014.

[43] M. R. Nelson, R. T. Hurst, S. F. Raslan, S. Cha, S. Wilansky, and S. J. Lester, "Echocardiographic measures of myocardial deformation by speckle-tracking technologies: the need for standardization?" *Journal of the American Society of Echocardiography*, vol. 25, no. 11, pp. 1189–1194, 2012.

[44] T. Y. Xu, J. P. Sun, A. P. Lee et al., "Three-dimensional speckle strain echocardiography is more accurate and efficient than 2D strain in the evaluation of left ventricular function," *International Journal of Cardiology*, vol. 176, no. 2, pp. 360–366, 2014.

[45] H.-K. Yu, W. Yu, D. K. L. Cheuk, S. J. Wong, G. C. F. Chan, and Y.-F. Cheung, "New three-dimensional speckle-tracking echocardiography identifies global impairment of left ventricular mechanics with a high sensitivity in childhood cancer survivors," *Journal of the American Society of Echocardiography*, vol. 26, no. 8, pp. 846–852, 2013.

[46] C. Mornoş, A. J. Manolis, D. Cozma, N. Kouremenos, I. Zacharopoulou, and A. Ionac, "The value of left ventricular global longitudinal strain assessed by three-dimensional strain imaging in the early detection of anthracycline-mediated cardiotoxicity," *The Hellenic Journal of Cardiology*, vol. 55, no. 3, pp. 235–244, 2014.

[47] M. Jarfelt, V. Kujacic, D. Holmgren, R. Bjarnason, and B. Lannering, "Exercise echocardiography reveals subclinical cardiac dysfunction in young adult survivors of childhood acute lymphoblastic leukemia," *Pediatric Blood and Cancer*, vol. 49, no. 6, pp. 835–840, 2007.

[48] M. Bountioukos, J. K. Doorduijn, J. R. Roelandt et al., "Repetitive dobutamine stress echocardiography for the prediction of anthracycline cardiotoxicity," *European Journal of Echocardiography*, vol. 4, no. 4, pp. 300–305, 2003.

[49] L. Lanzarini, G. Bossi, M. L. Laudisa, C. Klersy, and M. Aricò, "Lack of clinically significant cardiac dysfunction during intermediate dobutamine doses in long-term childhood cancer survivors exposed to anthracyclines," *American Heart Journal*, vol. 140, no. 2, pp. 315–323, 2000.

[50] E. T. H. Yeh, A. T. Tong, D. J. Lenihan et al., "Cardiovascular complications of cancer therapy: diagnosis, pathogenesis, and management," *Circulation*, vol. 109, no. 25, pp. 3122–3131, 2004.

[51] P. Thavendiranathan, B. J. Wintersperger, S. D. Flamm, and T. H. Marwick, "Cardiac MRI in the assessment of cardiac injury and toxicity from cancer chemotherapy a systematic review," *Circulation: Cardiovascular Imaging*, vol. 6, no. 6, pp. 1080–1091, 2013.

[52] R. Wassmuth, S. Lentzsch, U. Erdbruegger et al., "Subclinical cardiotoxic effects of anthracyclines as assessed by magnetic resonance imaging—a pilot study," *The American Heart Journal*, vol. 141, no. 6, pp. 1007–1013, 2001.

[53] N. Fallah-Rad, M. Lytwyn, T. Fang, I. Kirkpatrick, and D. S. Jassal, "Delayed contrast enhancement cardiac magnetic resonance imaging in trastuzumab induced cardiomyopathy," *Journal of Cardiovascular Magnetic Resonance*, vol. 10, article 5, 2008.

[54] B. C. Drafts, K. M. Twomley, R. D'Agostino Jr. et al., "Low to moderate dose anthracycline-based chemotherapy is associated with early noninvasive imaging evidence of subclinical cardiovascular disease," *Journal of the American College of Cardiology: Cardiovascular Imaging*, vol. 6, no. 8, pp. 877–885, 2013.

[55] T. G. Neilan, O. R. Coelho-Filho, D. Pena-Herrera et al., "Left ventricular mass in patients with a cardiomyopathy after treatment with anthracyclines," *The American Journal of Cardiology*, vol. 110, no. 11, pp. 1679–1686, 2012.

[56] T. Nakata, K. Miyamoto, A. Doi et al., "Cardiac death prediction and impaired cardiac sympathetic innervation assessed by MIBG in patients with failing and nonfailing hearts," *Journal of Nuclear Cardiology*, vol. 5, no. 6, pp. 579–590, 1998.

[57] G. S. Panjrath and D. Jain, "Monitoring chemotherapy-induced cardiotoxicity: role of cardiac nuclear imaging," *Journal of Nuclear Cardiology*, vol. 13, no. 3, pp. 415–426, 2006.

[58] S. Wakasugi, A. J. Fischman, J. W. Babich et al., "Metaiodobenzylguanidine: Evaluation of its potential as a tracer for monitoring doxorubicin cardiomyopathy," *Journal of Nuclear Medicine*, vol. 34, no. 8, pp. 1282–1286, 1993.

[59] I. Carrió, M. Estorch, L. Berná, J. López-Pousa, J. Tabernero, and G. Torres, "Indium-111-antimyosin and iodine-123-MIBG studies in early assessment of doxorubicin cardiotoxicity," *Journal of Nuclear Medicine*, vol. 36, no. 11, pp. 2044–2049, 1995.

TGFβ Signaling in Tumor Initiation, Epithelial-to-Mesenchymal Transition, and Metastasis

Panagiotis Papageorgis

Department of Health Sciences, Program in Biological Sciences, European University Cyprus, 6 Diogenes Street, Engomi, 1516 Nicosia, Cyprus

Correspondence should be addressed to Panagiotis Papageorgis; p.papageorgis@euc.ac.cy

Academic Editor: Apostolos Zaravinos

Retaining the delicate balance in cell signaling activity is a prerequisite for the maintenance of physiological tissue homeostasis. Transforming growth factor-beta (TGFβ) signaling is an essential pathway that plays crucial roles during embryonic development as well as in adult tissues. Aberrant TGFβ signaling activity regulates tumor progression in a cancer cell-autonomous or non-cell-autonomous fashion and these effects may be tumor suppressing or tumor promoting depending on the cellular context. The fundamental role of this pathway in promoting cancer progression in multiple stages of the metastatic process, including epithelial-to-mesenchymal transition (EMT), is also becoming increasingly clear. In this review, we discuss the latest advances in the effort to unravel the inherent complexity of TGFβ signaling and its role in cancer progression and metastasis. These findings provide important insights into designing personalized therapeutic strategies against advanced cancers.

1. Synthesis and Activation of TGFβ Family Members

The transforming growth factor-beta (TGFβ) and TGFβ-like molecules are members of a large superfamily of more than 40 secreted cytokines, including TGFβ, bone morphogenetic proteins (BMPs), activins, nodal, lefty, myostatin, anti-müllerian hormone (AMH), and growth differentiation factors (GDFs). These pleotropic cytokines control numerous biological functions such as proliferation, apoptosis, embryonic patterning, stem cell maintenance, cell differentiation, migration, and regulation of the immune system. Unraveling the complexity that underlies their mode of action has remained challenging because these effects are known to be highly cell type-specific and context-dependent [1–3]. The three TGFβ isoforms, TGFβ1, TGFβ2, and TGFβ3, are the most widely studied members of the family, mostly because they are ubiquitously expressed and can influence the majority of tissue types. On the other hand, the expression of other cytokines is limited to only a few tissues, such as myostatin, or particular developmental stages, such as the AMH [3, 4]. The TGFβ molecules are initially synthesized in an inactive pro-TGFβ form, which consists of TGFβ associated with latency associated proteins (LAPs). The TGFβ large latent complex (LLC) consists of the LAPs and the latency-TGFβ-binding proteins (LTBPs) assembled together with disulfide bridges between specific cysteine residues [5–8]. In turn, the LLC is covalently associated to the extracellular matrix (ECM) via the N-terminal region of LTBPs [9, 10]. The presence of the TGFβ ligand within the LLC complex maintains the cytokine in an inactive form by preventing the interaction with its receptors [11]. TGFβ can be activated in different ways. First, LAPs may undergo conformational changes induced by thrombospondin-1 (TSP-1) [12, 13] followed by cleavage mediated by proteases, including convertases, plasmins, or matrix metalloproteases (MMPs) [14–16]. Secondly, alpha v beta 6 ($\alpha_v\beta_6$) integrin, which becomes upregulated in response to wounding or inflammation, binds and activates latent TGFβ [17]. Furthermore, TGFβ can be activated by low pH levels in the local environment [18] or upon irradiation-induced reactive oxygen species (ROS) production [19]. Finally, mechanical contraction of myofibroblasts in the stroma can further activate latent TGFβ [20]. All these mechanisms result in the release of active TGFβ which can bind TGFβ receptors and propagate downstream signaling events. Overall, the bioavailability of active TGFβ ligand is greatly dependent on the maturation processes described above.

2. Sensing and Propagating TGFβ Signals

The SMAD family of proteins, comprised of eight structurally related human proteins, are the major effector molecules responsible for transducing intracellular signaling initiated by the TGFβ superfamily of cytokines [21–25]. Smads can be categorized in three functionally distinct groups: the receptor activated Smads (R-Smads), which include Smad1, Smad2, Smad3, Smad5, and Smad8; the common mediator Smad (co-Smad), Smad4; and the inhibitory Smads (I-Smads), Smad6 and Smad7 [25, 26]. They all have similar sizes and range in molecular weights from 42 to 60 kDa. Structurally, the R-Smads and the co-Smad consist of two MAD homology (MH) domains, MH1 and MH2, located at the amino- and carboxy-terminals ends of the protein, respectively, and are separated by a proline-rich acidic linker region. On the other hand, the I-Smads lack the MH1 domain [27–29]. While the MH2 domain is involved in protein complex formation, as well as transcriptional activation and repression, the MH1 domain exhibits DNA binding activity [27, 30]. In the absence of TGFβ ligand, the Smad proteins remain inactive because the MH1 and MH2 domains interact with each other resulting in their functional autoinhibition. TGFβ stimulation induces conformational changes to relieve this inhibition allowing the MH2 domain of R-Smads to interact with the TGFβ receptors [28, 31].

The TGFβ isoforms transduce signaling via three types of TGFβ receptors: TGFβRI, TGFβRII, and TGFβRIII. To date, seven TGFβRIs, five TGFβRIIs, and two TGFβRIIIs have been characterized: TGFβRIs include activin-like receptors 1–7 (ALK1–7); TGFβRIIs include the TGFβRII, BMPRII, ACTRII, ACTRIIB, and AMHRII; and betaglycan and endoglin belong to the TGFβRIIIs [32]. While TGFβRI and TGFβRII have been extensively studied during the last decade, the roles of TGFβRIII in physiology and disease have recently started to emerge. Betaglycan is considered to function as a coreceptor for TGFβ superfamily, primarily to enhance activin/inhibin signaling [33]. On the other hand, endoglin appears to be predominantly expressed in endothelial cells and acts to control angiogenesis [34–36]. However, in most tissues, TGFβ ligands function through heterotetrameric complex formation between two TGFβRIs and two TGFβRIIs. Both of these receptors exhibit Ser/Thr kinase activity but appear to have distinct roles; TGFβRIIs are able to activate the receptor complex while TGFβRIs propagate signaling to the R-Smads [37, 38]. TGFβRII-ALK5 complex formation can transduce signals from all three TGFβ isoforms in multiple tissues, whereas TGFβRII can specifically associate with ALK1 in endothelial cells and with ALK2 in cardiovascular tissues [39]. While ALK5 is the predominant type of TGFβRI which functionally transduces TGFβ signals, ALK2 and ALK4 are the ones which can bind activin with high affinity [38]. Also, alternative heteromeric receptor-ligand complexes can regulate distinct R-Smad family members. For example, ALK5 activates Smad2 and Smad3 (canonical TGFβ/Smad-dependent signaling pathway) whereas ALK2, ALK3, and ALK6 activate Smad1, Smad5, and Smad8 (BMP signaling pathway) [40–46].

2.1. Smad-Dependent Signaling. Mechanistically, all TGFβ isoforms initiate signaling in a similar manner. The active TGFβ1 ligand initially binds TGFβRII followed by recruitment of the ALK5 (TGFβRI) at the plasma membrane. With the heteromeric receptor-ligand complex formed, TGFβRII phosphorylates TGFβRI in a conserved Glycine-Serine (GS)-rich domain [47] leading to the dissociation of the inhibitory FKBP12 protein from TGFβRI [48]. This conformational switch allows activated TGFβRI to interact with R-Smads (Smad2/3) through their MH2 domain [49] resulting in their phosphorylation at the conserved SSXS C-terminal motif [31, 50]. SARA (Smad anchor for receptor activation) is a FYVE domain-containing protein which plays a central role in recruiting R-Smads to the activated TGFβRI to facilitate receptor-mediated phosphorylation. It preferentially associates with unphosphorylated Smad2 and is released upon Smad2 phosphorylation by TGFβRI [51]. This phosphorylation event triggers the formation of a heterotrimeric complex between phosphorylated R-Smads (Smad2/3) and co-Smad (Smad4), which can translocate into the nucleus to modulate gene expression (Figure 1) [3]. Smads act as transcription factors in cooperation with other coactivators, such as CBP/p300, P/CAF, SMIF, FoxO, Sp1, c-Jun/c-Fos, Sertad1, or corepressors, such as E2F4/5-p107, ATF3, TGIF, Ski, SnoN, FoxG1, EVI1, and CTBP [50, 52–68]. Furthermore, Smads can also indirectly regulate gene expression by controlling epigenetic processes, such as chromatin remodeling [69, 70] or by maintaining promoter DNA methylation, which is critical in silencing epithelial gene expression in cells that have undergone epithelial-to-mesenchymal transition (EMT) [71].

Importantly, the activity of TGFβ signaling is balanced by a negative feedback loop mediated by the inhibitory Smad7, a major target gene of the pathway [72]. Under basal conditions, Smad7 resides in the cell nucleus but it translocates to the cell membrane upon TGFβ-induced receptor complex formation [73]. Binding of Smad7 to the activated TGFβ receptor complex inhibits propagation of downstream signaling by blocking interactions between the R-Smads and the activated receptors [74]. Furthermore, Smad7 can interact with the E3-ubiquitin ligases Smurf1 or Smurf2 in the nucleus. Upon TGFβ activation, the Smad7-Smurf complex translocates to the plasma membrane where Smurf induces ubiquitination and proteasomal degradation of the TGFβ receptors [75, 76]. Furthermore, in some cases, Smad7 can inhibit TGFβ-mediated transcriptional events by directly binding to DNA, thus antagonizing the formation of a functional Smad-DNA complex [77].

It has also been shown that the R-Smads can regulate some cellular functions by partnering with factors other than Smad4. For example, TIF1γ (transcription intermediate factor 1γ) is able to compete against Smad4 for binding to Smad2/3 and plays a critical role in controlling erythroid differentiation [78]. Moreover, Smads2/3 can interact with IκB kinase α (IKKα), in a Smad4-independent manner, to regulate the expression of Mad1, an antagonist of the

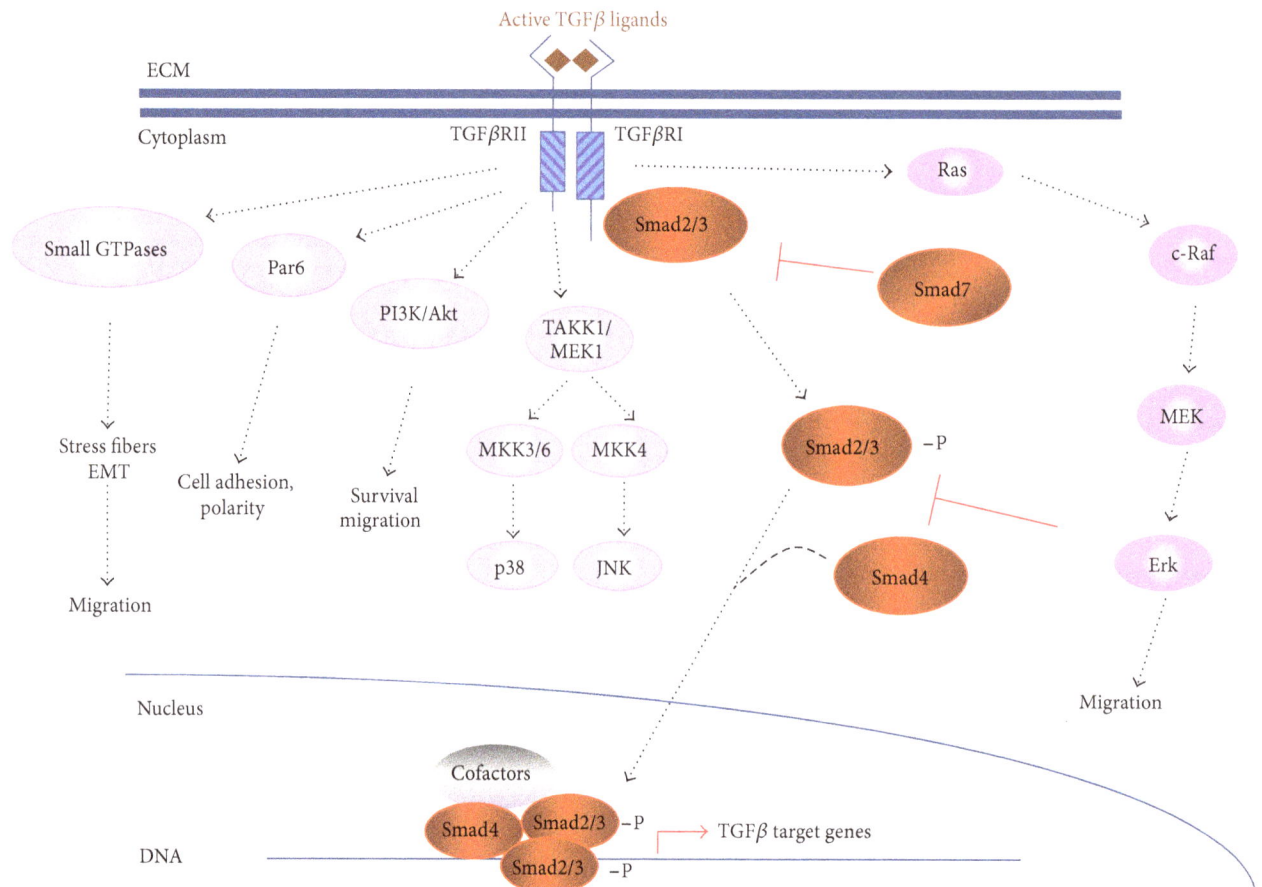

FIGURE 1: Smad-dependent and independent TGFβ pathways. Active TGFβ ligands initiate signaling by binding to TGFβRIs and TGFβRIIs. TGFβ receptors exhibit kinase activities that are necessary for transducing canonical TGFβ signaling by phosphorylating Smads2/3. Activated R-Smads can form a heterotrimeric complex with Smad4 which associates with other cofactors in the nucleus to regulate the expression of TGFβ target genes. Furthermore, downstream signaling can also be transduced via auxiliary pathways such as various brunches of the Mek/Erk, the Rho-like GTPases, and the PI3K/Akt and the p38/MAPK pathways to modulate biological responses including epithelial-to-mesenchymal transition, cell adhesion, migration, and survival.

Myc oncogene, and control keratinocyte differentiation [79]. These findings are consistent with the notion that Smad4 is essential for many, but not all, TGFβ-regulated Smad-dependent cellular responses.

2.2. Smad-Independent Signaling. Several studies have clearly demonstrated that TGFβ can also employ Smad-independent pathways as downstream effectors [80]. TGFβ induces activation of Erk signaling in multiple tissues including epithelial and endothelial cells, as well as in breast and colorectal cancer cells to promote the dissolution of adherens junctions and cell migration [81–87]. This induction is either indirect via activation of TGFα and FGF autocrine loops [84, 85] or can be direct by Src-mediated or autophosphorylation of TGFβRII at Tyr residues [88, 89]. Moreover, phosphorylation of TGFβRI at Tyr residues activates ShcA to promote the formation of a ShcA/Grb2/Sos complex. Subsequently, this complex can activate Ras on the plasma membrane, which in turn transduces downstream signaling via c-Raf, MEK, and Erk [90]. TGFβ can also promote activation of the JNK and p38-MAPK pathways to regulate apoptosis or cell

migration, depending on cellular context [91–93], via MKK4 and MKK3/6, respectively [94, 95]. Further upstream, these MKKs can be phosphorylated by either TRAF6-mediated recruitment of TAK1 [96–99], or by two other MAPKKKs, MEKK1, and MLK3 [100, 101]. Furthermore, the PI3K/Akt pathway has been implicated in mediating some of cellular functions of TGFβ. Studies have shown that TGFβ can rapidly induce PI3K activation followed by phosphorylation of its effector Akt to promote EMT, cell migration, and survival [102, 103]. Mechanistically, the p85 regulatory subunit of PI3K appears to be constitutively bound to the TGFβRII and, upon TGFβ stimulation, TGFβRI is recruited to the complex to activate PI3K and initiate downstream signaling [104]. The mammalian target of rapamycin (mTOR) acts as a major effector molecule of this pathway by controlling the phosphorylation of S6 kinase (S6K) and eukaryotic initiation factor 4E binding protein [105]. Activation of the mTOR pathway by TGFβ has been shown to be critically important for regulating protein synthesis, cell size, and EMT [106]. Finally, certain TGFβ functions, such as rearrangement of cytoskeletal organization, cell polarity, and cell migration, are mediated by the Rho-like family of small GTPases [107]. TGFβ can rapidly activate the RhoA and Cdc42/Rac1 pathways, in a Smad2/3-independent manner, to promote EMT, actin polymerization, and formation of stress fibers (Figure 1) [108, 109]. Conclusively, this evidence strongly supports that Smad-independent pathways play critical roles in regulating TGFβ-mediated cellular functions.

3. TGFβ Signaling in Cancer Initiation

It is unambiguously accepted that TGFβ plays fundamental roles in carcinogenesis and tumor progression. However, numerous studies have clearly demonstrated that TGFβ acts as a double-edge sword during this process. Initially, TGFβ is able to suppress growth in normal and premalignant epithelial cells. However, upon accumulation of genetic and epigenetic alterations in tumor cells, it switches to promotion of a proinvasive and prometastatic phenotype, accompanied by a progressive increase in the locally secreted TGFβ levels. The complexity of these functions is further increased due to the fact that these TGFβ functions may vary depending on the type and genetic background of tissues [110–113].

3.1. Regulation of Cell Proliferation and Apoptosis. Numerous *in vitro* studies using human cells as well as data from animal models provided concrete evidence for the role of TGFβ as a tumor suppressor in various normal tissues. It is well known that TGFβ has a growth-inhibitory effect on normal epithelial [114], endothelial [115, 116], and neuronal cells [117] as well as on cells of the immune system, such as T-cells [118]. Under physiological conditions, the cytostatic role of TGFβ is critical in order to prevent the generation of hyperproliferative disorders, such as fibrosis and cancer. Mechanistically, TGFβ can induce the expression of genes involved in opposing proliferative cell responses during all phases of the cell cycle, but it is primarily implicated in G1/S phase transition events [119]. Genome-wide transcriptional profiling studies using normal human epithelial cell lines from mammary gland, skin, and lung have identified a common set of genes that are transcriptionally regulated by TGFβ in order to mediate its cytostatic effects. This transcriptional program predominantly involves the activation of the G1/S phase checkpoint and cell cycle arrest by two main mechanisms. First, TGFβ induces the expression of the cyclin-dependent kinase inhibitors *CDKN2B* (encoding p15/INK4B) [120], *CDKN1A* (encoding p21/Cip/Waf1) [121], and p27/Kip1 [122]. In mammary epithelial cells, the induction of expression and protein stability of p15 enhances the formation of p15-CDK4/6 complexes and therefore inhibits cyclin D1-CDK4/6 association [123]. During early G1 phase and in the absence of TGFβ, cyclin D1-CDK4/6 complex formation is required for mitogen sensing and cell cycle progression through S phase. However, upon TGFβ-mediated p15 upregulation, p15 binds CDK4 and/or CDK6, inhibiting their catalytic activity and preventing their association with cyclin D1, resulting in cell cycle arrest. TGFβ can also inhibit G1/S phase progression by inhibiting the formation of cyclin E-CDK2 and cyclin A-CDK2 via induction of p21 and p27, which bind to these

cyclin-CDK complexes and similarly cause their functional inactivation [124, 125]. The second mechanism by which TGFβ inhibits cell cycle progression is by repressing the expression of the proliferation-inducing transcription factors c-Myc [126] and the family of inhibitor of DNA binding proteins ID1, ID2, and ID3 [57, 127]. In proliferating cells, c-MYC is recruited by the zinc-finger protein MIZ1 to the *CDKN2B* and *CDKN1A* gene promoters to suppress their transcription. Upon TGFβ stimulation, c-MYC expression is downregulated and the suppression of CDKN2B/CDKN1A is relieved [128, 129]. Suppression of ID family members also contributes to the cytostatic effects by TGFβ. The ID proteins are able to physically interact and inactivate the tumor suppressor retinoblastoma (Rb) protein to promote cell proliferation [130]. TGFβ promotes the formation of an ATF3-Smad3/Smad4 complex to transcriptionally repress ID1 expression [57], while downregulation of ID2 is achieved indirectly via suppression of the ID2-inducer c-MYC [130].

The growth inhibitory effects of TGFβ on epithelial tissues are also supported by gain or loss-of-function experiments using transgenic animal models. For examples, exogenous tissue-specific overexpression of TGFβ in the epidermis decreased keratinocyte proliferation and protected mice from carcinogen-induced hyperplasia and skin tumorigenesis [131]. Similarly, transgenic expression of a dominant-negative form of the TGFβRII in the mouse epidermis blocked TGFβ-induced growth inhibition [132]. In addition, Smad3-null mice exhibit increased keratinocyte proliferation and accelerated ability for wound healing [133]. Analogous findings were also reported for other tissues, such as the mammary gland and the colon. MMTV-driven overexpression of active TGFβ in the mammary gland of transgenic mice resulted in the formation of a hypoplastic virgin mammary gland and impaired alveolar development during pregnancy [134, 135]. Conversely, overexpression of dominant-negative TGFβRII in the mouse mammary gland resulted in increased side-branching, hyperplasia, and sensitivity to carcinogens [136, 137], whereas overexpression of the same transgene in the colon reduced TGFβ-mediated growth arrest [138].

In some cases, TGFβ is also known to induce apoptosis in these tissues even though the molecular mechanisms of this process remain poorly understood. Despite the fact that the induction of TGFβ-mediated apoptosis has yet to be established *in vivo*, studies using cell lines revealed a number of candidate proteins that may be implicated in this effect [139]. Initially, upregulation of the TGFβ-inducible early response gene-1 (TIEG1) by TGFβ was found to trigger apoptosis in pancreatic epithelial cells. Furthermore, TGFβ was shown to promote apoptosis of hepatoma cells via a Smad-dependent upregulation of the death-associated protein kinase DAPK [140]. Moreover, the adaptor protein Daxx has been implicated in mediating TGFβ apoptotic actions by enhancing JNK signaling [141]. Similarly, TGFβ is able to induce GADD45b expression which in turn stimulates p38-MAPK signaling, followed by caspase-8 and Bad activation to promote apoptosis [142]. Furthermore, TGFβ leads to ARTS translocation from the mitochondria to the nucleus where it physically interacts and suppresses the function of XIAP, a major inhibitor of apoptosis [143]. Finally, Bim was also shown to be another proapoptotic TGFβ target, which activates Bax to promote caspase-dependent apoptosis [144].

It is important to highlight that the effects of TGFβ in proliferation can be different, even opposing, depending on the tissue type. While TGFβ inhibits proliferation of normal epithelial, endothelial, neuronal, and T cells, it can also enhance the proliferation of fibroblasts [114]. In fact, 30 years ago, the initial experiments that led to the discovery of TGFβ and its naming as "transforming" growth factor were based on its ability to induce proliferation and transformation of fibroblasts [145]. This effect is mediated indirectly by TGFβ-induced connective tissue growth factor (CTGF) secretion, which is responsible for stimulating fibroblast proliferation [146]. Nonetheless, in most normal tissues TGFβ predominantly acts as an inhibitor of cell proliferation.

3.2. Smad Pathway Alterations in Human Cancers. One of the hallmarks of most cancer types is that the vast majority of cases exhibit insensitivity to TGFβ-mediated growth inhibition. Studies in human tumors have shown that TGFβ pathway components often become genetically inactivated in certain cancer types to explain, in part, the acquired insensitivity of TGFβ-mediated growth control. Loss of function or truncating mutations in *TGFβRI*, *TGFβRII*, *SMAD2*, and *SMAD4* genes have been detected in colorectal, pancreatic, gastric, and prostate tumors [21, 147–151]. Furthermore, 18q21 chromosome loss, harboring the Smad4 gene, is observed in 60% of pancreatic and 30% of colorectal cancers [152–155]. Subsequent functional studies further elucidated the role of Smad signaling inactivation in pancreatic and colorectal cancer progression. Restoration of Smad4 expression in pancreatic cancer cell lines suppresses tumor growth and angiogenesis by decreasing VEGF levels [156]. Similarly, homozygous Smad4 deletion accompanied by TGFβ overexpression induces VEGF expression via the MEK-Erk and p38 pathways in order to facilitate colon cancer progression and drug resistance [83].

Notably, these genetic alterations are not detected in all tumor types. For example, in breast cancers Smad gene mutations are rare [21, 150, 151] suggesting that additional mechanisms for acquiring resistance to TGFβ-mediated growth inhibition also exist. It has been shown that activation of the Ras oncogene and its downstream target Erk leads to the phosphorylation of Smad1, Smad2, and Smad3 in their linker region, thus inducing their retention in the cytoplasm and promoting their ubiquitin-dependent degradation [157–159]. In addition, metastatic breast cancer cells, isolated from pleural fluids of patients, exhibit intact Smad pathway components but were found to be unresponsive to TGFβ-mediated growth inhibition. In this study, the cytostatic responses to TGFβ appeared to be dependent on the transcription factor C/EBPβ which is essential for the induction of the cell cycle inhibitor p15/INK4b and the repression of c-MYC oncogene. Interestingly, cells from half of these patients overexpressed the dominant-negative C/EBPβ isoform LIP, which is able to bind and inhibit the transcriptionally active C/EBPβ isoform LAP in order to suppress TGFβ-mediated growth inhibition [160]. Another mechanism that TGFβ may exploit in order to switch from a tumor suppressive to a metastasis-promoting

factor is through differential regulation of *ID1* gene. While ID1 expression is suppressed by TGFβ in normal tissues, it was found to be induced in patient-derived metastatic breast cancer cells [161]. Importantly, high ID1 expression levels are correlated with relapse in patients with estrogen receptor negative (ER) breast tumors [162]. Also, the Tax oncoprotein, encoded by the Human T-cell leukemia virus type I (HTLV-I), is able to inhibit Smad-dependent transcription in T cells, thus contributing to the acquisition of resistance to growth inhibition [163]. Finally, the SKI and SKIL oncoproteins can interact with Smad3 and Smad4 to displace p300 and CBP from the active transcriptional complex in order to repress TGFβ-mediated growth inhibition [164].

4. TGFβ in Epithelial-to-Mesenchymal Transition (EMT)

EMT is a vital process for morphogenesis during embryonic development and was initially appreciated primarily by developmental biologists. During the last decade, however, it has become apparent that EMT can be abnormally reactivated in adult tissues during pathological conditions such as cancer and fibrosis [165]. EMT involves the induction of an orchestrated, reversible transcriptional program in which well-organized, tightly connected epithelial cells transdifferentiate into disorganized and motile mesenchymal cells. This process is characterized by disruption of tight junctions between epithelial cells due to downregulation and delocalization of tight junction proteins zonula occludens 1 (ZO-1), occludin, and claudins. Similarly, adherens cell junction complexes containing E-cadherin, p120, γ-catenin, and β-catenin also undergo dissolution. This is followed by loss of apical-basal cell polarity, dramatic remodeling of the cytoskeleton, and the formation of actin stress fibers. Concomitantly, cells acquire mesenchymal features such as spindle-shaped, fibroblast-like morphology and express mesenchymal components including N-cadherin, vimentin, fibronectin, and alpha smooth-muscle actin [166, 167]. TGFβ signaling plays an instrumental role in activating this transcriptional network by inducing the expression of several pleiotropically acting transcription factors, also known as "master regulators" of EMT. TGFβ-induced factors include the Snail family of proteins Snail [168] and Slug [169] as well as the two-handed zinc finger factors ZEB1/deltaEF1 [170] and ZEB2/SIP1 [171] while the basic helix-loop-helix (bHLH) protein Twist [172] can be upregulated by Wnt, EGFR, or STAT3 signaling [173, 174]. Other EMT transcription factors, also induced by the TGFβ-Smad pathway, such as HMGA2 [175] or Ets1 [176], act as upstream regulators in this network by upregulating the expression of Snail and ZEB family members, respectively. On the other hand, FOXC2 is a factor which functions downstream of Snail and Twist to promote EMT (Figure 2) [177]. In addition to these transcriptional mechanisms, recent studies indicate that overactive TGFβ-Smad2 signaling further contributes to the establishment of an EMT phenotype by maintaining the epigenetic silencing of key epithelial marker genes, such as E-cadherin, claudin-4, kallikrein-10, and cingulin. This appears to be mediated via Smad2-dependent regulation of DNA

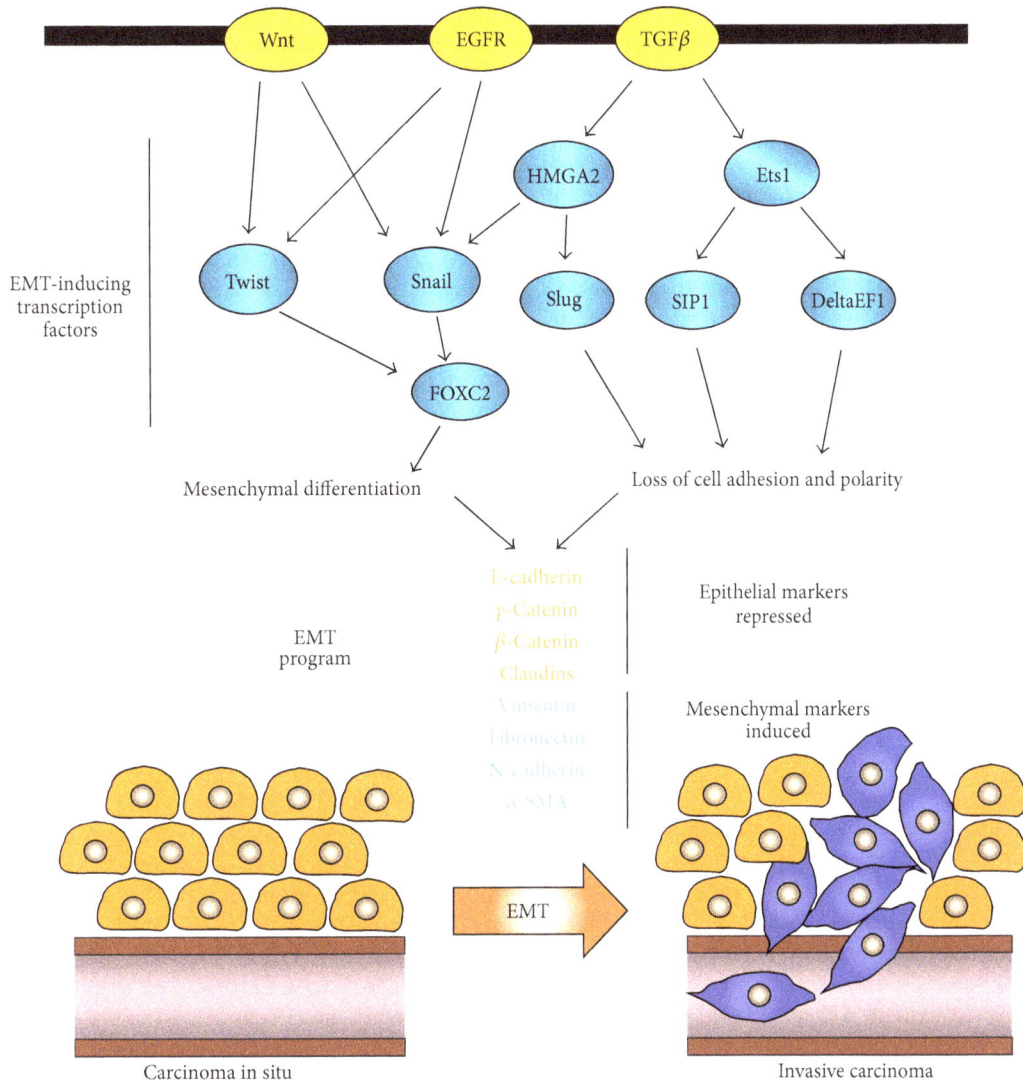

FIGURE 2: TGFβ signaling in epithelial-to-mesenchymal transition. TGFβ signaling mediated by Smad or non-Smad pathways can directly or indirectly induce the expression of different transcriptional "master regulators" of epithelial-to-mesenchymal transition. These factors, including Snail, Slug, ZEB1/delta EF1, and ZEB2/SIP1 are able to initiate a coordinated transcriptional network which results in suppression of epithelial and upregulation mesenchymal marker expression. As a result, epithelial cancer cells undergo dissolution of adherens and tight junctions along with dramatic remodeling of their cytoskeleton and acquire mesenchymal features. These fibroblast-like, spindle shaped tumor cells exhibit significantly enhanced migratory and invasive potential which allows them to enter the blood circulation through the basement membrane and initiate their metastatic dissemination to distal organs.

methyltransferase 1 (DNMT1) binding activity and DNA methylation of the corresponding gene promoter regions [71].

Therefore, one of the main mechanisms by which TGFβ promotes cell migration, invasion, and metastasis is through induction of EMT. Studies have shown that TGFβ stimulation of carcinoma-derived cell populations in culture can lead to the activation of this reversible process [45, 178, 179]. *In vivo* studies have further shown that expression of TGFβ1 in the skin of transgenic mice enhanced the conversion of benign skin tumors to carcinomas and highly invasive spindle-cell carcinomas [180]. Moreover, expression of a dominant-negative TGFβRII prevented squamous carcinoma cells from undergoing EMT in response to TGFβ *in vivo* [181]. Acquisition of an EMT phenotype results in cells with diminished

adhesive capacity that are highly migratory and invasive due to increased secretion of extracellular proteases. Therefore, EMT enhances intravasation of carcinoma *in situ* cells through the basement membrane in the circulation and facilitates extravasation at the distal tissues and formation of micrometastases in distal organs [165, 172, 182].

Besides Smads, other signaling molecules have also been implicated in TGFβ-mediated EMT, including Erk, PI3K-Akt, RhoA, and cofilin [183, 184]. Induction of Erk and p38-MAPK phosphorylation by TGFβ regulates the expression of genes involved in the remodeling of extracellular matrix and disruption of adherens and tight junctions to facilitate EMT [95, 185]. However, studies using Smad-binding defective TGFβRI constructs that can still mediate MAPK signal indicated that Smads are required for Erk-induced EMT process [95, 186]. Consistent with this evidence, other reports have demonstrated that cooperation between the TGFβ and Ras-Raf-MAPK pathways is involved in promoting EMT [178, 179, 187, 188]. Additional molecular evidence to support this synergistic effect resulted from studies showing that, under the influence of oncogenic Ras, formation of a mutant p53/Smad complex empowers TGFβ-induced metastasis by opposing p63 activity [189].

Finally, the microRNA 200 family members miR-200 and miR-205 have been shown to inhibit the E-cadherin repressors ZEB1 and ZEB2 to suppress EMT and promote an epithelial phenotype. Interestingly, loss of expression of these noncoding RNAs is observed in breast tumors and may facilitate EMT, invasion, and metastasis [190–193]. Furthermore, TGFβ suppresses miR-203 expression leading to upregulation of its target SLUG in order to promote EMT and metastasis [194]. In contrast, upregulation of miR-21 in some tumor types facilitates TGFβ-induced EMT and cancer cell migration [195]. In summary, it is becoming increasingly clear that TGFβ signaling controls a complex network of interconnected pathways to regulate EMT and, therefore, the metastatic properties of cancer cells.

5. TGFβ and "Cancer Stem Cells" (CSCs)

Evidence that emerged more than a decade ago strongly suggested that a subset of undifferentiated breast cancer cells that exhibit a CD44^{high}/CD24^{low} cell surface marker expression pattern possess stem cell-like properties and have a strong ability to initiate tumor formation, even at very low numbers [196]. According to the "cancer stem cell hypothesis," stem-like cancer cells are thought to represent a subpopulation of tumor cells that also promote cancer metastasis and resistance to therapy [197, 198]. Interestingly, TGFβ-induced EMT has been shown to generate cancer cells with stem-like properties through autocrine and paracrine loops [199, 200]. Therefore, aberrant activity of the TGFβ signaling pathway, in the vast majority of solid tumors, could be functionally linked to the development and maintenance of cancer stem cells, further supporting the notion that this pathway may represent an attractive target for cancer therapy. However, despite the numerous reports using experimental approaches showing the significance of EMT in cancer progression, the detection of this phenomenon and its importance in clinical histopathological samples has remained challenging. Recent findings convincingly demonstrated that circulating tumor cells (CTCs) from breast cancer patients exhibit dynamic changes between epithelial and mesenchymal characteristics during the course of therapy. Interestingly, the mesenchymal phenotype in CTCs correlated with expression of TGFβ and FOXC1 as well as with disease progression [201].

6. TGFβ in the Tumor Microenvironment

In many tumor types, excessive TGFβ secretion is often detected locally, in the microenvironment surrounding the tumor and within the stroma to promote invasion of the leading tumor front and facilitate metastasis [202–205]. TGFβ can be derived either from cancer cells [206] or from tumor infiltrating stromal cells, such as fibroblasts, macrophages, and leukocytes, as well as mesenchymal and myeloid precursor cells [207]. Also, TGFβ can be stored in the extracellular matrix (ECM) of the bone, becoming biologically activated during development of osteolytic metastatic lesions [208].

Within the tumor microenvironment, TGFβ exhibits a dynamic interaction with various stromal components. It plays a major role in the differentiation of mesenchymal progenitor cells into fibroblasts followed by conversion into myofibroblasts [209]. The latter, characterized by alpha-smooth muscle actin (α-SMA) expression, are highly contractile cells that further contribute to the secretion of TGFβ in the microenvironment. When stimulated by TGFβ in an autocrine or paracrine fashion, myofibroblasts produce extracellular matrix components, such as collagen, fibronectin, tenascin, osteopontin, osteonectin, and elastin, which create a desmoplastic ECM [210]. In this environment, myofibroblast contraction stimulates the release of active TGFβ from its latent form that is stored in the ECM [20, 211].

Furthermore, TGFβ elicits strong immunosuppressive effects by inhibiting the functions of different immune cell types. It has long been known that TGFβ inhibits the proliferation of and suppresses the antitumor functions of CD4+ or CD8+ T cells, both *in vitro* and *in vivo* [212, 213]; it is also capable of inducing apoptosis in B-cells [214]. TGFβ inhibits T-cell activation by suppressing antigen-presenting dendritic cells, which are responsible for the maturation and effective stimulation of T cells during immune responses [215]. In addition, TGFβ blocks the production of IFNγ by natural killer (NK) cells to weaken their ability to recognize and eliminate cancer cells [212]. Finally, TGFβ can promote tumor growth by inducing polarization of macrophages and neutrophils from the cancer cell-attacking type 1 to the type 2, which exhibits significantly reduced effector function and produces inflammatory cytokines, like IL-6, IL-11, and TGFβ [216, 217]. These studies collectively establish a critical role for TGFβ in suppressing host immune system to facilitate cancer progression.

7. Priming for Metastasis and Colonization

Dissemination of cancer cells is thought to represent a non-random, biologically active process which can be driven by specific genes, depending on the specific organs of metastasis [162, 218–220]. TGFβ has been shown to play a critical role in these processes, such as promoting breast cancer metastasis to the bone via the Smad pathway [221]. Also, TGFβ in the tumor microenvironment is able to prime breast cancer cells for pulmonary metastasis by inducing angiopoietin-like 4 (ANGPTL4) secretion which facilitates retention of cancer cells to the lungs [161].

Once cancer cells extravasate to a secondary tissue, they initially form micrometastatic lesions. However, since colonization of tumor cells in distal organs is a highly inefficient process, often described as the "rate-limiting step" of metastasis, cancer cells can remain in a dormant state which may last up to several years in cancer patients. Dormancy of cancer cells is a poorly understood condition which is largely responsible for local recurrence and metastatic growth even years or decades after therapy [222, 223]. While EMT is critical for the initiation of the metastatic cascade, colonization to distal tissues requires the reversal of this process which is described as mesenchymal-to-epithelial transition (MET) [224]. TGFβ has been shown to play a role during metastatic colonization by inducing ID1 expression only in cells that have already undergone EMT. In turn, ID1 upregulation promotes MET by suppressing Twist1 expression [225]. Interestingly, a recent study has identified that TGFβ may promote metastasis and organ colonization of hepatocellular carcinoma by upregulating the long noncoding RNA lncRNA-ATB [226]. Besides TGFβ, signaling via the closely related member of the superfamily bone morphogenetic growth factor (BMP) has been linked with metastatic colonization. Inhibition of BMP signaling by the secreted antagonist Coco was found to reactivate breast cancer cells at lung metastatic sites and promote their colonization [227].

8. Conclusions and Future Perspectives

It is unambiguously accepted that TGFβ signaling plays crucial roles during cancer progression and represents an attractive target for antimetastatic therapy. Several different promising therapeutic approaches are currently being tested in clinical trials or are still under preclinical investigation to evaluate their efficacy as antimetastatic molecules. These include blockers of TGFβ activation, ligand traps, neutralizing antibodies against TGFβ-receptor interaction, antisense oligonucleotides, or inhibitors of TGFβ receptor kinase activity [228]. However, since TGFβ exerts complex functions acting both as a tumor suppressor and a metastasis-promoting cytokine depending on cellular context, inhibition of TGFβ signaling as a therapeutic strategy must be approached with caution. The future use of such TGFβ signaling modulating drugs in the clinic must be carefully assessed, considering their effects on cancer cells and on cells of the tumor microenvironment in addition to potentially deleterious effects of these strategies on normal tissues.

Conflict of Interests

The author declares that there is no conflict of interests regarding the publication of this paper.

References

[1] R. Derynck and R. J. Akhurst, "Differentiation plasticity regulated by TGF-β family proteins in development and disease," *Nature Cell Biology*, vol. 9, no. 9, pp. 1000–1004, 2007.

[2] L. M. Wakefield and C. S. Hill, "Beyond TGFβ: roles of other TGFβ superfamily members in cancer," *Nature Reviews Cancer*, vol. 13, no. 5, pp. 328–341, 2013.

[3] J. Massagué, J. Seoane, and D. Wotton, "Smad transcription factors," *Genes and Development*, vol. 19, no. 23, pp. 2783–2810, 2005.

[4] J. Massagué and R. R. Gomis, "The logic of TGFβ signaling," *FEBS Letters*, vol. 580, no. 12, pp. 2811–2820, 2006.

[5] J. P. Annes, J. S. Munger, and D. B. Rifkin, "Making sense of latent TGFβ activation," *Journal of Cell Science*, vol. 116, no. 2, pp. 217–224, 2003.

[6] P.-E. Gleizes, R. C. Beavis, R. Mazzieri, B. Shen, and D. B. Rifkin, "Identification and characterization of an eight-cysteine repeat of the latent transforming growth factor-β binding protein-1 that mediates bonding to the latent transforming growth factor-β1," *Journal of Biological Chemistry*, vol. 271, no. 47, pp. 29891–29896, 1996.

[7] K. Miyazono, A. Olofsson, P. Colosetti, and C.-H. Heldin, "A role of the latent TGF-β1-binding protein in the assembly and secretion of TGF-β1," *The EMBO Journal*, vol. 10, no. 5, pp. 1091–1101, 1991.

[8] J. Saharinen, J. Taipale, and J. Keski-Oja, "Association of the small latent transforming growth factor-β with an eight cysteine repeat of its binding protein LTBP-1," *EMBO Journal*, vol. 15, no. 2, pp. 245–253, 1996.

[9] C. Unsöld, M. Hyytiäinen, L. Bruckner-Tuderman, and J. Keski-Oja, "Latent TGF-β binding protein LTBP-1 contains three potential extracellular matrix interacting domains," *Journal of Cell Science*, vol. 114, no. 1, pp. 187–197, 2001.

[10] I. Nunes, P.-E. Gleizes, C. N. Metz, and D. B. Rifkin, "Latent transforming growth factor-β binding protein domains involved in activation and transglutaminase-dependent cross-linking of latent transforming growth factor-β," *Journal of Cell Biology*, vol. 136, no. 5, pp. 1151–1163, 1997.

[11] D. A. Lawrence, R. Pircher, C. Kryceve-Martinerie, and P. Jullien, "Normal embryo fibroblasts release transforming growth factors in a latent form," *Journal of Cellular Physiology*, vol. 121, no. 1, pp. 184–188, 1984.

[12] S. E. Crawford, V. Stellmach, J. E. Murphy-Ullrich et al., "Thrombospondin-1 is a major activator of TGF-β1 in vivo," *Cell*, vol. 93, no. 7, pp. 1159–1170, 1998.

[13] S. M. F. Ribeiro, M. Poczatek, S. Schultz-Cherry, M. Villain, and J. E. Murphy-Ullrich, "The activation sequence of thrombospondin-1 interacts with the latency- associated peptide to regulate activation of latent transforming growth factor-β," *Journal of Biological Chemistry*, vol. 274, no. 19, pp. 13586–13593, 1999.

[14] C. M. Dubois, M.-H. Laprise, F. Blanchette, L. E. Gentry, and R. Leduc, "Processing of transforming growth factor β1 precursor by human furin convertase," *Journal of Biological Chemistry*, vol. 270, no. 18, pp. 10618–10624, 1995.

[15] Y. Sato and D. B. Rifkin, "Inhibition of endothelial cell movement by pericytes and smooth muscle cells: activation of a latent transforming growth factor-β1-like molecule by plasmin during co-culture," *Journal of Cell Biology*, vol. 109, no. 1, pp. 309–315, 1989.

[16] Q. Yu and I. Stamenkovic, "Cell surface-localized matrix metalloproteinase-9 proteolytically activates TGF-β and promotes tumor invasion and angiogenesis," *Genes and Development*, vol. 14, no. 2, pp. 163–176, 2000.

[17] J. S. Munger, X. Huang, H. Kawakatsu et al., "The integrin αvβ6 binds and activates latent TGFβ1: a mechanism for regulating pulmonary inflammation and fibrosis," *Cell*, vol. 96, no. 3, pp. 319–328, 1999.

[18] R. M. Lyons, J. Keski-Oja, and H. L. Moses, "Proteolytic activation of latent transforming growth factor-β from fibroblast-conditioned medium," *Journal of Cell Biology*, vol. 106, no. 5, pp. 1659–1665, 1988.

[19] M. H. Barcellos-Hoff, R. Derynck, M. L.-S. Tsang, and J. A. Weatherbee, "Transforming growth factor-β activation in irradiated murine mammary gland," *Journal of Clinical Investigation*, vol. 93, no. 2, pp. 892–899, 1994.

[20] P.-J. Wipff, D. B. Rifkin, J.-J. Meister, and B. Hinz, "Myofibroblast contraction activates latent TGF-β1 from the extracellular matrix," *The Journal of Cell Biology*, vol. 179, no. 6, pp. 1311–1323, 2007.

[21] G. J. Riggins, S. Thiagalingam, E. Rozenblum et al., "Mad-related genes in the human," *Nature Genetics*, vol. 13, no. 3, pp. 347–349, 1996.

[22] G. Lagna, A. Hata, A. Hemmati-Brivanlou, and J. Massague, "Partnership between DPC4 and SMAD proteins in TGF-β signalling pathways," *Nature*, vol. 383, no. 6603, pp. 832–836, 1996.

[23] A. Nakao, T. Imamura, S. Souchelnytskyi et al., "TGF-β receptor-mediated signalling through Smad2, Smad3 and Smad4," *EMBO Journal*, vol. 16, no. 17, pp. 5353–5362, 1997.

[24] R. Derynck, Y. Zhang, and X.-H. Feng, "Smads: transcriptional activators of TGF-β responses," *Cell*, vol. 95, no. 6, pp. 737–740, 1998.

[25] J. Massague, "TGF-beta signal transduction," *Annual Review of Biochemistry*, vol. 67, pp. 753–791, 1998.

[26] C.-H. Heldin, K. Miyazono, and P. ten Dijke, "TGF-β signalling from cell membrane to nucleus through SMAD proteins," *Nature*, vol. 390, no. 6659, pp. 465–471, 1997.

[27] M. P. De Caestecker, P. Hemmati, S. Larisch-Bloch, R. Ajmera, A. B. Roberts, and R. J. Lechleider, "Characterization of functional domains within Smad4/DPC4," *The Journal of Biological Chemistry*, vol. 272, no. 21, pp. 13690–13696, 1997.

[28] A. Hata, Y. Shi, and J. Massagué, "TGF-β signaling and cancer: structural and functional consequences of mutations in Smads," *Molecular Medicine Today*, vol. 4, no. 6, pp. 257–262, 1998.

[29] Y. Shi, Y.-F. Wang, L. Jayaraman, H. Yang, J. Massagué, and N. P. Pavletich, "Crystal structure of a Smad MH1 domain bound to DNA: insights on DNA binding in TGF-β signaling," *Cell*, vol. 94, no. 5, pp. 585–594, 1998.

[30] D. Wotton, R. S. Lo, S. Lee, and J. Massagué, "A smad transcriptional corepressor," *Cell*, vol. 97, no. 1, pp. 29–39, 1999.

[31] Y. Zhang, X.-H. Feng, R.-Y. Wu, and R. Derynck, "Receptor-associated Mad homologues synergize as effectors of the TGF-β response," *Nature*, vol. 383, no. 6596, pp. 168–172, 1996.

[32] B. Bierie and H. L. Moses, "Tumour microenvironment: TGFB: the molecular Jekyll and Hyde of cancer," *Nature Reviews Cancer*, vol. 6, no. 7, pp. 506–520, 2006.

[33] K. A. Lewis, P. C. Gray, A. L. Blount et al., "Betaglycan binds inhibin and can mediate functional antagonism of activin signalling," *Nature*, vol. 404, no. 6776, pp. 411–414, 2000.

[34] A. Gougos and M. Letarte, "Primary structure of endoglin, and RGD-containing glycoprotein of human endothelial cells," *The Journal of Biological Chemistry*, vol. 265, no. 15, pp. 8361–8364, 1990.

[35] S. H. Wong, L. Hamel, S. Chevalier, and A. Philip, "Endoglin expression on human microvascular endothelial cells association with betaglycan and formation of higher order complexes with TGF-β signalling receptors," *European Journal of Biochemistry*, vol. 267, no. 17, pp. 5550–5560, 2000.

[36] D. Y. Li, L. K. Sorensen, B. S. Brooke et al., "Defective angiogenesis in mice lacking endoglin," *Science*, vol. 284, no. 5419, pp. 1534–1537, 1999.

[37] J. L. Wrana, L. Attisano, R. Wieser, F. Ventura, and J. Massagué, "Mechanism of activation of the TGF-β receptor," *Nature*, vol. 370, no. 6488, pp. 341–347, 1994.

[38] P. ten Dijke, H. Yamashita, H. Ichijo et al., "Characterization of type I receptors for transforming growth factor-β and activin," *Science*, vol. 264, no. 5155, pp. 101–104, 1994.

[39] Y. Shi and J. Massagué, "Mechanisms of TGF-β signaling from cell membrane to the nucleus," *Cell*, vol. 113, no. 6, pp. 685–700, 2003.

[40] R. Derynck and Y. E. Zhang, "Smad-dependent and Smad-independent pathways in TGF-β family signalling," *Nature*, vol. 425, no. 6958, pp. 577–584, 2003.

[41] H. E. Olivey, N. A. Mundell, A. F. Austin, and J. V. Barnett, "Transforming growth factor-β stimulates epithelial-mesenchymal transformation in the proepicardium," *Developmental Dynamics*, vol. 235, no. 1, pp. 50–59, 2006.

[42] F. Lebrin, M. Deckers, P. Bertolino, and P. Ten Dijke, "TGF-β receptor function in the endothelium," *Cardiovascular Research*, vol. 65, no. 3, pp. 599–608, 2005.

[43] J. S. Desgrosellier, N. A. Mundell, M. A. McDonnell, H. L. Moses, and J. V. Barnett, "Activin receptor-like kinase 2 and Smad6 regulate epithelial-mesenchymal transformation during cardiac valve formation," *Developmental Biology*, vol. 280, no. 1, pp. 201–210, 2005.

[44] Y.-T. Lai, K. B. Beason, G. P. Brames et al., "Activin receptor-like kinase 2 can mediate atrioventricular cushion transformation," *Developmental Biology*, vol. 222, no. 1, pp. 1–11, 2000.

[45] P. J. Miettinen, R. Ebner, A. R. Lopez, and R. Derynck, "TGF-β induced transdifferentiation of mammary epithelial cells to mesenchymal cells: involvement of type I receptors," *The Journal of Cell Biology*, vol. 127, no. 6, pp. 2021–2036, 1994.

[46] K. Miyazono, S. Maeda, and T. Imamura, "BMP receptor signaling: Transcriptional targets, regulation of signals, and signaling cross-talk," *Cytokine and Growth Factor Reviews*, vol. 16, no. 3, pp. 251–263, 2005.

[47] S. Souchelnytskyi, P. Ten Dijke, K. Miyazono, and C.-H. Heldin, "Phosphorylation of ser165 in TGF-β type I receptor modulates TGF-β1-induced cellular responses," *The EMBO Journal*, vol. 15, no. 22, pp. 6231–6240, 1996.

[48] M. Huse, T. W. Muir, L. Xu, Y.-G. Chen, J. Kuriyan, and J. Massagué, "The TGFβ receptor activation process: an inhibitor-to substrate-binding switch," *Molecular Cell*, vol. 8, no. 3, pp. 671–682, 2001.

[49] R. S. Lo, Y. G. Chen, Y. Shi, N. P. Pavletich, and J. Massague, "The L3 loop: a structural motif determining specific interactions between SMAD proteins and TGF-β receptors," *EMBO Journal*, vol. 17, no. 4, pp. 996–1005, 1998.

[50] S. Abdollah, M. Macías-Silva, T. Tsukazaki, H. Hayashi, L. Attisano, and J. L. Wrana, "TβRI phosphorylation of Smad2 on Ser465 and Ser467 is required for Smad2-Smad4 complex formation and signaling," *Journal of Biological Chemistry*, vol. 272, no. 44, pp. 27678–27685, 1997.

[51] T. Tsukazaki, T. A. Chiang, A. F. Davison, L. Attisano, and J. L. Wrana, "SARA, a FYVE domain protein that recruits Smad2 to the TGFβ receptor," *Cell*, vol. 95, no. 6, pp. 779–791, 1998.

[52] X.-H. Feng, Y. Zhang, R.-Y. Wu, and R. Derynck, "The tumor suppressor Smad4/DPC4 and transcriptional adaptor CBP/p300 are coactivators for Smad3 in TGF-β-induced transcriptional activation," *Genes and Development*, vol. 12, no. 14, pp. 2153–2163, 1998.

[53] R. Janknecht, N. J. Wells, and T. Hunter, "TGF-β-stimulated cooperation of Smad proteins with the coactivators CBP/p300," *Genes and Development*, vol. 12, no. 14, pp. 2114–2119, 1998.

[54] S. Itoh, J. Ericsson, J. Nishikawa, C. H. Heldin, and P. ten Dijke, "The transcriptional co-activator P/CAF potentiates TGF-beta/Smad signaling," *Nucleic Acids Research*, vol. 28, pp. 4291–4298, 2000.

[55] R.-Y. Bai, C. Koester, T. Ouyang et al., "SMIF, a Smad4-interacting protein that functions as a co-activator in TGFβ signalling," *Nature Cell Biology*, vol. 4, no. 3, pp. 181–190, 2002.

[56] C.-R. Chen, Y. Kang, P. M. Siegel, and J. Massagué, "E2F4/5 and p107 as Smad cofactors linking the TGFβ receptor to c-myc repression," *Cell*, vol. 110, no. 1, pp. 19–32, 2002.

[57] Y. Kang, C.-R. Chen, and J. Massagué, "A self-enabling TGFβ response coupled to stress signaling: Smad engages stress response factor ATF3 for Id1 repression in epithelial cells," *Molecular Cell*, vol. 11, no. 4, pp. 915–926, 2003.

[58] D. Wotton, P. S. Knoepfler, C. D. Laherty, R. N. Eisenman, and J. Massagué, "The Smad transcriptional corepressor TGIF recruits mSin3," *Cell Growth and Differentiation*, vol. 12, no. 9, pp. 457–463, 2001.

[59] S. Akiyoshi, H. Inoue, J.-I. Hanai et al., "c-Ski acts as a transcriptional co-repressor in transforming growth factor-β signaling through interaction with Smads," *The Journal of Biological Chemistry*, vol. 274, no. 49, pp. 35269–35277, 1999.

[60] K. Luo, S. L. Stroschein, W. Wang et al., "The Ski oncoprotein interacts with the Smad proteins to repress TGFβsignaling," *Genes and Development*, vol. 13, no. 17, pp. 2196–2206, 1999.

[61] S. L. Stroschein, W. Wang, S. Zhou, Q. Zhou, and K. Luo, "Negative feedback regulation of TGF-β signaling by the SnoN oncoprotein," *Science*, vol. 286, no. 5440, pp. 771–774, 1999.

[62] Y. Sun, X. Liu, E. N. Eaton, W. S. Lane, H. F. Lodish, and R. A. Weinberg, "Interaction of the Ski oncoprotein with Smad3 regulates TGF-β signaling," *Molecular Cell*, vol. 4, no. 4, pp. 499–509, 1999.

[63] J. Seoane, H.-V. Le, L. Shen, S. A. Anderson, and J. Massagué, "Integration of smad and forkhead pathways in the control of neuroepithelial and glioblastoma cell proliferation," *Cell*, vol. 117, no. 2, pp. 211–223, 2004.

[64] K. Pardali, A. Kurisaki, A. Morén, P. Ten Dijke, D. Kardassis, and A. Moustakas, "Role of Smad proteins and transcription factor Sp1 in p21Waf1/Cip1 regulation by transforming growth factor-β," *Journal of Biological Chemistry*, vol. 275, no. 38, pp. 29244–29256, 2000.

[65] Y. Zhang, X.-H. Feng, and R. Derynck, "Smad3 and Smad4 cooperate with c-Jun/c-Fos to mediate TGF-β-induced transcription," *Nature*, vol. 394, no. 6696, pp. 909–913, 1998.

[66] X. Lin, Y.-Y. Liang, B. Sun et al., "Smad6 recruits transcription corepressor CtBP to repress bone morphogenetic protein-induced transcription," *Molecular and Cellular Biology*, vol. 23, no. 24, pp. 9081–9093, 2003.

[67] Y. Peng, S. Zhao, L. Song, M. Wang, and K. Jiao, "Sertad1 encodes a novel transcriptional co-activator of SMAD1 in mouse embryonic hearts," *Biochemical and Biophysical Research Communications*, vol. 441, no. 4, pp. 751–756, 2013.

[68] K. Izutsu, M. Kurokawa, Y. Imai, K. Maki, K. Mitani, and H. Hirai, "The corepressor CtBP interacts with Evi-1 to repress transforming growth factor β signaling," *Blood*, vol. 97, no. 9, pp. 2815–2822, 2001.

[69] Q. Xi, Z. Wang, A. Zaromytidou et al., "A poised chromatin platform for TGF-β access to master regulators," *Cell*, vol. 147, no. 7, pp. 1511–1524, 2011.

[70] S. Ross, E. Cheung, T. G. Petrakis, M. Howell, W. L. Kraus, and C. S. Hill, "Smads orchestrate specific histone modifications and chromatin remodeling to activate transcription," *The EMBO Journal*, vol. 25, no. 19, pp. 4490–4502, 2006.

[71] P. Papageorgis, A. W. Lambert, S. Ozturk et al., "Smad signaling is required to maintain epigenetic silencing during breast cancer progression," *Cancer Research*, vol. 70, no. 3, pp. 968–978, 2010.

[72] A. Nakao, M. Afrakhte, A. Morén et al., "Identification of Smad7, a TGFβ-inducible antagonist of TGF-β signalling," *Nature*, vol. 389, no. 6651, pp. 631–635, 1997.

[73] S. Itoh, M. Landström, A. Hermansson et al., "Transforming growth factor β1 induces nuclear export of inhibitory Smad7," *Journal of Biological Chemistry*, vol. 273, no. 44, pp. 29195–29201, 1998.

[74] H. Hayashi, S. Abdollah, Y. Qiu et al., "The MAD-related protein Smad7 associates with the TGFβ receptor and functions as an antagonist of TGFβ signaling," *Cell*, vol. 89, no. 7, pp. 1165–1173, 1997.

[75] T. Ebisawa, M. Fukuchi, G. Murakami et al., "Smurf1 interacts with transforming growth factor-β type I receptor through Smad7 and induces receptor degradation," *The Journal of Biological Chemistry*, vol. 276, no. 16, pp. 12477–12480, 2001.

[76] P. Kavsak, R. K. Rasmussen, C. G. Causing et al., "Smad7 binds to Smurf2 to form an E3 ubiquitin ligase that targets the TGFβ receptor for degradation," *Molecular Cell*, vol. 6, no. 6, pp. 1365–1375, 2000.

[77] S. Zhang, T. Fei, L. Zhang et al., "Smad7 antagonizes transforming growth factor β signaling in the nucleus by interfering with functional Smad-DNA complex formation," *Molecular and Cellular Biology*, vol. 27, no. 12, pp. 4488–4499, 2007.

[78] W. He, D. C. Dorn, H. Erdjument-Bromage, P. Tempst, M. A. S. Moore, and J. Massagué, "Hematopoiesis controlled by distinct TIF1gamma and Smad4 branches of the TGFβ pathway," *Cell*, vol. 125, no. 5, pp. 929–941, 2006.

[79] P. Descargues, A. K. Sil, Y. Sano et al., "IKKα is a critical coregulator of a Smad4-independent TGFβ-Smad2/3 signaling pathway that controls keratinocyte differentiation," *Proceedings of the National Academy of Sciences of the United States of America*, vol. 105, no. 7, pp. 2487–2492, 2008.

[80] Y. E. Zhang, "Non-Smad pathways in TGF-β signaling," *Cell Research*, vol. 19, no. 1, pp. 128–139, 2009.

[81] M. T. Hartsough and K. M. Mulder, "Transforming growth factor β activation of p44mapk in proliferating cultures of epithelial cells," *Journal of Biological Chemistry*, vol. 270, no. 13, pp. 7117–7124, 1995.

[82] R. S. Frey and K. M. Mulder, "TGFβ regulation of mitogen-activated protein kinases in human breast cancer cells," *Cancer Letters*, vol. 117, no. 1, pp. 41–50, 1997.

[83] P. Papageorgis, K. Cheng, S. Ozturk et al., "Smad4 inactivation promotes malignancy and drug resistance of colon cancer," *Cancer Research*, vol. 71, no. 3, pp. 998–1008, 2011.

[84] G. A. Finlay, V. J. Thannickal, B. L. Fanburg, and K. E. Paulson, "Transforming growth factor-β1-induced activation of the ERK pathway/activator protein-1 in human lung fibroblasts requires the autocrine induction of basic fibroblast growth factor," *Journal of Biological Chemistry*, vol. 275, no. 36, pp. 27650–27656, 2000.

[85] F. Viñals and J. Pouysségur, "Transforming growth factor β1 (TGF-β1) promotes endothelial cell survival during in vitro angiogenesis via an autocrine mechanism implicating TGF-α signaling," *Molecular and Cellular Biology*, vol. 21, no. 21, pp. 7218–7230, 2001.

[86] V. Ellenrieder, S. F. Hendler, W. Boeck et al., "Transforming growth factor β1 treatment leads to an epithelial-mesenchymal transdifferentiation of pancreatic cancer cells requiring extracellular signal-regulated kinase 2 activation," *Cancer Research*, vol. 61, no. 10, pp. 4222–4228, 2001.

[87] L. Xie, B. K. Law, A. M. Chytil, K. A. Brown, M. E. Aakre, and H. L. Moses, "Activation of the Erk pathway is required for TGF-β1-induced EMT *in vitro*," *Neoplasia*, vol. 6, no. 5, pp. 603–610, 2004.

[88] S. Lawler, X.-H. Feng, R.-H. Chen et al., "The type II transforming growth factor-β receptor autophosphorylates not only on serine and threonine but also on tyrosine residues," *Journal of Biological Chemistry*, vol. 272, no. 23, pp. 14850–14859, 1997.

[89] A. J. Galliher and W. P. Schiemann, "Src phosphorylates Tyr284 in TGF-β type II receptor and regulates TGF-β stimulation of p38 MAPK during breast cancer cell proliferation and invasion," *Cancer Research*, vol. 67, no. 8, pp. 3752–3758, 2007.

[90] M. K. Lee, C. Pardoux, M. C. Hall et al., "TGF-β activates Erk MAP kinase signalling through direct phosphorylation of ShcA," *EMBO Journal*, vol. 26, no. 17, pp. 3957–3967, 2007.

[91] J. H. Liao, J. S. Chen, M. Q. Chai, S. Zhao, and J. G. Song, "The involvement of p38 MAPK in transforming growth factor β1-induced apoptosis in murine hepatocytes," *Cell Research*, vol. 11, no. 2, pp. 89–94, 2001.

[92] N. Kimura, R. Matsuo, H. Shibuya, K. Nakashima, and T. Taga, "BMP2-induced apoptosis is mediated by activation of the TAK1-p38 kinase pathway that is negatively regulated by Smad6," *Journal of Biological Chemistry*, vol. 275, no. 23, pp. 17647–17652, 2000.

[93] A. V. Bakin, C. Rinehart, A. K. Tomlinson, and C. L. Arteaga, "p38 mitogen-activated protein kinase is required for TGFβ-mediated fibroblastic transdifferentiation and cell migration," *Journal of Cell Science*, vol. 115, no. 15, pp. 3193–3206, 2002.

[94] B. A. Hocevar, T. L. Brown, and P. H. Howe, "TGF-β induces fibronectin synthesis through a C-jun N-terminal kinase-dependent, Smad4-independent pathway," *EMBO Journal*, vol. 18, no. 5, pp. 1345–1356, 1999.

[95] L. Yu, M. C. Hébert, and Y. E. Zhang, "TGF-β receptor-activated p38 MAP kinase mediates smad-independent TGF-β responses," *The EMBO Journal*, vol. 21, no. 14, pp. 3749–3759, 2002.

[96] K. Yamaguchi, K. Shirakabe, H. Shibuya et al., "Identification of a member of the MAPKKK family as a potential Mediator of TGF-β signal transduction," *Science*, vol. 270, no. 5244, pp. 2008–2011, 1995.

[97] J.-H. Shim, C. Xiao, A. E. Paschal et al., "TAK1, but not TAB1 or TAB2, plays an essential role in multiple signaling pathways in vivo," *Genes and Development*, vol. 19, no. 22, pp. 2668–2681, 2005.

[98] M. Yamashita, K. Fatyol, C. Jin, X. Wang, Z. Liu, and Y. E. Zhang, "TRAF6 mediates Smad-independent activation of JNK and p38 by TGF-β," *Molecular Cell*, vol. 31, no. 6, pp. 918–924, 2008.

[99] A. Sorrentino, N. Thakur, S. Grimsby et al., "The type I TGF-β receptor engages TRAF6 to activate TAK1 in a receptor kinase-independent manner," *Nature Cell Biology*, vol. 10, no. 10, pp. 1199–1207, 2008.

[100] L. Zhang, W. Wang, Y. Hayashi et al., "A role for MEK kinase 1 in TGF-β/activin-induced epithelium movement and embryonic eyelid closure," *EMBO Journal*, vol. 22, no. 17, pp. 4443–4454, 2003.

[101] K.-Y. Kim, B.-C. Kim, Z. Xu, and S.-J. Kim, "Mixed lineage kinase 3 (MLK3)-activated p38 MAP kinase mediates transforming growth factor-β-induced apoptosis in hepatoma cells," *The Journal of Biological Chemistry*, vol. 279, no. 28, pp. 29478–29484, 2004.

[102] A. V. Bakin, A. K. Tomlinson, N. A. Bhowmick, H. L. Moses, and C. L. Arteaga, "Phosphatidylinositol 3-kinase function is required for transforming growth factor β-mediated epithelial to mesenchymal transition and cell migration," *Journal of Biological Chemistry*, vol. 275, no. 47, pp. 36803–36810, 2000.

[103] I. Shin, A. V. Bakin, U. Rodeck, A. Brunet, and C. L. Arteaga, "Transforming growth factor β enhances epithelial cell survival via Akt-dependent regulation of FKHRL1," *Molecular Biology of the Cell*, vol. 12, no. 11, pp. 3328–3339, 2001.

[104] Y. Y. Jae, I. Shin, and C. L. Arteaga, "Type I transforming growth factor β receptor binds to and activates phosphatidylinositol 3-kinase," *Journal of Biological Chemistry*, vol. 280, no. 11, pp. 10870–10876, 2005.

[105] M. Hidalgo and E. K. Rowinsky, "The rapamycin-sensitive signal transduction pathway as a target for cancer therapy," *Oncogene*, vol. 19, no. 56, pp. 6680–6686, 2000.

[106] S. Lamouille and R. Derynck, "Cell size and invasion in TGF-β-induced epithelial to mesenchymal transition is regulated by activation of the mTOR pathway," *Journal of Cell Biology*, vol. 178, no. 3, pp. 437–451, 2007.

[107] A. B. Jaffe and A. Hall, "Rho GTPases: biochemistry and biology," *Annual Review of Cell and Developmental Biology*, vol. 21, pp. 247–269, 2005.

[108] N. A. Bhowmick, M. Ghiassi, A. Bakin et al., "Transforming growth factor-β1 mediates epithelial to mesenchymal transdifferentiation through a RhoA-dependent mechanism," *Molecular Biology of the Cell*, vol. 12, no. 1, pp. 27–36, 2001.

[109] S. Edlund, M. Landström, C.-H. Heldin, and P. Aspenström, "Transforming growth factor-β-induced mobilization of actin cytoskeleton requires signaling by small GTPases Cdc42 and RhoA," *Molecular Biology of the Cell*, vol. 13, no. 3, pp. 902–914, 2002.

[110] B. Tang, M. Vu, T. Booker et al., "TGF-β switches from tumor suppressor to prometastatic factor in a model of breast cancer progression," *The Journal of Clinical Investigation*, vol. 112, no. 7, pp. 1116–1124, 2003.

[111] L. M. Wakefield and A. B. Roberts, "TGF-β signaling: positive and negative effects on tumorigenesis," *Current Opinion in Genetics and Development*, vol. 12, no. 1, pp. 22–29, 2002.

[112] P. M. Siegel, W. Shu, R. D. Cardiff, W. J. Muller, and J. Massagué, "Transforming growth factor β signaling impairs neu-induced mammary tumorigenesis while promoting pulmonary metastasis," *Proceedings of the National Academy of Sciences of the United States of America*, vol. 100, no. 14, pp. 8430–8435, 2003.

[113] A. B. Roberts and L. M. Wakefield, "The two faces of transforming growth factor β in carcinogenesis," *Proceedings of the National Academy of Sciences of the United States of America*, vol. 100, no. 15, pp. 8621–8623, 2003.

[114] P. M. Siegel and J. Massagué, "Cytostatic and apoptotic actions of TGF-β in homeostasis and cancer," *Nature Reviews Cancer*, vol. 3, no. 11, pp. 807–820, 2003.

[115] M. E. Choi and B. J. Ballermann, "Inhibition of capillary morphogenesis and associated apoptosis by dominant negative mutant transforming growth factor-β receptors," *The Journal of Biological Chemistry*, vol. 270, no. 36, pp. 21144–21150, 1995.

[116] K. M. Hyman, G. Seghezzi, G. Pintucci et al., "Transforming growth factor-β1 induces apoptosis in vascular endothelial cells

by activation of mitogen-activated protein kinase," *Surgery*, vol. 132, no. 2, pp. 173–179, 2002.

[117] J. N. Rich, M. Zhang, M. B. Datto, D. D. Bigner, and X.-F. Wang, "Transforming growth factor-β-mediated p15(INK4B) induction and growth inhibition in astrocytes is SMAD3-dependent and a pathway prominently altered in human glioma cell lines," *The Journal of Biological Chemistry*, vol. 274, no. 49, pp. 35053–35058, 1999.

[118] X. Yang, J. J. Letterio, R. J. Lechleider et al., "Targeted disruption of SMAD3 results in impaired mucosal immunity and diminished T cell responsiveness to TGF-β," *The EMBO Journal*, vol. 18, no. 5, pp. 1280–1291, 1999.

[119] M. Laiho, J. A. DeCaprio, J. W. Ludlow, D. M. Livingston, and J. Massagué, "Growth inhibition by TGF-β linked to suppression of retinoblastoma protein phosphorylation," *Cell*, vol. 62, no. 1, pp. 175–185, 1990.

[120] G. J. Hannon and D. Beach, "p15INK4B is a potential effector of TGF-β-induced cell cycle arrest," *Nature*, vol. 371, no. 6494, pp. 257–261, 1994.

[121] M. B. Datto, Y. Li, J. F. Panus, D. J. Howe, Y. Xiong, and X.-F. Wang, "Transforming growth factor β induces the cyclin-dependent kinase inhibitor p21 through a p53-independent mechanism," *Proceedings of the National Academy of Sciences of the United States of America*, vol. 92, no. 12, pp. 5545–5549, 1995.

[122] K. Polyak, J.-Y. Kato, M. J. Solomon et al., "P27Kip1, a cyclin-Cdk inhibitor, links transforming growth factor-β and contact inhibition to cell cycle arrest," *Genes and Development*, vol. 8, no. 1, pp. 9–22, 1994.

[123] C. Sandhu, J. Garbe, N. Bhattacharya et al., "Transforming growth factor β stabilizes p15(INK4B) protein, increases p15(INK4B)-cdk4 complexes, and inhibits cyclin D1-cdk4 association in human mammary epithelial cells," *Molecular and Cellular Biology*, vol. 17, no. 5, pp. 2458–2467, 1997.

[124] I. Reynisdottir, K. Polyak, A. Iavarone, and J. Massague, "Kip/Cip and Ink4 Cdk inhibitors cooperate to induce cell cycle arrest in response to TGF-β," *Genes and Development*, vol. 9, no. 15, pp. 1831–1845, 1995.

[125] I. Reynisdóttir and J. Massagué, "The subcellular locations of pl5(Ink4b) and p27(Kip1) coordinate their inhibitory interactions with cdk4 and cdk2," *Genes and Development*, vol. 11, no. 4, pp. 492–503, 1997.

[126] J. A. Pietenpol, R. W. Stein, E. Moran et al., "TGF-β1 inhibition of c-myc transcription and growth in keratinocytes is abrogated by viral transforming proteins with pRB binding domains," *Cell*, vol. 61, no. 5, pp. 777–785, 1990.

[127] J. D. Norton, "ID helix-loop-helix proteins in cell growth, differentiation and tumorigenesis," *Journal of Cell Science*, vol. 113, no. 22, pp. 3897–3905, 2000.

[128] J. Seoane, C. Pouponnot, P. Staller, M. Schader, M. Eilers, and J. Massagué, "TGFβ influences myc, miz-1 and smad to control the CDK inhibitor p15INK4b," *Nature Cell Biology*, vol. 3, no. 4, pp. 400–408, 2001.

[129] P. Staller, K. Peukert, A. Kiermaier et al., "Repression of p15INK4b expression by Myc through association with Miz-1," *Nature Cell Biology*, vol. 3, no. 4, pp. 392–399, 2001.

[130] A. Lasorella, M. Noseda, M. Beyna, Y. Yokota, and A. Iavarone, "Id2 is a retinoblastoma protein target and mediates signalling by Myc oncoproteins," *Nature*, vol. 407, pp. 592–598, 2000.

[131] X.-J. Wang, K. M. Liefer, S. Tsai, B. W. O'Malley, and D. R. Roop, "Development of gene-switch transgenic mice that inducibly express transforming growth factor β1 in the epidermis," *Proceedings of the National Academy of Sciences of the United States of America*, vol. 96, no. 15, pp. 8483–8488, 1999.

[132] X.-J. Wang, D. A. Greenhalgh, J. R. Bickenbach et al., "Expression of a dominant-negative type II transforming growth factor β (TGF-β) receptor in the epidermis of transgenic mice blocks TGF-β-mediated growth inhibition," *Proceedings of the National Academy of Sciences of the United States of America*, vol. 94, no. 6, pp. 2386–2391, 1997.

[133] G. S. Ashcroft, X. Yang, A. B. Glick et al., "Mice lacking Smad3 show accelerated wound healing and an impaired local inflammatory response," *Nature Cell Biology*, vol. 1, no. 5, pp. 260–266, 1999.

[134] D. F. Pierce Jr., M. D. Johnson, Y. Matsui et al., "Inhibition of mammary duct development but not alveolar outgrowth during pregnancy in transgenic mice expressing active TGF-β1," *Genes and Development*, vol. 7, no. 12, pp. 2308–2317, 1993.

[135] C. Jhappan, A. G. Geiser, E. C. Kordon et al., "Targeting expression of a transforming growth factor β1 transgene to the pregnant mammary gland inhibits alveolar development and lactation," *EMBO Journal*, vol. 12, no. 5, pp. 1835–1845, 1993.

[136] A. E. Gorska, H. Joseph, R. Derynck, H. L. Moses, and R. Serra, "Dominant-negative interference of the transforming growth factor β type II receptor in mammary gland epithelium results in alveolar hyperplasia and differentiation in virgin mice," *Cell Growth and Differentiation*, vol. 9, no. 3, pp. 229–238, 1998.

[137] E. P. Böttinger, J. L. Jakubczak, D. C. Haines, K. Bagnall, and L. M. Wakefield, "Transgenic mice overexpressing a dominant-negative mutant type II transforming growth factor β receptor show enhanced tumorigenesis in the mammary gland and lung in response to the carcinogen 7,12-dimethylbenz-[a]-anthracene," *Cancer Research*, vol. 57, no. 24, pp. 5564–5570, 1997.

[138] P. L. Beck, I. M. Rosenberg, R. J. Xavier, T. Koh, J. F. Wong, and D. K. Podolsky, "Transforming growth factor-β mediates intestinal healing and susceptibility to injury in vitro and in vivo through epithelial cells," *The American Journal of Pathology*, vol. 162, no. 2, pp. 597–608, 2003.

[139] K. Pardali and A. Moustakas, "Actions of TGF-β as tumor suppressor and pro-metastatic factor in human cancer," *Biochimica et Biophysica Acta—Reviews on Cancer*, vol. 1775, no. 1, pp. 21–62, 2007.

[140] C.-W. Jang, C.-H. Chen, C.-C. Chen, J.-Y. Chen, Y.-H. Su, and R.-H. Chen, "TGF-β induces apoptosis through Smad-mediated expression of DAP-kinase," *Nature Cell Biology*, vol. 4, no. 1, pp. 51–58, 2002.

[141] R. Perlman, W. P. Schiemann, M. W. Brooks, H. F. Lodish, and R. A. Weinberg, "TGF-β-induced apoptosis is mediated by the adapter protein Daxx that facilitates JNK activation," *Nature Cell Biology*, vol. 3, no. 8, pp. 708–714, 2001.

[142] J. Yoo, M. Ghiassi, L. Jirmanova et al., "Transforming growth factor-beta-induced apoptosis is mediated by Smad-dependent expression of GADD45b through p38 activation," *The Journal of Biological Chemistry*, vol. 278, no. 44, pp. 43001–43007, 2003.

[143] Y. Gottfried, A. Rotem, R. Lotan, H. Steller, and S. Larisch, "The mitochondrial ARTS protein promotes apoptosis through targeting XIAP," *EMBO Journal*, vol. 23, no. 7, pp. 1627–1635, 2004.

[144] M. Ohgushi, S. Kuroki, H. Fukamachi et al., "Transforming growth factor β-dependent sequential activation of Smad, Bim, and caspase-9 mediates physiological apoptosis in gastric

epithelial cells," *Molecular and Cellular Biology*, vol. 25, no. 22, pp. 10017–10028, 2005.

[145] A. B. Roberts, M. A. Anzano, L. M. Wakefield, N. S. Roche, D. F. Stern, and M. B. Sporn, "Type β transforming growth factor: a bifunctional regulator of cellular growth," *Proceedings of the National Academy of Sciences of the United States of America*, vol. 82, no. 1, pp. 119–123, 1985.

[146] G. R. Grotendorst, "Connective tissue growth factor: a mediator of TGf-β action on fibroblasts," *Cytokine and Growth Factor Reviews*, vol. 8, no. 3, pp. 171–179, 1997.

[147] K. Park, S.-J. Kim, Y.-J. Bang et al., "Genetic changes in the transforming growth factor β (TGF-β) type II receptor gene in human gastric cancer cells: correlation with sensitivity to growth inhibition by TGF-β," *Proceedings of the National Academy of Sciences of the United States of America*, vol. 91, no. 19, pp. 8772–8776, 1994.

[148] I. Y. Kim, H.-J. Ahn, D. J. Zelner et al., "Genetic change in transforming growth factor β (TGF-β) receptor type I gene correlates with insensitivity to TGF-β1 in human prostate cancer cells," *Cancer Research*, vol. 56, no. 1, pp. 44–48, 1996.

[149] S. Markowitz, J. Wang, L. Myeroff et al., "Inactivation of the type II TGF-β receptor in colon cancer cells with microsatellite instability," *Science*, vol. 268, no. 5215, pp. 1336–1338, 1995.

[150] G. J. Riggins, K. W. Kinzler, B. Vogelstein, and S. Thiagalingam, "Frequency of Smad gene mutations in human cancers," *Cancer Research*, vol. 57, no. 13, pp. 2578–2580, 1997.

[151] M. Schutte, R. H. Hruban, L. Hedrick et al., "DPC4 gene in various tumor types," *Cancer Research*, vol. 56, no. 11, pp. 2527–2530, 1996.

[152] K. Eppert, S. W. Scherer, H. Ozcelik et al., "MADR2 maps to 18q21 and encodes a TGFβ-regulated MAD-related protein that is functionally mutated in colorectal carcinoma," *Cell*, vol. 86, no. 4, pp. 543–552, 1996.

[153] S. A. Hahn, A. T. M. S. Hoque, C. A. Moskaluk et al., "Homozygous deletion map at 18q21.1 in pancreatic cancer," *Cancer Research*, vol. 56, no. 3, pp. 490–494, 1996.

[154] S. A. Hahn, M. Schutte, A. T. M. Shamsul Hoque et al., "DPC4, a candidate tumor suppressor gene at human chromosome 18q21.1," *Science*, vol. 271, no. 5247, pp. 350–353, 1996.

[155] S. Thiagalingam, C. Lengauer, F. S. Leach et al., "Evaluation of candidate tumour suppressor genes on chromosome 18 in colorectal cancers," *Nature Genetics*, vol. 13, no. 3, pp. 343–346, 1996.

[156] I. Schwarte-Waldhoff, O. V. Volpert, N. P. Bouck et al., "Smad4/DPC4-mediated tumor suppression through suppression of angiogenesis," *Proceedings of the National Academy of Sciences of the United States of America*, vol. 97, no. 17, pp. 9624–9629, 2000.

[157] M. Kretzschmar, J. Doody, I. Timokhina, and J. Massagué, "A mechanism of repression of TGFβ/Smad signaling by oncogenic Ras," *Genes and Development*, vol. 13, no. 7, pp. 804–816, 1999.

[158] M. Kretzschmar, J. Doody, and J. Massagué, "Opposing BMP and EGF signalling pathways converge on the TGF-β family mediator Smad1," *Nature*, vol. 389, no. 6651, pp. 618–622, 1997.

[159] J. Massagué, "Integration of Smad and MAPK pathways: a link and a linker revisited," *Genes and Development*, vol. 17, no. 24, pp. 2993–2997, 2003.

[160] R. R. Gomis, C. Alarcón, C. Nadal, C. Van Poznak, and J. Massagué, "C/EBPβ at the core of the TGFβ cytostatic response and its evasion in metastatic breast cancer cells," *Cancer Cell*, vol. 10, no. 3, pp. 203–214, 2006.

[161] D. Padua, X. H.-F. Zhang, Q. Wang et al., "TGFβ primes breast tumors for lung metastasis seeding through angiopoietin-like 4," *Cell*, vol. 133, no. 1, pp. 66–77, 2008.

[162] A. J. Minn, G. P. Gupta, P. M. Siegel et al., "Genes that mediate breast cancer metastasis to lung," *Nature*, vol. 436, no. 7050, pp. 518–524, 2005.

[163] N. Mori, M. Morishita, T. Tsukazaki et al., "Human T-cell leukemia virus type I oncoprotein Tax represses Smad-dependent transforming growth factor β signaling through interaction with CREB-binding protein/p300," *Blood*, vol. 97, no. 7, pp. 2137–2144, 2001.

[164] J. Deheuninck and K. Luo, "Ski and SnoN, potent negative regulators of TGF-β signaling," *Cell Research*, vol. 19, no. 1, pp. 47–57, 2009.

[165] J. P. Their, "Epithelial-mesenchymal transitions in tumor progression," *Nature Reviews Cancer*, vol. 2, no. 6, pp. 442–454, 2002.

[166] J. Xu, S. Lamouille, and R. Derynck, "TGF-β-induced epithelial to mesenchymal transition," *Cell Research*, vol. 19, no. 2, pp. 156–172, 2009.

[167] J. P. Thiery and J. P. Sleeman, "Complex networks orchestrate epithelial-mesenchymal transitions," *Nature Reviews Molecular Cell Biology*, vol. 7, no. 2, pp. 131–142, 2006.

[168] A. Cano, M. A. Pérez-Moreno, I. Rodrigo et al., "The transcription factor Snail controls epithelial-mesenchymal transitions by repressing E-cadherin expression," *Nature Cell Biology*, vol. 2, no. 2, pp. 76–83, 2000.

[169] P. Savagner, K. M. Yamada, and J. P. Thiery, "The zinc-finger protein slug causes desmosome dissociation, an initial and necessary step for growth factor-induced epithelial-mesenchymal transition," *Journal of Cell Biology*, vol. 137, no. 6, pp. 1403–1419, 1997.

[170] A. Eger, K. Aigner, S. Sonderegger et al., "DeltaEF1 is a transcriptional repressor of E-cadherin and regulates epithelial plasticity in breast cancer cells," *Oncogene*, vol. 24, no. 14, pp. 2375–2385, 2005.

[171] J. Comijn, G. Berx, P. Vermassen et al., "The two-handed E box binding zinc finger protein SIP1 downregulates E-cadherin and induces invasion," *Molecular Cell*, vol. 7, no. 6, pp. 1267–1278, 2001.

[172] J. Yang, S. A. Mani, J. L. Donaher et al., "Twist, a master regulator of morphogenesis, plays an essential role in tumor metastasis," *Cell*, vol. 117, no. 7, pp. 927–939, 2004.

[173] L. R. Howe, O. Watanabe, J. Leonard, and A. M. Brown, "Twist is up-regulated in response to Wnt1 and inhibits mouse mammary cell differentiation," *Cancer Research*, vol. 63, no. 8, pp. 1906–1913, 2003.

[174] H.-W. Lo, S.-C. Hsu, W. Xia et al., "Epidermal growth factor receptor cooperates with signal transducer and activator of transcription 3 to induce epithelial-mesenchymal transition in cancer cells via up-regulation of TWIST gene expression," *Cancer Research*, vol. 67, no. 19, pp. 9066–9076, 2007.

[175] S. Thuault, U. Valcourt, M. Petersen, G. Manfioletti, C.-H. Heldin, and A. Moustakas, "Transforming growth factor-β employs HMGA2 to elicit epithelial-mesenchymal transition," *Journal of Cell Biology*, vol. 174, no. 2, pp. 175–183, 2006.

[176] T. Shirakihara, M. Saitoh, and K. Miyazono, "Differential regulation of epithelial and mesenchymal markers by δEF1 proteins in epithelial-mesenchymal transition induced by TGF-β," *Molecular Biology of the Cell*, vol. 18, no. 9, pp. 3533–3544, 2007.

[177] S. A. Mani, J. Yang, M. Brooks et al., "Mesenchyme Forkhead 1 (FOXC2) plays a key role in metastasis and is associated with aggressive basal-like breast cancers," *Proceedings of the National Academy of Sciences of the United States of America*, vol. 104, no. 24, pp. 10069–10074, 2007.

[178] M. Oft, K.-H. Heider, and H. Beug, "TGFβ signaling is necessary for carcinoma cell invasiveness and metastasis," *Current Biology*, vol. 8, no. 23, pp. 1243–1252, 1998.

[179] M. Oft, J. Peli, C. Rudaz, H. Schwarz, H. Beug, and E. Reichmann, "TGF-β1 and Ha-Ras collaborate in modulating the phenotypic plasticity and invasiveness of epithelial tumor cells," *Genes and Development*, vol. 10, no. 19, pp. 2462–2477, 1996.

[180] W. Cui, D. J. Fowlis, S. Bryson et al., "TGFβ1 inhibits the formation of benign skin tumors, but enhances progression to invasive spindle carcinomas in transgenic mice," *Cell*, vol. 86, no. 4, pp. 531–542, 1996.

[181] G. Portella, S. A. Cumming, J. Liddell et al., "Transforming growth factor β is essential for spindle cell conversion of mouse skin carcinoma in vivo: implications for tumor invasion," *Cell Growth & Differentiation*, vol. 9, no. 5, pp. 393–404, 1998.

[182] Y. Kang and J. Massagué, "Epithelial-mesenchymal transitions: twist in development and metastasis," *Cell*, vol. 118, no. 3, pp. 277–279, 2004.

[183] J. Yang and R. A. Weinberg, "Epithelial-mesenchymal transition: at the crossroads of development and tumor metastasis," *Developmental Cell*, vol. 14, no. 6, pp. 818–829, 2008.

[184] S. Lamouille, J. Xu, and R. Derynck, "Molecular mechanisms of epithelial-mesenchymal transition," *Nature Reviews Molecular Cell Biology*, vol. 15, no. 3, pp. 178–196, 2014.

[185] J. Zavadil, M. Bitzer, D. Liang et al., "Genetic programs of epithelial cell plasticity directed by transforming growth factor-β," *Proceedings of the National Academy of Sciences of the United States of America*, vol. 98, no. 12, pp. 6686–6691, 2001.

[186] S. Itoh, M. Thorikay, M. Kowanetz et al., "Elucidation of Smad requirement in transforming growth factor-β type I receptor-induced responses," *The Journal of Biological Chemistry*, vol. 278, no. 6, pp. 3751–3761, 2003.

[187] E. Janda, K. Lehmann, I. Killisch et al., "Ras and TGFβ cooperatively regulate epithelial cell plasticity and metastasis: dissection of Ras signaling pathways," *Journal of Cell Biology*, vol. 156, no. 2, pp. 299–313, 2002.

[188] M. Oft, R. J. Akhurst, and A. Balmain, "Metastasis is driven by sequential elevation of H-ras and Smad2 levels," *Nature Cell Biology*, vol. 4, no. 7, pp. 487–494, 2002.

[189] M. Adorno, M. Cordenonsi, M. Montagner et al., "A Mutant-p53/Smad complex opposes p63 to empower TGFβ-induced metastasis," *Cell*, vol. 137, no. 1, pp. 87–98, 2009.

[190] U. Burk, J. Schubert, U. Wellner et al., "A reciprocal repression between ZEB1 and members of the miR-200 family promotes EMT and invasion in cancer cells," *EMBO Reports*, vol. 9, no. 6, pp. 582–589, 2008.

[191] M. Korpal, E. S. Lee, G. Hu, and Y. Kang, "The miR-200 family inhibits epithelial-mesenchymal transition and cancer cell migration by direct targeting of E-cadherin transcriptional repressors ZEB1 and ZEB2," *The Journal of Biological Chemistry*, vol. 283, no. 22, pp. 14910–14914, 2008.

[192] S.-M. Park, A. B. Gaur, E. Lengyel, and M. E. Peter, "The miR-200 family determines the epithelial phenotype of cancer cells by targeting the E-cadherin repressors ZEB1 and ZEB2," *Genes & Development*, vol. 22, no. 7, pp. 894–907, 2008.

[193] P. A. Gregory, A. G. Bert, E. L. Paterson et al., "The miR-200 family and miR-205 regulate epithelial to mesenchymal transition by targeting ZEB1 and SIP1," *Nature Cell Biology*, vol. 10, no. 5, pp. 593–601, 2008.

[194] X. Ding, S. I. Park, L. K. McCauley, and C. Y. Wang, "Signaling between transforming growth factor β (TGF-β) and transcription factor snai2 represses expression of microRNA miR-203 to promote epithelial-Mesenchymal transition and tumor metastasis," *Journal of Biological Chemistry*, vol. 288, no. 15, pp. 10241–10253, 2013.

[195] J. Zavadil, M. Narasimhan, M. Blumenberg, and R. J. Schneider, "Transforming growth factor-β and microRNA:mRNA regulatory networks in epithelial plasticity," *Cells Tissues Organs*, vol. 185, no. 1–3, pp. 157–161, 2007.

[196] M. Al-Hajj, M. S. Wicha, A. Benito-Hernandez, S. J. Morrison, and M. F. Clarke, "Prospective identification of tumorigenic breast cancer cells," *Proceedings of the National Academy of Sciences of the United States of America*, vol. 100, no. 7, pp. 3983–3988, 2003.

[197] P. B. Gupta, C. L. Chaffer, and R. A. Weinberg, "Cancer stem cells: mirage or reality?" *Nature Medicine*, vol. 15, no. 9, pp. 1010–1012, 2009.

[198] S. V. Sharma, D. Y. Lee, B. Li et al., "A chromatin-mediated reversible drug-tolerant state in cancer cell subpopulations," *Cell*, vol. 141, no. 1, pp. 69–80, 2010.

[199] C. Scheel, E. N. Eaton, S. H.-J. Li et al., "Paracrine and autocrine signals induce and maintain mesenchymal and stem cell states in the breast," *Cell*, vol. 145, no. 6, pp. 926–940, 2011.

[200] S. A. Mani, W. Guo, M.-J. Liao et al., "The epithelial-mesenchymal transition generates cells with properties of stem cells," *Cell*, vol. 133, no. 4, pp. 704–715, 2008.

[201] M. Yu, A. Bardia, B. S. Wittner et al., "Circulating breast tumor cells exhibit dynamic changes in epithelial and mesenchymal composition," *Science*, vol. 339, no. 6119, pp. 580–584, 2013.

[202] M. Pickup, S. Novitskiy, and H. L. Moses, "The roles of TGFβ in the tumour microenvironment," *Nature Reviews Cancer*, vol. 13, no. 11, pp. 788–799, 2013.

[203] H. Tsushima, S. Kawata, S. Tamura et al., "High levels of transforming growth factor in patients with colorectal cancer: association with disease progression," *Gastroenterology*, vol. 110, no. 2, pp. 375–382, 1996.

[204] B. I. Dalal, P. A. Keown, and A. H. Greenberg, "Immunocytochemical localization of secreted transforming growth factor-β1 to the advancing edges of primary tumors and to lymph node metastases of human mammary carcinoma," *The American Journal of Pathology*, vol. 143, no. 2, pp. 381–389, 1993.

[205] M. S. Steiner, Z.-Z. Zhou, D. C. Tonb, and E. R. Barrack, "Expression of transforming growth factor-β1 in prostate cancer," *Endocrinology*, vol. 135, no. 5, pp. 2240–2247, 1994.

[206] R. Derynck, R. J. Akhurst, and A. Balmain, "TGF-beta signaling in tumor suppression and cancer progression," *Nature Genetics*, vol. 29, pp. 117–129, 2001.

[207] D. F. Quail and J. A. Joyce, "Microenvironmental regulation of tumor progression and metastasis," *Nature Medicine*, vol. 19, no. 11, pp. 1423–1437, 2013.

[208] L. A. Kingsley, P. G. J. Fournier, J. M. Chirgwin, and T. A. Guise, "Molecular biology of bone metastasis," *Molecular Cancer Therapeutics*, vol. 6, no. 10, pp. 2609–2617, 2007.

[209] J. Massagué, "TGFβ in Cancer," *Cell*, vol. 134, no. 2, pp. 215–230, 2008.

[210] M. H. Branton and J. B. Kopp, "TGF-β and fibrosis," *Microbes and Infection*, vol. 1, no. 15, pp. 1349–1365, 1999.

[211] P. J. Wipff and B. Hinz, "Myofibroblasts work best under stress," *Journal of Bodywork and Movement Therapies*, vol. 13, no. 2, pp. 121–127, 2009.

[212] A. H. Rook, J. H. Kehrl, L. M. Wakefield et al., "Effects of transforming growth factor β on the functions of natural killer cells: depressed cytolytic activity and blunting of interferon responsiveness," *Journal of Immunology*, vol. 136, no. 10, pp. 3916–3920, 1986.

[213] L. Gorelink and R. A. Flavell, "Immune-mediated eradication of tumors through the blockade of transforming growth factor-β signaling in T cells," *Nature Medicine*, vol. 7, no. 10, pp. 1118–1122, 2001.

[214] S. Ramesh, G. M. Wildey, and P. H. Howe, "Transforming growth factor β (TGFβ)-induced apoptosis: the rise & fall of Bim," *Cell Cycle*, vol. 8, no. 1, pp. 11–17, 2009.

[215] F. Geissmann, P. Revy, A. Regnault et al., "TGF-β1 prevents the noncognate maturation of human dendritic Langerhans cells," *Journal of Immunology*, vol. 162, no. 8, pp. 4567–4575, 1999.

[216] A. Mantovani, S. Sozzani, M. Locati, P. Allavena, and A. Sica, "Macrophage polarization: tumor-associated macrophages as a paradigm for polarized M2 mononuclear phagocytes," *Trends in Immunology*, vol. 23, no. 11, pp. 549–555, 2002.

[217] Z. G. Fridlender, J. Sun, S. Kim et al., "Polarization of tumor-associated neutrophil phenotype by TGF-β: "N1" versus "N2" TAN," *Cancer Cell*, vol. 16, no. 3, pp. 183–194, 2009.

[218] P. D. Bos, X. H. Zhang, C. Nadal et al., "Genes that mediate breast cancer metastasis to the brain," *Nature*, vol. 459, no. 7249, pp. 1005–1009, 2009.

[219] Y. Kang, P. M. Siegel, W. Shu et al., "A multigenic program mediating breast cancer metastasis to bone," *Cancer Cell*, vol. 3, no. 6, pp. 537–549, 2003.

[220] D. X. Nguyen, P. D. Bos, and J. Massagué, "Metastasis: from dissemination to organ-specific colonization," *Nature Reviews Cancer*, vol. 9, no. 4, pp. 274–284, 2009.

[221] Y. Kang, W. He, S. Tulley et al., "Breast cancer bone metastasis mediated by the Smad tumor suppressor pathway," *Proceedings of the National Academy of Sciences of the United States of America*, vol. 102, no. 39, pp. 13909–13914, 2005.

[222] T. Shibue and R. A. Weinberg, "Metastatic colonization: settlement, adaptation and propagation of tumor cells in a foreign tissue environment," *Seminars in Cancer Biology*, vol. 21, no. 2, pp. 99–106, 2011.

[223] J. A. Aguirre-Ghiso, "Models, mechanisms and clinical evidence for cancer dormancy," *Nature Reviews Cancer*, vol. 7, no. 11, pp. 834–846, 2007.

[224] J. H. Tsai and J. Yang, "Epithelial-mesenchymal plasticity in carcinoma metastasis," *Genes & Development*, vol. 27, no. 20, pp. 2192–2206, 2013.

[225] M. Stankic, S. Pavlovic, Y. Chin et al., "TGF-β-Id1 signaling opposes twist1 and promotes metastatic colonization via a mesenchymal-to-epithelial transition," *Cell Reports*, vol. 5, no. 5, pp. 1228–1242, 2013.

[226] J.-H. Yuan, F. Yang, F. Wang et al., "A Long Noncoding RNA Activated by TGF-β promotes the invasion-metastasis cascade in hepatocellular carcinoma," *Cancer Cell*, vol. 25, no. 5, pp. 666–681, 2014.

[227] H. Gao, G. Chakraborty, A. P. Lee-Lim et al., "The BMP inhibitor Coco reactivates breast cancer cells at lung metastatic sites," *Cell*, vol. 150, no. 4, pp. 764–779, 2012.

[228] R. J. Akhurst and A. Hata, "Targeting the TGFbeta signalling pathway in disease," *Nature Reviews Drug Discovery*, vol. 11, pp. 790–811, 2012.

10

Dental Treatment in Patients with Leukemia

Caroline Zimmermann,[1] **Maria Inês Meurer,**[2,3]
Liliane Janete Grando,[2,3] **Joanita Ângela Gonzaga Del Moral,**[4]
Inês Beatriz da Silva Rath,[5] **and Silvia Schaefer Tavares**[6]

[1]*Graduate Program of Dentistry, Federal University of Santa Catarina, 88040-900 Florianópolis, SC, Brazil*
[2]*Department of Pathology, Federal University of Santa Catarina, 88040-900 Florianópolis, SC, Brazil*
[3]*Stomatology Clinic, University Hospital, Federal University of Santa Catarina, 88040-900 Florianópolis, SC, Brazil*
[4]*Hematology Service, University Hospital, Federal University of Santa Catarina, 88040-900 Florianópolis, SC, Brazil*
[5]*Department of Dentistry, Federal University of Santa Catarina, 88040-900 Florianópolis, SC, Brazil*
[6]*Integrated Multidisciplinary Health, Federal University of Santa Catarina, 88040-900 Florianópolis, SC, Brazil*

Correspondence should be addressed to Maria Inês Meurer; meurer.m.i@ufsc.br

Academic Editor: Bruce C. Baguley

Dental treatment of patients with leukemia should be planned on the basis of antineoplastic therapy which can be chemotherapy with or without radiotherapy and bone marrow transplantation. Many are the oral manifestations presented by these patients, arising from leukemia and/or treatment. In addition, performing dental procedures at different stages of treatment (before, during, or after) must follow certain protocols in relation to the haematological indices of patients, aimed at maintaining health and contributing to the effectiveness of the results of antineoplastic therapy. Through a literature review, the purpose of this study was to report the hematological abnormalities present in patients with leukemia, trying to correlate them with the feasibility of dental treatment at different stages of the disease. It is concluded in this paper that dental treatment in relation to haematological indices presented by patients with leukemia must follow certain protocols, mainly related to neutrophil and platelet counts, and the presence of the dentist in a multidisciplinary team is required for the health care of this patient.

1. Introduction

The insertion of dentistry in the multidisciplinary context of hematology-oncology is an important part of the success of cancer treatment. Oral complications can compromise the protocols of chemotherapy, possibly making it necessary to decrease the administered dose, the change in treatment protocol, or even discontinuation of antineoplastic therapy, directly affecting patient survival [1, 2].

The feasibility to perform certain dental procedures in leukemia patients depends on the overall state of health of the patient, as well as the stage of the disease and/or antineoplastic therapy or hematopoietic stem cell transplantation. Despite the expectation of finding a vast literature on the leukemia/dental relationship, the bibliographic survey conducted (PubMed, BIREME, Journals Portal CAPES, and SciELO) resulted in a few articles involving the amplitude of

this relationship. Facing the need to establish protocols for the dental care of oncohematological patients at University Hospital, Federal University of Santa Catarina, a simplified guide for the guidance of residents in dentistry in the evaluation and treatment of these patients was developed. The guide consists of tables correlating phases of chemotherapy and hematopoietic stem cell transplantation to the most common dental procedures (classification adapted from Sonis et al. [3]).

2. General Considerations regarding Leukemia

Leukemia is a malignant disease of the blood, where the uncontrolled proliferation of immature blood cells that originate from hematopoietic stem cell mutation occurs. Eventually these aberrant cells compete with normal cells for space in the bone marrow, causing bone marrow failure and death [4].

2.1. Classification. The most common leukemias are generally classified as (1) acute lymphocytic, (2) acute myeloid, (3) chronic lymphocytic, and (4) chronic myeloid. The classification criteria of leukemia is histological and is based on (a) the similarity between the leukemic cells and normal cells (myeloid versus lymphoid) and (b) the clinical course of the disease (acute versus chronic) [4].

The acute forms of leukemia result from the accumulation of immature and functionless cells in the bone marrow, with rapid progression [5], rapidly fatal in untreated patients [6]. Chronic leukemias, in turn, begin slow with uncontrolled proliferation of more mature and differentiated cells [5].

2.2. Treatment. The treatment of leukemia depends on factors such as type and subtype of the disease, risk factors, and age of the patient. In general, the recommended treatment is chemotherapy with or without adjuvant treatments. Hematopoietic stem cell transplantation (HSCT) is performed, in general, in the acute forms of the disease and some cases of chronic myeloid leukemia:

(i) acute lymphoblastic leukemia (ALL): prophase (initial reduction of leukemic cells), induction (achieve complete remission), consolidation (increase the quality of remission), intensification (postremission further reduction), and maintenance therapy (maintenance of consolidation); prophylactic central nervous system (CNS) therapeutic irradiation or irradiation if CNS is involved; the HSCT can be done in some cases [7];

(ii) acute myeloid leukemia (AML): induction (until complete remission), consolidation, and intensification [8];

(iii) chronic myeloid leukemia (CML): remission of leukemic cells and Philadelphia chromosome-positive with high doses of chemotherapy, monitoring of therapy, and HSCT [9];

(iv) chronic lymphocytic leukemia (CLL): conventional treatment is not curative; chemotherapy is performed as a control [10].

2.2.1. Special Considerations about HSCT. Treatment with HSCT aims to repopulate the marrow, previously destroyed with high doses of chemotherapy with or without radiation, for normal healthy cells. The HSCT can be of the autologous type (patient's own hematopoietic stem cells) or allogeneic (hematopoietic cells obtained from a donor) [4, 11] and consists of five phases: (1) preconditioning, (2) neutropenic phase conditioning, (3) engraftment to hematopoietic recovery, (4) immune reconstitution/recovery from systemic toxicity, and (5) long-term survival [1].

The main complications of HSCT are graft rejection (for failure in the patient's immunosuppression) and the graft-versus-host disease (GVHD), where immunocompetent donor cells attack the patient's antigens, which may lead to the depletion of T lymphocytes. Potentially fatal, GVHD can occur soon after HSCT (acute GVHD) or after a few months (chronic GVHD or cGVHD). With deep and long immunosuppression, the patient becomes susceptible to fungal and viral infections [4].

2.3. Oral Manifestations of Leukemia. In acute leukemias, gingival hyperplasia is generally observed, localized or generalized, mainly affecting the interdental papillae and the marginal gingiva caused by inflammation, or leukemic infiltration, and may be localized or generalized, the latter being the most frequent form [3, 5]. The infiltration of leukemic cells may also involve periapical tissues and simulate, both clinically and radiographically, periapical inflammatory lesions [6]. In chronic leukemia, the leukemic infiltrates in oral tissues is less frequent and can be observed: pallor of the mucosa, soft tissue infections, and generalized lymphadenopathy [5].

The manifestations of thrombocytopenia are more common when the platelet count is below 50,000 cells/mm³ [12] and may manifest as bruising, petechiae in the hard and soft palate, and also spontaneous gingival bleeding, especially if the platelet count is below 20,000 cells/mm³ [6].

Opportunistic infections with *Candida albicans* and Herpes viruses are common and can involve any area of the mucosa. Ulcers can also result from impaired immune defense in combating normal microbial flora [6].

2.4. Oral Manifestations Related to HSCT. The most common oral manifestations related to pre-, immediate post-, and late post-HSCT are summarized in Table 6.

The oral manifestations that may be present are correlated with the phases of HSCT [1]: (1) preconditioning: oral infections, ulceration, bleeding, and temporomandibular joint dysfunction; (2) neutropenic phase conditioning: mucositis, dysgeusia, xerostomia, bleeding, oral pain, opportunistic infections, neurotoxicity, and temporomandibular dysfunction, usually manifesting with high prevalence and severe forms; at this stage, the patient may develop hyperacute GVHD with further severe oral complications; (3) engraftment to hematopoietic recovery: opportunistic infections are common and acute GVHD becomes a concern; bleeding may be present, xerostomia, neurotoxicity, granulomas/papillomas, and temporomandibular dysfunction; (4) immune reconstitution/recovery from systemic toxicity: salivary dysfunction, late viral infections, craniofacial growth abnormalities, cGVHD, and squamous cell carcinoma; and (5) the long-term survival: in pediatric patients, particularly children under 6 years, one can observe complications in the development of bones and teeth; at this stage, recurrence and malignant neoplasms can be observed.

In the occurrence of GVHD, mucositis, gingivitis, erythema, and pain are usually observed. In cGVHD, the most common oral manifestations are lichen-type features, hyperkeratotic plaques, mucocele, atrophic mucosa, ulceration [13, 14], fibrosis with limited mouth opening, hyposalivation, and xerostomia [13–16]. In addition, secondary to cGVHD, the patients have a greater tendency to develop malignancies [14, 17, 18].

3. General Considerations regarding Dental Treatment

The dental management of patients with leukemia is necessarily embedded in a multidisciplinary context, because the medical complexity that this patient presents may interfere in the determination of priorities and the time available for dental treatment. For the US National Cancer Institute [2], the multidisciplinary team should have oncologists, nurses, dentists (general and stomatological practitioners), social workers, nutritionists, and other health professionals, which may contribute to the prevention and treatment of oral complications in these patients.

Sonis et al. [3] proposed the classification of patients into categories of high, moderate, and low risk for dental treatment, based on the type of leukemia (acute or chronic) and chemotherapy. Patients at high-risk are those with active leukemia, which have a high number of neoplastic cells in the bone marrow and peripheral blood; because of this, they are thrombocytopenic and neutropenic. This risk group also includes antileukemic patients under treatment, and as a result of therapy, present bone marrow suppression. Considered moderate risk patients are those who successfully completed the first phase of treatment (induction) and are undergoing the maintenance phase, thus not showing signs of malignancy in the bone marrow or peripheral blood; however, they present myelosuppression due to chemotherapy. In the low-risk category are patients who successfully completed treatment and present no evidence of malignancy or myelosuppression.

Basic health care should be part of the patient's routine during antineoplastic therapy and HSCT for maintaining good oral health and reducing the risk of systemic infections of oral origin. The objectives of care include prevention of infection, pain control, maintenance of oral functions, and management of complications of antineoplastic therapy, aimed at improving the quality of life of patients [19].

Little et al. [5] and Elad et al. [19] reinforce that the role of the dentist should occur at three different moments:

(1) pre-antineoplastic treatment evaluation and preparation of patients for this,

(2) guidelines and oral health care during treatment,

(3) posttreatment care.

3.1. Pre-Antineoplastic Treatment Assessment and Patient Preparation. Dental treatment at this stage is based on priorities and should be directed to the acute needs; elective treatment can be postponed to a time when the patient is appropriate for clinical and laboratory conditions [1, 2, 5, 19, 20].

The dental examination, if possible, should occur immediately after diagnosis and before initiation of chemotherapy so as to permit the removal of sources of infection of dental origin [3, 5, 20, 21], since expected neutropenia during chemotherapy predisposes patients to the spread of infection [5].

The objectives of the pre-antineoplastic treatment dental evaluation are as follows [1, 3, 5, 20–22]:

(1) identify and eliminate sources of existing or potential infection, without, however, promoting complications or delaying cancer therapy;

(2) educate the patient (or their relatives) about the importance of maintaining oral health in reducing problems and oral discomfort before, during, and after cancer treatment;

(3) warn about the possible effects of antineoplastic therapy in the oral cavity, such as mucositis;

(4) identify specific issues of the diagnosis of leukemia, such as leukemic infiltrates in oral tissues.

Injury prevention and oral infections is the focus of dental treatment in leukemic patients and the care with oral hygiene (brushing, use of fluoride, and noncariogenic diet) should be emphasized throughout treatment [1, 5, 19].

Data from the US National Cancer Institute [2] allege that some cancer centers encourage tooth brushing and flossing, while others indicate the interruption of brushing and flossing when blood components have a drop below specified limits (e.g., platelets <30,000 cells/mm^3). However, according to the institute itself, there is no evidence in the literature regarding the best approach. The centers providing strategy argue that the benefits of proper brushing and proper flossing outweigh the risks, because the interruption of routine oral hygiene increases the risk of infection, and this could promote bleeding as well as increase the risk of local and systemic infection. Elad et al. [23] agreed that dental treatment prior to HSCT is preferred to no dental intervention.

3.2. Oral Health Care during Antineoplastic Treatment. Patients undergoing chemotherapy have become immunosuppressed and therefore susceptible to systemic infections. They are classified as high-risk patients, not only by the possibility of developing infection, but the extent and severity of this potential, which can have quick course and be potentially fatal [24].

The objectives of dental care during chemotherapy are as follows [1]:

(1) maintain optimal oral health;

(2) treat side effects of antineoplastic therapy;

(3) reinforce to the patient the importance of oral health in reducing problems/discomforts arising from chemotherapy.

Apart from oral mucositis, the main oral complication of chemotherapy, other changes may occur, such as bleeding, increased rates of caries, infections (bacterial, viral, or fungal), gingival abscesses, recurrent herpetic stomatitis, candidiasis, salivary gland dysfunction, xerostomia, dysgeusia, and pain [2, 3, 20, 24]. It is important to realize that infections in the oral cavity can progress to systemic infections, worsening the health status of the patient, and the presence of a dentist and/or stomatologist provides important support to the medical staff [2, 3, 21, 25, 26].

3.3. Post-Antineoplastic Treatment Oral Health Care. In the post-antineoplastic treatment phase, patients are considered cured of leukemia and not having oral manifestations due to illness or chemotherapy, with the exception of those with sequelae of radiotherapy or children who received chemotherapy in the stage of tooth formation [3], which may present hypoplastic areas on tooth enamel (mineralization disorder) and changes in the development of dental roots (which are presented short and V-shaped) [27].

3.4. Special Considerations about Oral Health in HSCT Patients. Considerations regarding the oral health in HSCT patients in pre-, immediate post-, and late post-HSCT are summarized in Table 6.

The principles of dental care before HSCT are very similar to those discussed in Section 3.1 and must consider the following features: (1) In HSCT, the total dose of chemotherapy and/or irradiation of the body is performed a few days before transplantation and (2) immunosuppression will be long term after transplantation [1].

Even though common oral diseases such as periodontal disease can impact systemically in HSCT patients, the pre-HSCT assessment by a dentist is needed, and should include maintenance of the oral health guidelines.

All patients undergoing HSCT should receive specific care, particularly those who develop cGVHD. A complete dental evaluation should occur regularly, and special attention should be focused on early detection of oral cancer and precursor lesions [14, 17, 18, 28]; diagnosis and treatment of mucosal lesions [14, 28] and erythema or lichen-type features with symptomatology [18]; caries prevention [14, 28, 29]; reestablishment of oral health in case of rampant caries [14, 30], with the possibility of use of fluoride applications [14] or silver diamine fluoride for disease control and relief of hypersensitivity [30]; and pharmacological treatment [14, 28, 31] or nonpharmacological treatment [14, 28, 29] of hyposalivation and xerostomia.

The diagnosis of oral cGVHD depends on the patient's history, clinical findings, and early signs and symptoms [14] and it is generally not necessary to perform a biopsy [28].

Even after immunosuppressive therapy, patients who develop cGVHD require long term intensive care. In the care are the reduction of symptoms, resolution of painful injuries, and prevention and management of secondary complications, as well as guidelines for the maintenance of good oral hygiene [14].

4. Dental Procedures in Different Stages of the Disease and Treatment

Dental treatment should be planned according to the antineoplastic therapy [3] and HSCT [19]. The execution of some dental procedures—especially those of invasive character—depends on the overall health status of the patient and stage of antineoplastic treatment in which it lies. Considering the risk of bleeding and serious infections associated with invasive procedures in the oral cavity, there are already some protocols that emphasize the importance of evaluating certain hematological indices, mainly neutrophils and platelets. Variation

was observed among authors regarding the amounts considered minimal for invasive dental procedures in the pre- and transchemotherapy phases. Tables 1 and 2 show the variation as well as meeting the recommendations regarding the need for transfusions, antibiotic prophylaxis, and postponement of dental treatment [1–3, 5, 22, 32–34].

These explained variations will be presented and discussed in Tables 3, 4, and 5, constructed for each phase of treatment.

4.1. Dental Treatment in the Prechemotherapy Phase. Table 3 (prechemotherapy) summarizes the dental procedures and their limitations in the literature, concerning hematological indices and necessary precedence for the procedure considering the initiation of chemotherapy.

Initially, dental treatment should be directed to the acute needs [5]. Elective treatments should be postponed to an opportune time when the patient is in good clinical and hematological conditions [1, 2, 19, 20].

The US National Cancer Institute [2] argues that interventions at this stage should be directed to the treatment of lesions in the oral mucosa, carious and endodontic lesions, periodontal disease, poorly fitting dentures, orthodontic appliances, temporomandibular joint changes, and salivary dysfunction.

Elad et al. [19] recommend that the dentist should eliminate potential sources of trauma in the mucosa, such as orthodontic appliances, ill-fitting dentures, unsatisfactory restorations, traumatized teeth, and dental calculus. They also claim that nonrestorable teeth (with root exposure, severe periodontal involvement and impacted with pericoronitis signals) must be extracted. In the case of restorable teeth, it should be determined if there is enough time for proper treatment. Multiple extractions should be considered if teeth are neglected by the patient.

According to Sonis et al. [3], decayed teeth should be restored when there is no risk of pulpal involvement; if this risk exists, they should be removed or treated endodontically. They also state that any tooth with questionable prognosis should be removed, as well as teeth with periodontal involvement and partially erupted third molars which may prove to be the foci of pericoronitis.

The American Academy of Pediatric Dentistry [1] argues that when all dental needs cannot be addressed before the start of cancer therapy, priority should be eliminating sources of infection and trauma, as well as extractions and periodontal care. Endodontic treatment of symptomatic nonvital teeth should be done at least a week before the start of chemotherapy in order to have sufficient time to evaluate the success of treatment; if this is not possible, extraction is indicated. Teeth that cannot receive endodontic treatment in one session also have extraction as a treatment of choice, with antibiotic prophylaxis (penicillin or clindamycin) for about a week. In asymptomatic teeth, endodontic treatment should be delayed until the haematological indices of the patient stabilize (this includes endodontically treated teeth with periapical lesions, without signs and symptoms of infection). Teeth unable to be restored with periodontal pockets greater than 6 mm, with acute symptomatic infection, significant bone loss, furcation

TABLE 1: Minimum haematological values for performance of invasive dental procedures in prechemotherapy treatment patients according to different authors.

Authors	Platelet count	Neutrophil count
Eversole et al., 2001 [33]	**<50,000 cell/mm^3**: not perform dental or periodontal surgery in office setting.	—
Little et al., 2007 [5]	**<50,000 cell/mm^3**: avoid invasive procedures. **<40,000 cell/mm^3**: perform transfusions in invasive procedures.	**<500 cell/mm^3**: antimicrobial prophylaxis (or with leukocytes <2,000 cells/mm^3).
American Academy of Pediatric Dentistry, 2013 [1]	**>75,000 cell/mm^3**: without additional support. **40,000 to 75,000 cell/mm^3**: Platelet transfusion may be considered in the preoperative and postoperative (24 hours). **<40,000 cell/mm^3**: Postpone the dental treatment. In the case of dental emergency, contact the patient's physician before dental treatment to discuss supportive measures, such as platelet transfusion, control of bleeding, and need for hospitalization. Other coagulation tests may be necessary in some cases.	**>1,000 cell/mm^3**: no need for antibiotic prophylaxis. Some authors suggest that prophylaxis is performed with values between 1,000 and 2,000 cell/mm^3 (following recommendations of the American Heart Association). If infection is present or there is doubt, more aggressive antibiotic prophylaxis may be indicated and should be discussed with the medical team. **<1,000 cell/mm^3**: Postpone the dental treatment. In cases of emergency, discuss antibiotic coverage and endocarditis prophylaxis before treatment with the medical team. Hospitalization may be required.
US National Cancer Institute, 2011 [2]	**>60,000 cell/mm^3**: without additional support. **30,000 to 60,000 cell/mm^3**: optional transfusion for noninvasive procedure. **<30,000 cell/mm^3**: Platelets should be transfused 1 h before the procedure. Obtain immediate postinfusion platelet count; transfuse regularly to maintain counts >30,000–40,000 cell/mm^3 until the start of healing.	**>2,000 cell/mm^3**: without the need for antibiotic prophylaxis. **1,000 to 2,000 cell/mm^3**: antibiotic prophylaxis (low risk). **<1,000 cell/mm^3**: antibiotic prophylaxis with Amikacin 150 mg/m^2 1 h before surgery and Ticarcillin 75 mg/Kg IV 1 h before surgery. Repeat both 6 h postoperative.

TABLE 2: Minimum hematological values for performing invasive dental procedures in patients undergoing chemotherapy, according to different authors.

Authors	Platelet count	Neutrophil count
Sonis et al., 1995 [3]	**<100,000 cell/mm^3**: elective dental treatment should be postponed.	**<3,500 cell/mm^3** (leukocytes): elective dental treatment should be postponed.
Haytac et al., 2004 [32]	**<40,000 cell/mm^3**: periodontal probing and dental extractions contraindicated.	**<1,500 cell/mm^3**: periodontal probing and dental extractions contraindicated.
Brennan et al., 2008 [22]	**<50,000 cell/mm^3**: contraindication to perform invasive procedures.	**<1,000 cell/mm^3**: contraindication to perform invasive procedures.
Koulocheris et al., 2009 [34]	**>60,000 cell/mm^3**: acceptable for oral surgery.	**>1,000 cell/mm^3**: acceptable for oral surgery.

exposure, mobility, and impacted and residual roots should be removed. Ideally, extraction should occur two weeks before the start of the antineoplastic treatment or at least 7 to 10 days before. Finally, the academy recommends that surgical procedures should be as atraumatic as possible, without leaving remnant bone edges and with satisfactory suture of the wound. If there is infection associated with the tooth, antibiotic prophylaxis should be done for a week and by the drug ideally chosen by antibiogram.

According to Little et al. [5], the extraction should be made, preferably three weeks prior to chemotherapy or radiotherapy and at least 10 to 14 days earlier. If the platelet count is less than 50,000 cells/mm^3, invasive procedures should be avoided; when less than 40,000 cells/mm^3, this indicates performing transfusions. Antimicrobial prophylaxis is recommended when the leukocytes count is less than

2,000 cells/mm^3 or less than 500 cells/mm^3. Partially erupted molars can be a source of infection due to pericoronitis. If the gingival tissue which partially covers the tooth is a potential factor for infection, the tissue should be excised, if the hematological levels permit.

Toljanic et al. [35] conducted a prospective study aimed at assessing a minimum protocol for prechemotherapy dental treatment involving 48 patients with solid or hematological neoplasms, empirically classifying the chronic changes of odontogenic origin as mild, moderate, or severe, considering the probability of them developing into acute processes during chemotherapy. In acute diagnosed alterations based on signs (edema, purulent drainage, and compatible radiographic changes) and symptoms (pain, tenderness, and fever), the source of infection was removed before chemotherapy. In contrast, in chronic changes, the source

TABLE 3: Possibility of dental procedures in the prechemotherapy phase.

Procedure	Considerations and restrictions	Time before the start of CT
Type I		
Exam		
Clinical		
Radiographic	No restrictions.	—
Hygiene instructions		
Molding	Elective procedure, postpone	—
Type II		
Simple restorations (ART)	No restrictions.	—
Prophylaxis and supragingival scaling		
Orthodontics	Elective treatment, postpone. Consider removing orthodontic appliances.	—
Type III		
More complex restorations	Solely for adequacy of the oral environment. Consider use of provisional restorative materials (e.g., glass ionomer).	—
Scaling and root planning (subgingival)	Invasive procedure of high-risk carried out carefully. To evaluate hematological indices of platelets and neutrophils. Need for antibiotic prophylaxis.	—
Endodontics		
Symptomatic tooth	Evaluate hematological indices of platelets and neutrophils. Need for antibiotic prophylaxis. Consider extraction if endodontics fail.	At least 1 week [1]
Asymptomatic tooth	Postpone (tricresol formalin) OR Evaluate hematological indices of platelets and neutrophils. Need for antibiotic prophylaxis.	At least 1 week [1]
Type IV		
Simple extractions	Invasive procedure of high-risk. Evaluate hematological indices of platelets and neutrophils. Need for antibiotic prophylaxis.	3 weeks; minimum 10–14 days [5] 2 weeks; minimum 7–10 days [1]
Curettage (gingivoplasty)	Elective procedure, invasive and high-risk. Postpone.	—
Type V		
Multiple extractions	If for adequacy of the oral environment, evaluate hematological indices of platelets and neutrophils. Need for antibiotic prophylaxis. If elective, postpone.	3 weeks; minimum 10–14 days [5] 2 weeks; minimum 7–10 days [1]
Flap surgery/gingivectomy Extraction of impacted tooth Apicoectomy Single implant placement	Elective procedure, invasive and high-risk. Postpone.	—
Type VI		
Extraction of an entire arch or both	If adequacy of the oral environment, evaluate hematological indices of platelets and neutrophils. Need for antibiotic prophylaxis. If elective, postpone.	3 weeks; minimum 10–14 days [5] 2 weeks; minimum 7–10 days [1]
Extraction of multiple impacted teeth Flap surgery Orthognathic surgery Placement of multiple implants	Elective procedure, invasive and high-risk. Postpone.	—

TABLE 4: Possibility of dental procedures in transchemotherapy phase.

Procedure	Considerations or restrictions	Time between cycles
Type I		
Exam		
Clinical		
Radiographic	No restrictions.	—
Hygiene instructions		
Molding	Elective procedure. Postpone.	—
Type II		
Simple restorations (ART)	No restrictions.	—
Prophylaxis and supragingival scaling		
Orthodontics	Elective treatment. Consider removing orthodontic appliances.	—
Type III		
More complex restorations	Solely for adequacy of the oral environment. Consider use of provisional restorative materials (eg., Glass ionomer).	—
Scaling and root planning (subgingival)	Invasive treatment, of high-risk, perform carefully. Evaluate hematological indices of platelets and neutrophils. Need for antibiotic prophylaxis.	—
Endodontics		
Symptomatic tooth	Evaluate hematological indices of platelets and neutrophils. Need for antibiotic prophylaxis. Consider extraction if endodontics fails.	At least 1 week [1]
Asymptomatic tooth	Postpone (tricresol formalin). OR Evaluate hematological indices of platelets and neutrophils. Need for antibiotic prophylaxis.	At least 1 week [1]
Type IV		
Simple extractions	Invasive treatment of high-risk. Evaluate hematological indices of platelets and neutrophils. Need for antibiotic prophylaxis.	3 weeks; minimum 10–14 days [5] 2 weeks; minimum 7–10 days [1]
Curettage (gingivoplasty)	Elective treatment, invasive and high-risk. Postpone.	—
Type V		
Multiple extractions	If adequacy of the oral environment, evaluate hematological indices of platelets and neutrophils. Need for antibiotic prophylaxis. If elective, postpone.	3 weeks; minimum 10–14 days [5] 2 weeks; minimum 7–10 days [1]
Flap surgery/gingivectomy	Elective procedure, invasive and high-risk. Postpone.	—
Extraction of impacted tooth		
Apicoectomy		
Single implant placement		
Type VI		
Extraction of an entire arch or both	If adequacy of the oral environment, evaluate hematological indices of platelets and neutrophils. Need for antibiotic prophylaxis. If elective, postpone.	3 weeks; minimum 10–14 days [5] 2 weeks; minimum 7–10 days [1]
Extraction of multiple impacted teeth	Elective procedure, invasive and high-risk. Postpone.	—
Flap surgery		
Orthognathic surgery		
Placement of multiple implants		

TABLE 5: Possibility of dental procedures in postchemotherapy phase.

Intervention in postchemotherapy	Considerations and restrictions
Type I	
Exam	
Clinic	
Radiographic	No restrictions.
Hygiene instructions	
Molding	
Type II	
Simple restorations (ART)	No restrictions.
Prophylaxis and supragingival cell scaling	
Orthodontics	Completed chemotherapy and after two years free of disease, one can restart the orthodontic treatment
Type III	
More complex restorations	
Scaling and root planning cell (subgingival)	
Endodontics	No restrictions.
Symptomatic tooth	
Asymptomatic tooth	
Type IV	
Simple extractions	Need for antibiotic prophylaxis until six months after completion of chemotherapy.
Curettage (gingivoplasty)	
Type V	
Multiple extractions	
Flap surgery/gingivectomy	
Extraction of impacted tooth	Need for antibiotic prophylaxis until six months after completion of chemotherapy.
Apicoectomy	
Single implant placement	
Type VI	
Extraction of an entire arch or both	
Extraction of multiple impacted cell teeth	
Flap surgery	Need for antibiotic prophylaxis until six months after completion of chemotherapy.
Orthognathic surgery	
Placement of multiple implants	

of infection was not removed. Chronic lesions of odontogenic origin were identified in 79% of patients, where 44% were considered serious chronic illness; of these, only 4% had episodes of fever diagnosed as odontogenic in origin, which were treated with antibiotics without interruption of chemotherapy. For the authors, these results demonstrated that patients with chronic odontogenic lesions can safely undergo chemotherapy without dental procedures, since the conversion of chronic processes in acute cases was uncommon and when sharpening occurred it was effectively treated without interruption of therapy and without adversely affecting the oncological treatment. This strategy would significantly change the established protocols, which recommend a more aggressive prechemotherapy dental treatment. The authors reasoned that, depending on the severity of the cancer, there may be a need to quickly start chemotherapy to maximize its therapeutic effects and in that narrow window of time, the extraction of teeth without potential recovery may

be the only viable treatment option and still the possibility of infection after tooth extraction would delay the repair of the wound. It is concluded that the treatment of chronic odontogenic lesions can be safely postponed until the end of chemotherapy, considering the therapeutic benefits.

According to Haytac et al. [32] a neutrophil count of $1,500/mm^3$ and platelets of 40,000 cells/mm^3 are required for performing periodontal probing or extractions. The procedures must be performed under antibiotic cover and at least three days before the start of chemotherapy (approximately 10 days before the granulocyte count falls below 500 cells/mm^3); when not possible, dental treatment should be postponed until the haematological indices increase.

The American Academy of Pediatric Dentistry [1] argues that orthodontic appliances should be removed if the patient has deficient oral hygiene and/or in cases where the protocol of antineoplastic treatment confers risk for developing moderate or severe oral mucositis; simple devices that do not

TABLE 6: Special considerations regarding oral complications, oral health, and dental treatment in pre-, immediate post-, and late post-HSCT.

Special considerations	Pre-HSCT (preconditioning)	Immediate post-HSCT (neutropenic conditioning phase and engraftment to hematopoietic recovery)	Late post-HCST (immune reconstitution/recovery from systemic toxicity and long-term survival)
Oral manifestations	(i) Oral infections (ii) Soreness (iii) Bleeding (iv) Temporomandibular dysfunction.	(i) Mucositis (ii) Dysgeusia (iii) Xerostomia (iv) Hemorrhage (v) Oral pain (vi) Opportunistic infections (vii) Neurotoxicity (viii) Temporomandibular dysfunction (ix) Acute GVHD.	(i) Chronic GVHD (ii) Late viral infections (iii) Salivary dysfunction (iv) Squamous cell carcinoma (v) Craniofacial growth abnormalities (children) (vi) Impairment of bones and teeth (children).
Oral health	(i) Identify and eliminate sources of existing or potential infection. (ii) Orientate the patient about the importance of maintaining oral health. (iii) Warn about the possible effects of antineoplastic therapy in the oral cavity.	(i) Maintain and reinforce the importance of optimal oral health. (ii) Treat side effects of HSCT therapy. (iii) Pay attention to periodontitis and gingivitis as potential sources of bacteremia.	(i) Diagnosis and treatment of mucosal lesions and lichen-type features with symptoms (ii) Caries prevention and reestablishment of oral health in case of rampant caries (iii) Treatment of hyposalivation and xerostomia (iv) Early detection of oral cancer and precursor lesions.
Dental treatment	(i) Complete necessary dental treatment (ii) Elective treatment should be delayed until the re-establishment of immunity (at least 100 days after transplant, or more in the case of oral complications or other cGVHD).	*Neutropenic conditioning phase* (i) Dental procedures should not be performed at this stage (ii) If emergencies, perform the necessary dental approach, with the participation of medical staff. *Engraftment to hematopoietic recovery* (i) Monitoring and management of oral complications of HSCT (ii) Invasive procedures only with the approval of the medical team (iii) Strengthening the maintenance guidelines of good oral hygiene and noncariogenic diet (iv) Special attention to xerostomia and GVHD.	*Immune reconstitution/recovery from systemic toxicity* (i) Periodic dental evaluation (ii) Avoid invasive procedures (iii) Clarify risks and benefits of orthodontic appliances. *Long-term survival* (i) Periodic dental evaluation (ii) In the first 12 months after HSCT: (a) avoid routine dental care, including scaling and periodontal planning; (b) if emergencies, strategies to reduce inhalation of aerosols and antibiotic prophylaxis; (c) before invasive procedures, consider the use of IgG, antibiotics, corticosteroids, and/or platelet transfusion.

irritate the soft tissues, removable appliances, or retainers well adapted may be maintained provided that the patient has good oral hygiene. Sheller and Williams [36] defend that orthodontic appliances should be removed.

It is important that the dentist is aware of the signs and symptoms of periodontal disease, since these can be subtle when the patient is immunosuppressed [1, 37].

After treatment of acute needs, other procedures such as smoothing of rough restorations, rounding, or restoration of tooth fractures may be performed, in addition to the assessment of dentures. Scaling procedures and root planning should be performed to prevent periodontal infections, as well as enhancing oral hygiene instruction and the use of mouthwash with fluoride in preventing dental caries [3, 5].

4.2. Dental Treatment in the Transchemotherapy Phase.

Table 4 refers to the stage where the patient is undergoing chemotherapy and lists the dental procedures and restrictions assigned to it, referring to haematological indices and considering the period between cycles of chemotherapy.

In high-risk patients (active or under leukemia bone marrow suppression) dental intervention is limited to emergency care. However, oral hygiene must be maintained by the use of mouthwashes and mild antimicrobial and antiseptic solutions, in order to promote ulcer healing and minimize complications from infection. When there is evidence of oral infection, high-risk patients should receive broad-spectrum antibiotics intravenously [3, 5]. In UH/UFSC 0.12%, solution-based nonalcoholic chlorhexidine gluconate is used in the form of daily mouthwash or applied with gauze or swab.

In patients at moderate risk (maintenance phase), the myelosuppression peak is most evident, usually after 14 days of drug administration, and at this time, dental treatment should be avoided; before or 21 days after the start of chemotherapy the treatment can be performed; however, the doctor should be consulted. If the leucocyte count is below $3,500 \text{ cells/mm}^3$ or the platelet count is less than $100,000 \text{ cells/mm}^3$, elective dental treatment should be postponed [3]. According to these authors, type I procedures can be performed according to standard protocols, since in types II, III, and IV procedures, antimicrobial prophylaxis is recommended.

Tong and Rothwell [24] do not recommend routine antibiotic prophylaxis for dental procedures in patients undergoing chemotherapy; however, for invasive procedures such as tooth extractions and other deep periodontal scaling procedures that can cause significant bleeding and propagation of bacteria into the bloodstream, antibiotic coverage should be performed.

Koulocheris et al. [34], citing other authors, state that in oral surgical procedures during chemotherapy, the benefit/risk to the patient must be considered, as well as the consequences of chemotherapy cycles; these procedures should therefore be planned and agreed on an interdisciplinary level. Furthermore, the surgical procedure should be the most conservative possible, with trans and postantibiotic prophylaxis and postoperative platelet transfusion if necessary. It is claimed, in addition, that an absolute neutrophil count greater than 1000 cells/mm^3 and platelet count of at least $60,000 \text{ cells/mm}^3$ are acceptable rates for oral surgeries.

When there is spontaneous bleeding resulting from minor trauma, the dentist should strive to improve the oral hygiene of the patient and use local measures to control the bleeding. If these measures are not sufficient, platelet transfusion may be required [5].

The management for control of oral bleeding includes the use of vasoconstrictor agents, clots, and tissue guards. To reduce the flow of blood from bleeding vessels, one can use epinephrine; to organize and stabilize blood clots, topical thrombin and/or collagen hemostatic agents can be used; and to stanch the bleeding sites and protect organized clots, the application of the mucosa adhesive products, such as those based on cyanoacrylate, may be performed. The topical aminocaproic acid can be useful in patients with friable clots and intravenous administration may be considered, in some cases, to improve coagulation and the formation of stable clots [2]. Topical use of tranexamic acid is also cited as an effective hemostatic in reducing the incidence of postoperative bleeding in patients taking continuous use of oral anticoagulants [38, 39]. Coetzee [40] reports the empirical use of 500 mg crushed tablets ground in moist cotton at the site of the surgical wound after tooth extraction, or diluted in water for mouthwash, suggesting it as an option.

4.3. Dental Treatment after Chemotherapy.

Table 5 relates the postchemotherapy period and summarizes the considerations and constraints in the literature for performing dental procedures.

Patients who were cured of leukemia are considered to be of low risk and can be met with normal dental treatment regimens [3]. After completion of cancer therapy and only after two years free of disease, the orthodontic treatment that was interrupted can be restarted [36].

Koulocheris et al. [34] suggest that antibiotic prophylaxis during oral and maxillofacial surgical procedures should be performed for at least six months after the completion of chemotherapy.

4.4. Dental Treatment in Different Phases of Chemotherapy Treatment.

Table 7 shows, in summary form, the considerations and limitations related to dental procedures at different stages of antineoplastic treatment.

Noninvasive procedures do not require additional care and may be performed at any stage of the disease or chemotherapy. Fit in this situation the type I (clinical examination, radiographs, and oral hygiene instruction) and type II procedures (simple restorations, atraumatic restorative treatment—ART, supragingival scaling and prophylaxis) [3]. Since the priority is the treatment of leukemia before the diagnosis (prechemotherapy phase) or during antineoplastic treatment, some dental procedures, classified as type I (molding) and type II (orthodontic treatment), are considered elective for these patients, and even in the postchemotherapy phase, some restrictions must be considered when related to orthodontic treatment.

There are procedures, however, that are considered non-surgical (type III)—such as the realization of more complex restorations, scaling, root planning (subgingival), and endodontic treatment—but they require special care in the prechemotherapy and transchemotherapy phases, considering the general state of health and the risk versus benefit to the patient. Some authors suggest that periodontal procedures such as probing and periodontal scaling could cause bacteremia [41–44]. In addition, the endodontic treatment protocol for asymptomatic teeth, according to the literature, is not well established. Thus, the realization of endodontics has to justify the removal of infectious foci; however, some professionals prefer, in such situations, to adopt a radical behavior, performing the extraction of the dental element in question in order to avoid future complications. In the postchemotherapy period, these dental procedures can be performed without restrictions.

Invasive procedures such as simple extractions (type IV), multiple extractions (type V), or those of an entire arch or entire mouth (type VI) can be performed, but its execution is dependent on the patient's risk and should therefore the risk versus the benefit should be considered in specific situations [3]. We believe that gingivoplasty procedures, multiple extractions (no infectious foci) flap surgery (gingivectomy), extraction of single or multiple impacted teeth, apicoectomy, placing implants, and orthognathic surgery are considered elective treatments before the diagnosis and/or treatment of leukemia and should not be performed until the patient completes—and maintains—their antineoplastic treatment successfully.

4.5. Special Considerations about Dental Treatment in HSCT Patients. The considerations of the dental treatment in the pre-, immediate post-, and late post-HSCT are summarized in Table 6.

The American Academy of Pediatric Dentistry [1] recommends that dental treatment is made dependent on each phase of HSCT. In the preconditioning phase, all dental treatment should be completed before the patient becomes immunosuppressive. Elective treatment should be delayed until the reestablishment of immunity (at least 100 days after transplant, or more in the case of oral complications or other cGVHDs). In the neutropenic conditioning phase, the focus is the monitoring and management of oral complications, with reinforcement of maintenance guidelines of good oral hygiene. Dental procedures should not be performed at this stage; in the case of emergencies, dental approach should be developed with the participation of the medical staff. In the engraftment phase to hematopoietic recovery, a dental assessment should be performed, with special attention to xerostomia and GVHD. Invasive procedures should be made only with the approval of the medical staff; the patient should be encouraged to maintain good hygiene with a noncariogenic diet. In the immune reconstitution/recovery phase from systemic toxicity, a periodic evaluation with dental radiography can be performed; however, invasive procedures should still be avoided; clarifying the risks and benefits of the use of orthodontic appliances is recommended. Finally, in the long-term survival phase, a routine dental evaluation

TABLE 7: Possibility of dental procedures at various stages of chemotherapy.

Intervention	Pre	Trans	Post
Type I			
Exam			
Clinical	NR	NR	NR
Radiographic	NR	NR	NR
Oral hygiene instruction	NR	NR	NR
Molding	E	E	NR
Type II			
Simple restorations (ARTs)	NR	NR	NR
Prophylaxis and supragingival scaling	NR	NR	NR
Orthodontics	E	E	R
Type III			
More complex restorations	R	R	NR
Scaling and root planning (subgingival)	R HI, AP	R HI, AP	NR
Endodontics			
Symptomatic teeth	R HI, AP	R HI, AP	NR
Asymptomatic teeth	E, R HI, AP	E, R HI, AP	NR
Type IV			
Simple extractions	R, HI, AP	R, HI, AP	R
Curettage (gingivoplasty)	EIHR	EIHR	R
Type V			
Multiple extractions	R, HI, AP	R, HI, AP	R
Flap surgery/gingivectomy	EIHR	EIHR	R
Extraction of impacted tooth	EIHR	EIHR	R
Apicoectomy	EIHR	EIHR	R
Single implant placement	EIHR	EIHR	R
Type VI			
Extraction of an entire arch or both	R, HI, AP	R, HI, AP	R
Extraction of multiple impacted teeth	EIHR	EIHR	R
Flap surgery	EIHR	EIHR	R
Orthognathic surgery	EIHR	EIHR	R
Placement of multiple implants	EIHR	EIHR	R

NR: no restriction, R: with restriction, E: elective, EIHR: elective, invasive, and high-risk, HI: need for evaluation of hematological indices, and AP: antibiotic prophylaxis.

with interdisciplinary and multidisciplinary involvement is necessary.

The authors differ somewhat as to the best approach for a better dental protocol in HSCT patients, but are unanimous in stating that the assessment and dental care are needed.

Raber-Durlacher et al. [37] investigated the correlation between gingivitis/periodontitis and the development of bacteremia during the period of neutropenia after HSCT. Eighteen patients were examined and classified into two groups: (1) periodontally healthy (probing pocket depth: PPD

≤ 4 mm and bleeding on probing: BOP ≤ 10%) and (2) the presence of gingivitis (PPD ≤ 4 mm and BOP > 10%) or periodontitis (PPD > 4 mm and BOP ≥ 10%). Only 28% of the patients were considered periodontally healthy. Of the total, 67% of the patients developed bacteremia (diagnosed by blood samples collected 2 times per week), and group 2 had more frequent episodes during the neutropenia phase than group 1. The authors suggested that gingivitis and periodontitis may represent a risk factor for the development of bacteremia, which has also been shown in other studies [43, 44]. They further stated that the exacerbation of gingivitis and chronic periodontitis is rare, probably due to the institution of prophylactic therapy; on the other hand, common illnesses should not be overlooked, such as potential underdiagnosed of bacteremia source, particularly during periods of neutropenia.

Melkos et al. [45] conducted a prospective study of 58 patients undergoing HSCT and evaluated the preexisting odontogenic lesions, dental care, and the effect of both on the medical procedure. All patients were referred for a dental evaluation before the HSCT, being examined by two experienced dentists through clinical examination (soft and hard tissues) and radiographic (panoramic and occasionally for symptomatic periapical teeth). Infectious foci teeth were considered with periapical and periodontal infection and those semi-impacted. The type of pretransplant dental work and the occurrence of posttransplant complications (mucositis, infections, graft versus host disease (GVHD), and relapse of disease) were evaluated for an average of 50.45 weeks after the date of transplantation. The protocol for dental treatment included restoration of active caries and extraction of nonrestorable teeth and those with advanced periodontal disease; nonvital teeth were endodontically treated or extracted, whereas periapical lesions were treated endodontically, performing apicoectomy or extraction. Patients were divided into two groups: (I) no infectious foci or complete dental treatment before transplantation ($n = 36$) and (II) with infectious foci, submitted to transplantation without dental intervention ($n = 22$). Posttransplant complications were observed in 75% of patients in group I and 95.4% in group II. The impact of infectious outbreaks in the occurrence of posttransplant infections was not statistically significant, as well as correlations between decayed, impacted, and semierupted teeth, fever of unknown origin, mucositis, and the survival rate of patients with preexisting foci; however, the infectious foci were significant when associated with acute GVHD, mainly impacted teeth and periapical lesions. A higher rate of complications was found in group II, indicating the importance of evaluation and pretransplant dental work. It was concluded that dental treatment before HSCT should not be radical. Restorative and preventative techniques, however, must be individually adjusted for each patient.

Yamagata et al. [46] also conducted a prospective study of 41 patients who were undergoing HSCT using a conservative dental protocol. All patients were evaluated by clinical examination of the oral soft and hard tissues and, if necessary, radiographs were requested. Of the 41 patients, 36 required one or more dental interventions. The following diagnoses and procedures were performed: 101 carious lesions: 40 were restored and 61 were untreated; 5 pulpitis treated with endodontics; 10 teeth with apical periodontitis greater than 5 mm and 33 with less than 5 mm: 7 lesions were surgically removed, 5 teeth were endodontically treated (including two with symptomatology), and 31 teeth with lesions smaller than 5 mm and asymptomatic received no treatment; 94 teeth with periodontitis: 6 were extracted and 88 preserved, with survey monitoring and hygiene education; 21 partially erupted wisdom teeth: 3 presenting symptomatology were removed, the rest were untreated. All dental procedures were performed up to 10 days before HSCT, without change interruption or delay in the planning of the transplant. No patient had signs or symptoms of odontogenic infection during the immunosuppression period. The authors concluded that the conservative protocol appeared to be suitable for pre-HSCT patients.

Abdullah and Ahmad [47] conducted a study of 44 pediatric patients. Dental conditions were evaluated by clinical examination before HSCT. In the case of symptomatic tooth periapical radiographs were performed. Decayed teeth considered unviable were extracted, and the others were restored. In patients at high-risk of caries, sealant was applied. All patients received oral hygiene guidelines. The patients were evaluated after 1, 3, and 6 months after HSCT. Most patients (65.9%) needed some type of pre-HSCT dental treatment, having performed 101 restorations, 13 extractions, and 19 sealants. Within 6 months of monitoring, 10% of the patients who did not receive pre-HSCT dental treatment had odontogenic infection. No cases of odontogenic infection were observed in patients who previously received dental care. The authors concluded that the pre-HSCT dental treatment can reduce the occurrence of infection of dental origin, and it is important to prevent serious infections.

The US National Cancer Institute [48] points out that the time of reconstitution of the immune system in transplant patients can range from 6 to 12 months and that the dental care routine should not be done in this period, including scaling and periodontal planning. Procedures that produce aerosol, such as ultrasound equipment and high speed, can also present a risk of aspiration of debris and bacteria and cause pneumonia in these patients [19, 48]. If emergency treatment is required, strategies for reducing aerosol aspiration and antibiotic prophylaxis should be used. Finally, it is recommended that the use of IgG, antibiotics, corticosteroids, and/or platelet transfusion should be considered before implementing invasive procedures [48].

5. Final Considerations

From the literature review conducted, several oral manifestations in leukemic patients arose. These manifestations are often the first sign of leukemia and may present clinically as leukemic infiltration in oral tissues as well as simulating a periapical lesion. Other symptoms may occur such as pale mucosa, poor wound healing, bleeding (petechiae and ecchymoses), atypical or recurrent candidiasis, recurrent herpes infections, and ulcerations in the oral mucosa. During antineoplastic treatment (chemotherapy, mostly), the main complication is mucositis.

Other conditions that may also occur include bleeding, increase the rate of decay, infection, gum abscess, recurrent herpetic stomatitis, candidiasis, salivary gland dysfunction, xerostomia, dysgeusia, and pain. In the posttherapy period, patients are considered cured and usually present no sequelae of treatment.

Oral manifestations are similar in patients undergoing HSCT; however, generally these cases are due to long-term immunosuppression of the patient even after the transplantation. Special features are observed in patients undergoing allogeneic HSCT, such as cGVHD, which typically manifests as lichen-type features, hyperkeratotic plaques, mucocele, and fibrosis with limited mouth opening, and are more likely to develop malignancies such as squamous cell carcinoma.

Performing dental procedures can offer risk to the patient, depending on his state of health and phase of therapy. Furthermore, some procedures offer greater risk than others. Thus, noninvasive procedures (type I and type II) can be performed at any stage of the disease or treatment. Type III procedures may require special care. Finally, invasive procedures (types IV, V, and VI) offer higher risk. In emergency situations of risk considered, particularly those involving pain (acute cases), the patient should be assisted, if necessary, in a hospital setting, with the institution of measures to increase the hematological indices (transfusions) and, if applicable, with antibiotic coverage.

In assessing patients for dental procedures, two hematological indices are particularly important: neutrophil and platelet counts. At low levels of neutrophil counts, and when the procedure cannot be delayed, prophylactic antibiotic therapy protocols should be considered, being variable according to the degree of neutropenia; there is no strict consensus among authors, but most recommended antibiotic prophylaxis with values less than 1,000 cells/mm^3. In the case of the platelet count, the authors consider the need for transfusion from indices between 40,000 and 60,000 cells/mm^3.

Thus, we conclude, based on the literature review presented here, that the dental treatment in relation to haematological indices presented by patients with leukemia should follow some judicious protocols, mainly related to neutrophil and platelet counts. However, it is noteworthy that many of these studies are based on expert opinion. The presence of the dentist in a multidisciplinary team is essential, since we understand that maintaining oral health contributes significantly to the overall health and improved quality of life for patients through the use of dental approaches based on scientific evidence, preventive, curative, and palliative in nature.

Conflict of Interests

The authors declare that there is no conflict of interests regarding the publication of this paper.

References

[1] American Academy of Pediatric Dentistry, "Guideline on dental management of pediatric patients receiving chemotherapy, hematopoietic cell transplantation, and/or radiation," *Journal of Pediatric Dentistry*, vol. 35, no. 5, pp. E185–E193, 2013, http://www.ncbi.nlm.nih.gov/pubmed/24290549.

[2] US National Cancer Institute, *Oral Complications of Chemotherapy and Head/Neck Radiation*, US National Cancer Institute, 2011, http://www.cancer.gov/cancertopics/pdq/supportivecare/oralcomplications/HealthProfessional.

[3] S. T. Sonis, R. C. Fazio, and L. Fang, *Principles and Practice of Oral Medicine*, WB Saunders, 1995.

[4] M. R. Howard and P. J. Hamilton, "Leukaemia," in *Haematology*, pp. 33–66, Elsevier, Philadelphia, Pa, USA, 3rd edition, 2008.

[5] J. W. Little, D. A. Falace, C. S. Miller, and N. L. Rhodus, "Disorders of white blood cells," in *Dental Magenement of the Medically Compromised Patient*, pp. 373–395, 2007.

[6] B. Neville, D. Damm, C. Allem, and J. Bouquot, "Hematologic disorders," in *Oral and Maxillofacial Pathology*, pp. 573–613, Elsevier, 3rd edition, 2009.

[7] R. Wäsch, W. Digel, and M. Lübbert, "Acute lymphoblastic leukemia (ALL)," in *Concise Manual of Hematology and Oncology*, M. Andreeff, B. Koziner, H. Messner, and N. Thatcher, Eds., pp. 400–414, Springer, Berlin, Germany, 2008.

[8] K. Heining-Mikesch and M. Lübbert, "Acute myeloid leukemia (AML)," in *Concise Manual of Hematology and Oncology*, M. Andreeff, B. Koziner, H. Messner, and N. Thatcher, Eds., pp. 415–420, Springer, Berlin, Germany, 2008.

[9] W. Lange and C. Waller, "Chronic myeloid leukemia (CML)," in *Concise Manual of Hematology and Oncology*, pp. 432–438, Springer, Berlin, Germany, 2008.

[10] J. Burger and J. Finke, "Chronic lymphocytic leukemia (CLL)," in *Concise Manual of Hematology and Oncology*, pp. 470–476, Springer, Berlin, Germany, 2008.

[11] K. Durey, H. Patterson, and K. Gordon, "Dental assessment prior to stem cell transplant: treatment need and barriers to care," *British Dental Journal*, vol. 206, no. 9, article E19, 2009.

[12] J. B. Epstein, L. Vickars, J. Spinelli, and D. Reece, "Efficacy of chlorhexidine and nystatin rinses in prevention of oral complications in leukemia and bone marrow transplantation," *Oral Surgery Oral Medicine and Oral Pathology*, vol. 73, no. 6, pp. 682–689, 1992.

[13] A. H. Filipovich, D. Weisdorf, S. Pavletic et al., "National Institutes of Health consensus development project on criteria for clinical trials in chronic graft-versus-host disease: I. Diagnosis and staging working group report," *Biology of Blood and Marrow Transplantation*, vol. 11, no. 12, pp. 945–956, 2005.

[14] N. Treister, C. Duncan, C. Cutler, and L. Lehmann, "How we treat oral chronic graft-versus-host disease," *Blood*, vol. 120, no. 17, pp. 3407–3418, 2012.

[15] K. M. Hull, I. Kerridge, and M. Schifter, "Long-term oral complications of allogeneic haematopoietic SCT," *Bone Marrow Transplantation*, vol. 47, no. 2, pp. 265–270, 2012.

[16] H. S. Brand, C. P. Bots, and J. E. Raber-Durlacher, "Xerostomia and chronic oral complications among patients treated with haematopoietic stem cell transplantation," *British Dental Journal*, vol. 207, no. 9, article E17, 2009.

[17] R. A. Abdelsayed, T. Sumner, C. M. Allen, A. Treadway, G. M. Ness, and S. L. Penza, "Oral precancerous and malignant lesions associated with graft-versus-host disease: report of 2 cases," *Oral Surgery, Oral Medicine, Oral Pathology, Oral Radiology, and Endodontology*, vol. 93, no. 1, pp. 75–80, 2002.

[18] F. Demarosi, D. Soligo, G. Lodi, L. Moneghini, A. Sardella, and A. Carrassi, "Squamous cell carcinoma of the oral cavity associated with graft versus host disease: report of a case and review of the literature," *Oral Surgery, Oral Medicine, Oral Pathology, Oral Radiology and Endodontology*, vol. 100, no. 1, pp. 63–69, 2005.

[19] S. Elad, J. E. Raber-Durlacher, M. T. Brennan et al., "Basic oral care for hematology–oncology patients and hematopoietic

stem cell transplantation recipients: a position paper from the joint task force of the Multinational Association of Supportive Care in Cancer/International Society of Oral Oncology (MASCC/ISOO) and the European Society for Blood and Marrow Transplantation (EBMT)," *Supportive Care in Cancer*, vol. 23, no. 1, pp. 223–236, 2015.

[20] R. Albuquerque, V. Morais, and A. Sobral, "Protocolo de atendimento odontológico a pacientes oncológicos pediátricos—revisão de literatura," *Revista de Odontologia da UNESP*, vol. 36, no. 3, pp. 275–280, 2007.

[21] D. Martins, M. A. Martins, and L. Sêneda, "Suporte odontológico ao paciente oncológico: prevenção, diagnóstico, tratamento e reabilitação das sequelas bucais," *Prat Hosp*, vol. 7, no. 41, pp. 166–169, 2005.

[22] M. T. Brennan, S.-B. Woo, and P. B. Lockhart, "Dental treatment planning and management in the patient who has cancer," *Dental Clinics of North America*, vol. 52, no. 1, pp. 19–37, 2008.

[23] S. Elad, T. Thierer, M. Bitan, M. Y. Shapira, and C. Meyerowitz, "A decision analysis: the dental management of patients prior to hematology cytotoxic therapy or hematopoietic stem cell transplantation," *Oral Oncology*, vol. 44, no. 1, pp. 37–42, 2008.

[24] D. C. Tong and B. R. Rothwell, "Antibiotic prophylaxis in dentistry: a review and practice recommendations," *Journal of the American Dental Association*, vol. 131, no. 3, pp. 366–374, 2000.

[25] M. Paiva, J. Moraes, R. De Biase, O. Batista, and M. Honorato, "Estudo retrospectivo das complicações orais decorrentes da terapia antineoplásica em pacientes do Hospital Napoleão Laureano—PB," *Odontologia Clínico-Científica*, vol. 6, no. 1, pp. 51–55, 2007, http://www.scielo.br/scielo.php?script=sci_nlinks&ref=000139&pid=S1414-462X20130001000020002&lng=pt.

[26] C. Padmini and K. Y. Bai, "Oral and dental considerations in pediatric leukemic patient," *ISRN Hematology*, vol. 2014, Article ID 895721, 11 pages, 2014.

[27] A. Avşar, M. Elli, Ö. Darka, and G. Pinarli, "Long-term effects of chemotherapy on caries formation, dental development, and salivary factors in childhood cancer survivors," *Oral Surgery, Oral Medicine, Oral Pathology, Oral Radiology and Endodontology*, vol. 104, no. 6, pp. 781–789, 2007.

[28] S. Elad, S. B. Jensen, J. E. Raber-Durlacher et al., "Clinical approach in the management of oral chronic graft-versus-host disease (cGVHD) in a series of specialized medical centers," *Support Care Cancer*, 2014, http://www.ncbi.nlm.nih.gov/pubmed/25417041.

[29] J. B. Epstein, J. E. Raber-Durlacher, A. Wilkins, M.-G. Chavarria, and H. Myint, "Advances in hematologic stem cell transplant: an update for oral health care providers," *Oral Surgery, Oral Medicine, Oral Pathology, Oral Radiology, and Endodontology*, vol. 107, no. 3, pp. 301–312, 2009.

[30] C. Chu, A. H. Lee, L. Zheng, M. L. Mei, and G. C. Chan, "Arresting rampant dental caries with silver diamine fluoride in a young teenager suffering from chronic oral graft versus host disease post-bone marrow transplantation: a case report," *BMC Research Notes*, vol. 7, article 3, 2014.

[31] J. C. Atkinson, M. Grisius, and W. Massey, "Salivary hypofunction and xerostomia: diagnosis and treatment," *Dental Clinics of North America*, vol. 49, no. 2, pp. 309–326, 2005.

[32] M. C. Haytac, M. C. Dogan, and B. Antmen, "The results of a preventive dental program for pediatric patients with hematologic malignancies," *Oral Health & Preventive Dentistry*, vol. 2, no. 1, pp. 59–65, 2004.

[33] L. Eversole, "Bleeding disorders," in *Essentials of Oral Medicine*, S. Silverman, L. R. Eversole, and E. L. Truelove, Eds., pp. 61–66, BC Decker, London, UK, 2nd edition, 2001.

[34] P. Koulocheris, M. C. Metzger, M. R. Kesting, and B. Hohlweg-Majert, "Life-threatening complications associated with acute monocytic leukaemia after dental treatment," *Australian Dental Journal*, vol. 54, no. 1, pp. 45–48, 2009.

[35] J. A. Toljanic, J. F. Bedard, R. A. Larson, and J. P. Fox, "A prospective pilot study to evaluate a new dental assessment and treatment paradigm for patients scheduled to undergo intensive chemotherapy for cancer," *Cancer*, vol. 85, no. 8, pp. 1843–1848, 1999.

[36] B. Sheller and B. Williams, "Orthodontic management of patients with hematologic malignancies," *American Journal of Orthodontics and Dentofacial Orthopedics*, vol. 109, no. 6, pp. 575–580, 1996.

[37] J. E. Raber-Durlacher, A. M. G. A. Laheij, J. B. Epstein et al., "Periodontal status and bacteremia with oral viridans streptococci and coagulase negative staphylococci in allogeneic hematopoietic stem cell transplantation recipients: a prospective observational study," *Supportive Care in Cancer*, vol. 21, no. 6, pp. 1621–1627, 2013.

[38] F. W. G. Costa, R. R. Rodrigues, L. H. T. de Sousa et al., "Local hemostatic measures in anticoagulated patients undergoing oral surgery. A systematized literature review," *Acta Cirurgica Brasileira*, vol. 28, no. 1, pp. 78–83, 2013.

[39] G. Ramstrom, S. Sindet-Pedersen, G. Hall, M. Blomback, and U. Alander, "Prevention of postsurgical bleeding in oral surgery using tranexamic acid without dose modification of oral anticoagulants," *Journal of Oral and Maxillofacial Surgery*, vol. 51, no. 11, pp. 1211–1216, 1993.

[40] M. J. Coetzee, "The use of topical crushed tranexamic acid tablets to control bleeding after dental surgery and from skin ulcers in haemophilia," *Haemophilia*, vol. 13, no. 4, pp. 443–444, 2007.

[41] A. C. R. T. Horliana, L. Chambrone, A. M. Foz et al., "Dissemination of periodontal pathogens in the bloodstream after periodontal procedures: a systematic review," *PLoS ONE*, vol. 9, no. 5, Article ID e98271, 2014.

[42] C. G. Daly, D. H. Mitchell, J. E. Highfield, D. E. Grossberg, and D. Stewart, "Bacteremia due to periodontal probing: a clinical and microbiological investigation," *Journal of Periodontology*, vol. 72, no. 2, pp. 210–214, 2001.

[43] D. F. Kinane, M. P. Riggio, K. F. Walker, D. MacKenzie, and B. Shearer, "Bacteraemia following periodontal procedures," *Journal of Clinical Periodontology*, vol. 32, no. 7, pp. 708–713, 2005.

[44] C. Daly, D. Mitchell, D. Grossberg, J. Highfield, and D. Stewart, "Bacteraemia caused by periodontal probing," *Australian Dental Journal*, vol. 42, no. 2, pp. 77–80, 1997.

[45] A. B. Melkos, G. Massenkeil, R. Arnold, and P. A. Reichart, "Dental treatment prior to stem cell transplantation and its influence on the posttransplantation outcome," *Clinical oral investigations*, vol. 7, no. 2, pp. 113–115, 2003.

[46] K. Yamagata, K. Onizawa, H. Yoshida et al., "Dental management of pediatric patients undergoing hematopoietic stem cell transplant," *Pediatric Hematology and Oncology*, vol. 23, no. 7, pp. 541–548, 2006.

[47] S. Abdullah and Z. Ahmad, "Protocol for dental treatment before bone marrow transplantation (BMT) in paediatric patient," *Pakistan Oral & Dental Journal*, vol. 34, no. 3, pp. 399–405, 2014.

[48] National Cancer Institute (US), "Posttransplantation Dental Treatment," http://www.cancer.gov/cancertopics/pdq/supportivecare/oralcomplications/HealthProfessional/page11.

11

Hematopoietic Stem-Cell Transplantation in the Developing World: Experience from a Center in Western India

Chirag A. Shah, Arun Karanwal, Maharshi Desai, Munjal Pandya, Ravish Shah, and Rutvij Shah

Apollo Hospitals International Limited, Plot No. 1 A, Bhat GIDC Estate, Gandhinagar, Gujarat 382428, India

Correspondence should be addressed to Rutvij Shah; rutvij7555@yahoo.co.in

Academic Editor: Edward A. Copelan

We describe our experience of first 50 consecutive hematopoietic stem-cell transplants (HSCT) done between 2007 and 2012 at the Apollo Hospital, Gandhinagar, 35 autologous HSCT and 15 allogeneic HSCT. Indications for autologous transplant were multiple myeloma, non-Hodgkin lymphoma, Hodgkin lymphoma, and acute myeloid leukemia, and indications for allogeneic transplants were thalassemia major, aplastic anaemia, chronic myeloid leukemia, and acute lymphoblastic and myeloid leukaemia. The median age of autologous and allogeneic patient's cohort was 50 years and 21 years, respectively. Median follow-up period for all patients was 39 months. Major early complications were infections, mucositis, acute graft versus host disease, and venoocclusive disease. All of our allogeneic and autologous transplant patients survived during the first month of transplant. Transplant related mortality (TRM) was 20% ($N = 3$) in our allogeneic and 3% ($N = 1$) in autologous patients. Causes of these deaths were disease relapse, sepsis, hemorrhagic complications, and GVHD. 46% of our autologous and 47% of our allogeneic patients are in complete remission phase after a median follow-up of 39 months. 34% of our autologous patients and 13% of our allogeneic patients had disease relapse. Overall survival rate in our autologous and allogeneic patients is 65.7% and 57.1%, respectively. Our results are comparable to many national and international published reports.

1. Introduction

Trends of hematopoietic stem-cell transplantation (HSCT) evolved with the first successful transplantation done by Dr. E. Donnall Thomas in late 1950s, for which he received the Nobel Prize in Physiology or Medicine in 1990. That transplant was done between the identical twins in a case of leukemia [1]. In 1968, in Minnesota, the first successful nontwin (allogeneic) transplant was performed. In this case, the donor was a sibling of the patient. By this time, it was known that a key to a successful transplant was a specific type of genetic matching (known as HLA) of the donor to the patient [1]. The first successful unrelated donor transplant was done in 1973, when a young kid in New York with acute leukemia received multiple bone marrow transplants from a matched donor from Denmark [1]. The application of hematopoietic stem-cell transplantation is not new in India. India's first successful allogeneic bone marrow transplantation was done at Tata Memorial Hospital on March 20, 1983,

on a nine-year-old girl with acute myeloid leukemia [2]. Since then, many sophisticated hematopoietic stem-cell transplant centers (HSCT) have been established across the nation. Until September 2005, data from six transplant centres in India were collected and a total of 1540 transplants have been performed in a country of over one billion population [2]. In India, there are 11 centres currently reporting their data to CIBMTR (Center for International Blood and Marrow Transplant Research) [3]. However these numbers are not large, and centres which perform regular HSCT are low due to various reasons like lack of infrastructure and expertise and lack of knowledge of safety, efficacy, and cost of the procedure both in general population and in medical fraternity. Family genotype analysis in India reveals that 39.3% of the total numbers of patients have an HLA-matched sibling and that families with sibship size of more than or equal to 4 have a higher probability (68.8%) compared with those with sibship size of less than 4 (29.7%) [4]. Recently most of the transplant centres have started marrow unrelated donor (MUD)

TABLE 1: Baseline patient characteristics and transplant data of our autologous and allogeneic patients.

Characteristics	Autologous	Allogeneic
(1) Total numbers (N)	$N = 35$	$N = 15$
(2) Age (median)	50 years	21 years
(3) Gender (M : F)	28 : 7	13 : 2
(4) Indications	Multiple myeloma: 20 Non-Hodgkin lymphoma: 7 Hodgkin lymphoma: 5 Acute myeloid leukemia: 3	Chronic myeloid leukemia: 3 Aplastic anemia: 3 Thalassemia major: 3 Acute lymphoblastic leukemia: 2 Acute myeloid leukemia: 2 Myelodysplastic syndrome: 1 Non-Hodgkin lymphoma: 1
(5) Stem-cell source	All patients from peripheral blood	Peripheral blood: 11 Bone marrow: 4
(6) Stem-cell dose (median cell dose)	$2.56^\wedge 10^6$ cells	$5.15^\wedge 10^6$ cells
(7) Donor type	Not applicable	All siblings
(8) HLA matching	Not applicable	6/6 matched: $N = 14$ 4/6 matched: $N = 1$

transplants and a few centres have started doing haploidentical transplants. Apollo Hospital International Limited, Gandhinagar, is one of the registered institutes of CIBMTR. Apollo CBCC comprehensive cancer center is located in the capital city of Gujarat, Gandhinagar, and it is one of the largest and busiest private hospitals of Western India. It also is one of the few bone marrow transplant centers in the state of Gujarat, which has population of about 60 millions [5].

Description of Our Transplant Center. Apollo Hospital, Gandhinagar, is an NABH accredited hospital, part of India's largest and most reputed healthcare groups. Apollo CBCC Comprehensive Cancer Center is the first private comprehensive cancer center of Gujarat state, established in 2007, in collaboration with CBCC (Comprehensive Blood and Caner Center), USA. Our hematooncology ward consists of 14 beds, which includes 6 rooms with HEPA filters (neutropenic ward). Our transplant unit consists of 6 beds and is totally isolated from the other part of the hospital with restricted entry of personnel and very strict neutropenic precautions including HEPA filtered air and positive pressure ventilation. Our transplant team consists of a transplant physician (hematooncologist), adult intensivists, pediatric and neonatal intensivists, oncologists, an infectious disease specialist, a registrar, medical officers, skilled nursing staff, neutropenic dieticians, well-trained nursing assistants, and managing staff, which is a perfect example of a multidisciplinary team efforts.

2. Baseline Data

2.1. Materials and Methods. This is a retrospective analysis of first fifty consecutive patients who undergone transplant at our institute, 15 allogeneic and 35 autologous with M : F = 41 : 9, whom have been followed at least for 22 months to measure their parameters accurately with median follow-up of 39 months with range from 22 to 82 months. The data was obtained carefully from case sheets, medical records of the hospital, and statistically analyzed. We receive patients of all diseases in which bone marrow transplant may be necessary and/or indicated. Our majority of pool is from western and central states of India including Gujarat, Rajasthan, Maharashtra, Madhya Pradesh, and some other states too. We receive international patients from Africa, Asia, and Middle East countries. Baseline patients' characteristics are shown in Table 1.

2.2. Trends in Transplants by Type and Recipient Age. The median age of autologous BMT was 50 years and allogeneic BMT was 21 years. Majority of autologous transplants were done between the ages of 51 and 60 years and in patients with multiple myeloma, non-Hodgkin lymphoma, and Hodgkin lymphoma, which are more common in this age group. Major indications of allogeneic BMT in age group less than 20 years were thalassemia and aplastic anemia and for autologous BMT they were Hodgkin's lymphoma. Figures 1 and 2 show graphical presentation of age of distribution and major indications below age of 20.

2.3. Indications for Hematopoietic Stem-Cell Transplants. Common indications for autologous BMT were multiple myeloma (57%), non-Hodgkin's lymphoma (23%). Allogeneic BMTs were done in patients with acute lymphoblastic lymphoma relapse, chronic myeloid leukemia with imatinib failure, aplastic anemia, thalassemia, and myelodysplastic syndrome. Two AML relapse cases undergone allogeneic BMT whereas three AML patients undergone autologous BMT after induction and consolidation chemotherapy.

We started hematopoietic stem-cell transplantation in 2007. From the year 2007 till June 2012, numbers of transplants have gradually increased and in total we have completed 50 transplants.

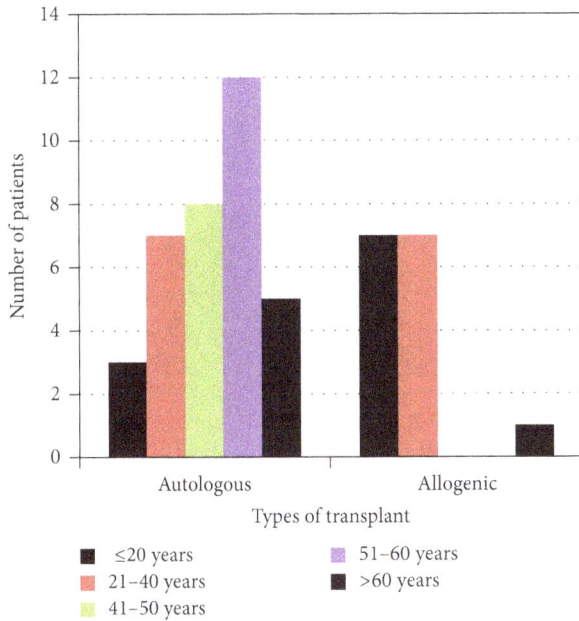

FIGURE 1: Age-wise distribution of transplant patients.

■ ≤20 years   ■ 51–60 years
■ 21–40 years   ■ >60 years
■ 41–50 years

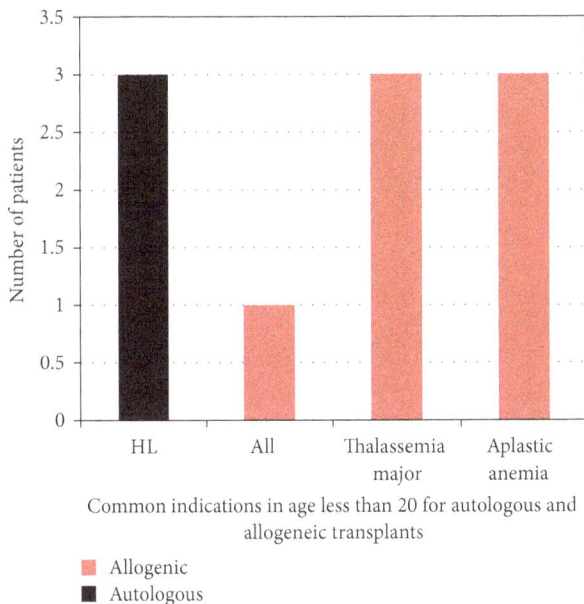

FIGURE 2: Major indications of transplant less than 20 years of age.

■ Allogenic
■ Autologous

2.4. Stem-Cell Collection. Stem cells were collected from peripheral blood in 92% [n = 46] of patients while in 8% [n = 4] patients bone marrow was the source. Till the date of analysis, we have not done allogeneic HSCT with stem-cells from cord blood, haploidentical donor, or marrow unrelated donor (MUD). All of the autologous stem-cells were collected from peripheral blood. All of our Allogeneic transplant patients were 6/6 HLA antigens matched according to standard protocols [12] except one patient in which we did transplant with 4/6 matched HLA antigens from

sibling. Stem-cells from peripheral blood were collected after mobilization therapy consisted of G-CSF stimulation in the dose of 10 mcg/kg/day for 4-5 days and from bone marrow collected by standard methods. Median stem-cell dose (CD34 cells/kg) transplanted for our allogeneic BMT is $5.15\hat{ }10^6$ and $2.56\hat{ }10^6$ for autologous transplant patients. Autologous HSC were cryopreserved in a preservative called DMSO and the cells were cooled very slowly in a controlled rate freezer to avoid cell loss by osmotic injury [13]. Cryopreservation is necessary especially in autologous transplants because HSC collections are usually done much in advance of its transplant. We preferred allogeneic HSC collection to be done very near to the transplant to avoid cell loss during freezing and thawing.

2.5. Transplant Conditioning Protocols. All patients were given myeloablative conditioning chemotherapy without the use of total body irradiation (TBI). We have not used non-myeloablative or reduced intensity regimens. Chemotherapy was given through central lines in all patients. BEAM regimen was used for Hodgkin and non-Hodgkin lymphomas. BuCy regimen was used for acute leukaemias. Melphalan was used for myelomas according to standard protocols [14]. Table 2 describes our major conditioning regimens.

2.6. Antimicrobial Prophylaxis. See Tables 4 and 5.

2.7. VOD Prophylaxis. This included tablets of Ursodeoxycholic acid 300 mg thrice daily to all allogeneic patients.

2.8. Graft versus Host Prophylaxis. Table 3 shows GVHD prophylaxis in our allogeneic HSCT patients.

3. Outcome Data

3.1. Posttransplant Complications: Early Complications within 100 Days after Transplant. The most common early post-transplant complications were mucositis, infections, venooc-clusive disease (VOD), graft versus host disease (GVHD), and hemorrhagic cystitis. We have taken references from CTCAE (Common Terminology Criteria for Adverse Events) to grade our posttransplant complications [15]. Table 6 shows major early posttransplant complications in our autologous and allogeneic patients.

3.1.1. Oral Mucositis. Oral mucositis was one of the most common complications of both allogeneic and autologous BMT. Four (27%) (two grade 2 and two grade 3) of our allogeneic transplant patients and five (15%) (one grade 1, two grade 2, and two grade 3) of our autologous transplant patients had mucositis [16]. Grade 2 mucositis patients were managed with dietary modification, analgesics, and oral care and patients with grade 3 required some kind of intervention like parental nutrition and/or feeding tube insertion. We use ice sucking during melphalan and fludarabine conditioning chemotherapy to prevent/reduce mucositis. Chemotherapy and HSCT were the probable causes of the mucositis [17].

TABLE 2

Conditioning regimens	Indications	Protocol
Autologous HSCT		
BEAM regimen	Hodgkin's lymphoma, non-Hodgkin's lymphoma	Day −6: Carmustine (BCNU) (300 mg/m^2) Days −5, −4, −3, −2: Etoposide (200 mg/m^2) immediately after Etoposide infusion Cytarabine (ara-c) (400 mg/m^2) Day −1: Melphalan (140 mg/m^2/dose) Day 0: stem-cell transplant
Melphalan regimen	Multiple myeloma	Day −1: Melphalan 200 mg/m^2 or Melphalan 140 mg/m^2 Day 0: stem-cell transplant
FluMel	NHL Follicular lymphoma	Fludarabine 30 mg/m^2 for 4 days, on days −7 to −4 Melphalan 70 mg/m^2 on days −3, −2
Allogenic HSCT		
BuCy regimen	AML, CML, ALL	Days −7, −6, −5, −4: Busulfan: 3.2 mg/kg/day IV Days −3, −2: Cyclophosphamide 60 mg/kg/day Day 0: stem-cell transplant
Cyclophosphamide + ATG	Aplastic anemia	Cyclophosphamide 200 mg/kg on days −5, −4, −3, −2; ATG 90 mg/kg on days −5, −4, −3
Cyclophosphamide + thiotepa + oral busulfan	Thalassemia	Days −10 to −2: oral Busulfan 4 mg/kg/day for 4 days; Thiotepa 10 mg/kg once; Cyclophosphamide 200 mg/kg over 4 days

TABLE 3: Graft versus host disease prophylaxis.

Day	Prophylaxis regimen
−1	Cyclosporine 2.5 mg/kg/dose twice daily
0	Peripheral stem-cell transplant
0	Cyclosporine 1.5 mg/kg/dose twice daily; continued till day +90 and then gradually taper the dose
+1, +3, +6, +11	Methotrexate 15 mg/m^2 on D +1, 10 mg/m^2 on rest of days [6]
+2, +4, +7, +12	Two doses of leucovorin 15 mg/kg/every six hours starting 24 hours after methotrexate

3.1.2. Infections

Allogeneic BMT. There were 22 febrile neutropenia incidences during the transplantation hospital stay, out of which in 17 (77%) infection was documented with culture positivity and 5 (23%) were culture negative. Major infections were bacterial followed by fungal and viral causes. Major bacteria were *Staphylococcus* (25%), *Pseudomonas* (20%), and *Bacillus* species (20%) and minor infections were *Streptococcus* (18%) and *E. coli*. Three incidences were fungal infections. *Candida* (66%) was the commonest cause followed by *Aspergillus* (33%). One *Cytomegalovirus* infection with significant viral copies was also noted which required Ganciclovir. Major sites of culture positivity were blood (40%) and respiratory tract (30%) and other were urine, stool, and CVP line.

Autologous BMT. There were 27 incidences of febrile neutropenia, out of which in 20 (74%) infection was documented with culture positivity. Major infections were bacterial followed by fungal and viral causes. Major bacterial infections were *Streptococcus* (25%), *E. coli* (22%), *S. aureus* (18%), and *Klebsiella* (18%) followed by other species like *Proteus*, *Pseudomonas*, and *Typhoid*. Major fungal infections were *Candida* (50%) followed by *Aspergillus* (25%), *Rhizopus*, and *Mucormycosis*. One incidence of *Cytomegalovirus* was noted with significant viral copies that required Ganciclovir and one incidence of Herpes zoster was noted. Major sites of culture positivity were respiratory tract (33%), blood (25%), and stool (25%) followed by urine, CVP/catheter tip, and wound.

3.1.3. Venoocclusive Disease (VOD).

Two incidences of VOD were noted in allogeneic BMT. They presented with gallbladder wall edema, hyperammonemia, and bilateral pleural effusion. Ultrasound in both cases showed loss of phasic variation in hepatic vein on spectral waveform. Biopsy was done in one patient to confirm the diagnosis while the other one was clinical diagnosis. No incidences of VOD were noted in autologous BMT.

TABLE 4: Our antimicrobial prophylaxis for autologous BMT is as follows.

Antibiotics	Dose	Duration
Trimethoprim-sulfamethoxazole single (double strength for adults) strength	1 tab. once daily	Stops on day −2 and is restarted after day 28 or engraftment and is continued for 6 months
Tab. of valacyclovir	500 mg twice daily	Starts on day −2 till discharge
Tab. of fluconazole	200 mg twice daily	Starts on day −7 till discharge
Tab. of levofloxacin	500 mg once daily	Starts on day −7 till discharge

TABLE 5: Our antimicrobial prophylaxis for allogeneic BMT is as follows.

Antibiotics	Dose	Duration/special comments
Tab. of levofloxacin	500 mg once daily	Day −3 till discharge
Capsule fluconazole	200 mg twice daily	From day −3 to day +75 or till patient is immunocompromised due to likely GVHD management as fungal prophylaxis or amphotericin B 0.5 to 1 mg/kg once daily or on alternate days after ANC becomes less than 200; antifungal prophylaxis stops after neutrophil engraftment
Tab. of valacyclovir	1000 mg once daily	From day −3 to day +30 or longer in case of GVHD as Varicella zoster virus and Herpes simplex virus prophylaxis
Trimethoprim/sulfamethoxazole	10 mg/kg/day	Double strength daily from day −8 till day −2; it is restarted twice weekly as soon as engraftment is achieved
Tab. of penicillin V	250 mg twice weekly	From day +28 for prophylaxis against encapsulated organisms or tab. of amoxicillin-clavulanate for *Pneumocystis carinii* prophylaxis

Febrile neutropenia episodes were managed as per standard protocols.

TABLE 6

Type of complication	All grades numbers = N	Grade 3 or 4 numbers = N
(1) Oral mucositis	Allogeneic: N = 4 Autologous: N = 5	Allogeneic: N = 2 (all grade 3, no grade 4) Autologous: N = 2 (all grade 3, no grade 4)
(2) Venoocclusive disease	Grades not applicable Allogeneic: N = 2 Autologous: N = 0	Grades not applicable
(3) Acute GVHD	Allogeneic: N = 4 Autologous: not applicable	Allogeneic: N = 2 (both grade 3 hepatic acute GVHD; no grade 4 GVHD noted) Autologous: not applicable
(4) Periengraftment syndrome	Grades not applicable Allogeneic: N = 1 Autologous: N = 4	Grades not applicable
(5) Diarrhoea	N = 12 in autologous and allogeneic	N = 7 in autologous and allogeneic

3.1.4. Acute Graft versus Host Disease (Acute GVHD). Four incidences of GVHD were noted in allogeneic BMT. Two patients have skin GVHD, one was grade 1 and the other was grade 2. Two were hepatic acute GVHD grade 2/3 with elevated SGPT, bilirubin, and LDH.

3.1.5. Periengraftment Syndrome. Five incidences (10%) (one allogeneic and four autologous) were noted. Common symptoms were weight gain, low grade fever, and electrolyte imbalances, which were treated with short courses of steroids.

3.1.6. Gastrointestinal Complications. These were twelve incidences of grade 2 and grade 3 diarrhoea. There were three incidences of oral and/or anal bleeding.

3.1.7. Renal Complications. Three incidences of acute renal failure (2 autologous and 1 allogeneic) were noted with rise in blood urea nitrogen and creatinine. One incidence of allergic acute kidney injury was noted.

3.1.8. Pulmonary Complications. Two incidences of restrictive lung disease were noted with reduced DLCO and were probably related to previous chemotherapy exposure.

3.1.9. Neurological Toxicity. This was one incidence of peripheral motor and sensory neuropathy.

3.2. Late Complications at 100 Days

3.2.1. Chronic GVHD. Two incidences of chronic GVHD (13%) were noted; both were hepatic (limited grade).

TABLE 7: Outcome parameters of our autologous and allogeneic patients till April 2014 after a median follow-up of 39 months.

Outcome data	Autologous	Allogeneic
(1) Median engraftment day (Range)	15 days (10–35 days)	14 days (9–34 days)
(2) Median posttransplant hospital stay (range)	18 days (10–80 days)	20 days (14–70 days)
(3) Mortality rate	30-day mortality: $N = 0$ 100-day mortality: $N = 1$ 1-year mortality: $N = 7$ 3-year mortality: $N = 12$ 39-month (median follow-up) mortality: $N = 12$ Current mortality: $N = 14$	30-day mortality: $N = 0$ 100-day mortality: $N = 3$ 1-year mortality: $N = 6$ 3-year mortality: $N = 6$ 39-month (median follow-up) mortality: $N = 6$ Current mortality: $N = 6$
(4) Current disease status	Complete remission: $N = 16$ Partial remission: $N = 2$ Relapse but alive: $N = 3$	Complete remission: $N = 7$ Partial remission: $N = 0$ Relapse but alive: $N = 2$
(5) OS at median (39 months) follow-up	65.7% ($N = 23$)	57.1% ($N = 8$)

TABLE 8: Outcomes of our autologous and allogeneic HSCT patients.

Outcomes of our transplant patients	Autologous HSCT ($n = 35$)		Allogeneic HSCT ($n = 15$)	
Complete remission	46% (16/35)		47% (7/15)	
Partial remission	6% (2/35)		0% (0/15)	
Relapse but alive	8% (3/35)		13% (2/15)	
Transplant related mortality (TRM)	3% (1/35)		20% (3/15)	
Non-TRM	37% (13/35)	Causes Disease relapse 9 Chronic GVHD 1 Sepsis with multiorgan failure 1 Haemorrhagic brain infarction 1 Chronic GVHD 1	20% (3/15)	Causes ARDS with multiorgan failure 1 Haemorrhagic cystitis 1 Resistant chronic GVHD 1

3.2.2. Infections. Three incidences of bacterial infections were noted. One incidence was bilateral fungal lung infection and was treated with oral voriconazole. One incidence of Herpes zoster was noted.

3.3. Engraftment (Table 7). By definition, WBC engraftment is absolute neutrophil count >500 for three consecutive days and the platelet engraftment is the platelet count >20,000 for three consecutive days without any external transfusion support [18]. The median engraftment for our autologous BMT was 15 days with range of 10–35 days. The median engraftment days for our allogeneic BMT are 14 days with range of 9–34 days. One allogeneic BMT patient had delayed engraftment because of graft rejection.

3.4. Duration of Hospital Stay after Transplant (Table 7). Average duration of hospital stay after autologous BMT is 18 days with a range of 10–80 days. Average duration of hospital stay after allogeneic BMT is 20 days with a range of 14–70 days.

3.5. Mortality, Survival, and Disease Status Statistics (Tables 7 and 8). Fourteen (40%) of the autologous transplant patients and six (40%) of our allogeneic patients died in the course of follow-up. All of them survived during the first month of

posttransplant period. Mortality at 100 days after transplant period also known as transplant related mortality (TRM) in autologous patients was very low with 3% (1/35) while, in allogeneic patients, it was 20% (3/15). Major causes of transplant related mortality were related to bleeding, infections, and acute GVHD. Mortality 1 year after transplant period in our autologous patients was 20% (7/35) and 40% (6/15) in our allogeneic patients. Sixteen (46%) out of our 35 autologous and seven (47%) out of 15 allogeneic patients are in complete remission. 2/35 (6%) autologous HSCT patients have partial remission of the disease while none of the allogeneic transplant patients are in partial remission phase now. 12 (34%) of the autologous transplant patients had disease relapse out of whom nine patients died during the course of follow-up and three patients are alive under some sort of second line management.

3.6. Diagnosis Based Mortality and Survival till April 2014. Figure 3 shows the alive and dead patients in various indications of transplants being performed.

Figure 4 shows number of patients alive at particular posttransplant follow-up period. All of our transplant patients survived during the first month after transplant. Transplant related mortality was four (3 allogeneic and 1 autologous). Major downfall in this graph comes between

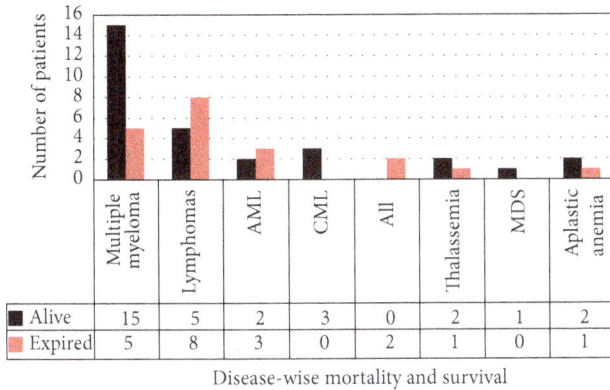

FIGURE 3

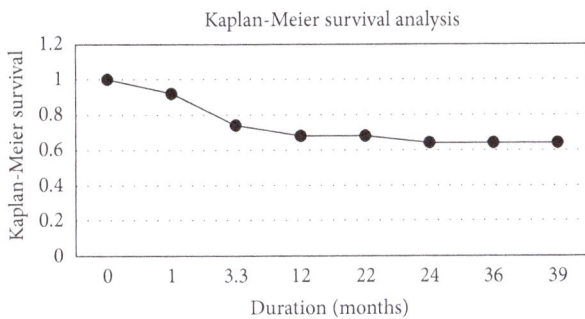

FIGURE 4: The figure shows Kaplan-Meier survival analysis.

100 days and 1 year after transplant period. The major causes of death in this period were neutropenic complications like sepsis, disease relapse, hemorrhagic complications, and GVHD. Our last transplant patient has been followed up for minimum of 22 months, so we can say that all of our patients have at least 22 months of follow-up. 34/50 (68%) patients survived during the first 22 months after transplant period. Number of patients alive at the median follow-up period was 32/50 (66%). The graph plateaus at 1 year of median follow-up after transplant. Two of our autologous patients died because of disease relapse after 39 months in the course of follow-up period.

4. Discussion

Apollo Hospital, Gandhinagar, is one of the major bone marrow transplant centres of India. The center is a registered transplant center of CIBMTR (Center for International Blood and Marrow Transplant Registry), USA. This hematopoietic stem-cell transplant data will be the first published data from Western India. The bone marrow/stem-cell transplant center at Apollo Hospital, Gandhinagar, is a new set-up compared to some other set-ups in India and across the world. The first successful autologous transplant was performed on July 5, 2007, in a six-year-old child with Hodgkin lymphoma and the first allogeneic transplant was performed on June 6, 2008, on a thirty-eight-year-old male with AML relapse. Within 5 years span, a total of 50 patients were treated with stem-cell transplants at Apollo Hospital, Gandhinagar. Majority of our

HSC collections were done from peripheral blood after G-CSF mobilization. We have not done cord blood transplants, haploidentical donor transplants, or marrow unrelated donor (MUD) transplants yet. We have followed all patients for at least 22 months with median follow-up of 39 months, which is comparable to many national and international studies. Although number of transplants performed is not big enough and data is for shorter duration, still the data is comparable with some national and international published data.

Mean duration of engraftment in our patients was 17 days for autologous BMT and 16 days for allogeneic BMT which is comparable to other standard international data [18]. Only one allogeneic BMT patient had delayed engraftment due to graft failure. Major risk factors of graft failure are disparity between recipient and donor within the major histocompatibility complex (MHC) [19]. We have only used myeloablative conditioning regimen in our transplant patients. One western study shows that the graft failure in myeloablative conditioning regimens is 1/34 compared to 6/24 in nonmyeloablative regimen with $P = 0.02$ [20].

Table 9 shows comparison of various parameters between Apollo Hospital, Gandhinagar, National Cancer Research Institute, Kolkata, Christian Medical College, Vellore, and western studies. Survival in patients of Apollo Hospital is parallel to most of the Indian published reports and many of the western countries.

Health Resources and Services Administration (HRSA), US Department of Health and Human Services, USA, publish their survival analysis data every year at 100 days, 1 year, and 3 years after transplant period [21]. Comparison of survival statistics are analogous to HRSA data from the United States of America but as the numbers of transplants in some of the categories are not sufficient, comparison can be misleading. There are some areas in our efforts, where our Apollo CBCC stem-cell transplant unit is behind some western studies.

For example, infection rates are comparable to other Indian centres but much higher than western studies, which report bacterial infection rate of 5%, viral infection rate of 7%, and fungal infection rate of 12% [8]. The possible risk factors of infections in our patients are aggressive myeloablative conditioning regimens at our center leading to prolonged neutropenia during preengraftment period and possible environmental factors in India [22]. Early posttransplant infection rates are higher in our allogeneic BMT patients probably because we use aggressive myeloablative conditioning regimens which produce very severe and prolonged neutropenia during preengraftment period. One western study demonstrates that, before neutrophil engraftment, the nonmyeloablative cohort had a 53% lower rate of bacterial infections, whereas after engraftment the density of bacterial infections was similar in myeloablative and nonmyeloablative groups. It also shows that, in the first month, both invasive fungal infections and viral infections were twofold less frequent in nonmyeloablative patients [23]. Incidence of viral infections is low (2 CMV and 1 HSV) as compared to two other published data of Indian centres. We do pretransplant evaluation for HIV, hepatitides B and C, and *Cytomegalovirus* (CMV). We also monitor CMV viral load in posttransplant period in all of our allogeneic HSCT patients. Other viruses

TABLE 9

	Apollo Hospital International Limited, Gandhinagar (N = 50)	Christian Medical College, Vellore (N = 221) [7]	National Cancer Research Institute, Kolkata (N = 22) [8]	Western studies
Bacterial infections	50%	34.9%	52%	5%
Viral infections	4%	42.9%	24%	7%
Fungal	14%	15.9%	12%	16%
Blood culture positivity	22%	53.8%	50%	12.5% [9]
Incidence of gram negative infection	22%	80%	80%	11.2% [9]
Graft versus host disease	Grade 1 skin GVHD in 6.7% (1/15), grade 2 skin GVHD in 6.7%, and acute hepatic GVHD grade 2-3 in 13.3% (2/15)	17% grade 3 and grade 4	Skin GVHD grade II in 18.2%, grade I GVHD of liver in 13.6%, and grades II-III gut GVHD in 9%	Data not available
Mortality rate	No mortality for the first month; 100 day mortality 8%; overall mortality 40% with the median follow-up of 39 months	Overall mortality is approximately 28%	Overall mortality was 13.7% at the median follow-up of 4.6 years	Mortality rate for allogeneic transplant is approximately 30% and for autologous transplant it is approximately 10% after 3 years of follow-up.(USA and Canada) [10]
Long term survival	Overall survival for thalassemia patients, autologous HSCT patients, and allogeneic HSCT patients was 66%, 65.7, and 57.1%, respectively, with median follow-up of 39 months	Overall survival 72.3 ± 3.1% of 218 patients of thalassemia at median follow-up of 5 years	Overall survival 86.3%; disease-free survival 68.2% seen at median follow-up of 22 patients for 4.6 years	50–70% in chronic leukaemias and 80–90% with aplastic anaemias (USA and Canada) [11]

like Epstein Barr virus and Herpes simplex virus are not monitored regularly.

Major complications during the transplant were GVHD, infections, mucositis, venoocclusive disease, disease related complications, and chemotherapy induced complications and complications related to other comorbidities. One of our myeloma patients required second transplant after the first one because of disease relapse.

Mortality rates are comparable to other Indian and western studies. Major causes of mortality in our patients were infections and disease relapse/progression. Transplant related mortality was found in 8% of our patients. By definition, transplant related mortality (TRM) means deaths occurring during the first 100 days after transplant due to complications of the transplant [24]. Majority of deaths occurred in the first year of posttransplant period. Common causes of non-TRM mortality in the first year after transplant period in our patients were disease relapse (45%), haemorrhagic complications (10%), GVHD (10%), and sepsis (10%).

Overall survival of our autologous and allogeneic HSCT transplant patients was 65.7% and 57.1%, respectively. 46% of our autologous and 47% of our allogeneic patients are in complete remission phase after a median follow-up of 39 months which is comparable to many national and international transplant centres as shown in Table 9. By definition,

complete remission means disappearance of all signs of cancer in response to treatment and does not always mean that the cancer has been cured. It is also called complete response [25].

In a developing country like India, there are very few centres, which perform regular HSCT due to various reasons like lack of infrastructure and expertise and lack of knowledge of safety, efficacy, and cost of the procedure both in general population and in medical fraternity. This study will help in sharing its outcomes with other hematology/oncology practitioners and will encourage other centres to start performing stem-cell transplantations or refer eligible patients for this important treatment option available.

5. Conclusion

With these encouraging results at our center, we can conclude that our data is comparable to national and international hematopoietic stem-cell transplantation centres in terms of complications, outcomes of treatment, and cost effectiveness. These results provide evidence that the stem-cell transplant, which is a recommended treatment option in various diseases, is possible in a nonuniversity hospital of developing country with excellent safety profile. We will continue to provide our services in the future and try to take them to the next level in terms of application of haplotransplantation, marrow unrelated donor transplantations, and cord blood as the stem-cell source. We will also try to make transplantation possible to some rare indications, nonaffording patients, reduce the complications, and improve the outcomes of the HSCT at our center.

Conflict of Interests

The authors declare that there is no conflict of interests regarding the publication of this paper.

Acknowledgments

This work would not have been possible without the active support of many departments in the Apollo Hospital: Blood Bank, Microbiology and Critical Care, Haematology, and Medical Records Department. The authors acknowledge the support from the Director of Oncology Department, Apollo Hospital, Gandhinagar, Dr. Bharat J. Parikh. They also acknowledge Shyam Hem-Onc Clinic for pre- and posttransplant assessment, counselling, and monitoring, and Supratech speciality laboratory for performing apheresis and CD 34 counts. The dedication and meticulous care provided by transplant nurses, registrars, and dietician and housekeeping staff are essential for success of a transplant program and are gratefully acknowledged.

References

[1] "History of Transplantation," Fred Hutchison Cancer Research Center, 2013, http://www.fredhutch.org/en/treatment/long-term-follow-up/FAQs/transplantation.html.

[2] M. Chandy, "Stem cell transplantation in India," *Bone Marrow Transplantation*, vol. 42, pp. S81–S84, 2008.

[3] "Participating Transplant Centers," CIBMTR, Center for International Blood & Marrow Transplant Research, 2013, http://www.cibmtr.org/About/WhoWeAre/Centers/Pages/index.aspx?country=India.

[4] U. Kanga, A. Panigrahi, S. Kumar, and N. K. Mehra, "Asian Indian donor marrow registry: all India Institute of Medical Sciences experience," *Transplantation Proceedings*, vol. 39, no. 3, pp. 719–720, 2007.

[5] Government of Gujarat, *Gujarat—Official Guajarat State Portal*, 2009, http://www.gujaratindia.com/state-profile/demography.htm.

[6] R. Storb, J. H. Antin, and C. Cutler, "Should methotrexate plus calcineurin inhibitors be considered standard of care for prophylaxis of acute graft-versus-host disease?" *Biology of Blood and Marrow Transplantation*, vol. 16, no. 1, pp. S18–S27, 2010.

[7] M. Chandy, A. Srivastava, D. Dennison, V. Mathews, and B. George, "Allogeneic bone marrow transplantation in the developing world: experience from a center in India," *Bone Marrow Transplantation*, vol. 27, no. 8, pp. 785–790, 2001.

[8] A. Mukhopadhyay, P. Gupta, J. Basak et al., "Stem cell transplant: an experience from Eastern India," *Indian Journal of Medical and Paediatric Oncology*, vol. 33, no. 4, pp. 203–209, 2012.

[9] W. Kruger, "Early infections in patients undergoing bone marrow or blood stem cell transplantation—a 7 year single centre investigation of 409 cases," *Bone Marrow Transplant*, vol. 23, no. 6, pp. 589–597, 1999, http://www.nature.com/bmt/journal/v23/n6/abs/1701614a.html.

[10] Encyclopedia of Surgery, *Bone Marrow Transplantation*, 2014, http://www.surgeryencyclopedia.com/A-Ce/Bone-Marrow-Transplantation.html.

[11] R. Chawla, *Infections after One Marrow Transplantation*, 2013, http://emedicine.medscape.com/article/1013470-overview.

[12] *Bone Marrow Transplantation and Peripheral Blood Stem Cell Transplantation*, 2013, http://www.cancer.gov/cancertopics/factsheet/Therapy/bone-marrow-transplant.

[13] "Practical aspects of stem cell collection-chapter 108," in *Hoffman: Hematology: Basic Principles and Practice*, Saunders, 2012, http://www.mdconsult.com/books/linkTo?type=bookPage&isbn=978-1-4377-2928-3&eid=4-u1.0-B978-1-4377-2928-3..00008-3.

[14] HemOnc.com, *Trnasplant Conditioning Regimens*, 2013, http://hemonc.org/Transplant_conditioning_regimens.

[15] Common Terminology Criteria for Adverse Events (CTCAE), *CTEP (Cancer Therapy Evaluation Trial)*, v4.0, 2013.

[16] C. Cutler, "Assesment and Grading of Oral Mucositis after Stem Cell Transplantation," http://www.cibmtr.org/Meetings/Materials/CRPDMC/Documents/2007/february/CutlerC_MucositisASB.pdf.

[17] National Cancer Institute, 2013, http://www.cancer.gov/cancertopics/pdq/supportivecare/oralcomplications/HealthProfessional/page5.

[18] Be The Match. (n.d.), Engraftment: 0-30 days, http://bethematch.org/For-Patients-and-Families/Getting-a-transplant/Engraftment–Days-0-30/.

[19] P. G. Beatty, R. A. Clift, E. M. Mickelson et al., "Marrow transplantation from related donors other than HLA-identical siblings," *The New England Journal of Medicine*, vol. 313, no. 13, pp. 765–771, 1985.

[20] K. le Blanc, M. Remberger, M. Uzunel, J. Mattsson, L. Barkholt, and O. Ringdén, "A comparison of nonmyeloablative and reduced-intensity conditioning for allogeneic stem-cell transplantation," *Transplantation*, vol. 78, no. 7, pp. 1014–1020, 2004.

[21] U.S. Department of Health and Human Services, *U.S. Patient Survival Report*, 2014, http://bloodcell.transplant.hrsa.gov/RESEARCH/Transplant_Data/US_Tx_Data/Survival_Data/survival.aspx.

[22] R. Chawla, "Infections after bone marrow transplantation," 2013, http://emedicine.medscape.com/article/1013470-overview.

[23] V. Bachanova, C. G. Brunstein, L. J. Burns et al., "Fewer infections and lower infection-related mortality following nonmyeloablative versus myeloablative conditioning for allotransplantation of patients with lymphoma," *Bone Marrow Transplantation*, vol. 43, no. 3, pp. 237–244, 2009.

[24] A. D. Schimmer, "Allogeneic or autologous bone marrow transplantation (BMT) for non-Hodgkin's lymphoma (NHL): results of a provincial strategy," *Bone Marrow Transplantation*, vol. 26, no. 8, pp. 859–864, 2000.

[25] "NCI Dictionary of Cancer Terms. (n.d.)," http://www.cancer.gov/dictionary?cdrid=45651.

12

Epithelial to Mesenchymal Transition in a Clinical Perspective

Jennifer Pasquier,[1,2] Nadine Abu-Kaoud,[1] Haya Al Thani,[1,2] and Arash Rafii[1,2]

[1]Stem Cell and Microenvironment Laboratory, Department of Genetic Medicine and Obstetrics and Gynecology,
  Weill Cornell Medical College in Qatar, Education City, Qatar Foundation, P.O. Box 24144, Doha, Qatar
[2]Department of Genetic Medicine, Weill Cornell Medical College, New York, NY 10021, USA

Correspondence should be addressed to Jennifer Pasquier; jep2026@qatar-med.cornell.edu
and Arash Rafii; jat2021@qatar-med.cornell.edu

Academic Editor: Sandra Cascio

Tumor growth and metastatic dissemination rely on cellular plasticity. Among the different phenotypes acquired by cancer cells, epithelial to mesenchymal transition (EMT) has been extensively illustrated. Indeed, this transition allows an epithelial polarized cell to acquire a more mesenchymal phenotype with increased mobility and invasiveness. The role of EMT is quite clear during developmental stage. In the neoplastic context in many tumors EMT has been associated with a more aggressive tumor phenotype including local invasion and distant metastasis. EMT allows the cell to invade surrounding tissues and survive in the general circulation and through a stem cell phenotype grown in the host organ. The molecular pathways underlying EMT have also been clearly defined and their description is beyond the scope of this review. Here we will summarize and analyze the attempts made to block EMT in the therapeutic context. Indeed, till today, most of the studies are made in animal models. Few clinical trials are ongoing with no obvious benefits of EMT inhibitors yet. We point out the limitations of EMT targeting such tumor heterogeneity or the dynamics of EMT during disease progression.

1. Introduction

Despite the improvement of treatment regimens, cancer remains a leading cause of death worldwide. Metastatic disease is responsible for the majority of cancer-induced mortality [1]. The development of new therapeutic strategies targeting key factors driving metastasis remains a challenging goal for both clinicians and scientists. Metastasis is artificially divided into a series of sequential highly organized and organ specific steps [2]. Among these steps is the acquisition of migratory and invasive proprieties by cancer cells, which can be achieved through epithelial-mesenchymal transition (EMT) [3–6].

First described in embryogenesis, EMT is a cellular reprogramming process in which epithelial cells acquire a mesenchymal phenotype [7]. During this transformation, epithelial cells lose their polygonal shape and ability to grow in colonies, but they acquire spindle-shaped morphology and exhibit a more motile and invasive behavior [8]. These phenotypic changes are associated with proteins and gene modifications in different interconnected families such as transcription factors, cadherins, catenins, matrix metalloproteases (MMPs), or growth receptors [9, 10].

While EMT has been well accepted and demonstrated *in vivo* during embryogenesis, its implication in the metastatic process is still debated [11–16]. Identifying the EMT process in neoplastic disease is difficult since cells undergoing EMT share many molecular and morphological characteristics with the surrounding stromal fibroblasts. Moreover, although primary carcinoma or circulating tumor cells (CTCs) display EMT features, cells present in the distant metastases site are generally epithelial [17]. In 2002, Their proposed an explanation to such observation by describing the reversible EMT metastasis model in which primary epithelial tumor cells activate EMT to invade distant sites, and, upon arriving, they undergo a MET (mesenchymal-epithelial transition) to form an epithelial metastatic lesion [18].

Numerous reviews have comprehensively described EMT in cancer as well as the molecular pathways implicated in EMT or MET [17, 19–21]. The description of such findings is beyond the scope of this review. Here, we focus on the latest research on EMT in the clinical context for prognostic or therapeutic or strategies.

2. Can We Use EMT to Predict Patient's Outcome?

Recently, the detection of circulating tumor cells above a defined cut-off has been associated with poor prognosis in different cancers such as breast or prostate tumors [22, 23]. Circulating tumor cells, as well as metastatic lesions, of many different cancers present EMT characteristic [24–30]. Many studies investigated whether the expression of EMT markers would be associated with poor patient prognosis. The aberrant expression of Snail is related to poor patient survival in breast [31–34], ovarian [33, 35, 36], hepatocellular [37–40], and colorectal carcinomas [41, 42]. Twist overexpression is associated with a poor clinical outcome in many cancers such as bladder cancer [43], breast cancer [34], oral squamous cell carcinoma [44], ovarian cancer [45, 46], or cervical cancer [47]. Vimentin overexpression in cancers and its correlation with growth and metastasis suggest that it might be an indicator of poor prognostic for many cancers [48]. In bladder cancer, a study of eleven different cell lines revealed that the loss of E-cadherin expression is a marker of poor response to the monoclonal antibody cetuximab, which blocks EGFR binding [49]. More recently, Twist-1 promoter hypermethylation, studied on 65 surgically resected specimens, was shown to be a useful molecular marker for predicting prognosis and contralateral cervical lymph node metastases in patients with tonsillar squamous cell carcinoma [50].

The increasing amount of data on single EMT indicators urged the investigation of the correlation between several markers on patients' prognosis. A 4-EMT genes signature (E-cadherin (CDH1), inhibitor of DNA binding 2 (ID2), matrix metalloproteinase 9 (MMP9), and transcription factor 3 (TCF3)) was used to predict clinical outcome in a cohort of 128 hepatocellular carcinoma patients and then validated in an independent cohort of 231 patients with hepatocellular carcinoma from three different institutions [51]. The authors claimed that this 4-gene signature could improve patients' survival prediction on the risk score and tumor stage. Recently, in a study including surgical specimens from 78 cases of esophageal squamous cell carcinoma resected without preoperative treatment between 2001 and 2013, Niwa et al. demonstrated that the vimentin/E-cadherin ratio was correlated with tumor invasion and can serve as an independent prognostic factor among chemonaive patients [52]. In an analysis of 100 surgically resected hepatic tumors, EMT markers Twist-1 and Zeb-2 were shown to be involved in early disease recurrence in hepatocellular carcinoma and served as good prognosis markers [53]. In a different study on paraffin-embedded hepatocellular carcinoma tissues (n = 113) and their corresponding peritumoral normal tissues (n = 106), although the expression of 3-EMT-related proteins, S100A4, vimentin, and E-cadherin was studied, the authors reported that E-cadherin alone can be used as a direct prognosticator

of negative outcome [54]. The prognostic significance of E-cadherin, twist, and vimentin was assayed in 121 patients with bladder cancer and, in this study, only vimentin appears as an independent predictor for cancer progression and survival [55].

Cancer stem cells have emerged as a particular entity within tumor cell plasticity. They have the ability to reinitiate the tumor in serial engraftment assays; they are more resistant to treatment than the bulk of the tumor and their role in the occurrence of metastasis has been suggested in several studies [1, 56–58]. Their identification relies on functional proprieties (spheroid formation in 3D media, asymmetric division, and serial passages in NOD/SCID mice) and specific markers. Several authors have described an increase of tumor stemness when cancer cells undergo EMT, leading to the study of stem cell associated markers combined with EMT-related markers as prognosis indicators. Luo et al. studied the correlation of SOX2, OCT4, and Nanog with E-cadherin, N-cadherin, and Snail in a nasopharyngeal carcinoma cohort of 122 patients [59]. They demonstrated that OCT4 and Nanog could be used as poor prognosis factor and are linked with the progression of the invasive front. In two different clinical studies, one on 119 human cholangiocarcinoma patients [60] and one on 276 consecutive primary gastric cancers and 54 matched lymph node metastases [61], the same team revealed that EMT markers (Snail-1, Zeb-1, E-cadherin, vimentin, and beta-catenin) and the CSC marker, CD44, are strongly correlated. Moreover, they revealed that the simultaneous expression of Snail-1, vimentin, E-cadherin, and CD44 was associated with advanced stage, metastasis, and invasion and was an independent indicator for disease-free survival.

Accumulating evidences in the literature are reflecting the regulatory roles of microRNAs (miRNAs) on EMT phenotype [62]. miRNAs can be optimal markers of specific disease or a patient' prognosis. Indeed, they can be found and quantified in many different biological fluids, including blood, urine, and cerebrospinal fluid; they also display great stability (even after boiling, freeze-thaw cycles, or low or high pH conditions). For instance, tumors with low expression of miR-335 and miR-126, 2 miRNA known to inhibit the first step of EMT, have been reported to present more probability to develop metastasis than tumors with higher expression of these miRNA [63]. In the blood, qPCR analysis of miR-10b, miR-34, and miR-155 allows the discrimination between patients with breast cancer metastasis and healthy controls. These miRNA play an important role in regulating EMT in response to TGFβ. A meta-analysis of 17 studies with various carcinomas uncovered the role of miR-21 (an oncomiR known to promote EMT through TGFβ pathway) as a poor prognosis biomarker in breast, squamous cell carcinoma, astrocytoma, and gastric cancer [64].

As described above, many EMT markers or their derivatives have been associated with patients' prognosis in different studies. However, while an EMT phenotype seems clearly associated with an increased metastatic phenotype, the use of such markers has not yet been translated into clinical practice. The requirements for an assay to be usable in clinical practice are quite stringent. Indeed, any prognosis marker has to first display great robustness. It should be reproducible among different laboratories and between pathologists. As prognostic markers will be used to give adjuvant therapy, their specificity should be quite high allowing the identification of patients who would not benefit from adjuvant treatment. While EMT markers have been independently associated with patients' prognosis, they have not yet been used in clinical practice for several reasons.

Tumor heterogeneity is one of the main reasons; the expression of EMT markers can vary at different locations of a tumor (usually increased mesenchymal phenotype at the periphery). Clear cut-offs are critical; most of the markers used in classical pathology have clear cut-offs (mitosis per field, Her2 overexpression, etc.). For EMT markers, defining the cut-offs might be difficult as different tumors display different levels of epithelial or mesenchymal phenotype and it is hard to clearly attribute a value for a particular marker. These are few difficulties among others including technical issues to do multiplex assays and the lack of large multicentric prospective trials.

One solution might be the advent of oncogenomic prognosis assays based on gene expression [65]. Currently, more than 100 clinical trials in cancer disease are ongoing using EMT as a keyword. Most of them study the prevalence of EMT markers in different cancers and their potential use as prognosis factor. The data from these studies will help us determine the clinical context where EMT could be used to tailor patients' treatment.

3. Can We Use EMT Effectors to Treat Patients?

EMT is an extremely well-organized process, activated in response to a combination of extracellular cues from the tumor microenvironment. EMT-inducing signals seem to be cell or tissue specific and require the cooperation between multiple signaling pathways and regulators. We considered the potential targets in three different groups classified based on their role during EMT: the molecular effectors executing EMT, the transcription factors acting as regulators to orchestrate EMT, and extracellular inducers that engage the cells in EMT.

3.1. Effectors. EMT effectors are mostly proteins that define the epithelial or mesenchymal phenotype of a cell. A key feature of EMT is the switch from E-cadherin (marker of epithelial cells) to N-cadherin (makers of mesenchymal cells) [9]. Targeting these cadherins in order to avoid a loss of E-cadherin or an upregulation of N-cadherin could therefore be a promising strategy.

Several groups studied the transfection of E-cadherin in highly mesenchymal and invasive cells and showed a reversion of the poorly differentiated carcinoma into a well-differentiated one with a minimally invasive epithelial phenotype [66–70]. In breast cancer, it has been demonstrated that salinomycin can selectively kill E-cadherin-negative breast epithelial cells as compared with E-cadherin-positive cells in NOD/SCID and Balb/c mice model [71]. Global gene expression analyses of breast tissues isolated directly from

patients display that salinomycin treatment results in the loss of cancer stem cell (CSC) expression. The tumor suppressor role of E-cadherin has been established in many cancers including hepatocellular carcinoma [72], esophagus [73], melanoma [74], breast cancer [75, 76], or squamous cell carcinoma of the skin, head, and neck [77, 78]. However, in ovarian tumors, E-cadherin is consistently upregulated and maintained in ovarian carcinoma cells that metastasize to the peritoneum and omentum [79]. E-cadherin expression has been found in patients with a family history of ovarian cancer, proposing a potential role of E-cadherin in tumor initiation and/or progression in this particular cancer [80]. Concordantly, several recent studies point to a promoting role of E-cadherin during tumor progression in different epithelial cancers such as ovarian, breast, or brain cancer (reviewed in [81]). An epithelial phenotype has been also correlated with an increase in cancer stemness and engraftment in host organs in prostate cancer [82]. Overall, targeting E-cadherin seems to be difficult due to its ambiguous role in carcinogenesis.

Inhibition of N-cadherin has been assessed in several studies [83, 84]. Shintani et al. reported that, in a mouse model of pancreatic cancer, the peptide ADH-1 is able to block N-cadherin and prevent tumor progression [85]. In head and neck cancer cell line, quercetin has been shown to significantly reduce the migration ability of sphere cells by decreasing N-cadherin production [86]. Recently, Sadler et al. demonstrated that targeting N-cadherin using a neutralizing antibody may be a good therapeutic strategy to treat multiple myeloma [87].

Vimentin is also a canonical marker of mesenchymal phenotype and therefore an important effector of EMT [48]. Few reports have shown a direct inhibition of vimentin. Lahat and collaborator suggested that the withaferin-A induces vimentin degradation in a panel of soft tissue sarcoma xenograft experiments, leading to the inhibition of growth, local recurrence, and metastasis [88]. In prostate tumors, both silibinin and flavonolignan inhibited invasion, motility, and migration of the cancer cells via downregulation of vimentin in cancer cell lines and mice models [89, 90]. Finally, salinomycin, an antibiotic, reduced significantly vimentin level and induced increase in E-cadherin expression in CD133$^+$ colorectal cancer cell lines HT29 and SW480 resulting in decreased malignant traits [91].

None of these strategies are currently tested in a clinical context. Indeed, EMT effectors have a complex role and their function might be time and context dependent during the metastatic process such as illustrated by the dual role of E-cadherin. Some additional key EMT effector molecules are proteins that promote cell migration and invasion during the process such as fibronectin, PDGF/PDGF receptor autocrine loop, Cd44, or integrin β6 [17]. Hence, these proteins might also be considered as potential targets to counter the EMT process.

3.2. Regulators. EMT regulators are a core of transcription factor such as Snail-1/Snail-1, basic helix-loop-helix family (E47, E2-2, and Twist-1/Twist-2), and Zeb-1/Zeb-1 [21, 92]. The role of these transcription factors in proliferation, invasion, and migration of epithelial tumors has been well described and their use as a target to block EMT process seems appealing [41, 93–95].

da Silva et al. reported that the inhibition of Twist-1 in metastatic oral squamous cell carcinoma (OSCC) induced a potent inhibition of cell invasiveness *in vitro* as well as *in vivo* using an orthotropic mouse model of metastatic OSCC [44]. The secreted frizzled-related protein (sFRP1 and sFRP2) two Wnt antagonists enhance the expression of E-cadherin through the inhibition of Twist-1 and suppress the invasiveness of cervical cancer *in vivo* in a xenograft animal model [96]. The bone morphogenetic protein 7 (BMP7) is a potential metastasis inhibitor that disrupts EMT through Twist-1 inhibition in melanoma WM-266-4 and HEK293T cell lines [97]. Arumugam et al. have shown using many different pancreatic cell lines that silencing Zeb-1 not only restored the expression of epithelial marker genes, but also increased cellular sensitivity to therapeutic reagents [98]. In a lung carcinoma cell line, the knockdown of Snail or Twist-1 is able to restore the cell chemosensitivity to cisplatin [99, 100].

The sulforaphane, an organosulfur compound, is able to downregulate Twist-1 as well as other EMT proteins like vimentin leading to a decrease of stemness properties in PANC-1, MIA PaCa-2, AsPC-1, and Bx PC-3 pancreatic cells lines [101]. Recently, moscatilin was shown to target the Akt-Twist-1 dependent pathway and decrease the migration and metastasis of MDA-MB-231 breast cancer cell line [102]. Fucoidan was also described to inhibit EMT in breast cancer cell lines such as 4T1 and MDA-MB-231 through the decreased Twist-1, Snail, and Slug expression [103]. In 2014, Myung and collaborators demonstrated that the knockdown of Snail with siRNA technique in three glioblastoma cell lines (KNS42, U87, and U373) suppresses the proliferation, viability, migration, and invasion of cells by disrupting the EMT process [104].

Despite the promising results in preclinical studies, overall, EMT core transcription factors remain technically challenging to target in a clinical setting. However, a clinical trial is currently investigating the molecular mechanism and clinical significance of the interplay between Twist-1 and other EMT regulators through microRNA-29 family in head and neck squamous cell carcinoma (NCT01927354).

3.3. Inducers. The principal inducers of EMT are proteins from the TGFβ (TGFβ1, TGFβ2, TGFβ3, inhibins, activin, anti-Müllerian hormone, bone morphogenetic protein, decapentaplegic, and Vg-1) and the growth factor (fgf, hgf, egf, and igf1) families [21]. High-throughput drug screening has been performed to identify potential inhibitors of EMT in response to various inducers. The majority of molecules selected inhibit specific EMT-inducing signals used in the screen. For instance, rapamycin and 17-AGG have been shown to inhibit TGFβ-induced EMT through the modification of TGFβ pathway itself as assessed by a global gene expression profile from a cell culture model of TGFβ-induced EMT [105]. Inhibitors of ALK5, MEK, and SRC are able to block EMT in response to EGF, HGF, and IGF-1 [105, 106]. In 2011, two different groups proposed c-MET as a potential therapeutic target in hepatocellular carcinoma

cell lines Huh7, Hep3B, MHCC97-L, and MHCC97-H [107] and BNL CL.2 (BNL) and BNL 1ME A. 7R.1 (1MEA) [108]. In prostate cancer, inhibition of c-Met expression and Met-mediated signaling by Frzb leads to the upregulation of epithelial markers and a decrease of the mesenchymal traits in a xenograft mouse model [109].

The most studied inducer of EMT remains TGFβ [110–112]. Targeting TGFβ pathway to alter EMT induced tumor cell invasion may be appropriate as metastasis prevention strategies in early stage carcinomas. SD-093 and LY-580276, two competitive inhibitors for the ATP-binding site of TGFβRI kinase, disrupt EMT and tumor cell migration in many cancers [113, 114]. EW-7203, EW-7195, and EW-7197, specific TGFβ/ALK5 inhibitors available as orally administered drugs [115, 116], have been shown to inhibit EMT in both TGFβ treated breast cancer cells and 4T1 orthotropic xenograft mice [117]. Bone morphogenetic protein 7 (BMP7) was revealed as a potential inhibitor of EMT induced by TGFβ in thirty liver tissue samples of patients with cholangiocarcinoma [118].

Currently, the only compounds interfering with EMT in clinical trial are the ones able to block EMT inducers. In 2008, already, the LY2157299, a clinical selective TGFβ1 receptor inhibitor, was undergoing a still unpublished phase I trial for colon, prostate, and adrenocortical or breast cancer and malignant melanoma patients [119]. That same year, another preclinical trial using human xenografts Calu6 (non-small-cell lung cancer) and MX1 (breast cancer) implanted subcutaneously in nude mice demonstrated that LY2157299 is able to reduce the tumor growth [120]. LY2157299 is now known to display antitumor effects in patients with glioblastoma and hepatocellular carcinoma [121]. LY2157299 is currently tested in four clinical trials, in patients recruiting state: Phase Ib/II in stages II–IV pancreatic cancer of LY2157299 combined with gemcitabine versus gemcitabine plus placebo (NCT01373164); Phase II in HCC patients with disease progression on sorafenib or who are not eligible to receive sorafenib (NCT01246986); Phase Ib/IIa study combining LY2157299 with standard temozolomide based radiochemotherapy in patients with newly diagnosed malignant glioma (NCT01220271); and Phase II Study of LY2157299 monotherapy or LY2157299 plus Lomustine therapy compared to Lomustine monotherapy in patients with recurrent glioblastoma (NCT01582269).

Erlotinib, an EGF receptor tyrosine kinase inhibitor, is approved for the treatment of second- and third-line advanced non-small-cell lung cancers [122, 123]. Interestingly, its efficacy is correlated with the EMT status of the cells; higher E-cadherin levels indicate sensitivity, whereas higher vimentin and Zeb-1 levels indicate resistance. Thus, in 2012, a randomized phase II trial on 132 patients with non-small-cell lung cancer evaluated the effect of erlotinib combined with the isoform selective histone deacetylase inhibitors, entinostat, known to prevent the resistance by reverting the cancer cell mesenchymal phenotype to an epithelial one [124]. Even if entinostat failed at improving the outcome of patients, the study revealed that E-cadherin expression levels at time of diagnosis could portray the sensitivity to

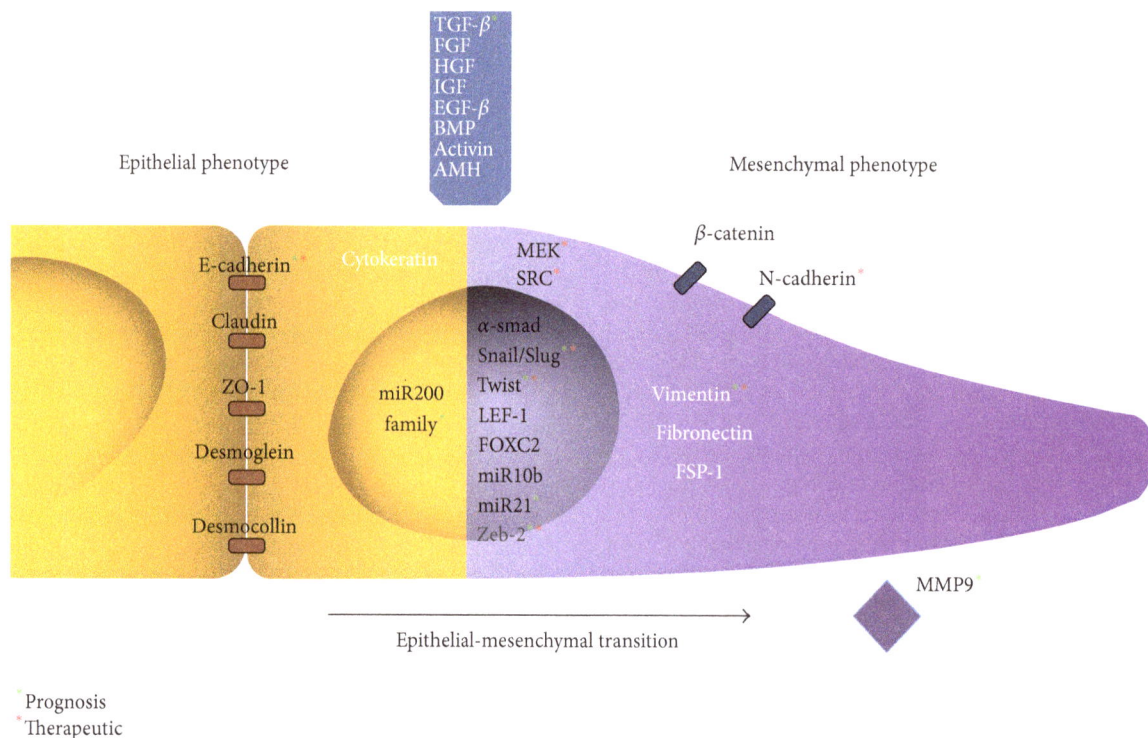

FIGURE 1: Epithelial to mesenchymal transition with effectors and inducers studied in the prognostic or therapeutic context. Green asterisk: implicated in prognosis. Red asterisk: targeted therapeutically.

HDACi/EGFR-TKI inhibition providing the basis for a biomarker-driven validation.

In 2014, the GC1008 (fresolimumab), a human anti-TGFβ monoclonal antibody, has undergone a phase I clinical trial in patients with advanced malignant melanoma or renal cell carcinoma [125]. 29 patients, 28 with malignant melanoma and 1 with renal cell carcinoma, were included and received intravenous GC1008 at 0.1, 0.3, 1, 3, 10, or 15 mg/kg on days 0, 28, 42, and 56. It demonstrated that GC1008 was presenting an acceptable safety and toxicity, and the maximum dose, 15 mg/kg, was determined. Multiple doses of GC1008 demonstrated only preliminary evidence of antitumor activity, allowing further studies of single agent and combination treatments in clinical trials. In fact, GC-1008 is currently tested in two clinical studies: fresolimumab and radiotherapy in metastatic breast cancer (NCT01401062) and safety and imaging study of GC1008 in glioma (NCT01472731).

4. A Moving Target

Despite the massive amount of preclinical data in most cancer types, there is still no clear cancer treatment specifically targeting EMT. Many aspects of tumor biology can explain the gap between the preclinical and clinical data.

In most preclinical studies an induced model of EMT is used to demonstrate the implication of EMT in tumor spread and then to demonstrate the efficacy of targeting EMT in achieving tumor response. These models are usually quite far from clinical reality. They do not perfectly reproduce tumor heterogeneity which is increased at the metastatic stage as

demonstrated by several studies of tumor phylogeny [126]. Such heterogeneity can be the result of cell intrinsic genomic differences or interaction with the microenvironment [127–133]. Tumor progression acquired through EMT can be transient and represent only a small timeframe in a patient's disease. Hence, targeting EMT will not have similar effect as in preclinical studies where EMT is constitutively activated. Many of the factors have dual or ambivalent roles. The recent demonstration of the role of MET in the establishment of metastasis in the host organ and its relationship to stemness in specific tumors adds a new degree of complexity to anti-EMT strategies. One could somehow potentially increase cancer stemness and improve host organ homing by inhibiting EMT.

5. Conclusion

Overall, despite the tremendous amount of preclinical data on the implication of EMT in cancer progression, there is still no routine clinical translation at both prognosis and therapeutic levels (Figure 1). Here, while we point out the different elements of the EMT cascades that could be targeted, we also underline the difficulties to translate the preclinical findings in routine clinic. However, we can hypothesize that as we enter the era of precision and personalized medicine, new technologies (next gene sequencing, circulating tumor cells, circulating tumor DNA, etc.) will help us better define patients' specific disease at precise time points during disease evolution. Such studies might then really illustrate whether EMT has a role in neoplastic evolution and point out the appropriate therapeutic window where EMT inhibition could lead to improved survival in patients.

Conflict of Interests

The authors declare that there is no conflict of interests regarding the publication of this paper.

Acknowledgment

The authors would like to acknowledge the Chalhoub Group for their support of cancer research.

References

[1] C. L. Chaffer and R. A. Weinberg, "A perspective on cancer cell metastasis," *Science*, vol. 331, no. 6024, pp. 1559–1564, 2011.

[2] T. J. Yeatman and G. L. Nicolson, "Molecular basis of tumor progression: mechanisms of organ-specific tumor metastasis," *Seminars in Surgical Oncology*, vol. 9, no. 3, pp. 256–263, 1993.

[3] R. Kalluri and R. A. Weinberg, "The basics of epithelial-mesenchymal transition," *The Journal of Clinical Investigation*, vol. 119, no. 6, pp. 1420–1428, 2009.

[4] K. Polyak and R. A. Weinberg, "Transitions between epithelial and mesenchymal states: acquisition of malignant and stem cell traits," *Nature Reviews Cancer*, vol. 9, no. 4, pp. 265–273, 2009.

[5] J. P. Thiery, H. Acloque, R. Y. J. Huang, and M. A. Nieto, "Epithelial-mesenchymal transitions in development and disease," *Cell*, vol. 139, no. 5, pp. 871–890, 2009.

[6] L. Wan, K. Pantel, and Y. Kang, "Tumor metastasis: moving new biological insights into the clinic," *Nature Medicine*, vol. 19, no. 11, pp. 1450–1464, 2013.

[7] D. C. Radisky, "Epithellial-mesenchymal transition," *Journal of Cell Science*, vol. 118, no. 19, pp. 4325–4326, 2005.

[8] J. P. Thiery and J. P. Sleeman, "Complex networks orchestrate epithelial-mesenchymal transitions," *Nature Reviews Molecular Cell Biology*, vol. 7, no. 2, pp. 131–142, 2006.

[9] U. Cavallaro and G. Christofori, "Cell adhesion and signalling by cadherins and Ig-CAMs in cancer," *Nature Reviews Cancer*, vol. 4, no. 2, pp. 118–132, 2004.

[10] B. M. Gumbiner, "Regulation of cadherin-mediated adhesion in morphogenesis," *Nature Reviews Molecular Cell Biology*, vol. 6, no. 8, pp. 622–634, 2005.

[11] M. H. Chui, "Insights into cancer metastasis from a clinico-pathologic perspective: Epithelial-Mesenchymal Transition is not a necessary step," *International Journal of Cancer*, vol. 132, no. 7, pp. 1487–1495, 2013.

[12] K. Garber, "Epithelial-to-mesenchymal transition is important to metastasis, but questions remain," *Journal of the National Cancer Institute*, vol. 100, no. 4, pp. 232–239, 2008.

[13] H. Ledford, "Cancer theory faces doubts," *Nature*, vol. 472, no. 7343, article 273, 2011.

[14] D. Tarin, E. W. Thompson, and D. F. Newgreen, "The fallacy of epithelial mesenchymal transition in neoplasia," *Cancer Research*, vol. 65, no. 14, pp. 5996–6000, 2005.

[15] S. Thomson, E. Buck, F. Petti et al., "Epithelial to mesenchymal transition is a determinant of sensitivity of non-small-cell lung carcinoma cell lines and xenografts to epidermal growth factor receptor inhibition," *Cancer Research*, vol. 65, no. 20, pp. 9455–9462, 2005.

[16] J. Zavadil, J. Haley, R. Kalluri, S. K. Muthuswamy, and E. Thompson, "Epithelial-mesenchymal transition," *Cancer Research*, vol. 68, no. 23, pp. 9574–9577, 2008.

[17] J. H. Tsai and J. Yang, "Epithelial-mesenchymal plasticity in carcinoma metastasis," *Genes and Development*, vol. 27, no. 20, pp. 2192–2206, 2013.

[18] J. P. Their, "Epithelial-mesenchymal transitions in tumor progression," *Nature Reviews Cancer*, vol. 2, no. 6, pp. 442–454, 2002.

[19] B. D. Craene and G. Berx, "Regulatory networks defining EMT during cancer initiation and progression," *Nature Reviews Cancer*, vol. 13, no. 2, pp. 97–110, 2013.

[20] H. Zheng and Y. Kang, "Multilayer control of the EMT master regulators," *Oncogene*, vol. 33, no. 14, pp. 1755–1763, 2014.

[21] S. Lamouille, J. Xu, and R. Derynck, "Molecular mechanisms of epithelial-mesenchymal transition," *Nature Reviews Molecular Cell Biology*, vol. 15, no. 3, pp. 178–196, 2014.

[22] C. Alix-Panabières, H. Schwarzenbach, and K. Pantel, "Circulating tumor cells and circulating tumor DNA," *Annual Review of Medicine*, vol. 63, pp. 199–215, 2012.

[23] A. Rafii, F. Vidal, G. Rathat, and C. Alix-Panabières, "Circulating tumor cells: cornerstone of personalized medicine," *Journal de Gynécologie Obstétrique et Biologie de la Reproduction*, vol. 43, no. 9, pp. 640–648, 2014.

[24] A. Bonnomet, L. Syne, A. Brysse et al., "A dynamic in vivo model of epithelial-to-mesenchymal transitions in circulating tumor cells and metastases of breast cancer," *Oncogene*, vol. 31, no. 33, pp. 3741–3753, 2012.

[25] N. P. A. D. Gunasinghe, A. Wells, E. W. Thompson, and H. J. Hugo, "Mesenchymal-epithelial transition (MET) as a mechanism for metastatic colonisation in breast cancer," *Cancer and Metastasis Reviews*, vol. 31, no. 3-4, pp. 469–478, 2012.

[26] D. Sarrió, S. M. Rodriguez-Pinilla, D. Hardisson, A. Cano, G. Moreno-Bueno, and J. Palacios, "Epithelial-mesenchymal transition in breast cancer relates to the basal-like phenotype," *Cancer Research*, vol. 68, no. 4, pp. 989–997, 2008.

[27] A. J. Trimboli, K. Fukino, A. de Bruin et al., "Direct evidence for epithelial-mesenchymal transitions in breast cancer," *Cancer Research*, vol. 68, no. 3, pp. 937–945, 2008.

[28] M. Yu, A. Bardia, B. S. Wittner et al., "Circulating breast tumor cells exhibit dynamic changes in epithelial and mesenchymal composition," *Science*, vol. 339, no. 6119, pp. 580–584, 2013.

[29] D. Entenberg, D. Kedrin, J. Wyckoff, E. Sahai, J. Condeelis, and J. E. Segall, "Imaging tumor cell movement in vivo," in *Current Protocols in Cell Biology*, chapter 19, unit 19.7, 2013.

[30] Y. Kang and K. Pantel, "Tumor cell dissemination: emerging biological insights from animal models and cancer patients," *Cancer Cell*, vol. 23, no. 5, pp. 573–581, 2013.

[31] M. J. Blanco, G. Moreno-Bueno, D. Sarrio et al., "Correlation of Snail expression with histological grade and lymph node status in breast carcinomas," *Oncogene*, vol. 21, no. 20, pp. 3241–3246, 2002.

[32] C. Côme, F. Magnino, F. Bibeau et al., "Snail and slug play distinct roles during breast carcinoma progression," *Clinical Cancer Research*, vol. 12, no. 18, pp. 5395–5402, 2006.

[33] S. Elloul, M. B. Elstrand, J. M. Nesland et al., "Snail, slug, and smad-interacting protein 1 as novel parameters of disease aggressiveness in metastatic ovarian and breast carcinoma," *Cancer*, vol. 103, no. 8, pp. 1631–1643, 2005.

[34] T. A. Martin, A. Goyal, G. Watkins, and W. G. Jiang, "Expression of the transcription factors snail, slug, and twist and their

clinical significance in human breast cancer," *Annals of Surgical Oncology*, vol. 12, no. 6, pp. 488–496, 2005.

[35] S. Elloul, I. Silins, C. G. Tropé, A. Benshushan, B. Davidson, and R. Reich, "Expression of E-cadherin transcriptional regulators in ovarian carcinoma," *Virchows Archiv*, vol. 449, no. 5, pp. 520–528, 2006.

[36] T. Imai, A. Horiuchi, C. Wang et al., "Hypoxia attenuates the expression of E-cadherin via up-regulation of SNAIL in ovarian carcinoma cells," *The American Journal of Pathology*, vol. 163, no. 4, pp. 1437–1447, 2003.

[37] M.-Y. Cai, R.-Z. Luo, J.-W. Chen et al., "Overexpression of ZEB2 in peritumoral liver tissue correlates with favorable survival after curative resection of hepatocellular carcinoma," *PLoS ONE*, vol. 7, no. 2, Article ID e32838, 2012.

[38] T. Li, Y. Zhu, W. Ren et al., "High co-expression of vascular endothelial growth factor receptor-1 and Snail is associated with poor prognosis after curative resection of hepatocellular carcinoma," *Medical Oncology*, vol. 29, no. 4, pp. 2750–2761, 2012.

[39] A. Miyoshi, Y. Kitajima, S. Kido et al., "Snail accelerates cancer invasion by upregulating MMP expression and is associated with poor prognosis of hepatocellular carcinoma," *British Journal of Cancer*, vol. 92, no. 2, pp. 252–258, 2005.

[40] K. Sugimachi, S. Tanaka, T. Kameyama et al., "Transcriptional repressor snail and progression of human hepatocellular carcinoma," *Clinical Cancer Research*, vol. 9, no. 7, pp. 2657–2664, 2003.

[41] C. Kahlert, S. Lahes, P. Radhakrishnan et al., "Overexpression of ZEB2 at the invasion front of colorectal cancer is an independent prognostic marker and regulates tumor invasion *in vitro*," *Clinical Cancer Research*, vol. 17, no. 24, pp. 7654–7663, 2011.

[42] C. Peña, J. M. Garciá, J. Silva et al., "E-cadherin and vitamin D receptor regulation by SNAIL and ZEB1 in colon cancer: clinicopathological correlations," *Human Molecular Genetics*, vol. 14, no. 22, pp. 3361–3370, 2005.

[43] H. Wallerand, G. Robert, G. Pasticier et al., "The epithelial-mesenchymal transition-inducing factor TWIST is an attractive target in advanced and/or metastatic bladder and prostate cancers," *Urologic Oncology*, vol. 28, no. 5, pp. 473–479, 2010.

[44] S. D. da Silva, M. A. Alaoui-Jamali, F. A. Soares et al., "TWIST1 is a molecular marker for a poor prognosis in oral cancer and represents a potential therapeutic target," *Cancer*, vol. 120, no. 3, pp. 352–362, 2014.

[45] S. Hosono, H. Kajiyama, M. Terauchi et al., "Expression of Twist increases the risk for recurrence and for poor survival in epithelial ovarian carcinoma patients," *British Journal of Cancer*, vol. 96, no. 2, pp. 314–320, 2007.

[46] H. Kajiyama, S. Hosono, M. Terauchi et al., "Twist expression predicts poor clinical outcome of patients with clear cell carcinoma of the ovary," *Oncology*, vol. 71, no. 5-6, pp. 394–401, 2007.

[47] K. Shibata, H. Kajiyama, K. Ino et al., "Twist expression in patients with cervical cancer is associated with poor disease outcome," *Annals of Oncology*, vol. 19, no. 1, pp. 81–85, 2008.

[48] A. Satelli and S. Li, "Vimentin in cancer and its potential as a molecular target for cancer therapy," *Cellular and Molecular Life Sciences*, vol. 68, no. 18, pp. 3033–3046, 2011.

[49] P. C. Black, G. A. Brown, T. Inamoto et al., "Sensitivity to epidermal growth factor receptor inhibitor requires E-cadherin expression in urothelial carcinoma cells," *Clinical Cancer Research*, vol. 14, no. 5, pp. 1478–1486, 2008.

[50] M. J. Kwon, J. H. Kwon, E. S. Nam et al., "TWIST1 promoter methylation is associated with prognosis in tonsillar squamous cell carcinoma," *Human Pathology*, vol. 44, no. 9, pp. 1722–1729, 2013.

[51] J. Kim, S. J. Hong, J. Y. Park et al., "Epithelial - mesenchymal transition gene signature to predict clinical outcome of hepatocellular carcinoma," *Cancer Science*, vol. 101, no. 6, pp. 1521–1528, 2010.

[52] Y. Niwa, S. Yamada, M. Koike et al., "Epithelial to mesenchymal transition correlates with tumor budding and predicts prognosis in esophageal squamous cell carcinoma," *Journal of Surgical Oncology*, vol. 110, no. 6, pp. 764–769, 2014.

[53] S. Yamada, N. Okumura, L. Wei et al., "Epithelial to mesenchymal transition is associated with shorter disease-free survival in hepatocellular carcinoma," *Annals of Surgical Oncology*, vol. 21, no. 12, pp. 3882–3890, 2014.

[54] X. Zhai, H. Zhu, W. Wang, S. Zhang, Y. Zhang, and G. Mao, "Abnormal expression of EMT-related proteins, S100A4, vimentin and E-cadherin, is correlated with clinicopathological features and prognosis in HCC," *Medical Oncology*, vol. 31, no. 6, article 970, 2014.

[55] J. Zhao, D. Dong, L. Sun, G. Zhang, and L. Sun, "Prognostic significance of the epithelial-tomesenchymal transition markers e-cadherin, vimentin and twist in bladder cancer," *International Brazilian Journal of Urology*, vol. 40, no. 2, pp. 179–189, 2014.

[56] T. Brabletz, A. Jung, S. Spaderna, F. Hlubek, and T. Kirchner, "Migrating cancer stem cells—an integrated concept of malignant tumour progression," *Nature Reviews Cancer*, vol. 5, no. 9, pp. 744–749, 2005.

[57] G. Ghiaur, J. Gerber, and R. J. Jones, "Concise review: cancer stem cells and minimal residual disease," *Stem Cells*, vol. 30, no. 1, pp. 89–93, 2012.

[58] J. Pasquier and A. Rafii, "Role of the microenvironment in ovarian cancer stem cell maintenance," *BioMed Research International*, vol. 2013, Article ID 630782, 10 pages, 2013.

[59] W. Luo, S. Li, B. Peng, Y. Ye, X. Deng, and K. Yao, "Embryonic stem cells markers SOX2, OCT4 and Nanog expression and their correlations with epithelial-mesenchymal transition in nasopharyngeal carcinoma," *PLoS ONE*, vol. 8, no. 2, Article ID e56324, 2013.

[60] H. S. Ryu, D. J. Park, H. H. Kim, W. H. Kim, and H. S. Lee, "Combination of epithelial-mesenchymal transition and cancer stem cell-like phenotypes has independent prognostic value in gastric cancer," *Human Pathology*, vol. 43, no. 4, pp. 520–528, 2012.

[61] H. S. Ryu, J.-H. Chung, K. Lee et al., "Overexpression of epithelial-mesenchymal transition-related markers according to cell dedifferentiation: clinical implications as an independent predictor of poor prognosis in cholangiocarcinoma," *Human Pathology*, vol. 43, no. 12, pp. 2360–2370, 2012.

[62] Y. Wang, S. Kim, and I. M. Kim, "Regulation of metastasis by microRNAs in ovarian cancer," *Frontiers in Oncology*, vol. 4, article 143, 2014.

[63] S. F. Tavazoie, C. Alarcón, T. Oskarsson et al., "Endogenous human microRNAs that suppress breast cancer metastasis," *Nature*, vol. 451, no. 7175, pp. 147–152, 2008.

[64] X. Fu, Y. Han, Y. Wu et al., "Prognostic role of microRNA-21 in various carcinomas: a systematic review and meta-analysis," *European Journal of Clinical Investigation*, vol. 41, no. 11, pp. 1245–1253, 2011.

[65] A. Rafii, C. Touboul, H. Al Thani, K. Suhre, and J. A. Malek, "Where cancer genomics should go next: a clinician's perspective," *Human Molecular Genetics*, vol. 23, no. R1, pp. R69–R75, 2014.

[66] U. H. Frixen, J. Behrens, M. Sachs et al., "E-cadherin-mediated cell-cell adhesion prevents invasiveness of human carcinoma cells," *The Journal of Cell Biology*, vol. 113, no. 1, pp. 173–185, 1991.

[67] J. Luo, D. M. Lubaroff, and M. J. C. Hendrix, "Suppression of prostate cancer invasive potential and matrix metalloproteinase activity by E-cadherin transfection," *Cancer Research*, vol. 59, no. 15, pp. 3552–3556, 1999.

[68] S. E. Witta, R. M. Gemmill, F. R. Hirsch et al., "Restoring E-cadherin expression increases sensitivity to epidermal growth factor receptor inhibitors in lung cancer cell lines," *Cancer Research*, vol. 66, no. 2, pp. 944–950, 2006.

[69] A. S. T. Wong and B. M. Gumbiner, "Adhesion-independent mechanism for suppression of tumor cell invasion by E-cadherin," *The Journal of Cell Biology*, vol. 161, no. 6, pp. 1191–1203, 2003.

[70] M. Yanagisawa and P. Z. Anastasiadis, "p120 catenin is essential for mesenchymal cadherin-mediated regulation of cell motility and invasiveness," *Journal of Cell Biology*, vol. 174, no. 7, pp. 1087–1096, 2006.

[71] P. B. Gupta, T. T. Onder, G. Jiang et al., "Identification of selective inhibitors of cancer stem cells by high-throughput screening," *Cell*, vol. 138, no. 4, pp. 645–659, 2009.

[72] B. Zhai, H.-X. Yan, S.-Q. Liu, L. Chen, M.-C. Wu, and H.-Y. Wang, "Reduced expression of E-cadherin/catenin complex in hepatocellular carcinomas," *World Journal of Gastroenterology*, vol. 14, no. 37, pp. 5665–5673, 2008.

[73] Z.-Q. Ling, P. Li, M.-H. Ge et al., "Hypermethylation-modulated down-regulation of CDH1 expression contributes to the progression of esophageal cancer," *International Journal of Molecular Medicine*, vol. 27, no. 5, pp. 625–635, 2011.

[74] I. Molina-Ortiz, R. A. Bartolomé, P. Hernández-Varas, G. P. Colo, and J. Teixidó, "Overexpression of E-cadherin on melanoma cells inhibits chemokine-promoted invasion involving p190RhoGAP/p120ctn-dependent inactivation of RhoA," *The Journal of Biological Chemistry*, vol. 284, no. 22, pp. 15147–15157, 2009.

[75] G. Berx and F. Van Roy, "The E-cadherin/catenin complex: an important gatekeeper in breast cancer tumorigenesis and malignant progression," *Breast Cancer Research*, vol. 3, no. 5, pp. 289–293, 2001.

[76] K. Strumane, G. Berx, and F. van Roy, "Cadherins in Cancer," in *Cell Adhesion*, vol. 165 of *Handbook of Experimental Pharmacology*, pp. 69–103, Springer, Berlin, Germany, 2004.

[77] J. K. Field, "Oncogenes and tumour-suppressor genes in squamous cell carcinoma of the head and neck," *European Journal of Cancer Part B: Oral Oncology*, vol. 28, no. 1, pp. 67–76, 1992.

[78] B. Ruggeri, J. Caamano, T. J. Slaga, C. J. Conti, W. J. Nelson, and A. J. P. Klein-Szanto, "Alterations in the expression of uvomorulin and Na+,K(+)-adenosine triphosphatase during mouse skin tumor progression," *The American Journal of Pathology*, vol. 140, no. 5, pp. 1179–1185, 1992.

[79] M. Köbel, D. Turbin, S. E. Kalloger, D. Gao, D. G. Huntsman, and C. B. Gilks, "Biomarker expression in pelvic high-grade serous carcinoma: comparison of ovarian and omental sites," *International Journal of Gynecological Pathology*, vol. 30, no. 4, pp. 366–371, 2011.

[80] A. S. Wong, S. L. Maines-Bandiera, B. Rosen et al., "Constitutive and conditional cadherin expression in cultured human ovarian surface epithelium: influence of family history of ovarian cancer," *International Journal of Cancer*, vol. 81, no. 2, pp. 180–188, 1999.

[81] F. J. Rodriguez, L. J. Lewis-Tuffin, and P. Z. Anastasiadis, "E-cadherin's dark side: possible role in tumor progression," *Biochimica et Biophysica Acta*, vol. 1826, no. 1, pp. 23–31, 2012.

[82] T. Celià-Terrassa, Ó. Meca-Cortés, F. Mateo et al., "Epithelial-mesenchymal transition can suppress major attributes of human epithelial tumor-initiating cells," *The Journal of Clinical Investigation*, vol. 122, no. 5, pp. 1849–1868, 2012.

[83] A. Gheldof and G. Berx, "Cadherins and epithelial-to-mesenchymal transition," *Progress in Molecular Biology and Translational Science*, vol. 116, pp. 317–336, 2013.

[84] M. J. Wheelock, Y. Shintani, M. Maeda, Y. Fukumoto, and K. R. Johnson, "Cadherin switching," *Journal of Cell Science*, vol. 121, no. 6, pp. 727–735, 2008.

[85] Y. Shintani, Y. Fukumoto, N. Chaika et al., "ADH-1 suppresses N-cadherin-dependent pancreatic cancer progression," *International Journal of Cancer*, vol. 122, no. 1, pp. 71–77, 2008.

[86] W.-W. Chang, F.-W. Hu, C.-C. Yu et al., "Quercetin in elimination of tumor initiating stem-like and mesenchymal transformation property in head and neck cancer," *Head and Neck*, vol. 35, no. 3, pp. 413–419, 2013.

[87] N. M. Sadler, B. R. Harris, B. A. Metzger, and J. Kirshner, "N-cadherin impedes proliferation of the multiple myeloma cancer stem cells," *The American Journal of Blood Research*, vol. 3, no. 4, pp. 271–285, 2013.

[88] G. Lahat, Q.-S. Zhu, K.-L. Huang et al., "Vimentin is a novel anti-cancer therapeutic target; insights from *In Vitro* and *In Vivo* mice xenograft studies," *PLoS ONE*, vol. 5, no. 4, Article ID e10105, 2010.

[89] R. P. Singh, K. Raina, G. Sharma, and R. Agarwal, "Silibinin inhibits established prostate tumor growth, progression, invasion, and metastasis and suppresses tumor angiogenesis and epithelial-mesenchymal transition in transgenic adenocarcinoma of the mouse prostate model mice," *Clinical Cancer Research*, vol. 14, no. 23, pp. 7773–7780, 2008.

[90] K. J. Wu, J. Zeng, G. D. Zhu et al., "Silibinin inhibits prostate cancer invasion, motility and migration by suppressing vimentin and MMP-2 expression," *Acta Pharmacologica Sinica*, vol. 30, no. 8, pp. 1162–1168, 2009.

[91] T.-T. Dong, H.-M. Zhou, L.-L. Wang, B. Feng, B. Lv, and M.-H. Zheng, "Salinomycin selectively targets 'CD133+' cell subpopulations and decreases malignant traits in colorectal cancer lines," *Annals of Surgical Oncology*, vol. 18, no. 6, pp. 1797–1804, 2011.

[92] Y. Teng and X. Li, "The roles of HLH transcription factors in epithelial mesenchymal transition and multiple molecular mechanisms," *Clinical and Experimental Metastasis*, vol. 31, no. 3, pp. 367–377, 2014.

[93] S.-P. Han, J.-H. Kim, M.-E. Han et al., "SNAI1 is involved in the proliferation and migration of glioblastoma cells," *Cellular and Molecular Neurobiology*, vol. 31, no. 3, pp. 489–496, 2011.

[94] S. A. Mikheeva, A. M. Mikheev, A. Petit et al., "TWIST1 promotes invasion through mesenchymal change in human glioblastoma," *Molecular Cancer*, vol. 9, article 194, 2010.

[95] M. Xia, M. Hu, J. Wang et al., "Identification of the role of Smad interacting protein 1 (SIP1) in glioma," *Journal of Neuro-Oncology*, vol. 97, no. 2, pp. 225–232, 2010.

[96] M.-T. Chung, H.-C. Lai, H.-K. Sytwu et al., "SFRP1 and SFRP2 suppress the transformation and invasion abilities of

cervical cancer cells through Wnt signal pathway," *Gynecologic Oncology*, vol. 112, no. 3, pp. 646–653, 2009.

[97] Y.-R. Na, S.-H. Seok, D.-J. Kim et al., "Bone morphogenetic protein 7 induces mesenchymal-to-epithelial transition in melanoma cells, leading to inhibition of metastasis," *Cancer Science*, vol. 100, no. 11, pp. 2218–2225, 2009.

[98] T. Arumugam, V. Ramachandran, K. F. Fournier et al., "Epithelial to mesenchymal transition contributes to drug resistance in pancreatic cancer," *Cancer Research*, vol. 69, no. 14, pp. 5820–5828, 2009.

[99] W. Zhuo, Y. Wang, X. Zhuo, Y. Zhang, X. Ao, and Z. Chen, "Knockdown of Snail, a novel zinc finger transcription factor, via RNA interference increases A549 cell sensitivity to cisplatin via JNK/mitochondrial pathway," *Lung Cancer*, vol. 62, no. 1, pp. 8–14, 2008.

[100] W.-L. Zhuo, Y. Wang, X.-L. Zhuo, Y.-S. Zhang, and Z.-T. Chen, "Short interfering RNA directed against TWIST, a novel zinc finger transcription factor, increases A549 cell sensitivity to cisplatin via MAPK/mitochondrial pathway," *Biochemical and Biophysical Research Communications*, vol. 369, no. 4, pp. 1098–1102, 2008.

[101] R. K. Srivastava, S.-N. Tang, W. Zhu, D. Meeker, and S. Shankar, "Sulforaphane synergizes with quercetin to inhibit self-renewal capacity of pancreatic cancer stem cells," *Frontiers in Bioscience, Elite*, vol. 3, no. 2, pp. 515–528, 2011.

[102] H.-C. Pai, L.-H. Chang, C.-Y. Peng et al., "Moscatilin inhibits migration and metastasis of human breast cancer MDA-MB-231 cells through inhibition of Akt and Twist signaling pathway," *Journal of Molecular Medicine*, vol. 91, no. 3, pp. 347–356, 2013.

[103] H.-Y. Hsu, T.-Y. Lin, P.-A. Hwang et al., "Fucoidan induces changes in the epithelial to mesenchymal transition and decreases metastasis by enhancing ubiquitin-dependent TGF-beta receptor degradation in breast cancer," *Carcinogenesis*, vol. 34, no. 4, pp. 874–884, 2013.

[104] J. K. Myung, S. A. Choi, S. K. Kim, K. C. Wang, and S. H. Park, "Snail plays an oncogenic role in glioblastoma by promoting epithelial mesenchymal transition," *International Journal of Clinical and Experimental Pathology*, vol. 7, no. 5, pp. 1977–1987, 2014.

[105] A. K. Reka, R. Kuick, H. Kurapati, T. J. Standiford, G. S. Omenn, and V. G. Keshamouni, "Identifying inhibitors of epithelial-mesenchymal transition by connectivity map-based systems approach," *Journal of Thoracic Oncology*, vol. 6, no. 11, pp. 1784–1792, 2011.

[106] K.-N. Chua, W.-J. Sim, V. Racine, S.-Y. Lee, B. C. Goh, and J. P. Thiery, "A cell-based small molecule screening method for identifying inhibitors of epithelial-mesenchymal transition in carcinoma," *PLoS ONE*, vol. 7, no. 3, Article ID e33183, 2012.

[107] H. You, W. Ding, H. Dang, Y. Jiang, and C. B. Rountree, "c-Met represents a potential therapeutic target for personalized treatment in hepatocellular carcinoma," *Hepatology*, vol. 54, no. 3, pp. 879–889, 2011.

[108] O. O. Ogunwobi and C. Liu, "Hepatocyte growth factor upregulation promotes carcinogenesis and epithelial-mesenchymal transition in hepatocellular carcinoma via Akt and COX-2 pathways," *Clinical and Experimental Metastasis*, vol. 28, no. 8, pp. 721–731, 2011.

[109] Y. Guo, J. Xie, E. Rubin et al., "Frzb, a secreted Wnt antagonist, decreases growth and invasiveness of fibrosarcoma cells associated with inhibition of Met signaling," *Cancer Research*, vol. 68, no. 9, pp. 3350–3360, 2008.

[110] H. Ikushima and K. Miyazono, "TGFB 2 signalling: a complex web in cancer progression," *Nature Reviews Cancer*, vol. 10, no. 6, pp. 415–424, 2010.

[111] Y. Katsuno, S. Lamouille, and R. Derynck, "TGF-β signaling and epithelial-mesenchymal transition in cancer progression," *Current Opinion in Oncology*, vol. 25, no. 1, pp. 76–84, 2013.

[112] J. Xu, S. Lamouille, and R. Derynck, "TGF-B-induced epithelial to mesenchymal transition," *Cell Research*, vol. 19, no. 2, pp. 156–172, 2009.

[113] H. Peng, O. A. Carretero, N. Vuljaj et al., "Angiotensin-converting enzyme inhibitors: a new mechanism of action," *Circulation*, vol. 112, no. 16, pp. 2436–2445, 2005.

[114] G. Subramanian, R. E. Schwarz, L. Higgins et al., "Targeting endogenous transforming growth factor β receptor signaling in Smad4-deficient human pancreatic carcinoma cells inhibits their invasive phenotype," *Cancer Research*, vol. 64, no. 15, pp. 5200–5211, 2004.

[115] C. Y. Park, D. K. Kim, and Y. Y. Sheen, "EW-7203, a novel small molecule inhibitor of transforming growth factor-beta (TGF-beta) type I receptor/activin receptor-like kinase-5, blocks TGF-betal-mediated epithelial-to-mesenchymal transition in mammary epithelial cells," *Cancer Science*, vol. 102, no. 10, pp. 1889–1896, 2011.

[116] C.-Y. Park, J.-Y. Son, C. H. Jin, J.-S. Nam, D.-K. Kim, and Y. Y. Sheen, "EW-7195, a novel inhibitor of ALK5 kinase inhibits EMT and breast cancer metastasis to lung," *European Journal of Cancer*, vol. 47, no. 17, pp. 2642–2653, 2011.

[117] Y. Y. Sheen, M.-J. Kim, S.-A. Park, S.-Y. Park, and J.-S. Nam, "Targeting the transforming growth factor-β signaling in cancer therapy," *Biomolecules and Therapeutics*, vol. 21, no. 5, pp. 323–331, 2013.

[118] K. Duangkumpha, A. Techasen, W. Loilome et al., "BMP-7 blocks the effects of TGF-β-induced EMT in cholangiocarcinoma," *Tumor Biology*, vol. 35, no. 10, pp. 9667–9676, 2014.

[119] A. R. Tan, G. Alexe, and M. Reiss, "Transforming growth factor-β signaling: emerging stem cell target in metastatic breast cancer?" *Breast Cancer Research and Treatment*, vol. 115, no. 3, pp. 453–495, 2009.

[120] L. Bueno, D. P. de Alwis, C. Pitou et al., "Semi-mechanistic modelling of the tumour growth inhibitory effects of LY2157299, a new type I receptor TGF-beta kinase antagonist, in mice," *European Journal of Cancer*, vol. 44, no. 1, pp. 142–150, 2008.

[121] J. Rodon, R. Dienstmann, V. Serra, and J. Tabernero, "Development of PI3K inhibitors: lessons learned from early clinical trials," *Nature Reviews Clinical Oncology*, vol. 10, no. 3, pp. 143–153, 2013.

[122] F. Cappuzzo, T. Ciuleanu, L. Stelmakh et al., "Erlotinib as maintenance treatment in advanced non-small-cell lung cancer: a multicentre, randomised, placebo-controlled phase 3 study," *The Lancet Oncology*, vol. 11, no. 6, pp. 521–529, 2010.

[123] F. A. Shepherd, J. R. Pereira, T. Ciuleanu et al., "Erlotinib in previously treated non-small-cell lung cancer," *The New England Journal of Medicine*, vol. 353, no. 2, pp. 123–132, 2005.

[124] S. E. Witta, R. M. Jotte, K. Konduri et al., "Randomized phase II trial of erlotinib with and without entinostat in patients with advanced non-small-cell lung cancer who progressed on prior chemotherapy," *Journal of Clinical Oncology*, vol. 30, no. 18, pp. 2248–2255, 2012.

[125] J. C. Morris, A. R. Tan, T. E. Olencki et al., "Phase I study of GC1008 (Fresolimumab): a human anti-transforming growth factor-beta (TGFβ) monoclonal antibody in patients with

advanced malignant melanoma or renal cell carcinoma," *PLoS ONE*, vol. 9, no. 3, Article ID e90353, 2014.

[126] J. A. Malek, E. Mery, Y. A. Mahmoud et al., "Copy number variation analysis of matched ovarian primary tumors and peritoneal metastasis," *PLoS ONE*, vol. 6, no. 12, Article ID e28561, 2011.

[127] R. Lis, J. Capdet, P. Mirshahi et al., "Oncologic trogocytosis with Hospicells induces the expression of N-cadherin by breast cancer cells," *International Journal of Oncology*, vol. 37, no. 6, pp. 1453–1461, 2010.

[128] R. Lis, C. Touboul, N. M. Halabi et al., "Mesenchymal cell interaction with ovarian cancer cells induces a background dependent pro-metastatic transcriptomic profile," *Journal of Translational Medicine*, vol. 12, article 59, 2014.

[129] R. Lis, C. Touboul, C. M. Raynaud et al., "Mesenchymal cell interaction with ovarian cancer cells triggers pro-metastatic properties," *PLoS ONE*, vol. 7, no. 5, Article ID e38340, 2012.

[130] J. A. Malek, A. Martinez, E. Mery et al., "Gene expression analysis of matched ovarian primary tumors and peritoneal metastasis," *Journal of Translational Medicine*, vol. 10, no. 1, article 121, 2012.

[131] J. Pasquier, B. S. Guerrouahen, H. Al Thawadi et al., "Preferential transfer of mitochondria from endothelial to cancer cells through tunneling nanotubes modulates chemoresistance," *Journal of Translational Medicine*, vol. 11, no. 1, article 94, 2013.

[132] J. Pasquier, H. A. Thawadi, P. Ghiabi et al., "Microparticles mediated cross-talk between tumoral and endothelial cells promote the constitution of a pro-metastatic vascular niche through Arf6 up regulation," *Cancer Microenvironment*, vol. 7, no. 1-2, pp. 41–59, 2014.

[133] C. Touboul, R. Lis, H. Al Farsi et al., "Mesenchymal stem cells enhance ovarian cancer cell infiltration through IL6 secretion in an amniochorionic membrane based 3D model," *Journal of Translational Medicine*, vol. 11, no. 1, article 28, 2013.

13

Role of Rebiopsy in Relapsed Non-Small Cell Lung Cancer for Directing Oncology Treatments

Antti P. Jekunen

Clinical Cancer Research Center, Vaasa Oncology Clinic, Turku University, Hietalahdenkatu 2-4, 65100 Vaasa, Finland

Correspondence should be addressed to Antti P. Jekunen; antti.jekunen@vshp.fi

Academic Editor: James L. Mulshine

Background. Currently, few rebiopsies are performed in relapses of advanced non-small cell lung cancer. They are not customary in clinical practice of lung cancer. However, it is not possible to properly target treatments in cases of relapse without knowing the nature of new lesions. *Design.* This paper comprehensively summarizes the available literature about rebiopsy and broadly discusses the importance of rebiopsy in advanced non-small cell lung cancer. *Results.* Altogether 560 abstracts were used as material for further analysis. 19 articles were about clinical rebiopsy in lung cancer and were reviewed in detailed manner. *Conclusions.* This review shows that rebiopsy is feasible in non-small cell lung cancer, and success rates can be high if rebiopsy is accompanied by adequate evaluation before biopsy. Its use may resolve the difficulties in sampling bias and detecting changes in cancer characteristics. In cases where treatment was selected based on tissue characteristics that then change, the treatment selection process must be repeated while considering new characteristics of the tumor. Rebiopsy may be used to predict therapeutic resistance and consequently redirect targeted therapies. Such knowledge may resolve the difficulties in sampling bias and also in selecting preexisting clones or formulating drug-resistant ones. Rebiopsy should be performed more often in non-small cell lung cancer.

1. Introduction

1.1. Imaging. Lung cancer is usually suspected in individuals who have an abnormal chest radiograph results or symptoms caused by either local or systemic tumor effects [1]. An initial diagnosis relies on imaging examinations when patients seek help for symptoms. Today, more tumor lesions are found secondarily in routine checkups. Chest X-ray and computer tomography (CT) scans are widely used. Positron emission tomography (PET) is a golden standard for staging of lung cancer. Additionally, it is used when doctors require more information about metabolic activity in certain lesions or when seeking lymph nodes or lesions for biopsy, in case of relapses and metastases.

1.2. Methods of Tumor Biopsy. In cases of peripheral tumor, ultrasound- or CT-guided percutaneous fine-needle aspiration or core biopsy is performed (Table 1). Video-assisted thoracoscopy (VATS) is used for wedge excisions and needle aspirations. A thoracotomy is usually an option when a lobectomy is being considered. Central tumors, often with symptoms such as repeated pneumonias and hemoptysis, can be diagnosed by sputum cytology. Bronchoscopy provides better samples with a brush, a fine-needle biopsy, and a core biopsy. Percutaneous-core needle biopsies, when it is possible to perform them, give larger samples of tissue material for further studies. However, a thoracotomy would be the best option when tissue sample size is important. Based on a recent meta-analysis, endobronchial ultrasound (EBUS) and electromagnetic navigation (EMN) bronchoscopy have the potential to increase the diagnostic yield of peripheral lung tumors [1]. A thoracoscopic biopsy of the pleura had the highest yield for diagnosing metastatic pleural effusion in a patient with lung cancer. When stereotactic high dose radiotherapy is considered tissue samples need to be taken before radiation, because afterwards there is nothing to be biopsied for. Acquiring adequate tissue samples for histological and molecular characterization of non-small cell lung cancer (NSCLC) is considered paramount.

TABLE 1: Techniques for obtaining tissue.

Method	Nature of sample	Size	Suitable for
Sputum	Cytology	50 mg	Limited immunohistology
Bronchoscopy brushing	Cytology	50 mg	Limited immunohistology
Fine needle biopsy	Cytology	100 mg	Immunohistology and PCR
Core needle biopsy	Histology	200–400 mg	Plus gene mutation testing, FISH, and DNA tests
Resection	Histology	>1 g	Plus exome tests, large immunohistology panels, and RNA tests (−70°C)

Biopsy is used to characterize tumors. Here in this study, rebiopsy means biopsy after cancer progression on initial therapy and repeated biopsy is used for conditions where an initial biopsy was not adequate for diagnosis and a new biopsy is performed. Basic staining and immunohistochemistry are routine in pathological diagnosis and also useful in rebiopsy. Table 1 lists various means of obtaining tissue and gives estimation of tissue yields.

TABLE 2: Information from rebiopsy.

Standard of care	Experimental
Histologic	Proteomics
Immunohistochemistry	RNAsequencing
Molecular information	Exome analysis
EGFR/KRAS/ALK	

1.3. Risks of Biopsy. Taking sputum samples is without safety issues, while all others have some risk for complications. As needle size increases, risk level increases also for biopsy complications. Clearly, it is of importance to determine what risks are coming from the location of biopsy target. The most serious complications include pneumothorax and bleeding. Of course, in resections overall risk of general anesthesia needs to be calculated before operation.

1.4. Molecular Pathology. Molecular methods are becoming more common in the pathological diagnosis (Table 2). Molecular biology techniques, particularly gene-expression microarrays, proteomics, and next-generation sequencing, have recently been developed to facilitate molecular classification [2]. Proteomics can further characterize tissue with two-dimensional gels. Third-generation immunoassays and protein pathway circuit arrays are also being used experimentally. DNA is quite stable and can be genotyped by different oligonucleotide arrays, based on PCR or sequencing. RNA is more difficult to extract, as it is rapidly destroyed by ribonucleases if samples are not quickly frozen to −70°C after biopsy. RNA provides opportunities to measure gene expression by complementary DNA microarrays or microRNAs by sequencing. Many analyses are already part of a standard care (Table 2). Protein analysis by immunohistochemistry is routine and widely available. Gene testing is becoming a regular practice, and preparations for sending adequate tissue samples with sufficient numbers of malignant cells to central laboratories are becoming common practice in all clinical pathology laboratories. This process depends upon determining gene changes that are related to drug activity.

1.5. Changing Therapies on Genetic Mutations. Consequently, measurements are needed to direct therapies, thus justifying collecting biopsy samples. In NSCLC-type adenocancer, two mutations are widely used to direct treatments: an epidermal growth factor receptor- (EGFR-) activating mutation indicating use of gefitinib erlotinib and afatinib [3] and

an ALK (anaplastic lymphoma kinase) gene rearrangement, indicating use of critsonitib [4, 5].

1.6. Mutations. In NSCLC, there are many variations and mutations in DNA, and it is only a matter of time and successful research before there are more predictive mutations available to clinical practice. The most frequent mutations in adenocarcinomas are in TP53, KRAS, and STK11 and EGFR genes. ALK mutations are measured in 3% to 5% of all lung adenocarcinomas. Genomic pathology provides an opportunity to stratify patients, based on genomic predictive features after successful rebiopsy, and consider changing treatment.

A common clonal origin indicates intrapulmonary multifocal metastases in almost two-thirds of cases, while 36% of multifocal NSCLC display unique molecular profiles, which suggests separate primary tumors. Divergent KRAS and/or EGFR mutations have been observed in 8% of cases [6]. The same research studied the clonal relationship of multifocal NSCLC with indistinguishable histomorphology in 78 patients by polymorphic short tandem repeated markers and mutation testing of KRAS and EGFR [6]. This could provide remarkably increased response rates and better treatment outcomes, compared to ordinary histopathology-based stratification. This increased response rate is already the case with tyrosine kinase inhibitors (TKIs) and ALK inhibitors.

1.7. Histology. Diagnosis of lung cancer is challenging. Resected tumors provide histological tissue, and diagnosis can almost always be obtained. However, there are a lot of situations where obtaining adequate material for diagnosis is challenging in initial biopsies, and a lot of tumors are not operated on at all. An additional challenge is presented by known intratumor heterogeneity, which must be considered, especially when histological material is limited and not representative of the entire tumor. However, there can be small lesions or a situation that does not require an operation. In those clinical cases with small lesions requiring biopsies, histological tumor sampling remains difficult, and obtaining

TABLE 3: PubMed literature search for rebiopsy.

Rebiopsy	309
+ Colon cancer	2
+ Lung cancer	16
+ Breast cancer	23
+ Prostate cancer	104
Rebiopsy histology	235
Rebiopsy DNA	12
Rebiopsy mutations	11

biopsy samples for thorough pathological assessments is difficult. Often, molecular pathology is simply not done. In some cases, only cytology is available, and further sampling is not possible because of the lesion location or the patient's low lung function. Treatment will begin, based on a fine-needle biopsy, or even a sputum sample, but there must be evidence of cancer. At the very least, lesions should behave like lung cancer. Different lung cancer types and different NSCLC cell clones behave differently and require different treatments.

There must be clinical confirmation of cancer, since oncology treatments generate so many side effects that clinical indication is required for their use. For a proper diagnosis, adequate histological or cytological material is required for morphological assessments, immunohistochemistry, and gene testing in cases of adenocancer. Here rebiopsy means biopsy after cancer progression on initial therapy and its role will be comprehensively summarized and broadly discussed in lung cancer.

2. Materials and Methods

This review is based on a PubMed search for the terms *rebiopsy* and *lung cancer* (Table 3). Publications in languages other than English and trials involving non-human subjects were excluded. Fourteen publications were reviewed, and a classification was performed with the predetermined variables listed in Table 3. The number of publications and trial protocols cited are as researched in March 2014. Additionally, *recurrent lung cancer* and *relapsed lung cancer* search terms were used resulting in 5225 and 1182 hits, but no additional articles were found by combining them with a *rebiopsy* search term. In order to check other articles and validate the search procedure, a repeated search was performed with the terms *repeated biopsy*, *lung cancer*, and *clinical*. It produced 544 hits from year 1975 to date. All abstracts were reviewed, and adequate articles that focused on rebiopsy were selected and included in this literature review. Two articles and two letters to the editor were evaluated for additional adequate information, and were subsequently incorporated into the analysis as additional articles.

3. Results

A PubMed search of the term *cancer diagnosis* produced almost 2 million hits. With the term *clinical biopsy*, there were 152,197 hits. This number dramatically decreased when

the search was conducted for both *cancer diagnosis* and *clinical biopsy* or with lung cancer terms (see Table 3). Combining the term *rebiopsy* with *colon cancer*, *lung cancer*, *breast cancer*, and *prostate cancer* produced two, 16, 23, and 14 hits, respectively (Table 3). Of the articles with all indications, abstract analysis revealed that DNA and mutations were central to 12 and 11 articles, respectively, while histology was discussed in 235 of 309 articles with the term *rebiopsy*. No review articles were found in the area of rebiopsy in lung cancer.

Eighteen articles with the search terms *rebiopsy* and *lung cancer* were targeted for further analysis (Table 3). These articles were used to find more suitable works, which were then referenced. Four articles dealt with other cancers and were excluded from further analysis. The remaining 14 articles focused on NSCLC (Table 4). Details of major findings are given for each article. Four were case reports. One was about the pharmacoeconomic aspects of rebiopsy, and ten were original articles. Of these ten articles, one was a prospective clinical trial report, and one reported extensive mutation genotyping. Two articles focused on a specific gene expression, while the remaining six focused on tyrosine kinase (TK) resistance and mainly discussed the most frequent secondary mutation T790M.

3.1. Chemotherapy and Gene Expression. The prospective study assessed if chemotherapy selection based on *in situ* excision repair cross-completion group 1 (ERCC1) and ribonucleotide reductase M1 (RRM1) protein levels would improve survival in patients with advanced NSCLC [7]. A total of 275 eligible patients were randomly assigned to the control arm with gemcitabine/carboplatin or the trial's experimental arm. Chemotherapy therapy was given based on protein levels at repeated biopsy: if RRM1 and ERCC1 were low, gemcitabine/carboplatin were given; if RRM1 was high and ERCC1 was low then docetaxel/carboplatin were given; if RRM1 was low and ERCC1 was high then gemcitabine/docetaxel were given; if both were high then docetaxel/vinorelbine were given. While no statistically significant differences were observed between the experimental and control arms in PFS (progression free survival) (6.1 months versus 6.9 months) or overall survival (11 months versus 11.3 months), a subset analysis revealed that patients with low levels of both proteins who received the same treatment in both treatment arms had a statistically better PFS ($P = 0.02$) in the control arm (8.1 months) than in the experimental arm (five months). This study was in newly diagnosed patients with advanced-stage NSCLC. However, a repeated tumor biopsy without complications was needed in 17% of cases to ensure enough material for protein-level measurements [7]. This study gives a prospective setup for repeated biopsies, and even in the chemotherapy context may warrant conducting proper justification and direct chemotherapy.

Jakobsen et al. published two studies about specific gene expressions at the protein level obtained using immunohistochemistry. They discovered that thymidylate synthase (TS), which was a potential predictive marker for treatment efficacy with pemetrexed, did not significantly change in rebiopsied lung tumors compared to primary tumors in

65 NSCLC patients taking after preoperative carboplatin and paclitaxel [8]. In another study, 65 NSCLC patients taking preoperative carboplatin and paclitaxel and a group of 53 NSCLC patients treated with surgery alone showed no statistically significant change between primary and rebiopsy material of lung tumors in class-III-beta-tubulin expression, which may be a potential predictive factor for microtubule interfering cytotoxic drug treatment [9]. In these situations, the biomarker was not valid and thus rebiopsies were not justified. However, there was intratumoral heterogeneity in both studies, which highlighted the need for sufficient representative material for diagnosis.

3.2. Tyrosine Kinase Inhibitors and Resistance. Understandably, the main area for rebiopsies is among TKIs in adenocancers of NSCLC. All patients with EGFR-mutant lung cancers eventually develop acquired resistance to EGFR TKIs. This is associated with second-site mutations in the EGFR kinase gene (e.g., T790M), amplification of alternative kinases (e.g., mesenchymal-epithelial transition factor, MET), histologic transformation to small cell lung cancer (SCLC), and epithelial to mesenchymal transition. Various mechanisms have been identified to account for resistance, and many methods have been proposed to overcome resistance, especially caused by T790M [4, 10, 11]. The EGFR mutation T790M is reported in approximately half of adenocancers with acquired resistance to EGFR inhibitors and is a potential prognostic, predictive biomarker. Patients with EGFR-mutant lung adenocarcinoma develop acquired resistance to EGFR TKIs after a median of 10 to 16 months. In half of these cases, a second EGFR mutation, T790M, underlies acquired resistance. However, rebiopsy to confirm T790M status can be challenging due to limited tissue availability and procedural feasibility. Furthermore, little is known of the differences among patients with or without T790M mutation. Here, various rebiopsy studies reporting the frequency of T790M, reporting analysis for EGFR/ALK mutations and reporting responses to EGFR TKI are described. When there is a mechanism of resistance found, that is potentially actionable, new drug development could be initiated. So that for T790 mutations found, a T790M mutant specific inhibitors could be developed and, for MET amplification, a MET inhibitor could be tested.

A mutation genotype was investigated in a large, 155-patient study reported by Yu et al. [12]. Adequate tumor samples from rebiopsies for molecular analysis were obtained in lung adenocarcinoma tumors with acquired resistance to erlotinib or gefitinib. Sample material included fine-needle aspirations, core biopsies, surgical samples, and cytology from malignant effusions. There was one recorded complication of pneumothorax requiring a catheter placement. Furthermore, sites of rebiopsies included lung tumor (82), pleural effusions (14), bone (9), liver (13), lymph nodes (9), peritoneal fluid (1) and central nervous fluid (1), and other organs (9). The tissue samples were obtained via operational procedures in 17 cases, including 10 brain resections, 5 lymph node excisions and 3 adrenalectomies and two autopsies. Of these 155 patients, 98 had second-site EGFR T790M mutations (63%; 95% confidence interval [CI], 55%–70%). Four

samples had small cell transformation. MET amplification was seen in four of 75 samples, and HER2 amplification was seen in three of 24 samples. No acquired mutations were observed in PIK3CA, AKT1, BRAF, HER2, KRAS, MEK1, or NRAS genes (0 of 88). The study identified EGFR T790M as the most common mechanism of acquired resistance, whereas MET amplification, HER2 amplification, and small cell histologic transformation occurred less frequently. The authors concluded that more rebiopsy studies were needed to characterize molecular alterations in situations of acquired resistance to EGFR TKIs [12].

Using a highly sensitive, locked nucleic-acid (LNA) PCR/sequencing assay with an analytical sensitivity of approximately 0.1%, T790M was detected in as many as 68% of patients with acquired resistance presenting either relapses or metastases. Tumor samples (153 samples in 121 patients) included the samples from clinically required procedures in 84 cases (e.g., 11 VATS biopsies, 6 lung resections, 3 image guided lung biopsies, and 2 fine-needle biopsies and 26 pleural effusions). In addition, the samples were obtained from other organs than lung in resections (14), biopsies (12), and fluid aspirations (8). The samples were studied for sensitizing EGFR mutations [13]. A total of 121 patients were rebiopsied and samples underwent tissue sampling. Of these, 104 (86%) samples were successfully analyzed for sensitizing EGFR mutations. Most failures were related to low tumor cell content. All patients (61) with matched pretreatment and resistance specimens showed susceptibility to the original sensitizing EGFR mutation. Standard T790M mutation analysis of 99 patients detected 51 (51%) mutations. Retesting of 30 EGFR-negative patients by the LNA-based method detected 11 additional mutations, for an estimated prevalence of 68%. MET was amplified in 11% of cases (4/37). The authors concluded that rebiopsy of lung cancer patients with acquired resistance was feasible and provided sufficient material for mutation analysis in most patients [13].

Of 126 patients referred for rebiopsy with NSCLC that was resistant to conventional chemotherapy or EGFR TKIs, 94 patients were selected for rebiopsy [14]. CT chest images excluded 32 patients. Percutaneous transthoracic lung biopsy was performed with a CT-guided, C-arm cone-beam, which had a technical success rate of 100%. In 75 (80%) of the 94 patients, specimens were adequate for mutational analysis. Thirty-five specimens were tested for EGFR mutation, 34 for ALK rearrangement, and six for both. The results were positive for EGFR-sensitizing mutation (exon 19 or 21) in 20 patients, EGFR T790M mutation in five, and ALK rearrangement in 11. Rebiopsy complications occurred in 13 (14%) patients. The study concluded that rebiopsies are feasible and safe when applying rigorous CT criteria and provide adequate material for gene analysis [14].

A study of 93 patients with EGFR-mutant lung cancer and acquired resistance to EGFR TKIs compared T790M status in terms of postprogression survival and characteristics of disease progression [15]. Mutation of T790M was observed in the initial rebiopsy specimens from 58 patients (62%, 95% CI: 52–72). T790M was more common in biopsies of lung/pleura tissue and lymph nodes than in other sites and it was more likely to progress in an existing site of disease than in new sites. Patients with T790M had a significantly longer postprogression survival time than patients without. Additionally, patients without T790M more often progressed to tumors in new, uninvolved organs and had a poorer performance status at time of progression. This study suggested that T790M serves a prognostic value that can be found by rebiopsy. Among patients with acquired resistance to EGFR TKIs, the presence of T790M defines a clinical subset with a relatively favorable prognosis and slower progression. The authors concluded that knowing T790M status was essential for clinical treatment decision making and understanding results of clinical trials after TKI use [15].

A study investigated 78 EGFR-mutant patients who underwent rebiopsy after TKI failure [16]. A sensitive, peptide nucleic acid-LNA polymerase chain-reaction clamp method was used in EGFR mutational analyses. The study found that patients with T790M after TKI failure had better prognoses than those without T790M. The T790M mutation was only identified rarely in four (17%) of 24 central nervous-system lesions and 22 (41%) of 54 other lesions ($P = 0.0417$). Median PFS was 31.4 months in 26 patients with T790M, and 11.4 months in 52 patients without T790M ($P = 0.0017$). In the multivariate analysis, statistically significant factors for longer PFS included positive for T790M, good performance status, and no carcinomatous meningitis [16].

Postprogression tumor specimens were prospectively collected for T790M mutation analysis in 70 NSCLC patients with acquired resistance to initial EGFR TKIs [17]. Thirty-six patients (51%) had T790M mutation in the rebiopsy specimen. There was no difference between the pattern of disease progression, PFS for initial TKIs (12.8 and 11.3 months), post-progression survival (14.7 and 14.1 months), or overall survival (43.5 and 36.8 months) in patients with and without T790M. After rebiopsy, 34 patients received afatinib treatment. The response rate was 18%, and the median PFS with afatinib was 3.7 months for the entire group and 3.2 and 4.6 months, respectively, for the subgroups with and without T790M. This means that there might be benefits for directing subsequent TKI therapies according to T790M status. Although T790M had no prognostic or predictive role in this study, identifying T790M as an acquired resistance mechanism was clinically feasible. Further research was felt to be necessary to identify patients with T790M-mutant tumors who might benefit from new T790M-specific TKIs currently in development [17].

3.3. Pharmacoeconomic Study.

One report evaluated rebiopsy in NSCLC by cost-benefit modeling [18]. A decision-analysis model compared the costs and effects of platinum combination chemotherapy (carboplatin and paclitaxel; carboplatin and pemetrexed; and carboplatin, pemetrexed, and bevacizumab) with erlotinib therapy in patients with EGFR mutation-positive tumors. Compared with a combined carboplatin paclitaxel regimen, targeted therapy based on testing available tissue yielded an incremental cost-effectiveness ratio (ICER) of $110,644 per quality-adjusted life year (QALY). The rebiopsy strategy yielded an ICER of $122,219 per QALY. With a willingness to pay of $100,000 per QALY, the testing strategy was cost-effective 58% of the time, and the rebiopsy strategy was cost-effective 54% of the time. Compared with carboplatin, pemetrexed, and bevacizumab, ICERs were $25,547 per QALY for the testing strategy and $44,036 per QALY for the rebiopsy strategy. Personalized therapy with an EGFR-TKI was more favorable when the nontargeted chemotherapy regimen was more expensive. The authors concluded that cost-effectiveness analysis supports testing for EGFR mutations in patients with Stage IV or recurrent lung adenocarcinomas, performing rebiopsy if insufficient tissue is available for testing and treating patients with EGFR mutations with erlotinib as a first-line therapy. However, this study assumed that erlotinib offered a PFS benefit, and total costs greatly depended on costs of nontargeted chemotherapy, which could also depend on the health care system. QALY costs were much higher in the erlotinib group, and rebiopsy increased costs. In practice, patients tend to receive both targeted therapy and chemotherapy as the cancer evolves, so crossover is evident, and it is difficult to extract a single therapy element.

3.4. Case Reports.

Four case reports were identified. Two of the reports dealt with rebiopsies on cancer progression and two additional ones were about insufficient initial biopsy and the necessity to perform repeated biopsy to obtain sufficient material for a proper diagnosis. The first case highlighted acquired EGFR-TKI resistance through transformation to the high-grade neuroendocrine carcinoma spectrum and that such transformation might not be evident at time of progression on TKI therapy [21]. A case of relapsed, EGFR exon-19 deletion, lung adenocarcinoma was treated with erlotinib and cisplatin-pemetrexed after resistance. Liver rebiopsy on progression identified an afatinib-resistant cancer with combined SCLC and NSCLC within neuroendocrine morphology, retaining the EGFR exon-19 deletion. Several acquired resistance mechanisms of EGFR-mutant lung adenocarcinoma to EGFR-TKI therapy were described, the most recent being transformation to SCLC [21].

The second case report demonstrated repeated responses to EGFR TKIs in a woman with adenocarcinoma and no history of smoking [20]. After six cycles of gemcitabine and cisplatin, the patient was treated by gefitinib for four months until progression. Following six cycles of third-line pemetrexed, gefitinib retreatment was initiated, with partial response for six months. After progression, the patient was recruited for an irreversible EGFR inhibitor trial. Time to progression was 11 months. Although EGFR direct sequencing on the initial diagnostic specimen revealed a wild type (nonmutated), rebiopsy of a progressed subcarinal node was performed at the end of the trial. Analysis showed an EGFR of mutation of L858R/L861Q [20].

The third study addressed the problem of tumor heterogeneity encountered in small bronchoscopic biopsies and the difficulties of evaluating the histological subtype in poorly differentiated carcinomas [19]. Initial diagnosis of squamous cell cancer (SCC) of the lung obtained by bronchoscopic biopsy was based on immunohistochemical staining only by positive results for cytokeratin (CK) 5/6 and p63 because morphological diagnosis was not possible. However, bronchoscopic repeated biopsy showed a mixed squamous/glandular immunophenotype with nests of undifferentiated tumor cells. There was weak immunoreactivity of some tumor cells for CK5/6 and p63 and no positivity of some tumor cells for thyroid transcription factor-1. In addition, an EGFR mutation was found in exon 21 (L858R). This was missed on initial biopsy. The patient achieved TKI and prolonged clinical benefit from treatment. The authors concluded that initial bronchoscopy should be performed by an experienced pulmonologist to obtain sufficient material from different areas of the tumor. In the era of targeted therapy, a patient having a history of remote smoking in cases of not-otherwise-specified (NOS) NSCLC that favors SCC should also provoke EGFR mutation testing [19]. Similarly, the fourth study also addressed the importance of adequate material for pathological evaluation in a report of five cases of regenerative, atypical squamous metaplasia at the site of a previous bronchial biopsy that was unnecessarily resected based on erroneous diagnosis of squamous cell carcinoma on repeated biopsy [22].

3.5. Additional Articles. In order to check for other articles and validate the search procedure, the search terms *repeated biopsy, lung cancer,* and *clinical* were entered, generating 544 hits. All abstracts were reviewed, and four additional articles were selected for this review: one case report about rebiopsy and three others dealing with repeated biopsy: two original articles and one letter to the editor.

A case report in a letter discussed an 80-year-old male with relapsed EGFR exon-19 deletion lung adenocarcinoma treated with EGFR-TKI. There were poor response and rapid increase of serum neuron-specific enolase [23]. Rebiopsy characterized transformation from NSCLS adenocancer to SCLC, and the EGFR mutation remained.

Three additional articles were about repeated biopsy rather than rebiopsy. Welker et al. [24] studied 118 patients with a solitary lung nodule (4 cm or smaller) who underwent transbronchial biopsy, percutaneous needle aspiration, clinical observation, repeat CT scans, and repeated biopsies. The mean follow-up was four years. The incidence of malignancy was 61%, and the positive predictive value, negative predictive value, sensitivity, specificity, and accuracy were all 100%. Moreover, this procedure reduced the incidence of unnecessary surgical excision of benign nodules from 60% to 5% [24]. Another letter to the editor stated that repeated needle biopsies were recognized to be safe and accurate in the management of a solitary pulmonary nodule [25]. The second original article was a retrospective study of 836 cases. Ninety-five cases with fine-needle aspiration +/− core biopsies over a five-year period were identified initially as nonmalignant [26]. Of these, 21 were confirmed later benign, and the remaining 74 included 53 initially benign and 21 nondiagnostic specimens. Seven of the 53 benign (13%) and six of 21 nondiagnostic specimens (29%) were malignant at excisional biopsy during radiologic follow-up. Sixteen of 95 cases (17%) had postprocedural pneumothorax that required a chest tube [26]. Therefore, repeated biopsy or resection is necessary for benign nonspecific and nondiagnostic biopsy results due to an unacceptably high rate of malignancy.

3.6. Safety. Serious complications in rebiopsy are rare. As there is already an initial diagnosis available, additional biopsies are carefully considered. Patients with lung cancer tend to develop metastases and especially liver and lymph node lesions are highly accessible for a biopsy. Probably a selection of biopsy sites has impact on low number of reported complications. One serious complication among 155 rebiopsies patients (12) and 13 minor complications in 94 patients (14) were reported in articles of this review. Additionally, no complications in 47 biopsied patients were reported by Bepler et al. in their repeated biopsy article [7]. In conclusion, rebiopsy appears to be safe when biopsy sites are carefully selected and the risk evaluation is made before rebiopsy.

4. Discussion

PubMed results reflect a lack of activity in rebiopsy for many indications, such as colon and lung cancers. Only 14 articles were found about rebiopsy in lung cancer by the search terms *rebiopsy* and *lung cancer* (Table 4). Prostate cancer had more hits (104) on the term *rebiopsy*. This reflects the attitude among urologists of actively performing repeated biopsies in follow-up and rebiopsies on relapses on prostate cancer patients. Of course, in the first place, it needs to recognize that the multiple biopsies are easier to do in prostate cancer than in lung cancer because of anatomical accessibility, lesion location, and minimal risk of complications. The situation with breast cancer is similar. The location of tumor relapse in breast tissue is usually accessible, but enlarged lymph nodes may be situated in places where performing a rebiopsy would pose too great a risk.

Solid tumors have a heterogeneous histological background, which makes it impossible to cover all metastases, even with only one highly targeted agent, which can only block one-cell clone at a time. In tumor growth and spread, cancer clones are probably randomly selected to survive, some of which may be resistant to given therapies, having an edge over other cell clones [27]. Furthermore, metastasizing involves one cell type and originates from one cell clone. New therapies block certain cell clones but miss others that develop based on other mutations [28, 29]. Therefore therapy fails, and redirection is needed.

In the optimal situation, therapeutic effect should be constantly monitored by repeating the histological examination, as the primary tumor can change. One clone or two clones may become resistant to a given therapy and dominate. In the metastasizing process, a limited number of cells fix themselves on remote places in the body. Some of these cells can avoid immunoreaction and start forming metastases. So a metastasis of a solid tumor can be very different from its parent tumor. Rebiopsy of lung cancer patients with acquired resistance is feasible and could provide sufficient material for mutation analysis in most patients [13]. Using a highly sensitivity method, a LNA PCR/sequencing assay, T790M, was detected in up to 68% of these patients, which was 12% more than with ordinary analysis methods.

Rebiopsies are widely used in cancers other than those in the lung. In prostate cancer, repeated biopsies and rebiopsies

TABLE 4: Rebiopsy and lung cancer.

	Number of articles	Number of patients	Content	Reference
Case reports	4	8		[17–20]
Pharmacoeconomic analysis	1			[16]
Original articles	9			
		53	TS expression	[9]
		65	Beta tubulin	[8]
		70	T790 mutation	[15]
		78	T790 mutation	[14]
		93	T790 mutation	[13]
		94	EGFR mutations ALK rearrangement	[12]
		121	T790 mutation	[11]
		155	Mutation genotyping	[10]
		331	ECCI and RRMI proteins	[7]

are readily performed, when prostate specific antigen (PSA) is increased, because doing so is easy, as there are no vital organs in the neighborhood of the prostate [30]. Similarly, rebiopsies are often performed in breast cancer to confirm cancer relapse and provide characteristics of a new breast cancer lesion. This will direct treatments, such as hormonal treatment in hormone receptor-positive cases. It will also confirm if the mutation in the HER2 oncogene and the elevated levels of HER2 protein are present, which triggers use of targeted therapies [31, 32]. It is difficult to access bone lesions and to retrieve good histological samples, and consequently bone lesions are normally not biopsied. The metastatic lesions were rebiopsied by core needle aspiration, or CT- or ultrasound-guided biopsy with no major complications. Additionally, rebiopsies may show a second malignancy [32, 33].

In neuroendocrine lung cancers, rebiopsy is widely used to pick up transformations to more aggressive types of cancer, such as small cell cancers. Transformation is also highly important to uncover in cases of suspected lymphoma relapse, for example, in thoracic area. There is also increased risk of secondary cancer in areas that have been radiated in Hodgkin's disease. The risk increases remarkably after decades from given radiotherapy. In certain cases, rebiopsy is not recommended. Schneider et al. [34] recommended omitting rebiopsy from clinical practice in esophageal cancer for objective response evaluation, based on his prospective study of 80 patients [34]. Table 5 summarizes the general reasons for not performing rebiopsy. The common reasons for not doing rebiopsy are that it is not routine practice, the anatomical location for the target tumor may make the operation too risky, and general perceptions that there is high risk involved.

One clear benefit from rebiopsy in treatment of NSCLC is that it provides an updated look at tumor characteristics, which can be used to redirect treatments [4]. This was demonstrated in the case reports addressing individualized approaches to lung cancer treatment. There was tumor

TABLE 5: Why rebiopsy is not done in NSCLC.

(i) Not part of clinical routine

(ii) Anatomical location is difficult for biopsy

(iii) Sense of risk involved in rebiopsy

(iv) Limited number of drugs that can be directed by rebiopsy

(v) Only a few reports available in the literature

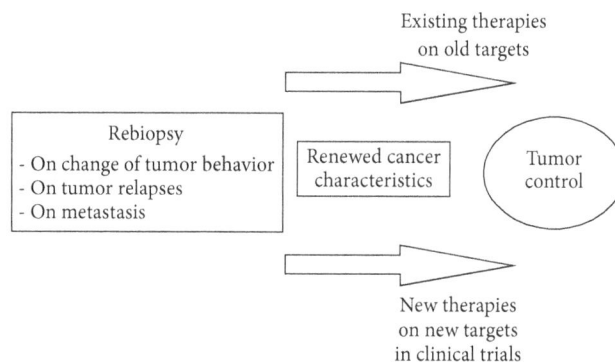

FIGURE 1: Role of rebiopsy in NSCLC treatment selection. Rebiopsy will renew tumor characteristics and give opportunity to act on changes of tumor behavior. Rebiopsy can confirm old existing targets when current therapies are allowed, or it can find new targets that need to be treated with new drug molecules in clinical trials. Thus changes in treatment facilitate better tumor control.

heterogeneity in small bronchoscopic biopsies and challenges in histological subtyping of poorly differentiated carcinomas, repeated responses to EGFR TKIs based on EGFR mutation (in spite of initial wild-type characterization), and acquired EGFR-TKI resistance through transformation to the high-grade neuroendocrine carcinoma spectrum. All these cases highlight a need for rebiopsy.

Figure 1 summarizes the potential benefits of rebiopsy in reassessing treatment options. Table 5 lists main reasons not

TABLE 6: Recommendation for rebiopsy in NSCLC.

When rebiopsy should not be performed:

(i) Too difficult a location for safe biopsy

(ii) Result will not change treatment

When rebiopsy should be performed:

(i) If the prior specimen is too small for adequate tumor characterization, including genetic testing for predictive alterations

(ii) If relapse happens a long time (six months) after CR treatment result

(iii) If the new tumor behaves in a different way than expected from the primary tumor

(iv) If new molecules entering clinical trials in the near future is foreseeable, such as adenocancer relapses

to perform rebiopsy, while Table 6 gives recommendation for rebiopsy in management of NSCLC. It can be important in treatment control when tumor behavior changes, as happens in a transformation into a more aggressive cancer type. It is important to get a look at changed tumor characteristics to determine the proper action. For example, neuroendocrine lung cancer can switch to SCLC type, which could be detected by rebiopsy. Tumor characteristics are important in directing treatments. Old targets can validate the choice to use existing and previous therapies. Moreover, material from rebiopsy makes it possible to explore a new target and to conduct clinical trials on new molecules [35]. When a TKI is used in NSCLC, there is a resistance tendency that becomes evident within two years. Some patients develop treatment resistance quicker than others, and rebiopsy is needed to confirm progression and look at new molecules that are being developed to overcome resistance. Without doing a rebiopsy to investigate the type of resistance and new targets, it would not be possible to use therapies against resistance in a controlled manner. One obstacle to drug development is that second-line patients with adequate tumor recharacterization to indicate gene alteration are difficult to find because rebiopsies are not customarily performed. However, nearly all clinical study protocols in relapsed adenocancer NSCLC now require a rebiopsy option to gather histological samples.

Novel immunotherapy strategy is pending on histological definition of targets in tumor, and those targets can change in time [36, 37]. So it is essential to search, for example, PD-L1 positivity for confirming reactivity of lung cancer on nivolumab before initiating treatment [38, 39]. PD-1 is expressed by activated T cells and down modulates T-cell effector functions on antigen-presenting cells; and in cancer patients, its expression on tumor-infiltrating lymphocytes and its interaction with the ligands on tumor and immune cells in the tumor microenvironment undermine antitumor immunity [40]. As PD-L1 measurement is done regularly in clinical trials that will be used in registration purposes, future treatment instructions after approval by drug agencies will include PD-L1 check before starting nivolumab. PD-L1 can be measured at protein level by immunohistochemistry, but there are only centralized measurements available at this

early stage. This makes it necessary to send samples first for EGFR and ALK testing and then if negative send them to different central laboratory for PD-L1 testing, and less than 40% of samples will turn negative. This adds time for treatment decision-making and may slow down remarkably clinical trials. In addition, in case of relapses, patients cannot be entered into the trial if there are no rebiopsies done at relapse, as is usually the case. At the end, there will be no possibility to include patients in the treatment after the drug is approved by drug agencies, if a fresh rebiopsy is missing.

Rather than performing rebiopsies, some researchers have proposed analyzing serum for tumor DNA. Recent studies show that genomic alterations in solid cancers can be characterized by massively parallel sequencing of circulating, cell-free tumor DNA released from cancer cells into plasma. This represents a noninvasive liquid biopsy [38–40]. Cell-free DNA fragments from multiple lesions in the same individual all mix together in the peripheral blood. Therefore, serum tumor DNA is likely to contain a wider representation of the genomes from multiple metastatic sites, whereas a single biopsy may miss them [41]. Furthermore, intratumor heterogeneity in renal cell cancer makes it difficult to fully characterize primary tumor material and metastases that may be derived from a subclone missed in the primary tumor biopsy [42]. Similar situations were found in breast cancer [43] and probably in other solid cancers, including lung cancer [42]. When this new technology is clinically available, it will revolutionize NSCLC treatment with TKIs, as the development of resistance could be followed frequently and without rebiopsy restrictions, and further treatments could be properly redirected. Exceptions may occur where this approach may not work, as in immunotherapy. However, more research is needed, along with development of a methodology to suit clinical practice, which will certainly take many years. Meanwhile, it is important to use available methods in all clinical practices and to bridge new methodology with the old data, which will require rebiopsy material.

5. Conclusions

This review shows that rebiopsy is feasible in NSCLC, and success rates can be high if rebiopsy is accompanied by adequate evaluation before biopsy. As rebiopsy can be valuable method in clinical practice to help in selecting more efficient therapies for NSCLC patients, it should be performed more often (Table 6). However, before performing rebiopsy, adequate evaluation of risks for complications should be performed including anatomic and technical aspects of accessing tumor. A patient overall condition should also be taken in account. In situations where no possibility for active oncological interventions can be considered, rebiopsy is not indicated. Use of rebiopsy may resolve the difficulties in sampling bias and selecting preexisting or forming new drug-resistant clones. In cases where treatment was selected based on tissue characteristics that change, the treatment selection process must be repeated while considering new characteristics of the tumor. In the near future, rebiopsy will be used to predict therapeutic resistance and consequently redirect targeted therapies. Rebiopsy is done after the initial biopsy that provided the diagnosis. It is important to remember that metastases may behave differently, and have remarkable differences in histology content. Primary tumors can develop in such a way that the original histological content will change. This can be enhanced by efficient cancer therapy that usually influences nearly all cells. However, those cancer cells that do not die can develop into resistant clones. It would be critical to know when this development occurs. Even with the development of promising, new noninvasive methods for following cancer characteristics in serum samples, rebiopsy material will be urgently needed to identify and ensure those characteristics. Rebiopsies should be performed on lung lesions that were inadequately sampled by an initial biopsy when new metastatic lesions or relapses occur, in order to confirm the nature of the lesions and select the optimal targeted therapy.

Accordingly, some clinical practice guidelines already include this recommendation. For example, the ESMO 2012 guideline of advanced NSCLC states that obtaining adequate tissue material for histological diagnosis and molecular testing is important to individual treatment decisions and that rebiopsy at disease progression should be considered [44]. Clinical treatment will benefit from accurate histological diagnosis, and patients will be offered more focused therapies. Figure 1 addresses the importance of rebiopsy in NSCLC, in which treatment control can be received by recharacterization of tumor and selecting proper treatment on defined targets. If there is no tumor tissue available from a relapsed or progressed primary tumor, changed tumor behavior and cancer transformation are missed, and the molecularly guided stratification of patients into redirected treatments fails to happen.

Abbreviations

CT: Computer tomography
PET: Positron emission tomography
VATS: Video-assisted tomography
EBUS: Endobronchial untrasound
EMN: Electromagnetic navigation
NSCLC: Non-small cell lung cancer
DNA: Deoxyribonucleic acid
RNA: Ribonucleic acid
EGFR: Epidermal growth factor receptor
ALK: Anaplastic lymphoma kinase gene
TP53: Tumor protein p53
KRAS: Kirsten rat sarcoma viral oncogen homolog
STK1: Serological thymidine kinase 1
TKI: Tyrosine kinase inhibitor
PubMed: An Internet site for biomedical literature
TK: Tyrosine kinase
T790M: A gatekeeper mutation in EGFR
ERCCI: DNA excision repair protein
RPMI: Disease resistance protein
PFS: Progression free survival
TS: Thymidylate synthetase
SCLC: Small cell lung cancer
MET: Mesenchymal-epithelial transition factor

PIK3CA: Phosphatidylinositol-4,5-biphosphate 3-kinase, catalytic subunit alpha
AKT1: RAC-alpha serine/threonine-protein kinase
BRAF: v-Raf murine sarcoma viral oncogene homolog B
NRAS: Neuroblastoma RAS viral oncogene homolog
HER2: Human epidermal growth factor receptor 2
LNA: Locked nucleic acid
PCR: Polymerase chain reaction
QALY: Quality adjusted life year
ICER: Oncremental cost-effectiveness ratio
CK: Cytokeratin
NOS: Not otherwise specified
PSA: Prostate specific antigen
ER: Estrogen receptor
PR: Progesterone receptor
PD-L1: Programmed death-ligand 1
T-cell: Lymphocytes maturing in thymus
ESMO: European Society of Medical Oncology.

Conflict of Interests

The author declares that there is no conflict of interests regarding the publication of this paper.

Acknowledgment

This study was financially supported by the Competitive State Research Financing of the Expert Responsibility area of Tampere University Hospital, Grant no. 1009.

References

[1] M. P. Rivera, A. C. Mehta, and M. M. Wahidi, "Establishing the diagnosis of lung cancer: diagnosis and management of lung cancer, 3rd ed: American college of chest physicians evidence-based clinical practice guidelines," *Chest*, vol. 143, no. 5, supplement, pp. e142S–e165S, 2013.

[2] Y. Yu and J. He, "Molecular classification of non-small-cell lung cancer: diagnosis, individualized treatment, and prognosis," *Frontiers of Medicine*, vol. 7, no. 2, pp. 157–171, 2013.

[3] S. H. Lim, J. Y. Lee, J.-M. Sun, J. S. Ahn, K. Park, and M.-J. Ahn, "Comparison of clinical outcomes following gefitinib and erlotinib treatment in non-small-cell lung cancer patients harboring an epidermal growth factor receptor mutation in either exon 19 or 21," *Journal of Thoracic Oncology*, vol. 9, no. 4, pp. 506–511, 2014.

[4] P. Bordi, M. Tiseo, B. Bortesi, N. Naldi, S. Buti, and A. Ardizzoni, "Overcoming T790M-driven acquired resistance to EGFR-TKIs in NSCLC with afatinib: a case report," *Tumori*, vol. 100, no. 1, pp. 20e–23e, 2014.

[5] C. Gridelli, F. de Marinis, F. Cappuzzo et al., "Treatment of advanced non-small-cell lung cancer with epidermal growth factor receptor (EGFR) mutation or ALK gene rearrangement: results of an International expert panel meeting of the Italian association of thoracic oncology," *Clinical Lung Cancer*, vol. 15, no. 3, pp. 173–181, 2014.

[6] A. Warth, S. Macher-Goeppinger, T. Muley et al., "Clonality of multifocal nonsmall cell lung cancer: implications for staging and therapy," *European Respiratory Journal*, vol. 39, no. 6, pp. 1437–1442, 2012.

[7] G. Bepler, C. Williams, M. J. Schell et al., "Randomized international phase III trial of ERCC1 and RRM1 expression-based chemotherapy versus gemcitabine/carboplatin in advanced non-small-cell lung cancer," *Journal of Clinical Oncology*, vol. 31, no. 19, pp. 2404–2412, 2013.

[8] J. N. Jakobsen, E. Santoni-Rugiu, and J. B. Sørensen, "Longitudinal assessment of TUBB3 expression in non-small cell lung cancer patients," *Cancer Chemotherapy and Pharmacology*, vol. 73, no. 1, pp. 43–51, 2014.

[9] J. N. Jakobsen, E. Santoni-Rugiu, and J. B. Sørensen, "Thymidylate synthase protein expression levels remain stable during paclitaxel and carboplatin treatment in non-small cell lung cancer," *Journal of Cancer Research and Clinical Oncology*, vol. 140, no. 4, pp. 645–652, 2014.

[10] T. Yoshida, G. Zhang, M. A. Smith et al., "Tyrosine phosphoproteomics identifies both codrivers and cotargeting strategies for T790M-related EGFR-TKI resistance in non-small cell lung cancer," *Clinical Cancer Research*, vol. 20, no. 15, pp. 4059–4074, 2014.

[11] C. Rolfo, E. Giovannetti, D. S. Hong et al., "Novel therapeutic strategies for patients with NSCLC that do not respond to treatment with EGFR inhibitors," *Cancer Treatment Reviews*, vol. 40, no. 8, pp. 990–1004, 2014.

[12] H. A. Yu, M. E. Arcila, N. Rekhtman et al., "Analysis of tumor specimens at the time of acquired resistance to EGFR-TKI therapy in 155 patients with EGFR-mutant lung cancers," *Clinical Cancer Research*, vol. 19, no. 8, pp. 2240–2247, 2013.

[13] M. E. Arcila, G. R. Oxnard, K. Nafa et al., "Rebiopsy of lung cancer patients with acquired resistance to EGFR inhibitors and enhanced detection of the T790M mutation using a locked nucleic acid-based assay," *Clinical Cancer Research*, vol. 17, no. 5, pp. 1169–1180, 2011.

[14] H. J. Yoon, H. Y. Lee, K. S. Lee et al., "Repeat biopsy for mutational analysis of non-small cell lung cancers resistant to previous chemotherapy: adequacy and complications," *Radiology*, vol. 265, no. 3, pp. 939–948, 2012.

[15] G. R. Oxnard, M. E. Arcila, C. S. Sima et al., "Acquired resistance to EGFR tyrosine kinase inhibitors in EGFR-mutant lung cancer: distinct natural history of patients with tumors harboring the T790M mutation," *Clinical Cancer Research*, vol. 17, no. 6, pp. 1616–1622, 2011.

[16] A. Hata, N. Katakami, H. Yoshioka et al., "Rebiopsy of non-small cell lung cancer patients with acquired resistance to epidermal growth factor receptor-tyrosine kinase inhibitor: comparison between T790M mutation-positive and mutation-negative populations," *Cancer*, vol. 119, no. 24, pp. 4325–4332, 2013.

[17] J.-M. Sun, M.-J. Ahn, Y.-L. Choi, J. S. Ahn, and K. Park, "Clinical implications of T790M mutation in patients with acquired resistance to EGFR tyrosine kinase inhibitors," *Lung Cancer*, vol. 82, no. 2, pp. 294–298, 2013.

[18] E. A. Handorf, S. McElligott, A. Vachani et al., "Cost effectiveness of personalized therapy for first-line treatment of stage IV and recurrent incurable adenocarcinoma of the lung," *Journal of Oncology Practice*, vol. 8, no. 5, pp. 267–274, 2012.

[19] M. Schwitter, R. Rodriguez, T. Schneider, T. Kluckert, M. Brutsche, and M. Früh, "Epidermal growth factor receptor mutation in a patient with squamous cell carcinoma of the lung:

who should be tested?" *Case Reports in Oncology*, vol. 6, no. 2, pp. 263–268, 2013.

[20] E. Y. Kim, Y. H. Kim, H. J. Ban et al., "Repeated favorable responses to epidermal growth factor receptor-tyrosine kinase inhibitors in a case of advanced lung adenocarcinoma," *Tuberculosis and Respiratory Diseases*, vol. 74, no. 3, pp. 129–133, 2013.

[21] S. Popat, A. Wotherspoon, C. M. Nutting, D. Gonzalez, A. G. Nicholson, and M. O'Brien, "Transformation to 'high grade' neuroendocrine carcinoma as an acquired drug resistance mechanism in EGFR-mutant lung adenocarcinoma," *Lung Cancer*, vol. 80, no. 1, pp. 1–4, 2013.

[22] E. A. Chandraratnam, D. W. Henderson, D. J. Meredith, and S. Jain, "Regenerative atypical squamous metaplasia in fibreoptic bronchial biopsy sites—a lesion liable to misinterpretation as carcinoma on rebiopsy: report of 5 cases," *Pathology*, vol. 19, no. 4, pp. 419–424, 1987.

[23] Y. Zhang, X.-Y. Li, Y. Tang et al., "Rapid increase of serum neuron specific enolase level and tachyphylaxis of EGFR-tyrosine kinase inhibitor indicate small cell lung cancer transformation from EGFR positive lung adenocarcinoma?" *Lung Cancer*, vol. 81, no. 2, pp. 302–305, 2013.

[24] J. A. Welker, M. Alattar, and S. Gautam, "Repeat needle biopsies combined with clinical observation are safe and accurate in the management of a solitary pulmonary nodule," *Cancer*, vol. 103, no. 3, pp. 599–607, 2005.

[25] D. Sortini, K. Maravegias, C. V. Feo, A. Sortini, and J. A. Welker, "Repeat needle biopsies combined with clinical observation are safe and accurate in the management of a solitary pulmonary nodule," *Cancer*, vol. 104, no. 3, pp. 664–665, 2005.

[26] C. Savage, E. M. Walser, V. Schnadig, K. J. Woodside, E. Ustuner, and J. B. Zwischenberger, "Transthoracic image-guided biopsy of lung nodules: when is benign really benign?" *Journal of Vascular and Interventional Radiology*, vol. 15, no. 2, pp. 161–164, 2004.

[27] P. Workman and J. Travers, "Cancer: drug-tolerant insurgents," *Nature*, vol. 464, no. 7290, pp. 844–845, 2010.

[28] S. Carrera, A. Buque, E. Azkona et al., "Epidermal growth factor receptor tyrosine-kinase inhibitor treatment resistance in non-small cell lung cancer: biological basis and therapeutic strategies," *Clinical and Translational Oncology*, vol. 16, no. 4, pp. 339–350, 2014.

[29] N. Yamaguchi, A. R. Lucena-Araujo, S. Nakayama et al., "Dual ALK and EGFR inhibition targets a mechanism of acquired resistance to the tyrosine kinase inhibitor crizotinib in ALK rearranged lung cancer," *Lung Cancer*, vol. 83, no. 1, pp. 37–43, 2014.

[30] K.-P. Braun, S. Brookman-Amissah, M. May et al., "The significance of rebiopsy in the diagnosis of prostate cancer," *Urologe A*, vol. 48, no. 2, pp. 163–169, 2009.

[31] E. Alba, J. Albanell, J. de la Haba et al., "Trastuzumab or lapatinib with standard chemotherapy for HER2-positive breast cancer: results from the GEICAM/2006-14 trial," *The British Journal of Cancer*, vol. 110, no. 5, pp. 1139–1147, 2014.

[32] Q. Qu, C. Xu, X.-S. Chen et al., "Use of rebiopsy for clinically diagnosed metastatic lesion in patients with breast cancer," *Zhonghua Yi Xue Za Zhi*, vol. 93, no. 35, pp. 2820–2822, 2013.

[33] C. Wiratkapun, B. Wibulpholprasert, S. Wongwaisayawan, and K. Pulpinyo, "Nondiagnostic core needle biopsy of the breast under imaging guidance: result of rebiopsy," *Journal of the Medical Association of Thailand*, vol. 88, no. 3, pp. 350–357, 2005.

[34] P. M. Schneider, R. Metzger, H. Schaefer et al., "Response evaluation by endoscopy, rebiopsy, and endoscopic ultrasound

does not accurately predict histopathologic regression after neoadjuvant chemoradiation for esophageal cancer," *Annals of Surgery*, vol. 248, no. 6, pp. 902–908, 2008.

[35] Y. Kim, J. Ko, Z. Cui et al., "The EGFR T790M mutation in acquired resistance to an irreversible second-generation EGFR inhibitor," *Molecular Cancer Therapeutics*, vol. 11, no. 3, pp. 784–791, 2012.

[36] P. M. Forde, K. A. Reiss, A. M. Zeidan, and J. R. Brahmer, "What lies within: novel strategies in immunotherapy for non-small cell lung cancer," *Oncologist*, vol. 18, no. 11, pp. 1203–1213, 2013.

[37] H. Suzuki, Y. Owada, Y. Watanabe et al., "Recent advances in immunotherapy for non-small-cell lung cancer," *Human Vaccines & Immunotherapeutics*, vol. 10, no. 2, pp. 352–357, 2014.

[38] R. Sundar, R. Soong, B.-C. Cho, J. R. Brahmer, and R. A. Soo, "Immunotherapy in the treatment of non-small cell lung cancer," *Lung Cancer*, vol. 85, no. 2, pp. 101–109, 2014.

[39] D. Heigener and M. Reck, "Exploring the potential of immuno-oncology-based treatment for patients with non-small cell lung cancer," *Expert Review of Anticancer Therapy*, vol. 15, no. 1, pp. 69–83, 2015.

[40] C. Wang, K. B. Thudium, M. Han et al., "In vitro characterization of the anti-pd-1 antibody nivolumab, BMS-936558, and in vivo toxicology in non-human primates," *Cancer Immunology Research*, vol. 2, no. 9, pp. 846–856, 2014.

[41] K. C. A. Chan, P. Jiang, Y. W. L. Zheng et al., "Cancer genome scanning in plasma: detection of tumor-associated copy number aberrations, single-nucleotide variants, and tumoral heterogeneity by massively parallel sequencing," *Clinical Chemistry*, vol. 59, no. 1, pp. 211–224, 2013.

[42] T. Forshew, M. Murtaza, C. Parkinson et al., "Noninvasive identification and monitoring of cancer mutations by targeted deep sequencing of plasma DNA," *Science Translational Medicine*, vol. 4, no. 136, Article ID 136ra68, 2012.

[43] R. J. Leary, M. Sausen, I. Kinde et al., "Detection of chromosomal alterations in the circulation of cancer patients with whole-genome sequencing," *Science Translational Medicine*, vol. 4, no. 162, Article ID 162ra154, 2012.

[44] M. Murtaza, S. J. Dawson, D. W. Y. Tsui et al., "Non-invasive analysis of acquired resistance to cancer therapy by sequencing of plasma DNA," *Nature*, vol. 497, no. 7447, pp. 108–112, 2013.

14

Exercise Prevention of Cardiovascular Disease in Breast Cancer Survivors

Amy A. Kirkham[1] **and Margot K. Davis**[2]

[1]*Rehabilitation Sciences, University of British Columbia, 212–2177 Wesbrook Mall, Vancouver, BC, Canada V6T 1Z3*
[2]*Division of Cardiology, University of British Columbia, Diamond Health Care Centre, 9th Floor, 2775 Laurel Street, Vancouver, BC, Canada V5Z 1M9*

Correspondence should be addressed to Margot K. Davis; margot.davis@ubc.ca

Academic Editor: Christine Brezden-Masley

Thanks to increasingly effective treatment, breast cancer mortality rates have significantly declined over the past few decades. Following the increase in life expectancy of women diagnosed with breast cancer, it has been recognized that these women are at an elevated risk for cardiovascular disease due in part to the cardiotoxic side effects of treatment. This paper reviews evidence for the role of exercise in prevention of cardiovascular toxicity associated with chemotherapy used in breast cancer, and in modifying cardiovascular risk factors in breast cancer survivors. There is growing evidence indicating that the primary mechanism for this protective effect appears to be improved antioxidant capacity in the heart and vasculature and subsequent reduction of treatment-related oxidative stress in these structures. Further clinical research is needed to determine whether exercise is a feasible and effective nonpharmacological treatment to reduce cardiovascular morbidity and mortality in breast cancer survivors, to identify the cancer therapies for which it is effective, and to determine the optimal exercise dose. Safe and noninvasive measures that are sensitive to changes in cardiovascular function are required to answer these questions in patient populations. Cardiac strain, endothelial function, and cardiac biomarkers are suggested outcome measures for clinical research in this field.

1. Introduction

Breast cancer is the most common malignancy among women worldwide [1], and an estimated 1% of the population are survivors of breast cancer [2]. Advances in breast cancer therapy have contributed to dramatic improvements in survival, but many of these therapies, particularly anthracycline chemotherapy, left-sided radiotherapy, and trastuzumab targeted therapy, are associated with cardiovascular toxicities [3]. Breast cancer survivors are at increased risk of cardiovascular disease-related death compared to women without breast cancer [4], likely due in part to these toxicities. An increased prevalence of traditional cardiovascular risk factors in this population at diagnosis, and lifestyle perturbations associated with cancer treatment also contribute to this increased risk [3]. Chemotherapy for breast cancer will induce menopause in one- to two-thirds of women [5], further increasing cardiovascular risk [1, 6]. As breast cancer survival rates rise, cardiovascular disease becomes an increasingly important competing risk [7]. Combined, these factors contribute to the recent finding that cardiovascular disease has surpassed breast cancer as the leading cause of death in older women diagnosed with breast cancer [8].

Current strategies to mitigate cardiotoxicity associated with anthracycline treatment include dose reduction, modified administration methods, liposomal formulations, and administration of cardioprotective medications [9]. However, dose modification may be associated with reduced oncological benefit [10], and pharmacological interventions may be associated with additional side effects.

Aerobic exercise training and other forms of physical activity are effective in primary and secondary prevention of cardiovascular disease and cardiovascular disease-related death [11]. For breast cancer survivors, exercise training is safe and effective in improving cardiorespiratory fitness, strength, body composition, fatigue, anxiety, depression, and quality of life, and is recommended during and after treatment [12]. However, the effect of aerobic exercise on cardiovascular function and outcomes during or after breast cancer treatment is not well established in humans.

The purpose of this paper is to (1) review the potential mechanisms mediating exercise prevention of cardiovascular toxicity; (2) review the available evidence for the role of exercise in prevention of cardiovascular disease in breast cancer survivors, including predominantly preclinical studies of the heart and clinical studies of cardiovascular risk factors; and (3) suggest outcome measures for translation of the preclinical findings to clinical studies.

2. Potential Mechanisms Mediating Exercise Prevention of Cardiovascular Toxicity

The vast majority of studies investigating exercise prevention of direct cardiovascular toxicity are in rodent models utilizing the anthracycline agent doxorubicin and compare an exercise-trained treated group to a sedentary treated group. The discussion of mechanisms and preclinical evidence refers to studies with this design unless otherwise noted. The mechanism underlying the cardioprotective effects of aerobic exercise before or during treatment with doxorubicin has not been fully elucidated but is likely to be multifactorial with summative effects and feedback from diverse processes. Potential mechanisms by which exercise may act in opposition to the negative effects of doxorubicin to protect the heart and vasculature are listed in Table 1. There is available evidence for exercise protection mechanisms related to reduced oxidative stress, interruption of topoisomerase-mediated pathways, cardiomyocyte contractile protein isoform shifts, and upregulation of heat shock proteins (HSP), endothelial nitric oxide (NO), and endothelial progenitor cells.

The most widely supported mechanism by which exercise may prevent doxorubicin cardiotoxicity is through its antioxidant effects. The production of reactive oxygen species (ROS) is one of the possible mechanisms for doxorubicin cardiotoxicity [13, 14]. Although cells are equipped with an endogenous antioxidant system to protect against ROS, cardiomyocytes have only one fourth of the antioxidative capacity of the liver and other tissues [15], making them particularly vulnerable to oxidative stress. Exercise-induced enhancement of cardiomyocyte antioxidant capacity may prevent ROS-induced damage associated with doxorubicin treatment [16]. Compared with untrained animals, exercise-trained rodents have increased levels of antioxidant activity and reduced levels of oxidative stress markers following doxorubicin exposure [17–22]. However this mechanism may not play a role in cardioprotection when exercise is of low intensity and duration [23]. Reduced levels of protein turnover via the ubiquitin-proteasome pathway, an important mechanism for degradation of cellular proteins with oxidative damage, have been demonstrated in exercise-trained rodents compared to sedentary rodents [24]. This finding provides further support for exercise protection via reduced oxidative stress.

Anthracycline-induced ROS cause lipid peroxidation [25] and downregulate expression of the sarcoplasmic reticulum calcium pump, SERCA2a [14]. Decreased calcium uptake by SERCA2a then leads to an increase in cytosolic calcium [14]. These two changes result in opening of the mitochondrial permeability transition pore, allowing release of calcium from the mitochondrial matrix, downregulation of mitochondrial respiration, and leaking of proapoptotic mitochondrial proteins into the cytosol [26, 27]. A single submaximal exercise session 24 hours before doxorubicin treatment prevented opening of the mitochondria permeability transition pore, mitigating the downstream effects [26]. This hypothesis is supported indirectly by several other studies demonstrating attenuation of doxorubicin-associated increases in the proapoptotic proteins caspase-9 and 3 in exercise trained rodents [18, 23, 24, 26]. These findings may be related to modulation of defense systems including stress chaperones like HSPs, or antioxidants, but may not be related to exercise-induced upregulation of SERCA2a [28, 29].

There is emerging evidence implicating topoisomerase 2β, an enzyme regulating DNA unwinding, in doxorubicin-induced cardiomyocyte mitochondrial dysfunction [30], secondary to downregulation of peroxisome proliferator-activated receptor-γ coactivator (PGC)-1α, a transcriptional coactivator of mitochondrial biogenesis [31]. Exercise training upregulates expression of PGC-1α in skeletal muscle, although a similar response in cardiomyocytes has not been observed [32, 33]. Two recent preclinical studies investigating the role of PGC-1α in exercise cardioprotection did not demonstrate an interaction between exercise and doxorubicin [22, 34]. However, the capacity of exercise to impact topoisomerase 2β and PGC-1α in cardiomyocytes requires further investigation before this mechanism can be dismissed.

In the rodent heart, doxorubicin causes disruption of cardiac bioenergetics and an associated shift from the α isoform of the contractile protein, myosin heavy chain (MHC), to the β isoform which has reduced contractile power [35]. Exercise training before [28, 35] and during doxorubicin treatment [36, 37] conserves the α isoform in rats. However, healthy human hearts express 7% of the α isoform on average, while this is the predominant isoform expressed in the rat heart [38]. Therefore the extent and subsequent impact of a doxorubicin-induced shift in MHC isoform distribution may be smaller for human myocardium. Clinical research is required to clarify the role of prevention of MHC isoform shifts in exercise cardioprotection.

HSPs control protein folding and unfolding, and are upregulated in cardiomyocytes during times of oxidative stress [24]. An exercise-induced increase in HSP expression is hypothesized to play a role in cardioprotection against doxorubicin by preserving the integrity and activity of mitochondrial respiratory complexes and thereby attenuating mitochondrial dysfunction [39]. Although there is some evidence supporting HSP-mediated cardioprotection [17, 19, 23], there are also conflicting results [19, 24, 40].

Breast cancer therapies, including chemotherapy, targeted therapies, and radiotherapy, may be associated with endothelial dysfunction, a disease process involving impaired

TABLE 1: Potential mechanisms for exercise prevention of doxorubicin-related cardiovascular toxicity.

Myocardial target	Role of target	Direction of exercise-induced change*	Direction of doxorubicin-induced change*	Evidence of exercise prevention of doxorubicin-induced change
Mechanisms with evidence for their role in exercise prevention				
Antioxidant to oxidative stress ratio	Prevention of oxidative damage	↑ [15]	↓ [13]	√ [17–21, 52] × [23]
Expression of $\alpha : \beta$ myosin heavy chain isoform in rodents	Motor protein required for muscular contraction; in a healthy rodent heart there is a much higher concentration of the α isoform	↑ [154]	↓ [155]	√ [28, 35–37] × [23]
Caspase 3 and 9 activity	Markers for apoptotic signaling	↓ [156]	↑ [14]	√ [18, 23, 24, 26]
HSP 60 expression	Controls protein folding and unfolding in response to stress	↑ [18]	↑↑ [19]	√ [17, 19]
Mitochondrial permeability transition pore opening	Regulation of calcium handling and apoptosis	↓ [157]	↑ [158]	√ [26]
Ubiquitin-proteasome activation	Maintains protein function and quality control	↓ [159]	↑ [160]	√ [24]
Endothelial progenitor cell level	Physiologic and pathologic vessel formation	↑ [54]	↓ [161]	√ [55]
HSP72 expression	Controls protein folding and unfolding in response to stress	↑ [18, 162]	= [163]	√ [23] × [24, 40]
SERCA2a expression	Calcium recycling from the cytosol into the sarcoplasmic reticulum	↑ [164]	↓ [165]	√ [166] × [28, 29]
Mechanisms with evidence against their role in exercise prevention				
HSP 70 expression	Controls protein folding and unfolding in response to stress	↑ [167]	↓ [168]	× [19]
AMPK activation	Senses and regulates energy homeostasis	↑ [169]	↓ [170]	× [166]
Cardiac progenitor cell level/heart mass	Physiological turnover of cardiomyocytes	↑ [171]	↓ [172]	× [29]
Expression of PGC-1α	Transcription coactivator that regulates mitochondrial biogenesis and angiogenesis	= [32, 33]	↓ [173]	× [22, 34]
Potential mechanisms for exercise prevention lacking investigation				
Neuregulin-1/ErbB4 signalling	Cardiac cell survival growth factor	↑ [60]	↓ [174]	∅
Expression of GATA-4	Transcription factor involved in cardiac survival, hypertrophic growth of the heart	↑ [58]	↓ [175]	∅

↑: increase; ↓: decrease; =: no change; √: evidence available in favor of this mechanism; ×: evidence available against this mechanism; ∅: no evidence available.
HSP: heat shock protein; SERCA: sarcoplasmic reticulum calcium pump; AMPK: AMP-activated protein kinase; PGC: peroxisome proliferator-activated receptor-γ coactivator.
*Note: Where possible reference cited provides evidence for the cardiomyocyte response, which may differ from other cell types.

regulation of vascular tone and loss of atheroprotection [41]. Flow-mediated dilatation is triggered by shear stress from increased blood flow through a vessel, resulting in NO-mediated vasodilation [42]. Doxorubicin impairs both endothelium-dependent (i.e., flow-mediated) and endothelium-independent vasodilation [41, 43, 44]. Breast radiation impairs endothelium-dependent vasodilation in exposed axillary arteries, causes ultrastructural damage to myocardial capillaries, and can induce atherosclerosis in coronary arteries [45–48]. Trastuzumab may cause endothelial dysfunction through reductions in NO [49].

Exercise training improves endothelial dysfunction, predominantly through increased NO production as a result of chronic periods of pulsatile blood flow [50]. In the presence of the superoxide ROS, NO reacts to form a reactive molecule that can damage DNA, and this reaction also decreases the bioavailability of NO [51]. The upregulation of antioxidative enzymes associated with exercise training may therefore promote NO bioavailability by scavenging ROS [51]. Hayward et al. provided evidence that exercise preconditioning prior to 5-fluorouracil chemotherapy exposure increased NO production in rodents [52].

Endothelial progenitor cells (EPCs) contribute to maintaining the integrity of the endothelial cell layer, and lower levels of circulating EPCs are associated with an increased risk of cardiovascular events and death [53]. Exercise stimulates EPC mobilization from the bone marrow [54]. In human breast cancer survivors receiving doxorubicin-containing chemotherapy, exercise has been associated with an increase in circulating EPCs relative to usual care controls [55].

There are other proposed mechanisms for cardiotoxicity where exercise training could counteract the doxorubicin-induced molecular response that have not yet been investigated as mechanisms for exercise cardioprotection. For example, pharmacological α1-adrenoceptor activation of the cardiac transcription factor GATA-4 has demonstrated cardioprotective capacity against doxorubicin [56]. Therefore, exercise training, which appears to enhance both α1-adrenoceptor responsiveness [57], and GATA-4 mRNA level in the heart [58] may also exert a cardioprotective effect via a GATA-4 pathway. Another example includes doxorubicin and trastuzumab downregulation of neuregulin-1/ErbB4 receptor tyrosine kinase signaling in cardiomyocytes. Neuregulin-1/ErbB4 signaling plays a critical role in cardiac development and cardiomyocyte survival and organization [59]. Intriguingly, exercise training upregulates expression of neuregulin-1 in rodent cardiomyocytes [60], indicating a potential mechanism for exercise prevention of doxorubicin- and trastuzumab-related cardiotoxicity. Readers are referred to a more comprehensive review of potential mechanisms for exercise prevention of targeted cancer therapy-related cardiotoxicity [61].

In summary, although evidence exists for several different mechanisms through which exercise protects the heart and vasculature from doxorubicin-related toxicity, the unifying feature appears to be increased antioxidant capacity and reduction of oxidative stress. Several potential mechanisms, including exercise-induced upregulation of topoisomerase

2β/PGC-1α, GATA-4, and neuregulin-1/ErbB4 warrant further investigation to determine their role in cardioprotection.

3. Evidence for Exercise Prevention of Cardiovascular Disease

3.1. Cardiotoxicity Prevention

3.1.1. Acute Exercise. In animal models, doxorubicin-related cardiotoxicity can be attenuated by a single exercise session in close proximity to time of exposure. In the seminal study in this area, a 30-minute exercise session completed half an hour after doxorubicin exposure reduced mortality [62]. These findings were extended to demonstrate that an exhaustive exercise session half an hour after doxorubicin exposure attenuated markers of cardiomyocyte mitochondrial dysfunction [63]. Sixty minutes of submaximal exercise performed 24 hours prior to doxorubicin prevented or attenuated left ventricular (LV) systolic and diastolic dysfunction, cardiomyocyte mitochondrial apoptosis and dysfunction, and lipid peroxidation at 5 days post-treatment in rodents [26, 64].

The potential of a single exercise session to provide cardioprotection is particularly appealing, as regular, supervised exercise training during chemotherapy may not be feasible for all patients due to distance from home to exercise centers, difficulty with treatment symptoms, scheduling conflict with work, or family obligations. Ongoing research by our group is investigating the cardioprotective benefit of an acute exercise session 24 hours prior to doxorubicin administration in women with breast cancer.

3.1.2. Exercise Training before Treatment. In animals receiving high-dose bolus doxorubicin, exercise preconditioning prevents or attenuates acute (~24 hour post) increases in cardiac troponin I [17, 18], markers of oxidative stress [17–21, 24, 65], cardiomyocyte mitochondrial dysfunction [18, 19, 24], morphological and histological damage [16], markers of apoptosis [18, 24, 66], and decreases in HSP expression [17, 19] and LV systolic function [40, 65]. Similar findings have been reported in studies that extended the follow-up time to 5–10 days after doxorubicin exposure [35, 40, 67, 68]. Findings exclusive to studies with longer follow-up include attenuation of deficits in coronary flow [40], transmitral, and transaortic flow [35, 67], as well as transformation to the β-MHC isoform [35]. Even at four weeks after doxorubicin exposure, the beneficial effects of exercise preconditioning on β-MHC transformation, LV wall thickness, mass and systolic function, and transmitral/transaortic flow were still apparent [28].

The feasibility of exercise preconditioning in humans has been questioned, as the interval between breast cancer diagnosis and treatment is shorter than the length of most training programs that have been studied (8 to 14 weeks). However, cardioprotective effects have been reported after as little as 5 days to 3 weeks of training in rodents [21, 24, 66]. It should be noted that administered doxorubicin doses in these studies were higher than comparable human doses. It is unclear whether similar benefits would be seen in patients receiving standard treatment doses.

3.1.3. Exercise Training during Treatment.

Exercise training concurrent to chronic doxorubicin treatment in rodents has been associated with attenuation of LV systolic and diastolic dysfunction [23, 29, 37, 69, 70], cardiomyocyte apoptosis [23], transformation to β-MHC [36, 37], reductions in LV wall thickness [69] and heart mass [22], and deficits in coronary [23], transmitral, and transaortic flow [29, 37, 69].

Exercise training in humans during chemotherapy treatment for breast cancer is feasible and prevents the decrease in cardiorespiratory fitness seen in usual care controls [70–72]. Preliminary clinical studies of the effects of exercise training on cardiac function in humans undergoing breast cancer treatment have had disappointing results, however. A small randomized control trial of exercise training compared to usual care during doxorubicin-containing chemotherapy for breast cancer found no change in LV ejection fraction (LVEF) in either group [70]. A single-arm study investigated the effects of four months of exercise training in 17 breast cancer survivors receiving adjuvant trastuzumab therapy. Despite exercise training, trastuzumab was associated with LV dilatation and reduced LVEF [73]. However the exercise training dose may have been insufficient, as participants did not attend 41% of exercise sessions. More sensitive measures of cardiac function and a higher exercise dose are likely required in order to demonstrate a cardioprotective benefit in clinical studies.

3.1.4. Exercise Training after Treatment.

Although Héon et al. have reported reduced markers of cardiomyocyte apoptosis and oxidative stress in rodents undergoing exercise training two weeks after the completion of doxorubicin administration [74], to our knowledge the effects of post-treatment exercise on cardiac function have not been studied.

3.1.5. Summary of Cardiotoxicity Prevention Evidence.

In summary, acute and chronic exercise before, during or after doxorubicin treatment in rodents consistently results in prevention or attenuation of doxorubicin-induced deleterious effects to cardiomyocyte morphology and biochemistry, as well as cardiac function. Preclinical experimental research is needed to determine whether exercise can provide cardioprotection from cancer therapies other than doxorubicin.

3.2. Vascular Toxicity Prevention.

Few studies have investigated the effects of exercise on vascular function during breast cancer treatment. Six weeks of exercise training, initiated four weeks after doxorubicin treatment, was associated with improved endothelium-independent but not endothelium-dependent vasodilation, and with reduced mortality in rats with cardiac dysfunction [75]. Similarly, eight, but not four weeks of exercise training prior to exposure to 5-fluorouracil chemotherapy was associated with enhanced endothelium-dependent vasodilation in rats [52]. In humans, two small randomized trials of the effect of exercise training during doxorubicin-containing chemotherapy on endothelial function have had conflicting results [55, 70]. To advance understanding of exercise prevention of cardiovascular disease in breast cancer survivors, future exercise cardioprotection studies should include measurement of vascular function in addition to the cardiac measures.

3.3. Cardiovascular Risk Factors Modification.

Traditional cardiovascular risk factors should be monitored and managed in breast cancer patients who receive cardiotoxic cancer therapies to prevent additional injury [76]. Exercise can favorably improve a number of cardiovascular risk factors including hypertension, raised cholesterol/lipids, overweight and obesity, raised blood glucose or diabetes, and cardiorespiratory fitness [77].

Hypertension is more than twice as prevalent among breast cancer survivors aged 55 and older as it is among the general population [78], and may be caused by chemotherapy agents used to treat breast cancer including cyclophosphamide, cisplatin and carboplatin [79]. Chemotherapy for breast cancer is also associated with elevations in triglyceride levels [80], while tamoxifen treatment may reduce levels of protective high density lipoprotein (HDL) [81]. Prior to treatment, breast cancer survivors may already have a suboptimal lipid profile including higher total cholesterol, triglyceride, and low density lipoprotein levels, and lower HDL levels than healthy controls [82–86]. A similar pattern occurs with overweight or obesity, where overweight, a risk factor for development of breast cancer [87], is often an issue prior to treatment, and chemotherapy treatment perpetuates the problem via its association with greater weight gains than other treatments in the year following diagnosis [88]. Therefore, it is not surprising that almost half of breast cancer survivors are overweight or obese [89]. Treatment also has lasting adverse effects on peak oxygen consumption (VO_2), the gold standard measurement of cardiorespiratory fitness [90]. Chemotherapy causes a 6–10% reduction in peak VO_2 [71, 91], and following breast cancer treatment completion, remains an average of 22% lower than that of healthy sedentary controls [92]. Furthermore, the level of cardiorespiratory fitness amongst breast cancer survivors appears to mediate incidence of cardiovascular disease and risk factors [93]. Lastly, breast cancer survivors are at an increased risk for diabetes from two up to 10 years following diagnosis [94], and its presence increases the risk of mortality in this population [95]. In early stage breast cancer survivors, high blood insulin levels, indicative of insulin resistance, are associated with obesity, poor lipid profiles [96], distant recurrence and death [97].

A number of exercise intervention studies in human breast cancer survivors have included cardiovascular risk factors as outcome measures. Exercise interventions in breast cancer survivors have consistently reported decreases in systolic blood pressure of 3–5 mmHg both during [98–100] and after [99, 101–105] treatment. Reported effects on blood lipids following an exercise intervention with or without dietary intervention include significant positive effects on triglycerides [102, 105], and HDL [105], or no effect [104, 106,

107]. Numerous exercise interventions have measured weight or body composition change with mixed results, showing either no effect or weight reduction [12]. Small feasibility studies have demonstrated that the combination of exercise with a diet intervention could be more effective in reducing weight in breast cancer survivors [106, 107]. Exercise training during chemotherapy or radiation treatment for breast cancer at minimum can prevent the peak VO$_2$ decline occurring in usual care controls [71], or improve peak VO$_2$ [70, 72, 91, 108, 109]. Exercise training following completion of breast cancer treatment improves peak VO$_2$ [106, 110, 111]. Only one [105] of six randomized controlled trials to examine the effect of an exercise intervention on insulin and/or insulin resistance demonstrated statistically significant changes [104, 107, 112–114]. This same study also reported improvements in fasting blood glucose [105].

In summary, exercise interventions appear to have clinically meaningful effects on blood pressure and peak VO$_2$, whereas the effects on blood lipids, weight, and insulin/glucose and potential development of diabetes are less clear. The strong established relationships between both blood pressure and peak VO$_2$ and cardiovascular disease development and mortality in noncancer populations [6, 115–117] provide convincing support for the role of exercise in prevention of cardiovascular disease in human breast cancer survivors.

4. Translation of Preclinical Findings to Clinical Studies

Substantial preclinical evidence supports the role of exercise in prevention of cardiovascular disease toxicity, and there is some evidence for modification of cardiovascular risk factors in clinical trials. Further clinical research is warranted to determine whether exercise is a feasible and effective method for the reduction of cardiovascular morbidity and mortality in breast cancer survivors. Barriers to the translation of preclinical findings to human models include the need for more sensitive outcome measures and uncertainty regarding the optimal exercise dose.

Demonstration of the cardioprotective benefits of exercise in rodents has typically required euthanasia. One of the greatest barriers to this research in humans is identification of a noninvasive and sensitive outcome measure. Three-dimensional echocardiography-derived LVEF has emerged as a more reliable measure of LV function in patients receiving chemotherapy compared to traditional two-dimensional imaging [118], although this does not necessarily imply greater sensitivity to early changes in function. Echocardiography-derived LV global longitudinal strain and strain rate are able to detect changes in cardiac function during chemotherapy, radiation and trastuzumab treatment before changes in LVEF are detectable [119]. In noncancer populations, cardiac strain responds to exercise training [120]. Our research group is conducting an ongoing study to determine whether exercise training can prevent the doxorubicin-related decline in cardiac strain parameters in women with breast cancer. These parameters are widely available in conjunction with standard echocardiography [121]; with acceptable inter- and intra-observer variability (5% and 3.5%, resp.) [122]. Global longitudinal strain is predictive of all-cause mortality for a number of other cardiac conditions [123–126], and may be a stronger predictor of outcomes than LVEF [123, 126], but its relationship with clinical outcomes other than LVEF in breast cancer survivors is unknown.

Endothelial function is another attractive clinical outcome measure because dysfunction is an early process in the development of cardiovascular disease, and in noncancer populations, responds to pharmacological [42, 127] and exercise [50] interventions. Endothelial function can be easily measured in humans with a reactive hyperemia test, in which a cuff is inflated around the arm to occlude blood flow for 5 minutes. With release, the sudden increase in blood flow causes vasodilatation, which can be measured with ultrasound or peripheral arterial tonometry [127].

Cardiac biomarkers may play a role in predicting and identifying cardiotoxicity [128]. N-terminal prohormone brain natriuretic peptide (NT-proBNP) is frequently elevated during and after anthracycline treatment in adults [129–131]. There is mixed evidence regarding its ability to predict cardiac dysfunction following anthracycline treatment [130–132], as several studies where trastuzumab treatment followed anthracycline treatment, do not report a predictive ability of NT-proBNP [122, 133–135]. Due to inter-individual variations in kinetics, several measurements may be required to capture an elevation in cardiac troponins in patients receiving anthracyclines [122, 129, 130, 133, 134, 136–146], but the occurrence of an elevation in troponin I is predictive of chemotherapy and trastuzumab-related decreases in LVEF [139, 147], and cardiac events [140]. Exercise in heart failure patients does not change levels of NT-proBNP [148] or cardiac troponin I [149], but chronic heart failure has a different pathophysiology than the acute effects of cardiotoxic cancer therapies. Nonetheless, cardiac biomarkers may prove to be an effective outcome measure for exercise cardioprotection interventions due to their accessibility and reliability as a marker of cardiotoxicity.

Another important factor in the effective translation of preclinical findings to humans is the exercise intervention design. While preclinical and clinical experimental studies demonstrate that high intensity aerobic exercise results in greater cardiac benefits than moderate or low intensity [150, 151], the strenuous exercise prescription applied in most preclinical studies (five days a week, moderate to high intensity, 20–90 minutes) would likely not be tolerable for humans undergoing chemotherapy treatment [152]. One rodent study implemented a more clinically feasible and practical exercise prescription and doxorubicin treatment protocol involving 20 minutes of low intensity exercise, performed five days per week during chronic low dose doxorubicin treatment [23]. Although the lower doxorubicin dose failed to induce the MHC isoform shift and lipid peroxidation reported with higher doses, the lower exercise dose was protective against LV dysfunction and cardiomyocyte apoptosis [23]. In heart failure patients, moderate intensity exercise performed three days per week has been shown to improve systolic function [153]. Therefore, the required exercise dose for cardioprotection likely involves three to five days per week of moderate to high intensity aerobic exercise of at least 20 minutes in duration, but greater benefits will likely occur with higher doses. The optimal prescription requires a balance of patient tolerance with protective efficacy.

5. Conclusion

Breast cancer therapy has efficacious antitumor effects, but is associated with increased risk of cardiovascular disease. A considerable body of research, including preclinical studies and clinical trials, indicates that exercise may be an effective nonpharmacological method of attenuating the harmful effects of breast cancer therapies on the heart and vasculature, of modifying cardiovascular risk factors, and potentially reducing cardiovascular morbidity and mortality in this vulnerable population. The mechanisms for exercise prevention appear to be predominantly related to an increase in antioxidant capacity and associated reduction in oxidative stress. Clinical trials are needed to investigate the role of exercise in the prevention of direct cardiovascular toxicity of breast cancer treatment and the effect on cardiovascular events and mortality. The role of exercise in the prevention of cardiovascular disease in other cancer populations also warrants further research, as the detrimental combination of a high incidence of baseline risk factors combined with cancer treatment cardiovascular toxicity may be common to multiple cancer types. Echocardiographic quantification of LV global longitudinal strain and strain rate, endothelial function quantification, and measurement of circulating cardiac biomarkers are safe, noninvasive measures that may be sensitive and effective outcome measures for clinical studies of exercise prevention of breast cancer treatment-related cardiovascular toxicity. The exercise frequency, intensity, and duration demonstrating cardioprotection in most preclinical studies may need to be modified to accommodate human patient tolerability during ongoing cancer treatment.

Conflict of Interests

The authors declare that there is no conflict of interests regarding the publication of this paper.

Acknowledgments

Amy Kirkham is supported by a Canada Graduate Scholarship from the Canadian Institute of Health Research. Margot Davis is supported by a Vancouver Coastal Health Research Institute Mentored Clinician Scientist award.

References

[1] P. Boyle and B. Levin, Eds., *World Cancer Report*, International Agency for Research on Cancer, Lyon, France, 2008.

[2] Canadian Cancer Society/National Cancer Institute of Canada, *Canadian cancer statistics 2007*, Canadian Cancer Society/ National Cancer Institute of Canada, Toronto, Canada, 2007.

[3] L. W. Jones, M. J. Haykowsky, J. J. Swartz, P. S. Douglas, and J. R. Mackey, "Early breast cancer therapy and cardiovascular injury,"
Journal of the American College of Cardiology, vol. 50, no. 15, pp. 1435–1441, 2007.

[4] M. Riihimäki, H. Thomsen, A. Brandt, J. Sundquist, and K. Hemminki, "Death causes in breast cancer patients," *Annals of Oncology*, vol. 23, no. 3, pp. 604–610, 2012.

[5] S. E. Minton and P. N. Munster, "Chemotherapy-induced amenorrhea and fertility in women undergoing adjuvant treatment for breast cancer," *Cancer Control*, vol. 9, no. 6, pp. 466–472, 2002.

[6] World Heart Federation, *Cardiovascular Disease Risk Factors*, World Heart Federation, Geneva, Switzerland, 2013.

[7] M. S. Ewer and S. Glück, "A woman's heart: the impact of adjuvant endocrine therapy on cardiovascular health," *Cancer*, vol. 115, no. 9, pp. 1813–1826, 2009.

[8] J. L. Patnaik, T. Byers, C. DiGuiseppi, D. Dabelea, and T. D. Denberg, "Cardiovascular disease competes with breast cancer as the leading cause of death for older females diagnosed with breast cancer: a retrospective cohort study," *Breast Cancer Research*, vol. 13, no. 3, article R64, 2011.

[9] A. R. Lehenbauer Ludke, A. A.-R. S. Al-Shudiefat, S. Dhingra, D. S. Jassal, and P. K. Singal, "A concise description of cardioprotective strategies in doxorubicin-induced cardiotoxicity," *Canadian Journal of Physiology and Pharmacology*, vol. 87, no. 10, pp. 756–763, 2009.

[10] J. Chang, "Chemotherapy dose reduction and delay in clinical practiceevaluating the risk to patient outcome in adjuvant chemotherapy for breast cancer," *European Journal of Cancer*, vol. 36, no. 1, pp. 11–14, 2000.

[11] D. E. R. Warburton, C. W. Nicol, and S. S. D. Bredin, "Health benefits of physical activity: the evidence," *Canadian Medical Association Journal*, vol. 174, no. 6, pp. 801–809, 2006.

[12] K. H. Schmitz, K. S. Courneya, C. Matthews et al., "American college of sports medicine roundtable on exercise guidelines for cancer survivors," *Medicine and Science in Sports and Exercise*, vol. 42, no. 7, pp. 1409–1426, 2010.

[13] D. A. Gewirtz, "A critical evaluation of the mechanisms of action proposed for the antitumor effects of the anthracycline antibiotics adriamycin and daunorubicin," *Biochemical Pharmacology*, vol. 57, no. 7, pp. 727–741, 1999.

[14] G. Minotti, P. Menna, E. Salvatorelli, G. Cairo, and L. Gianni, "Anthracyclines: molecular advances and pharmacologie developments in antitumor activity and cardiotoxicity," *Pharmacological Reviews*, vol. 56, no. 2, pp. 185–229, 2004.

[15] K. Husain and S. M. Somani, "Response of cardiac antioxidant system to alcohol and exercise training in the rat," *Alcohol*, vol. 14, no. 3, pp. 301–307, 1997.

[16] A. Ascensão, J. Magalhães, J. Soares et al., "Endurance exercise training attenuates morphological signs of cardiac muscle damage induced by doxorubicin in male mice," *Basic and Applied Myology*, vol. 16, pp. 27–35, 2006.

[17] A. Ascensão, J. Magalhães, J. Soares et al., "Endurance training attenuates doxorubicin-induced cardiac oxidative damage in mice," *International Journal of Cardiology*, vol. 100, no. 3, pp. 451–460, 2005.

[18] A. Ascensão, J. Magalhães, J. M. C. Soares et al., "Moderate endurance training prevents doxorubicin-induced in vivo mitochondriopathy and reduces the development of cardiac apoptosis," *American Journal of Physiology—Heart and Circulatory Physiology*, vol. 289, no. 2, pp. H722–H731, 2005.

[19] A. Ascensão, R. Ferreira, P. J. Oliveira, and J. Magalhães, "Effects of endurance training and acute doxorubicin treatment on rat

heart mitochondrial alterations induced by in vitro anoxia-reoxygenation," *Cardiovascular Toxicology*, vol. 6, no. 3-4, pp. 159–172, 2006.

[20] J. Ashrafi, V. D. Roshan, and S. Mahjoub, "Cardioprotective effects of aerobic regular exercise against doxorubicin-induced oxidative stress in rat," *African Journal of Pharmacy and Pharmacology*, vol. 6, pp. 2380–2388, 2012.

[21] J. Ashrafi and V. D. Roshan, "Is short-term exercise a therapeutic tool for improvement of cardioprotection against DOX-induced cardiotoxicity? An experimental controlled protocol in rats," *Asian Pacific Journal of Cancer Prevention*, vol. 13, no. 8, pp. 4025–4030, 2012.

[22] I. Marques-Aleixo, E. Santos-Alves, D. Mariani et al., "Physical exercise prior and during treatment reduces sub-chronic doxorubicin-induced mitochondrial toxicity and oxidative stress," *Mitochondrion*, vol. 20, pp. 22–33, 2015.

[23] A. J. Chicco, D. S. Hydock, C. M. Schneider, and R. Hayward, "Low-intensity exercise training during doxorubicin treatment protects against cardiotoxicity," *Journal of Applied Physiology*, vol. 100, no. 2, pp. 519–527, 2006.

[24] A. N. Kavazis, A. J. Smuder, K. Min, N. Tümer, and S. K. Powers, "Short-term exercise training protects against doxorubicin-induced cardiac mitochondrial damage independent of HSP72," *American Journal of Physiology—Heart and Circulatory Physiology*, vol. 299, no. 5, pp. H1515–H1524, 2010.

[25] C. A. Geisberg and D. B. Sawyer, "Mechanisms of anthracycline cardiotoxicity and strategies to decrease cardiac damage," *Current Hypertension Reports*, vol. 12, no. 6, pp. 404–410, 2010.

[26] A. Ascensão, J. Lumini-Oliveira, N. G. Machado et al., "Acute exercise protects against calcium-induced cardiac mitochondrial permeability transition pore opening in doxorubicin-treated rats," *Clinical Science*, vol. 120, no. 1, pp. 37–49, 2011.

[27] M. R. Duchen, "Mitochondria and calcium: from cell signalling to cell death," *Journal of Physiology*, vol. 529, no. 1, pp. 57–68, 2000.

[28] D. S. Hydock, C.-Y. Lien, B. T. Jensen, C. M. Schneider, and R. Hayward, "Exercise preconditioning provides long-term protection against early chronic doxorubicin cardiotoxicity," *Integrative Cancer Therapies*, vol. 10, no. 1, pp. 47–57, 2011.

[29] R. Hayward, C.-Y. Lien, B. T. Jensen, D. S. Hydock, and C. M. Schneider, "Exercise training mitigates anthracycline-induced chronic cardiotoxicity in a juvenile rat model," *Pediatric Blood and Cancer*, vol. 59, no. 1, pp. 149–154, 2012.

[30] S. Zhang, X. Liu, T. Bawa-Khalfe et al., "Identification of the molecular basis of doxorubicin-induced cardiotoxicity," *Nature Medicine*, vol. 18, no. 11, pp. 1639–1642, 2012.

[31] P. Vejpongsa and E. T. H. Yeh, "Topoisomerase 2β: a promising molecular target for primary prevention of anthracycline-induced cardiotoxicity," *Clinical Pharmacology & Therapeutics*, vol. 95, no. 1, pp. 45–52, 2014.

[32] A. Botta, I. Laher, J. Beam et al., "Short term exercise induces PGC-1α, ameliorates inflammation and increases mitochondrial membrane proteins but fails to increase respiratory enzymes in aging diabetic hearts," *PLoS ONE*, vol. 8, no. 8, Article ID e70248, 2013.

[33] L. Li, C. Mühlfeld, B. Niemann et al., "Mitochondrial biogenesis and PGC-1α deacetylation by chronic treadmill exercise: differential response in cardiac and skeletal muscle," *Basic Research in Cardiology*, vol. 106, no. 6, pp. 1221–1234, 2011.

[34] A. N. Kavazis, A. J. Smuder, and S. K. Powers, "Effects of short-term endurance exercise training on acute doxorubicin-induced FoxO transcription in cardiac and skeletal muscle," *Journal of Applied Physiology*, vol. 117, no. 3, pp. 223–230, 2014.

[35] D. S. Hydock, C.-Y. Lien, C. M. Schneider, and R. Hayward, "Exercise preconditioning protects against doxorubicin-induced cardiac dysfunction," *Medicine and Science in Sports and Exercise*, vol. 40, no. 5, pp. 808–817, 2008.

[36] D. S. Hydock, K. Y. Wonders, C. M. Schneider, and R. Hayward, "Voluntary wheel running in rats receiving doxorubicin: effects on running activity and cardiac myosin heavy chain," *Anticancer Research*, vol. 29, no. 11, pp. 4401–4407, 2009.

[37] D. S. Hydock, C.-Y. Lien, B. T. Jensen, T. L. Parry, C. M. Schneider, and R. Hayward, "Rehabilitative exercise in a rat model of doxorubicin cardiotoxicity," *Experimental Biology and Medicine*, vol. 237, no. 12, pp. 1483–1492, 2012.

[38] S. Miyata, W. Minobe, M. R. Bristow, and L. A. Leinwand, "Myosin heavy chain isoform expression in the failing and nonfailing human heart," *Circulation Research*, vol. 86, no. 4, pp. 386–390, 2000.

[39] A. Ascensão, R. Ferreira, and J. Magalhães, "Exercise-induced cardioprotection—biochemical, morphological and functional evidence in whole tissue and isolated mitochondria," *International Journal of Cardiology*, vol. 117, no. 1, pp. 16–30, 2007.

[40] A. J. Chicco, C. M. Schneider, and R. Hayward, "Exercise training attenuates acute doxorubicin-induced cardiac dysfunction," *Journal of Cardiovascular Pharmacology*, vol. 47, no. 2, pp. 182–189, 2006.

[41] J. T. Kuvin, A. R. Patel, K. A. Sliney et al., "Assessment of peripheral vascular endothelial function with finger arterial pulse wave amplitude," *American Heart Journal*, vol. 146, no. 1, pp. 168–174, 2003.

[42] M. Kelm, "Flow-mediated dilatation in human circulation: diagnostic and therapeutic aspects," *The American Journal of Physiology —Heart and Circulatory Physiology*, vol. 282, no. 1, pp. H1–H5, 2002.

[43] R. Hayward, D. Hydock, N. Gibson, S. Greufe, E. Bredahl, and T. Parry, "Tissue retention of doxorubicin and its effects on cardiac, smooth, and skeletal muscle function," *Journal of Physiology and Biochemistry*, vol. 69, no. 2, pp. 177–187, 2013.

[44] D. S. Celermajer, "Reliable endothelial function testing: at our fingertips?" *Circulation*, vol. 117, no. 19, pp. 2428–2430, 2008.

[45] J. A. Beckman, A. Thakore, B. H. Kalinowski, J. R. Harris, and M. A. Creager, "Radiation therapy impairs endothelium-dependent vasodilation in humans," *Journal of the American College of Cardiology*, vol. 37, no. 3, pp. 761–765, 2001.

[46] B. W. Corn, B. J. Trock, and R. L. Goodman, "Irradiation-related ischemic heart disease," *Journal of Clinical Oncology*, vol. 8, no. 4, pp. 741–750, 1990.

[47] A. M. Gaya and R. F. U. Ashford, "Cardiac complications of radiation therapy," *Clinical Oncology*, vol. 17, no. 3, pp. 153–159, 2005.

[48] R. Virmani, A. Farb, A. J. Carter, and R. M. Jones, "Pathology of radiation-induced coronary artery disease in human and pig," *Cardiovascular Radiation Medicine*, vol. 1, no. 1, pp. 98–101, 1999.

[49] A. Sandoo, G. D. Kitas, and A. R. Carmichael, "Endothelial dysfunction as a determinant of trastuzumab-mediated cardiotoxicity in patients with breast cancer," *Anticancer Research*, vol. 34, no. 3, pp. 1147–1151, 2014.

[50] D. J. Green, A. Spence, J. R. Halliwill, N. T. Cable, and D. H. J. Thijssen, "Exercise and vascular adaptation in asymptomatic humans," *Experimental Physiology*, vol. 96, no. 2, pp. 57–70, 2011.

[51] S. Gielen, G. Schuler, and V. Adams, "Cardiovascular effects of exercise training: molecular mechanisms," *Circulation*, vol. 122, no. 12, pp. 1221–1238, 2010.

[52] R. Hayward, R. Ruangthai, C. M. Schneider, R. M. Hyslop, R. Strange, and K. C. Westerlind, "Training enhances vascular relaxation after chemotherapy-induced vasoconstriction," *Medicine & Science in Sports & Exercise*, vol. 36, no. 3, pp. 428–434, 2004.

[53] N. Werner, S. Kosiol, T. Schiegl et al., "Circulating endothelial progenitor cells and cardiovascular outcomes," *The New England Journal of Medicine*, vol. 353, no. 10, pp. 999–1007, 2005.

[54] U. Laufs, A. Urhausen, N. Werner et al., "Running exercise of different duration and intensity: effect on endothelial progenitor cells in healthy subjects," *European Journal of Cardiovascular Prevention and Rehabilitation*, vol. 12, no. 4, pp. 407–414, 2005.

[55] L. W. Jones, D. R. Fels, M. West et al., "Modulation of circulating angiogenic factors and tumor biology by aerobic training in breast cancer patients receiving neoadjuvant chemotherapy," *Cancer Prevention Research*, vol. 6, no. 9, pp. 925–937, 2013.

[56] A. Aries, P. Paradis, C. Lefebvre, R. J. Schwartz, and M. Nemer, "Essential role of GATA-4 in cell survival and drug-induced cardiotoxicity," *Proceedings of the National Academy of Sciences of the United States of America*, vol. 101, no. 18, pp. 6975–6980, 2004.

[57] D. H. Korzick and R. L. Moore, "Chronic exercise enhances cardiac α1-adrenergic inotropic responsiveness in rats with mild hypertension," *American Journal of Physiology—Heart and Circulatory Physiology*, vol. 271, no. 6, pp. H2599–H2608, 1996.

[58] J. Xiao, T. Xu, J. Li et al., "Exercise-induced physiological hypertrophy initiates activation of cardiac progenitor cells," *International Journal of Clinical and Experimental Pathology*, vol. 7, pp. 663–669, 2014.

[59] D. B. Sawyer, X. Peng, B. Chen, L. Pentassuglia, and C. C. Lim, "Mechanisms of anthracycline cardiac injury: can we identify strategies for cardioprotection?" *Progress in Cardiovascular Diseases*, vol. 53, no. 2, pp. 105–113, 2010.

[60] C. D. Waring, C. Vicinanza, A. Papalamprou et al., "The adult heart responds to increased workload with physiologic hypertrophy, cardiac stem cell activation, and new myocyte formation," *European Heart Journal*, vol. 35, no. 39, pp. 2722–2731, 2014.

[61] J. M. Scott, S. Lakoski, J. R. Mackey, P. S. Douglas, M. J. Haykowsky, and L. W. Jones, "The potential role of aerobic exercise to modulate cardiotoxicity of molecularly targeted cancer therapeutics," *Oncologist*, vol. 18, no. 2, pp. 221–231, 2013.

[62] A. B. Combs, S. L. Hudman, and H. W. Bonner, "Effect of exercise stress upon the acute toxicity of adriamycin in mice," *Research Communications in Chemical Pathology and Pharmacology*, vol. 23, no. 2, pp. 395–398, 1979.

[63] E. W. Mitchell, "Effects of adriamycin on heart mitochondrial function in rested and exercised rats," *Biochemical Pharmacology*, vol. 47, no. 5, pp. 877–885, 1994.

[64] K. Y. Wonders, D. S. Hydock, C. M. Schneider, and R. Hayward, "Acute exercise protects against doxorubicin cardiotoxicity," *Integrative Cancer Therapies*, vol. 7, no. 3, pp. 147–154, 2008.

[65] A. J. Chicco, C. M. Schneider, and R. Hayward, "Voluntary exercise protects against acute doxorubicin cardiotoxicity in the isolated perfused rat heart," *American Journal of Physiology—Regulatory Integrative and Comparative Physiology*, vol. 289, no. 2, pp. R424–R431, 2005.

[66] C. Werner, M. Hanhoun, T. Widmann et al., "Effects of physical exercise on myocardial telomere-regulating proteins, survival pathways, and apoptosis," *Journal of the American College of Cardiology*, vol. 52, no. 6, pp. 470–482, 2008.

[67] B. T. Jensen, *The effect of exercise on cardiac function and doxorubicin accumulation in left ventricular tissue of rats [Ph.D. dissertation]*, University of Northern Colorado, Greeley, Colo, USA, 2011.

[68] K. Y. Wonders, D. S. Hydock, S. Greufe, C. M. Schneider, and R. Hayward, "Endurance exercise training preserves cardiac function in rats receiving doxorubicin and the HER-2 inhibitor GW2974," *Cancer Chemotherapy and Pharmacology*, vol. 64, no. 6, pp. 1105–1113, 2009.

[69] D. S. Hydock, T. L. Parry, B. T. Jensen, C.-Y. Lien, C. M. Schneider, and R. Hayward, "Effects of endurance training on combined goserelin acetate and doxorubicin treatment-induced cardiac dysfunction," *Cancer Chemotherapy and Pharmacology*, vol. 68, no. 3, pp. 685–692, 2011.

[70] L. Jones, V. Dolinsky, M. Haykowsky et al., "Effects of aerobic training to improve cardiovascular function and prevent cardiac remodeling after cytotoxic therapy in early breast cancer," in *Proceedings of the American Association for Cancer Research 102nd Annual Meeting*, Orlando, Fla, USA, April 2011, abstract 5024.

[71] K. S. Courneya, R. J. Segal, J. R. Mackey et al., "Effects of aerobic and resistance exercise in breast cancer patients receiving adjuvant chemotherapy: a multicenter randomized controlled trial," *Journal of Clinical Oncology*, vol. 25, no. 28, pp. 4396–4404, 2007.

[72] A. L. Schwartz, K. Winters-Stone, and B. Gallucci, "Exercise effects on bone mineral density in women with breast cancer receiving adjuvant chemotherapy," *Oncology Nursing Forum*, vol. 34, no. 3, pp. 627–633, 2007.

[73] M. J. Haykowsky, J. R. Mackey, R. B. Thompson, L. W. Jones, and D. I. Paterson, "Adjuvant trastuzumab induces ventricular remodeling despite aerobic exercise training," *Clinical Cancer Research*, vol. 15, no. 15, pp. 4963–4967, 2009.

[74] S. Héon, M. Bernier, N. Servant et al., "Dexrazoxane does not protect against doxorubicin-induced damage in young rats," *American Journal of Physiology—Heart and Circulatory Physiology*, vol. 285, no. 2, pp. H499–H506, 2003.

[75] C. Matsuura, T. M. C. Brunini, L. C. M. M. Carvalho et al., "Exercise training in doxorubicin-induced heart failure: effects on the L-arginine-NO pathway and vascular reactivity," *Journal of the American Society of Hypertension*, vol. 4, no. 1, pp. 7–13, 2010.

[76] M. M. Abu-Khalaf and L. Harris, "Anthracycline-induced cardiotoxicity: risk assessment and management," *Oncology*, vol. 23, no. 3, pp. 239–252, 2009.

[77] G. F. Fletcher, G. Balady, S. N. Blair et al., "Statement on exercise: benefits and recommendations for physical activity programs for all Americans: a statement for health professionals by the committee on exercise and cardiac rehabilitation of the Council on Clinical Cardiology, American Heart Association," *Circulation*, vol. 94, no. 4, pp. 857–862, 1996.

[78] R. Yancik, R. J. Havlik, M. N. Wesley et al., "Cancer and comorbidity in older patients: a descriptive profile," *Annals of Epidemiology*, vol. 6, no. 5, pp. 399–412, 1996.

[79] E. Mouhayar and A. Salahudeen, "Hypertension in cancer patients," *Texas Heart Institute Journal*, vol. 38, no. 3, pp. 263–265, 2011.

[80] C. G. Alexopoulos, S. Pournaras, M. Vaslamatzis, A. Avgerinos, and S. Raptis, "Changes in serum lipids and lipoproteins in

cancer patients during chemotherapy," *Cancer Chemotherapy and Pharmacology*, vol. 30, no. 5, pp. 412–416, 1992.

[81] R. R. Love, D. A. Wiebe, P. A. Newcomb et al., "Effects of tamoxifen on cardiovascular risk factors in postmenopausal women," *Annals of Internal Medicine*, vol. 115, no. 11, pp. 860–864, 1991.

[82] W. Thompat, S. Sukarayodhin, A. Sornprom, Y. Sudjaroen, and P. Laisupasin, "Comparison of serum lipid profiles between normal controls and breast cancer patients," *Journal of Laboratory Physicians*, vol. 5, no. 1, p. 38, 2013.

[83] K. Hasija and H. K. Bagga, "Alterations of serum cholesterol and serum lipoprotein in breast cancer of women," *Indian Journal of Clinical Biochemistry*, vol. 20, no. 1, pp. 61–66, 2005.

[84] E. Kökoğlu, I. Karaarslan, H. Mehmet Karaarslan, and H. Baloğlu, "Alterations of serum lipids and lipoproteins in breast cancer," *Cancer Letters*, vol. 82, no. 2, pp. 175–178, 1994.

[85] J.-B. Lopez-Saez, J. A. Martinez-Rubio, M. M. Alvarez et al., "Metabolic profile of breast cancer in a population of women in southern Spain," *Open Clinical Cancer Journal*, vol. 2, pp. 1–6, 2008.

[86] N. K. Yadav, B. Poudel, C. Thanpari, and B. C. Koner, "Assessment of biochemical profiles in premenopausal and postmenopausal women with breast cancer," *Asian Pacific Journal of Cancer Prevention*, vol. 13, no. 7, pp. 3385–3388, 2012.

[87] A. R. Carmichael and T. Bates, "Obesity and breast cancer: a review of the literature," *Breast*, vol. 13, no. 2, pp. 85–92, 2004.

[88] P. J. Goodwin, M. Ennis, K. I. Pritchard et al., "Adjuvant treatment and onset of menopause predict weight gain after breast cancer diagnosis," *Journal of Clinical Oncology*, vol. 17, no. 1, pp. 120–129, 1999.

[89] K. S. Courneya, P. T. Katzmarzyk, and E. Bacon, "Physical activity and obesity in Canadian cancer survivors: population-based estimates from the 2005 Canadian Community Health Survey," *Cancer*, vol. 112, no. 11, pp. 2475–2482, 2008.

[90] L. W. Jones, N. D. Eves, M. Haykowsky, S. J. Freedland, and J. R. Mackey, "Exercise intolerance in cancer and the role of exercise therapy to reverse dysfunction," *The Lancet Oncology*, vol. 10, no. 6, pp. 598–605, 2009.

[91] S. G. Lakoski, N. D. Eves, P. S. Douglas, and L. W. Jones, "Exercise rehabilitation in patients with cancer," *Nature Reviews Clinical Oncology*, vol. 9, no. 5, pp. 288–296, 2012.

[92] L. W. Jones, K. S. Courneya, J. R. Mackey et al., "Cardiopulmonary function and age-related decline across the breast cancer: survivorship continuum," *Journal of Clinical Oncology*, vol. 30, no. 20, pp. 2530–2537, 2012.

[93] J. B. Peel, X. Sui, S. A. Adams, J. R. HIbert, J. W. Hardin, and S. N. Blair, "A prospective study of cardiorespiratory fitness and breast cancer mortality," *Medicine and Science in Sports and Exercise*, vol. 41, no. 4, pp. 742–748, 2009.

[94] L. L. Lipscombe, W. W. Chan, L. Yun, P. C. Austin, G. M. Anderson, and P. A. Rochon, "Incidence of diabetes among postmenopausal breast cancer survivors," *Diabetologia*, vol. 56, no. 3, pp. 476–483, 2013.

[95] R. Yancik, M. N. Wesley, L. A. G. Ries, R. J. Havlik, B. K. Edwards, and J. W. Yates, "Effect of age and comorbidity in postmenopausal breast cancer patients aged 55 years and older," *Journal of the American Medical Association*, vol. 285, no. 7, pp. 885–892, 2001.

[96] P. J. Goodwin, M. Ennis, M. Bahl et al., "High insulin levels in newly diagnosed breast cancer patients reflect underlying insulin resistance and are associated with components of the insulin resistance syndrome," *Breast Cancer Research and Treatment*, vol. 114, no. 3, pp. 517–525, 2009.

[97] P. J. Goodwin, M. Ennis, K. I. Pritchard et al., "Fasting insulin and outcome in early-stage breast cancer: results of a prospective cohort study," *Journal of Clinical Oncology*, vol. 20, no. 1, pp. 42–51, 2002.

[98] G. G. Kolden, T. J. Strauman, A. Ward et al., "A pilot study of group exercise training (GET) for women with primary breast cancer: feasibility and health benefits," *Psycho-Oncology*, vol. 11, no. 5, pp. 447–456, 2002.

[99] C. M. Schneider, C. C. Hsieh, L. K. Sprod, S. D. Carter, and R. Hayward, "Effects of supervised exercise training on cardiopulmonary function and fatigue in breast cancer survivors during and after treatment," *Cancer*, vol. 110, no. 4, pp. 918–925, 2007.

[100] C.-J. Kim, D.-H. Kang, B. A. Smith, and K. A. Landers, "Cardiopulmonary responses and adherence to exercise in women newly diagnosed with breast cancer undergoing adjuvant therapy," *Cancer Nursing*, vol. 29, no. 2, pp. 156–165, 2006.

[101] C. C. Hsieh, L. K. Sprod, D. S. Hydock, S. D. Carter, R. Hayward, and C. M. Schneider, "Effects of a supervised exercise intervention on recovery from treatment regimens in breast cancer survivors," *Oncology Nursing Forum*, vol. 35, no. 6, pp. 909–915, 2008.

[102] A. S. Fairey, K. S. Courneya, C. J. Field et al., "Effect of exercise training on C-reactive protein in postmenopausal breast cancer survivors: a randomized controlled trial," *Brain, Behavior, and Immunity*, vol. 19, no. 5, pp. 381–388, 2005.

[103] B. M. Pinto, M. M. Clark, N. C. Maruyama, and S. I. Feder, "Psychological and fitness changes associated with exercise participation among women with breast cancer," *Psycho-Oncology*, vol. 12, no. 2, pp. 118–126, 2003.

[104] E. Guinan, J. Hussey, J. M. Broderick et al., "The effect of aerobic exercise on metabolic and inflammatory markers in breast cancer survivors: a pilot study," *Supportive Care in Cancer*, vol. 21, no. 7, pp. 1983–1992, 2013.

[105] R. Nuri, M. R. Kordi, M. Moghaddasi et al., "Effect of combination exercise training on metabolic syndrome parameters in postmenopausal women with breast cancer," *Journal of Cancer Research and Therapeutics*, vol. 8, no. 2, pp. 238–242, 2012.

[106] K. L. Campbell, C. L. Van Patten, S. E. Neil et al., "Feasibility of a lifestyle intervention on body weight and serum biomarkers in breast cancer survivors with overweight and obesity," *Journal of the Academy of Nutrition and Dietetics*, vol. 112, no. 4, pp. 559–567, 2012.

[107] W. Demark-Wahnefried, L. D. Case, K. Blackwell et al., "Results of a diet/exercise feasibility trial to prevent adverse body composition change in breast cancer patients on adjuvant chemotherapy," *Clinical Breast Cancer*, vol. 8, no. 1, pp. 70–79, 2008.

[108] M. G. MacVicar, M. L. Winningham, and J. L. Nickel, "Effects of aerobic interval training on cancer patients' functional capacity," *Nursing Research*, vol. 38, no. 6, pp. 348–351, 1989.

[109] J. S. Drouin, T. J. Young, J. Beeler et al., "Random control clinical trial on the effects of aerobic exercise training on erythrocyte levels during radiation treatment for breast cancer," *Cancer*, vol. 107, no. 10, pp. 2490–2495, 2006.

[110] K. S. Courneya, J. R. Mackey, G. J. Bell, L. W. Jones, C. J. Field, and A. S. Fairey, "Randomized controlled trial of exercise training in postmenopausal breast cancer survivors: cardiopulmonary and quality of life outcomes," *Journal of Clinical Oncology*, vol. 21, no. 9, pp. 1660–1668, 2003.

[111] F. Herrero, A. F. San Juan, S. J. Fleck et al., "Combined aerobic and resistance training in breast cancer survivors: a randomized, controlled pilot trial," *International Journal of Sports Medicine*, vol. 27, no. 7, pp. 573–580, 2006.

[112] A. S. Fairey, K. S. Courneya, C. J. Field, G. J. Bell, L. W. Jones, and J. R. Mackey, "Effects of exercise training on fasting insulin, insulin resistance, insulin-like growth factors, and insulin-like growth factor binding proteins in postmenopausal breast cancer survivors: a randomized controlled trial," *Cancer Epidemiology, Biomarkers & Prevention*, vol. 12, no. 8, pp. 721–727, 2003.

[113] J. A. Ligibel, N. Campbell, A. Partridge et al., "Impact of a mixed strength and endurance exercise intervention on insulin levels in breast cancer survivors," *Journal of Clinical Oncology*, vol. 26, no. 6, pp. 907–912, 2008.

[114] M. L. Irwin, K. Varma, M. Alvarez-Reeves et al., "Randomized controlled trial of aerobic exercise on insulin and insulin-like growth factors in breast cancer survivors: the yale exercise and survivorship study," *Cancer Epidemiology Biomarkers and Prevention*, vol. 18, no. 1, pp. 306–313, 2009.

[115] S. N. Blair, H. W. Kohl III, C. E. Barlow, R. S. Paffenbarger Jr., L. W. Gibbons, and C. A. Macera, "Changes in physical fitness and all-cause mortality: a prospective study of healthy and unhealthy men," *Journal of the American Medical Association*, vol. 273, no. 14, pp. 1093–1098, 1995.

[116] J. Stamler, R. Stamler, and J. D. Neaton, "Blood pressure, systolic and diastolic, and cardiovascular risks: US population data," *Archives of Internal Medicine*, vol. 153, no. 5, pp. 598–615, 1993.

[117] J. Stamler, G. Rose, R. Stamler, P. Elliott, A. Dyer, and M. Marmot, "INTERSALT study findings. Public health and medical care implications," *Hypertension*, vol. 14, no. 5, pp. 570–577, 1989.

[118] P. Thavendiranathan, A. D. Grant, T. Negishi, J. C. Plana, Z. B. Popović, and T. H. Marwick, "Reproducibility of echocardiographic techniques for sequential assessment of left ventricular ejection fraction and volumes: application to patients undergoing cancer chemotherapy," *Journal of the American College of Cardiology*, vol. 61, no. 1, pp. 77–84, 2013.

[119] P. Thavendiranathan, F. Poulin, K.-D. Lim, J. C. Plana, A. Woo, and T. H. Marwick, "Use of myocardial strain imaging by echocardiography for the early detection of cardiotoxicity in patients during and after cancer chemotherap: a systematic review," *Journal of the American College of Cardiology*, vol. 63, no. 25, pp. 2751–2768, 2014.

[120] A. L. Baggish, K. Yared, F. Wang et al., "The impact of endurance exercise training on left ventricular systolic mechanics," *American Journal of Physiology—Heart and Circulatory Physiology*, vol. 295, no. 3, pp. H1109–H1116, 2008.

[121] R. A. Argyle and S. G. Ray, "Stress and strain: double trouble or useful tool?" *European Journal of Echocardiography*, vol. 10, no. 6, pp. 716–722, 2009.

[122] N. Fallah-Rad, J. R. Walker, A. Wassef et al., "The utility of cardiac biomarkers, tissue velocity and strain imaging, and cardiac magnetic resonance imaging in predicting early left ventricular dysfunction in patients with human epidermal growth factor receptor II-positive breast cancer treated with adjuvant trastuzumab therapy," *Journal of the American College of Cardiology*, vol. 57, no. 22, pp. 2263–2270, 2011.

[123] G.-Y. Cho, T. H. Marwick, H.-S. Kim, M.-K. Kim, K.-S. Hong, and D.-J. Oh, "Global 2-dimensional strain as a new prognosticator in patients with heart failure," *Journal of the American College of Cardiology*, vol. 54, no. 7, pp. 618–624, 2009.

[124] M. Bertini, A. C. T. Ng, M. L. Antoni et al., "Global longitudinal strain predicts long-term survival in patients with chronic ischemic cardiomyopathy," *Circulation: Cardiovascular Imaging*, vol. 5, no. 3, pp. 383–391, 2012.

[125] M. Iacoviello, A. Puzzovivo, P. Guida et al., "Independent role of left ventricular global longitudinal strain in predicting prognosis of chronic heart failure patients," *Echocardiography*, vol. 30, no. 7, pp. 803–811, 2013.

[126] T. Stanton, R. Leano, and T. H. Marwick, "Prediction of all-cause mortality from global longitudinal speckle strain: comparison with ejection fraction and wall motion scoring," *Circulation: Cardiovascular Imaging*, vol. 2, no. 5, pp. 356–364, 2009.

[127] J. Lekakis, P. Abraham, A. Balbarini et al., "Methods for evaluating endothelial function: a position statement from the European Society of Cardiology Working Group on Peripheral Circulation," *European Journal of Cardiovascular Prevention and Rehabilitation*, vol. 18, no. 6, pp. 775–789, 2011.

[128] A. Dolci, R. Dominici, D. Cardinale, M. T. Sandri, and M. Panteghini, "Biochemical markers for prediction of chemotherapy-induced cardiotoxicity systematic review of the literature and recommendations for use," *The American Journal of Clinical Pathology*, vol. 130, no. 5, pp. 688–695, 2008.

[129] F. J. F. Broeyer, S. Osanto, H. J. Ritsema Van Eck et al., "Evaluation of biomarkers for cardiotoxicity of anthracyclin-based chemotherapy," *Journal of Cancer Research and Clinical Oncology*, vol. 134, no. 9, pp. 961–968, 2008.

[130] S. Romano, S. Fratini, E. Ricevuto et al., "Serial measurements of NT-proBNP are predictive of not-high-dose anthracycline cardiotoxicity in breast cancer patients," *British Journal of Cancer*, vol. 105, no. 11, pp. 1663–1668, 2011.

[131] M. T. Sandri, M. Salvatici, D. Cardinale et al., "N-terminal pro-B-type natriuretic peptide after high-dose chemotherapy: a marker predictive of cardiac dysfunction?" *Clinical Chemistry*, vol. 51, no. 8, pp. 1405–1410, 2005.

[132] A. Kittiwarawut, Y. Vorasettakarnkij, S. Tanasanvimon, S. Manasnayakorn, and V. Sriuranpong, "Serum NT-proBNP in the early detection of doxorubicin-induced cardiac dysfunction," *Asia-Pacific Journal of Clinical Oncology*, vol. 9, no. 2, pp. 155–161, 2013.

[133] H. Sawaya, I. A. Sebag, J. C. Plana et al., "Assessment of echocardiography and biomarkers for the extended prediction of cardiotoxicity in patients treated with anthracyclines, taxanes, and trastuzumab," *Circulation: Cardiovascular Imaging*, vol. 5, no. 5, pp. 596–603, 2012.

[134] H. Sawaya, I. A. Sebag, J. C. Plana et al., "Early detection and prediction of cardiotoxicity in chemotherapy-treated patients," *The American Journal of Cardiology*, vol. 107, no. 9, pp. 1375–1380, 2011.

[135] B. Ky, M. Putt, H. Sawaya et al., "Early increases in multiple biomarkers predict subsequent cardiotoxicity in patients with breast cancer treated with doxorubicin, taxanes, and trastuzumab," *Journal of the American College of Cardiology*, vol. 63, no. 8, pp. 809–816, 2014.

[136] H. W. Auner, C. Tinchon, W. Linkesch et al., "Prolonged monitoring of troponin T for the detection of anthracycline cardiotoxicity in adults with hematological malignancies," *Annals of Hematology*, vol. 82, no. 4, pp. 218–222, 2003.

[137] F. Dodos, T. Halbsguth, E. Erdmann, and U. C. Hoppe, "Usefulness of myocardial performance index and biochemical markers for early detection of anthracycline-induced cardiotoxicity in adults," *Clinical Research in Cardiology*, vol. 97, no. 5, pp. 318–326, 2008.

[138] C. Nisticò, E. Bria, F. Cuppone et al., "Troponin-T and myoglobin plus echocardiographic evaluation for monitoring early

cardiotoxicity of weekly epirubicin-paclitaxel in metastatic breast cancer patients," *Anti-Cancer Drugs*, vol. 18, no. 2, pp. 227–232, 2007.

[139] D. Cardinale, M. T. Sandri, A. Martinoni et al., "Myocardial injury revealed by plasma troponin I in breast cancer treated with high-dose chemotherapy," *Annals of Oncology*, vol. 13, no. 5, pp. 710–715, 2002.

[140] D. Cardinale, M. T. Sandri, A. Colombo et al., "Prognostic value of troponin I in cardiac risk stratification of cancer patients undergoing high-dose chemotherapy," *Circulation*, vol. 109, no. 22, pp. 2749–2754, 2004.

[141] M. T. Sandri, D. Cardinale, L. Zorzino et al., "Minor increases in plasma troponin I predict decreased left ventricular ejection fraction after high-dose chemotherapy," *Clinical Chemistry*, vol. 49, no. 2, pp. 248–252, 2003.

[142] M. Feola, O. Garrone, M. Occelli et al., "Cardiotoxicity after anthracycline chemotherapy in breast carcinoma: effects on left ventricular ejection fraction, troponin I and brain natriuretic peptide," *International Journal of Cardiology*, vol. 148, no. 2, pp. 194–198, 2011.

[143] B. C. Drafts, K. M. Twomley, R. D'Agostino Jr. et al., "Low to moderate dose anthracycline-based chemotherapy is associated with early noninvasive imaging evidence of subclinical cardiovascular disease," *JACC: Cardiovascular Imaging*, vol. 6, no. 8, pp. 877–885, 2013.

[144] B. Erkus, S. Demirtas, A. A. Yarpuzlu, M. Can, Y. Genc, and L. Karaca, "Early prediction of anthracycline induced cardiotoxicity," *Acta Paediatrica, International Journal of Paediatrics*, vol. 96, no. 4, pp. 506–509, 2007.

[145] G. Mercuro, C. Cadeddu, A. Piras et al., "Early epirubicin-induced myocardial dysfunction revealed by serial tissue Doppler echocardiography: correlation with inflammatory and oxidative stress markers," *Oncologist*, vol. 12, no. 9, pp. 1124–1133, 2007.

[146] S. Polena, M. Shikara, S. Naik et al., "Troponin I as a marker of doxorubicin induced cardiotoxicity," *Proceedings of the Western Pharmacology Society*, vol. 48, pp. 142–144, 2005.

[147] D. Cardinale, A. Colombo, R. Torrisi et al., "Trastuzumab-induced cardiotoxicity: clinical and prognostic implications of troponin I evaluation," *Journal of Clinical Oncology*, vol. 28, no. 25, pp. 3910–3916, 2010.

[148] T. Ahmad, M. Fiuzat, D. B. Mark et al., "The effects of exercise on cardiovascular biomarkers in patients with chronic heart failure," *American Heart Journal*, vol. 167, no. 2, pp. 193.e1–202.e1, 2014.

[149] O. Schulz and A. Kromer, "Cardiac troponin I: a potential marker of exercise intolerance in patients with moderate heart failure," *American Heart Journal*, vol. 144, no. 2, pp. 351–358, 2002.

[150] U. Wisløff, Ø. Ellingsen, and O. J. Kemi, "High-intensity interval training to maximize cardiac benefits of exercise training?" *Exercise and Sport Sciences Reviews*, vol. 37, no. 3, pp. 139–146, 2009.

[151] U. Wisløff, A. Støylen, J. P. Loennechen et al., "Superior cardiovascular effect of aerobic interval training versus moderate continuous training in heart failure patients: a randomized study," *Circulation*, vol. 115, no. 24, pp. 3086–3094, 2007.

[152] C. A. Emter and D. K. Bowles, "Curing the cure: utilizing exercise to limit cardiotoxicity," *Medicine and Science in Sports and Exercise*, vol. 40, no. 5, pp. 806–807, 2008.

[153] M. J. Haykowsky, Y. Liang, D. Pechter, L. W. Jones, F. A. McAlister, and A. M. Clark, "A Meta-analysis of the effect of exercise training on left ventricular remodeling in heart failure patients: the benefit depends on the type of training performed," *Journal of the American College of Cardiology*, vol. 49, no. 24, pp. 2329–2336, 2007.

[154] K. M. Baldwin and F. Haddad, "Invited review: effects of different activity and inactivity paradigms on myosin heavy chain gene expression in striated muscle," *Journal of Applied Physiology*, vol. 90, no. 1, pp. 345–357, 2001.

[155] E. L. de Beer, A. E. Bottone, J. van der Velden, and E. E. Voest, "Doxorubicin impairs crossbridge turnover kinetics in skinned cardiac trabeculae after acute and chronic treatment," *Molecular Pharmacology*, vol. 57, no. 6, pp. 1152–1157, 2000.

[156] H.-B. Kwak, W. Song, and J. M. Lawler, "Exercise training attenuates age-induced elevation in Bax/Bcl-2 ratio, apoptosis, and remodeling in the rat heart," *The FASEB Journal*, vol. 20, no. 6, pp. 791–793, 2006.

[157] M. Marcil, K. Bourduas, A. Ascah, and Y. Burelle, "Exercise training induces respiratory substrate-specific decrease in Ca^{2+}-induced permeability transition pore opening in heart mitochondria," *The American Journal of Physiology—Heart and Circulatory Physiology*, vol. 290, no. 4, pp. H1549–H1557, 2006.

[158] D. Montaigne, X. Marechal, S. Preau et al., "Doxorubicin induces mitochondrial permeability transition and contractile dysfunction in the human myocardium," *Mitochondrion*, vol. 11, no. 1, pp. 22–26, 2011.

[159] V. Adams, A. Linke, S. Gielen, S. Erbs, R. Hambrecht, and G. Schuler, "Modulation of Murf-1 and MAFbx expression in the myocardium by physical exercise training," *European Journal of Cardiovascular Prevention and Rehabilitation*, vol. 15, no. 3, pp. 293–299, 2008.

[160] Y. Shi, M. Moon, S. Dawood, B. McManus, and P. P. Liu, "Mechanisms and management of doxorubicin cardiotoxicity," *Herz*, vol. 36, no. 4, pp. 296–305, 2011.

[161] S. Hamed, I. Barshack, G. Luboshits et al., "Erythropoietin improves myocardial performance in doxorubicin-induced cardiomyopathy," *European Heart Journal*, vol. 27, no. 15, pp. 1876–1883, 2006.

[162] H. A. Demirel, K. L. Hamilton, R. A. Shanely, N. Tümer, M. J. Koroly, and S. K. Powers, "Age and attenuation of exercise-induced myocardial HSP72 accumulation," *American Journal of Physiology: Heart and Circulatory Physiology*, vol. 285, no. 4, pp. H1609–H1615, 2003.

[163] T. Ohtsuboa, E. Kanob, K. Uedac et al., "Enhancement of heat-induced heat shock protein (hsp)72 accumulation by doxorubicin (Dox) in vitro," *Cancer Letters*, vol. 159, no. 1, pp. 49–55, 2000.

[164] O. J. Kemi, M. Ceci, G. Condorelli, G. L. Smith, and U. Wisloff, "Myocardial sarcoplasmic reticulum Ca^{2+} ATPase function is increased by aerobic interval training," *European Journal of Cardiovascular Prevention and Rehabilitation*, vol. 15, no. 2, pp. 145–148, 2008.

[165] R. D. Olson, H. A. Gambliel, R. E. Vestal, S. E. Shadle, H. A. Charlier Jr., and B. J. Cusack, "Doxorubicin cardiac dysfunction: effects on calcium regulatory proteins, sarcoplasmic reticulum, and triiodothyronine," *Cardiovascular Toxicology*, vol. 5, no. 3, pp. 269–283, 2005.

[166] V. W. Dolinsky, K. J. Rogan, M. M. Sung et al., "Both aerobic exercise and resveratrol supplementation attenuate doxorubicin-induced cardiac injury in mice," *American Journal of Physiology—Endocrinology and Metabolism*, vol. 305, no. 2, pp. E243–E253, 2013.

[167] P. M. Siu, R. W. Bryner, J. K. Marty, and S. E. Alway, "Apoptotic adaptations from exercise training in skeletal and cardiac muscles," *The FASEB Journal*, vol. 18, no. 10, pp. 1150–1152, 2004.

[168] S. H. Kim, D. Kim, G. S. Jung, J. H. Um, B. S. Chung, and C. D. Kang, "Involvement of c-Jun NH_2-terminal kinase pathway in differential regulation of heat shock proteins by anticancer drugs," *Biochemical and Biophysical Research Communications*, vol. 262, no. 2, pp. 516–522, 1999.

[169] D. L. Coven, X. Hu, L. Cong et al., "Physiological role of AMP-activated protein kinase in the heart: graded activation during exercise," *American Journal of Physiology - Endocrinology and Metabolism*, vol. 285, no. 3, pp. E629–E636, 2003.

[170] M. Tokarska-Schlattner, M. Zaugg, R. da Silva et al., "Acute toxicity of doxorubicin on isolated perfused heart: response of kinases regulating energy supply," *American Journal of Physiology—Heart and Circulatory Physiology*, vol. 289, no. 1, pp. H37–H47, 2005.

[171] P. Boström, N. Mann, J. Wu et al., "C/EBPβ controls exercise-induced cardiac growth and protects against pathological cardiac remodeling," *Cell*, vol. 143, no. 7, pp. 1072–1083, 2010.

[172] A. de Angelis, E. Piegari, D. Cappetta et al., "Anthracycline cardiomyopathy is mediated by depletion of the cardiac stem cell pool and is rescued by restoration of progenitor cell function," *Circulation*, vol. 121, no. 2, pp. 276–292, 2010.

[173] Y. Yang, H. Zhang, X. Li, T. Yang, and Q. Jiang, "Effects of PPARα/PGC-1α on the myocardial energy metabolism during heart failure in the doxorubicin induced dilated cardiomyopathy in mice," *International Journal of Clinical and Experimental Medicine*, vol. 7, pp. 2435–2442, 2014.

[174] D. B. Sawyer, C. Zuppinger, T. A. Miller, H. M. Eppenberger, and T. M. Suter, "Modulation of anthracycline-induced myofibrillar disarray in rat ventricular myocytes by neuregulin-1β and anti-erbB2: potential mechanism for trastuzumab-induced cardiotoxicity," *Circulation*, vol. 105, no. 13, pp. 1551–1554, 2002.

[175] Y. Kim, A.-G. Ma, K. Kitta et al., "Anthracycline-induced suppression of GATA-4 transcription factor: implication in the regulation of cardiac myocyte apoptosis," *Molecular Pharmacology*, vol. 63, no. 2, pp. 368–377, 2003.

15

Evolving Concepts: Immunity in Oncology from Targets to Treatments

Hina Khan,[1] Rasim Gucalp,[2] and Iuliana Shapira[3]

[1]*Department of Hematology Oncology, Montefiore Medical Center, Albert Einstein School of Medicine, 1300 Morris Park Avenue, Bronx, NY 10461, USA*

[2]*Department of Oncology, Montefiore Medical Center, Albert Einstein School of Medicine, 1300 Morris Park Avenue, Bronx, NY 10461, USA*

[3]*Department of Hematology Oncology, Hofstra North Shore LIJ School of Medicine, Hempstead, NY 11549, USA*

Correspondence should be addressed to Hina Khan; hkhan@montefiore.org

Academic Editor: Bruno Vincenzi

Cancer is associated with global immune suppression of the host. Malignancy-induced immune suppressive effect can be circumvented by blocking the immune checkpoint and tip the immune balance in favor of immune stimulation and unleash cytotoxic effects on cancer cells. Human antibodies directed against immune checkpoint proteins: cytotoxic T lymphocytes antigen-4 (CTLA-4) and programmed death-1 (PD-1), programmed death-ligand 1 (PD-L1), have shown therapeutic efficacy in advanced melanoma and non-small-cell lung cancer and other malignancies. Immune check point blockade antibodies lead to diminished tolerance to self and enhanced immune ability to recognize and eliminate cancer cells. As a class these agents have immune-related adverse events due to decreased ability of effector immune cells to discriminate between self and non-self. Seventy percent of patients participating in clinical trials have experienced anticancer activities and varying degrees of immune mediated dose-limiting side effects.

1. Background

Global Immune Suppression Precedes the Development of Overt Malignancy: Mechanisms. Developing malignancies evade immune detection due to failure of T lymphocytes to recognize and respond to tumor specific antigens. Patients with advanced metastatic disease and large tumor burdens manifest a global immune suppression as evidenced by decrease response to challenge with common antigens and diminished T-cell function [1–5].

Epidemiological studies suggest occult malignancy is associated with global immune suppression and diminished immune surveillance with manifestations such as zoster, tuberculosis, and viral reactivation. Clinical reactivation of herpes zoster precedes overt cancer by more than 800 days [6–8].

T-cells are able to recognize and eliminate foreign antigens when presented to T-cell receptor (TCR) in the context of self-major histocompatibility complex (MHC), to activate immune responses following TCR binding a second, more adhesive, signal to create immune synapse necessary for T-cell activation. The second signal comes from cell-cell interaction between CD28 on T-cell and B-7 receptors (either CD80 or CD86) on antigen presenting cells (APC). Once T-cell is activated it becomes CD8+, effector T-cell capable of recognizing and eliminating cells marked by foreign antigen and generating intracellular signals producing interleukin-2 (IL-2) a cytokine that promotes T-cell proliferation [9].

Activated T-cells start expressing CTLA-4 receptor, an immune check point receptor, which has a higher binding affinity for B-7 ligand than CD28. CTLA4 displaces CD28 from B7 receptors leading to termination of effector immune responses and establishment of tolerance for the antigen presented minimizing the danger of autoimmunity. In activated T-cells CTLA4 is induced by ligation of CD28 to B7 ligands while T-regulatory cells (CD4+ CD25+) constitutively express CTLA4.

Table 1: B-7 family of receptor ligands expressed by antigen presenting cells and various malignancies: CD cluster derivation; B7.1 known as CD80; B7.2 known as CD86; CD-28 and CD-152 present on T-naïve cells; ICOS inducible costimulatory ligand; (+) with and (−) without; CD152 also known as CTLA4 cytotoxic T lymphocytes antigen-4; PD-1 programmed death-1 also known as CD279; PD-L1 programmed death-ligand 1 known as B7-H1 or CD274; PD-L2 programmed death-ligand 2, known as CD273 or B7-DC B-7 dendritic cell; IFN-γ interferon gamma; IL-2 interleukin 2; Ref reference.

B-7 family molecules	CD-designation	Major ligands on immune cells	Role immunity activation versus immune suppression	Malignancies expressing B-7 molecules	Ref
B7.1	CD80	CD28; CTLA4 (CD152)	(+) 2nd signal activation (−) second signal anergy	CD-80 on acute myeloid leukemia cells	[37]
B7.2	CD86	CD28; CTLA4 (CD152)	(+) 2nd signal activation (−) second signal anergy	CD-86 on chronic lymphatic leukemia cells	[46]
B7-H1 (PD-L1)	CD274	PD-1 (CD279)	Ligating PD-1 on T-cells suppresses CD8+ response	None	[47]
B7-H2; B7-H3; B7-H6; ICOS	CD275	CD278	Immune suppression	Dendritic cells infiltrating malignancies; cancer cells: hematologic malignancies, breast, gastrointestinal, lung, melanoma, bladder, and genitourinary cancers	[48]
PD-L2 B7-DC	CD273	PD-1 (CD279)	Immune suppression reduces IL-2 and IFN-γ secretion, decreases proliferation and cytotoxicity, and induces apoptosis in activated T-cells	Primary mediastinal (thymic) large B-cell lymphoma	[49]

In addition interactions between B-7 on APC and immune check point receptors PD-1 and or CTLA4 lead to production of arginase and indolamine dioxygenase (IDO) [9]. IDO decreases T-cell access to tryptophan starvation, transforms tryptophan to N formyl-kynurenine inducing T-cell apoptosis [10] further decreasing cytotoxic effector T-cell responses to tumor associated antigens (TAA). High IDO expression is an independent prognostic variable for reduced overall survival in cancer patients [11]. Arginase depletes tumor microenvironment from the essential amino acid arginine needed for zeta chain synthesis of the T-cell [12], the principal signal-transduction element of the T-cell receptor (TCR), without arginine T-cells becoming anergic [13, 14]. Arginase and indolamine dioxygenase deplete the microenvironment from arginine and tryptophan, two essential amino acids critical for CD8+ T-cell survival; absence of these amino acids leads to CD8+ cell anergy and death [15].

Programmed death-1 (PD-1) is a protein that belongs to CD-28 family and is expressed on T-cells, dendritic cells, natural killer cells, macrophages, and B-cells [16]. PD-1 is not expressed on resting T-cells but is inducible, appearing within 24 h after stimulation and T-cell activation [17] (Table 1).

PD-1 has three known ligands PD-L1 (programmed death ligand-1), PD-L2 (programmed death ligand-2), and B7-1 (CD80) [18]. PD-L1 can be expressed by T-cells, B-cells, myeloid dendritic cells, and at very low levels tissue macrophages in the lung, kidney, liver, heart, and placenta [19, 20]. PD-L1 is constitutively expressed on many solid and hematological malignancies [21–30] (Table 1). When PD-1 binds to PD-L1 and PD-L2 (programmed death ligand), the immune responses are dampened and T-cell becomes unresponsive [31]. PD-L1 binding to B7-1 on antigen reactive

T-cells inhibits late stage T-cell responses [18] and limits the response to inflammation [30, 32–34]. Blockade of PD-1 on regulatory T-cells (CD4+, CD25+) inhibits their ability to mediate tolerance [35–37] (Table 1).

Blocking humanized monoclonal antibodies against cytotoxic T lymphocyte antigen-4-mediated PD-1, PD-L1, and PD-L2 prevents binding to (CD80/CD86) allowing them to be available for CD28 binding and T-cell activation and decreasing immune tolerance to tumor associated antigens [38, 39] (Figure 2).

Malignant cells express members of B7 family of receptors such as CD80, CD86, PD-L1, PD-L2, and ICOS (Table 1), with high affinity for CTLA4 and or PD-1 converting T-cells into anergic and tolerant regulatory T-cells (T-regs).

In various cancer types high expression of PD-L1 on tumor cells and to a lesser extent of PD-L2 has been found to correlate with poor prognosis and survival [40].

Levels of circulating immune suppressor cells are three to five times higher in patients with advanced head and neck, non-small-cell lung cancer, pancreatic cancer, and colon and breast cancer, when compared to normal controls [41] supporting the conclusion that immune anergy, tolerance, and suppression are central not only to cancer development but also to cancer progression [42].

The initial research attempts to manipulating immune response by stimulating effector T-cells in antigen-independent fashion were done using a humanized CD-28 molecule TGN1412. TGN1412 activated CD28 positive effector T-cells with antitumor activity in animal models of cancer including in primates. In a phase I clinical trial TGN1412 induced a "cytokine storm" in all six enrolled participants leading to life-threatening multiorgan failure in normal human volunteers.

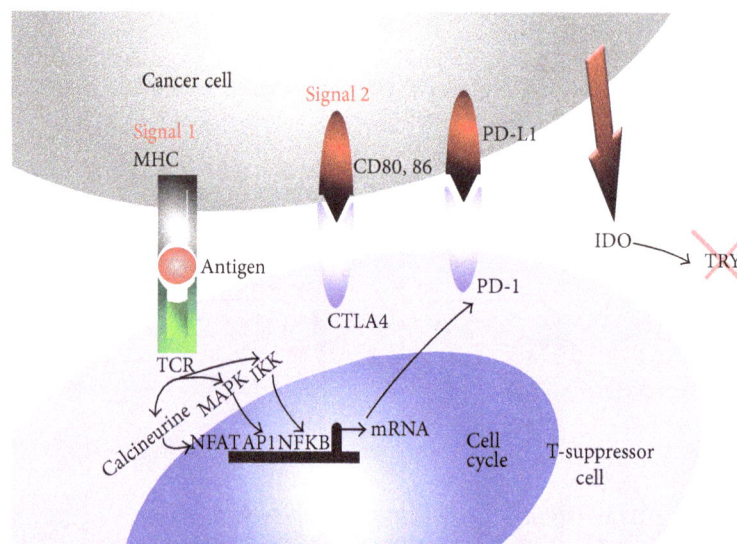

FIGURE 1: Cancer cell mediated immune suppression: upon ligation CTLA4 or PD-1 on suppressor cells, cancer cells produce 2,3 indolamine dioxygenase (IDO) and others (arginase, nitric oxide synthase) degrading amino acids arginine and tryptophan necessary for immune detection and elimination function of the effector CD8+ T-cells. Cancer cells undergo phenotypic or genomic modification under immune attack resulting in the survival and selection of variants that are capable of escaping immune attack. These modifications include HLA class 1, loss of tumor antigens, lack of death receptor signaling, regulatory T-cells, inhibitory cytokines, and immune check point molecules. Ligation of PD-L1 on the tumor cell surface results in tumor protection from cell death [82]. Interactions between PD-L1 and PD-1 in the tumor microenvironment protect the tumor through several distinct pathways including the ligation of PD-1 by PD-L1 on antigen specific T-cells leading to functional anergy and/or apoptosis of these effector T-cells [19, 83]. Effector T cells are further inhibited by PD-L1:CD80 interactions [18]. While PD-L1 interactions with PD-1 on cytotoxic CD8 T-cells dampen tumor specific effector immunity, PD-L1 PD1 interaction on T-regulatory cells (CD4+, CD25+) increases their suppressive function [35–37]. IDO: indolamine 2,3 deoxygenase; TCR: T cell receptor; MHC: major histocompatibility antigen; IL-2: interleukin-2; CTLA4 cytotoxic T lymphocytes antigen-4; PD-1: programmed death-1 also known as CD279; PD-L1 programmed death-ligand 1 known as B7-H1 or CD274; PD-L2 programmed death-ligand 2, known as CD273 or B7-DC B-7 dendritic cell; IFN-γ: interferon gamma; IL-2: interleukin-2; APC: antigen presenting cells; TRY: tryptophan, AP-1: activator protein-1; NFAT: nuclear factor of activated T-cells; NFKB: nuclear factor kappa B; MAPK: mitogen activated protein kinase; IKK: I kappa B kinase; PI3K: phosphatidylinositol-4,5-biphosphate 3-kinase; CDK: cyclin dependant kinase; JAK3: Janus kinase 3; mTOR: mammalian target of rapamycin.

Current immune check point inhibitors anti-CTLA-4, anti-PD-1, and anti-PDL1 therapies are not antigen specific thus able to bind common molecular epitopes that are expressed on the targeted as well as on the nontargeted T-cells [43].

2. Immune Check Point Inhibitors in Use and Clinical Trials

(1) Ipilimumab. A fully humanized IgG1 monoclonal antibody [BMS-734016] recognizing CTLA-4 interferes with CTLA-B7 interactions on the surface of antigen presenting cells, permitting CD28-B7 complex formation. Since 2011, Ipilimumab is approved for the treatment of unresectable or metastatic melanoma at 3 mg/kg intravenous every 3 weeks for a total of 4 doses. It is currently undergoing trials for the treatment of non-small-cell lung carcinoma, bladder cancer, and metastatic castrate resistant prostate cancer (Table 2).

(2) Tremelimumab. A CTLA-4 blocking Ig G2 monoclonal antibody showed durable responses in advanced melanoma patients in early phase studies; however in phase III trial at dose of 15 mg/kg versus standard chemotherapy, Tremelimumab showed no survival benefits. It is being investigated in colorectal, gastric, and NSCLC patients (Table 2).

(3) Nivolumab. [BMS-936558, MDX-1106] A humanized IgG4 monoclonal antibody blocking PD-1. In phase I clinical trials, doses from 1 to 10 mg/kg every 2 weeks showed objective responses in 20–25% of patients with non-small-cell carcinoma (NSCLC), melanoma, and RCC [44]. Phase III trials are currently underway at 3 mg/kg dosing every 2 weeks, to evaluate its efficacy in renal cell carcinoma (RCC), NSCLC, and melanoma (Table 2).

(4) Pembrolizumab. Formerly known as Lambrolizumab [MK-3475], a humanized IgG4 monoclonal antibody binding to PD-1 it is the first anti-PD-1 agent approved by FDA. It is used in relapsed or refractory malignant melanoma following treatment with Ipilimumab or after treatment with Ipilimumab and a BRAF inhibitor in patients who carry a BRAF mutation at doses from 2 mg/kg to 10 mg/kg (Table 2).

(5) MPDL3280. It is a humanized IgG1 monoclonal antibody blocking PD-L1. In phase I setting, with doses ranging from 1 to 20 mg/kg every 3 weeks, an overall response (ORR) of 21% was seen in locally advanced or metastatic solid tumors such as melanoma, RCC, NSCLC, colon cancer, gastric cancer, head and neck squamous cell carcinoma (HNSCC), and lymphomas. Currently ongoing trials are evaluating its use in advanced melanoma, NSCLC, metastatic RCC, and metastatic urothelial bladder cancer (Table 2).

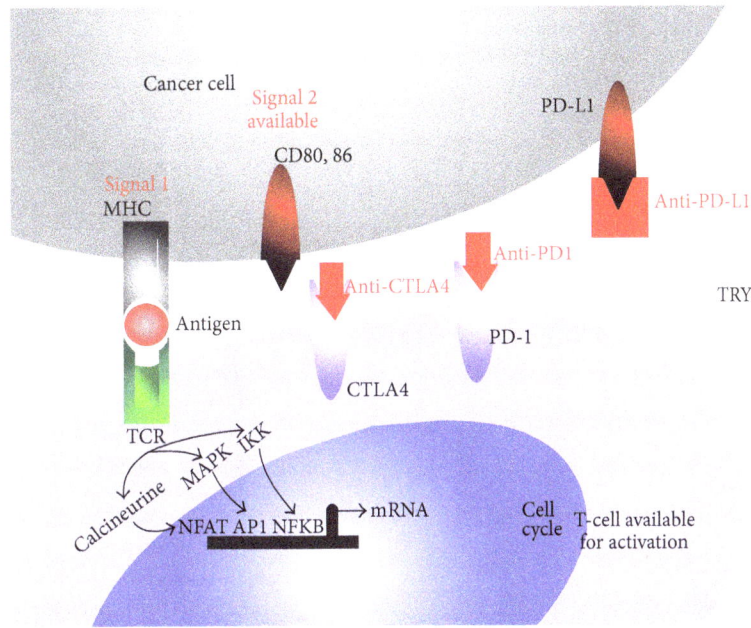

FIGURE 2: Immune therapy in cancer: blocking CTLA4-B7 interactions to enhance T-cell activation could help overcome tumor antigen tolerance and consequently potentiate enhanced antitumoral responses. Blocking PD-1, PD-L1 allows for more B7 family members on immune cells such as CD80/CD86 to be available and bind CD28 (Figure 1) allowing for more activated effector T-cells capable to recognize and eliminate cells bearing cancer antigens. TCR: T-cell receptor; MHC: major histocompatibility antigen; IL-2: interleukin-2; CTLA4: cytotoxic T lymphocytes antigen-4; PD-1: programmed death-1 also known as CD279; PD-L1: programmed death-ligand 1 known as B7-H1 or CD274; PD-L2: programmed death-ligand 2, known as CD273 or B7-DC B-7 dendritic cell; IFN-γ: interferon gamma; IL-2: interleukin-2; APC: antigen presenting cells; TRY: tryptophan; AP-1: activator protein-1; NFAT: nuclear factor of activated T-cells; NFKB: nuclear factor kappa B; MAPK: mitogen activated protein kinase; IKK: I kappa B kinase; PI3K: phosphatidylinositol-4,5-biphosphate 3-kinase; CDK: cyclin dependant kinase; JAK3: Janus kinase 3; mTOR: mammalian target of rapamycin; anti-CTLA4: antibody blocking CTLA4; anti-PD-1: antibody blocking PD-1; anti-PD-L1: antibody blocking PD-L1.

(6) MS-936559. A humanized PD-L1 Ig-G4 blocking monoclonal antibody [MDX-1105] blocks binding of PD-L1 to PD-1. Phase I studies in metastatic melanoma and NSCLC at doses ranging from 0.1 to 10 mg/kg every 2 weeks for up to 16 cycles, with 3 doses in each cycle being discontinued due to excellent results seen with Nivolumab.

(7) Pidilizumab. A humanized monoclonal IgG1 antibody [CT-011] blocks PD-1, the binding of PD-1 to PD-L1 and PD-L2. Early phases I-II trials are underway at doses of 0.2–0.6 mg/kg intravenously in diffuse large B-cell lymphoma (DLBCL) and metastatic colorectal cancer.

In animal studies, combination of immune check point inhibitors such as combining anti-CTLA4 and anti-PD1 antibodies enhanced effectory T-cell infiltration in tumor lesions resulting in decreased regulatory T-cell density [45]. There are clinical trials described below that use combination of immune check point inhibitors.

3. Malignancies Treated with Immune Checkpoint Blocking Monoclonal Antibodies

3.1. Malignant Melanoma. Stage IV melanoma treated with Dacarbazine for many years had dismal outcome with a median overall survival of 6–10 months and a 5-year survival

rate of 10% [84, 85]. Immune therapy for melanoma focused on recombinant cytokines interferon alpha-2b (IFN α-2b) and interleukin-2 (IL-2). High dose IL-2 for advanced disease reported overall responses (ORR) of 5–27% and complete responses of up to 4% of patients [86]. High doses of IFN α-2b prolonged disease-free survival by 5% and, when used in the adjuvant setting, increased overall survival (OS) in high-risk patients by 3% [87].

Melanoma cells evade immune detection by downregulating surface HLA class I antigens with concomitant upregulation of nonclassical HLA-G antigen. Melanoma cells constitutively overexpress Fas receptor (FAS-R). FAS-ligand (FAS-L) is overexpressed on activated effector CD8+ T cells. Binding of FAS-R on the surface of melanoma cells to the FAS-L leads to apoptotic death of activated T-cells. Melanoma cells upregulate immune coinhibitory signals the PD-L1 (B7-H1) ligand and upon binding of these ligands on PD-1 receptor on T-cells immune suppressive cytokines are released from the malignant cell further impairing immune detection.

Ipilimumab, anti-CTLA4 human IgG1 antibody, showed sustained responses for longer than 2 years in metastatic malignant melanoma patients. A randomized, double-blind, dose-ranging clinical study with 88 patients of unresectable stage III or IV melanoma showed response rates as high as 11.1% and survival data of up to 30%. Grade 3 or 4 adverse events such as colitis, rash, and liver function abnormalities were observed in 19% of patients [39, 50, 88].

TABLE 2: Currently available immune check point inhibitors in clinical use. CD152 also known as CTLA4 cytotoxic T lymphocytes antigen-4; PD-1: programmed death-1 also known as CD279; PD-L1: programmed death-ligand 1 known as B7-H1 or CD274; PD-L2: programmed death-ligand 2, known as CD273 or B7-DC B-7 dendritic cell; IFN-γ: interferon gamma; IL-2: interleukin-2; AE: adverse events; NSCLC: non-small-cell carcinoma; RCC: renal cell carcinoma, ORR: overall response; HNSCC: head and neck squamous cell carcinoma; OS: overall survival; PFS: progression-free survival; RECIST: response evaluation criteria in solid tumors; vs: versus; gp100: vaccine glycoprotein 100 vaccine; FIGO: Federation International for Gynecologic Oncology; RCC: renal cell carcinoma; CRPC: castrate resistant prostate cancer; SCC: squamous cell carcinoma.

Type of cancer	Drug	Target	Clinical trial, Phase	Outcome	Ref
Malignant melanoma	Ipilimumab (FDA approved in 2011)	CTLA-4	NCT00094653, III	676 unresectable stage III or IV melanoma treated with Ipilimumab vs gp100 vaccine. Improved survival with Ipilimumab, with median OS 10 months. Grades 3-4 AEs seen only in 10–15% patients.	[38]
	Ipilimumab	CTLA-4	I/II	Among 88 patients with unresectable stage III/IV melanoma treated with Ipilimumab at different dose levels, 7 had stable disease and 2 had response. Grades 3-4 AEs were only seen in 14% patients.	[50]
	Ipilimumab + Dacarbazine vs Dacarbazine	CTLA-4	NCT00324155, III	502 patients with untreated metastatic melanoma were given Ipilimumab + Dacarbazine vs Dacarbazine alone. Median OS was 11 months in combination arm vs 9 months with Dacarbazine only arm.	[51]
	Ipilimumab + Dacarbazine vs Ipilimumab	CTLA-4	NCT00050102, II	72 patients with unresectable, metastatic melanoma received Ipilimumab with Dacarbazine or Ipilimumab alone. ORR was 14.3% with median OS 14.3 months in first arm vs ORR of 5.4% with median OS 11.4 months in second arm.	[52]
	Tremelimumab	CTLA-4	NCT00086489, I/II	28 patients with metastatic melanoma received escalating (3, 6, and 10 mg/kg) doses of Tremelimumab. Durable antitumor responses were seen and drug was well tolerable.	[53]
	Tremelimumab	CTLA-4	NCT00257205, III	In 534 patients with treatment naïve, unresectable stage III or IV melanoma, median OS was 12.6 months in Tremelimumab arm vs 10.7 months in Temozolamide or Dacarbazine arm. ORR was similar in both arms but response duration was 35.8 months vs 13.7 months. No significant survival advantage was seen.	[54]
	Nivolumab	PD-1	NCT00441337, I	10 patients with advanced metastatic melanoma showed evidence of antitumor activity with Nivolumab and drug was well tolerated.	[55]
	Nivolumab	PD-1	NCT00730639, I	Among 107 advanced melanoma patients treated with Nivolumab, 33 had objective tumor regression, with a response duration of 2 years, and median OS was 16.8 months.	[56]
	Pembrolizumab (MK-3475)	PD-1	NCT01295827, I	MK-3475 was used in 173 patients with advanced melanoma who progressed after Ipilimumab. ORR was 26% and treatment was well tolerated.	[57–59]
	MPDL3280A	PD-L1	NCT01375842, I	In 45 melanoma patients, MPDL3280A was well tolerated and an ORR of 26% was observed. 24-week PFS was 25%.	[60]
	BMS-936559	PD-L1	NCT00729664, I	Among 55 melanoma patients, durable tumor responses and prolonged stable disease were seen.	[61]

TABLE 2: Continued.

Type of cancer	Drug	Target	Clinical trial, Phase	Outcome	Ref
Lung	Ipilimumab	CTLA-4	II	An objective response rate of 19% for NSCLC patients with squamous histology and 15% with nonsquamous histology. Patients who received phased Ipilimumab and Carboplatin and Paclitaxel showed improved PFS as compared to Carboplatin/Paclitaxel alone.	[62]
	Nivolumab	PD-1	I	Among 6 heavily pretreated patients with NSCLC, one had partial remission for over 14 months and other 5 had stable disease.	[55]
	Nivolumab	PD-1	I	Among 129 NSCLC patients, 17% had objective responses. Best response of 24% was seen at 3 mg/kg dose and median OS was 14.9 months. Durable and rapid responses, with OS 42% at 1 year and 24% at 2 years, across all histological subtypes. Median OS was 9.2 m in squamous and 10.1 m in nonsquamous.	[63–65]
	Pembrolizumab (MK-3475)	PD-1	I	Among 38 patients with advanced NSCLC who received >2 prior therapies, responses as early as 9 weeks were seen in 24% patients, both in squamous and non-squamous histologies. Median OS was 51 weeks.	[66]
	BMS-936559	PD-L1	I	Among 49 patients with advanced NSCLC, objective responses were seen in 6 patients and another 6 with stable disease (both squamous and nonsquamous subtypes).	[61]
	MPDL-3280A	PD-L1	NCT01375842, I	85 patients with NSCLC were evaluated for safety and 53 for efficacy. ORR was 21% with higher rates in PD-L1 positive tumors. Responses were sustained and dramatic response was seen in the smoking cohort.	[67, 68]
	MEDI-4736	PD-L1	NCT01693562, I	In 13 heavily retreated NSCLC patients (median 4 lines of prior treatment), 3 patients achieved PR and 2 with response not reaching PR as early as 6 weeks. Response was durable. Acceptable safety profile at all doses.	[69]
	Tremelimumab vs best supportive care	CTLA-4	NCT00312975, II	Among 87 patients with locally advanced or metastatic NSCLC, no superiority in PFS was seen in study arm over BSC. 4.8% ORR was seen.	[70]
Metastatic CRPC	Ipilimumab	CTLA-4	NCT00323882, I/II	50 CRPC patients received Ipilimumab 10 mg/kg and RT and had manageable AEs. Eight patients had PSA decline >50%, 1 had CR and 6 had stable disease.	[71]
	Ipilimumab	CTLA-4	III	No difference in OS with Ipilimumab vs placebo in post-Docetaxel CRPC and bone metastasis following radiation therapy. PFS advantage was seen with Ipilimumab.	[72]
	Nivolumab (BMS-936558)	PD-1	NCT00730639, I	No objective responses were seen in 17 CRPC enrolled.	[63]

Type of cancer	Drug	Target	Clinical trial, Phase	Outcome	Ref
Metastatic RCC	Nivolumab	PD-1	NCT01354431, II	168 patients with metastatic clear cell RCC, median duration of response was 15.7 months and median OS was 18.2 months. 54% of responses lasted >12–20+ months.	[44]
	Nivolumab	PD-1	NCT01358721, I	91 patients with metastatic RCC, Nivolumab showed clinical activity in previously treated and untreated metastatic RCC [ORR 16%]. Median duration of response was 15 months. Responses were higher in PD-L1+ patients (ORR 22%) but also seen in PD-L1 patients (ORR 8%).	[73]
	Nivolumab + Sunitinib or Pazopanib	PD-1	NCT01472081, I	Seven patients with metastatic RCC received Nivolumab in combination with Sunitinib (S) (33 patients) or Pazopanib (P) (20 patients). 41% had responses as early as 6 weeks, with ORR 52% in (S) arm; 56% has responses as early as 6 weeks, with ORR 45% in (P) arm PFS at 24 weeks was 78% for S arm and 55% for (P) arm.	[74]
	MPDL3280A	PD-L1	NCT01375842, I	53 patients with metastatic RCC were evaluated for efficacy and safety. RECIST responses were observed across all doses and some has prolonged stable disease prior to RECIST response. 24-month PFS was 50%.	[75]
	Nivolumab + Ipilimumab	CTLA-4	NCT01472081, I	ORR was 29% in Nivolumab (N) and Ipilimumab (I) (N-3 mg/kg and I-1 mg/kg) arm. ORR was 39% in N-1 mg/kg and I-3 mg/kg arm. Stable disease was seen in 33% in N3 + I1 arm and 39% in N1 + I3 arm.	[76]
Urothelial bladder	MPDL3280A	PD-L1	NCT01375842, I	ORR was 50% with a median time to response of 43 days, among 31 metastatic urothelial bladder cancer patients, including visceral metastases.	[71]
Ovarian	Ipilimumab	CTLA-4	I	Among 2 pretreated advanced ovarian cancer patients, CA-125 level stabilization was seen in one and reduction in the other.	[77]
	Ipilimumab	CTLA-4	I	Among 11 patients with FIGO stage IV ovarian cancer, who previously received GVAX-antitumor activity was seen in one with dramatic fall in CA-125 and regression of metastatic lesions. Another 5 patients had stable disease per CA-125 and imaging.	[78]
	MDX-1105 (BMS-936559)	PD-L1	NCT00729664, I	Among 17 patients with ovarian cancer, 1 has partial response and 3 had stable disease lasting at least 24 weeks, all at 10 mg/kg dose.	[61]
SCC head and neck	MPDL3280A	PD-L1	NCT01375842, I/II	One patient with metastatic head and neck cancer had response by second cycle of therapy.	[79]
	MK3475	PD-1	NCT01848834, IB	On interim analysis of 60 patients with metastatic or recurrent head and neck cancer, drug was well tolerated. Tumor shrinkage was seen in many patients, but protocol specific analysis is pending.	[80]
	MEDI4736	PD-L1	NCT01693562, I	Preliminary data suggests that even in heavily pretreated patients of head and neck cancer, tumor shrinkage was detectable as early as 6 weeks.	[81]

In combination with Dacarbazine, Ipilimumab increased response rates of 10% were seen with combination treatment when compared with single treatment controls [51, 52].

A phase III randomized trial showed that, at a dose level of 3 mg/kg, a median overall survival of 10 months was seen. When Ipilimumab was combined with an HLA-A*0201-restricted gp100 vaccine peptide the median OS was 10.1 months; gp100 peptide treatment alone showed a median overall survival of 6.4 months [38]. Ipilimumab is FDA approved at dose of 3 mg/kg once every 3 weeks for 4 times for the treatment of unresectable or metastatic melanoma (stages III and IV disease). Of note, patients who experience immune-related adverse events are more likely to benefit from treatment with Ipilimumab.

Phase III study comparing Tremelimumab with chemotherapy (Dacarbazine and Temozolomide), indicated no increase in OS (12.6 m versus 10.7 m) and had similar ORR (10.7% versus 9.8%) except significantly longer response duration after Tremelimumab [54]. About 40% patients develop immune-related adverse events through the universal activation of T-cells, leading to tissue-specific inflammation and autoimmune related side effects, such as dermatitis, colitis and hepatitis, and panhypophysitis. The immune adverse events are best managed by systemic steroid treatment, without decrease in antibody therapy benefit [54].

Ten patients with metastatic melanoma treated with Nivolumab had benefit in a phase I study: one had partial response and one had tumor regression not meeting partial response (PR) criteria. Frequent side effects were decreased CD4+ count, lymphopenia, fatigue, and musculoskeletal events. Immune mediated events: inflammatory colitis, hypothyroidism, and polyarticular arthropathies were under 10% [55]. A phase I/II clinical trial with Nivolumab in 107 patients with stage IV melanoma showed sustained clinical response, which persisted even after cessation of therapy and a median OS of 16.8 months, 62% 1-year and 43% 2-year survival rates. Grades 3 and 4 toxicities were seen in only 5% of patients [56, 89].

Pembrolizumab (MK-3475, formerly called Lambrolizumab) was FDA approved in September 2014 for use in relapsed or refractory malignant melanoma following treatment with Ipilimumab or after treatment with Ipilimumab and a BRAF inhibitor in patients who carry a BRAF mutation. In early phase trial of a total of 135 patients with advanced melanoma, using doses from 2 mg/kg to 10 mg/kg response rates up to 38% were seen and a median progression-free survival >7 months [57]. There was a durable antitumor effect seen, with 87% of responders with ongoing response for more than 13 months of follow-up. At one year 81% of patients treated survived. Low grade fatigue, pruritus, and rash were common. If the tumors were PD-L1 positive an improved ORR and PFS by RECIST were seen (51% versus 6% in PD-L1 negative). One-year OS rate was 84% in PD-L1 positive and 69% in PD-L1 negative [58]. Baseline tumor size appears to be the strongest independent prognostic factor in metastatic melanoma patients treated with MK3475 [90]. Tumor size >90 mm was associated with a worse prognosis though these patients derived a benefit from MK-3475 achieving a median OS of 14 months.

A phase I trial Nivolumab (BMS-936559) of 207 advanced solid tumor patients included 55 patients with advanced melanoma; disease control was seen as early as 6 weeks in 46%. It induced durable tumor regression (ORR 6–17%) and prolonged stabilization of disease (12–41% at 24 weeks) was seen for all melanoma patients. Grade 3 or 4 toxic effects were seen in about 9% of patients [61].

A phase I clinical trial of Nivolumab (BMS-936559 IgG4 antibody to PD-1) in combination with Ipilimumab (IgG1 antibody to CTLA4) in 86 patients with stage III or IV melanoma (53 received concurrent therapy and 33 received sequential therapy) showed a 53% objective response rate at 2.5-year follow-up; in the concurrent treatment group there were marked tumor reductions of over 80% compared to 20% objective response rate (ORR) for sequenced treatments. While the combination therapy offers higher chances of response, increased ORR, and durable responses; toxicity with concurrent treatment was high with more than 50% of treated patients experiencing grades 3 and 4 toxicities [91]. Several phase III trials are currently underway to examine the safety and efficacy of combination regimens (Table 2).

3.2. Non-Small-Cell Lung Cancer. Metastatic non-small-cell lung cancer has dismal outcome with current treatments with only 4% of patients alive at 5 years despite intense multidisciplinary treatment. In metastatic lung cancer the tumor microenvironment favors the development of tolerant dendritic cells that drive the differentiation of T-cells towards immunosuppressive regulatory T-cells that release TGF-B [92]. TGF-B causes tolerance to tumor antigens. The presence of CD4+/CD8+ tumor-infiltrating lymphocytes in pathologic specimen has been associated with improved survival in [93] while it elevated levels of infiltrating immunosuppressive regulatory T-cells (CD4+ CD25+ FOXP3+) with increased risk of relapse [94].

A phase II randomized double-blind trial Ipilimumab in 204 stage IIIB and stage IV or recurrent NSCLC chemotherapy-naïve, randomized to carboplatin and paclitaxel, with placebo or Ipilimumab as either a concurrent or phased regimen was recently completed. The dose of Ipilimumab was 10 mg/kg in both arms. The concurrent arm used Ipilimumab with first 4 cycles and placebo with the last 2 cycles. The phased Ipilimumab arm assigned patients to placebo during the first 2 cycles of carboplatin and paclitaxel with Ipilimumab added with cycle #3 and continued for a total of 4 cycles [95]. Chemotherapy induces cancer cell death with release of tumor-associated antigens (TAA). TAA are able to amplify immune responses in the presence of immune check point inhibitors. Having more TAA to stimulate T-cells before Ipilimumab treatment seemed reasonable. The phased Ipilimumab had a significant increase in PFS: 5.1 months for phased regimen, 4.2 months for control regimen, and 4.1 months for concurrent regimen. Squamous histology was predictive of better outcomes in the phased arm. In currently ongoing phase III trial, NCT01285609 aims to validate these results and assess any change in OS.

In phase I clinical trial of 76 NSCLC patients treated with Nivolumab (BMS-936559 IgG4 antibody to PD-1) had response rates ranging from 6 to 32% when using doses of

1 mg/kg, 3 mg/kg, or 10 mg/kg every 2 weeks [63]. Thirty-three percent of patients with squamous cell histology and 12% of patients with nonsquamous cell histology showed an objective response, overall ORR 17%. PFS was 33% at 24 weeks with a median response duration of 74 weeks [64, 96]. More than half of the patients had a sustained response and had an OS of 42% at 1 year and 14% at 2 years. Among the 3 dose levels used, 3 mg/kg had highest objective response rate of 24%. Therapy was well tolerated, with only 9% grades 3-4 toxicities mainly fatigue, diarrhea, decreased appetite, nausea, and anemia.

In phase I clinical study of 38 patients with metastatic and locally advanced non-small-cell lung cancer who had previously been treated with two systemic chemotherapy regimens, Pembrolizumab (MK-3475) was given at 10 mg/kg every 3 weeks [66]. A 24% objective response rate was noted, including both squamous and nonsquamous subtypes and pretreatment PD-1 tumor expression was a predictor of response. Common adverse events were grades 1 and 2 fatigue, rash, pruritus, and diarrhea.

In a phase I clinical trial, 85 patients with heavily pre-treated locally advanced and metastatic NSCLC patients were treated with MPDL-3280A, a humanized IgG1 monoclonal antibody against PD-L1. Twenty-four percent of patients had objective response in squamous and nonsquamous cell histologies and at 24 weeks PFS rate was 46% [67]. One hundred percent of patients with PDL-1 positive tumors had treatment response. Response rates were different according to smoking status, the former or current smokers had 25% versus 16% in never-smoker, indicating that immune stimulation may detect cancer cells after carcinogen exposure.

3.3. Renal Cell Carcinoma.
A phase I clinical trial of 34 patients with metastatic renal cell carcinoma Nivolumab (BMS-936559 IgG4 antibody to PD-1) at doses of 1 mg/kg and 10 mg/kg achieved objective responses in 9 patients and stable disease lasting >24 weeks in another 9 patients [63].

A double-blinded phase II randomized trial of Nivolumab (BMS-936559 IgG4 antibody to PD-1) dose-ranging monotherapy, at 0.3, 2, or 10 mg/kg intravenously every 3 weeks until progression or toxicity in 168 heavily pretreated (four or less lines of therapy) metastatic clear-cell RCC patients showed an objective response in 20 to 22% of patients and median OS of 18.2 months in the lowest dose group [44]. The responses were durable, lasting longer than 12–20 months. Nivolumab was overall well tolerated, with grades 3-4 CTCAE adverse events in less than 17% patients. The median PFS ranged from 2.7 to 4.2 months. No clear dose-response relationship was seen, suggesting that even low doses of anti-PD1 may elicit significant clinical benefit likely due to binding affinity of these antibodies to their targets.

Phase I clinical trials of combinations Nivolumab (BMS-936559 IgG4 antibody to PD-1) with the VEGF receptor TKIs, Pazopanib, and Sunitinib were based on the rationale that PD-1 and VEGF inhibition may have additive benefit for intratumoral immune environment by decreasing immune suppressive cell populations and suppressing effects of VEGF on dendritic cell function [74]. Among the 33 patients in the Nivolumab (2 mg/kg every 3 weeks and 5 mg/kg every 3

weeks) and Sunitinib arm (at dose 50 mg/kg, 4 weeks on and 2 weeks off), objective response was seen in 52% patients, most as early as 6 weeks. In this arm, the PFS rate was 78% at 24 weeks and the median PFS was 12 months, but this included mostly treatment of naïve patients. The combination of Sunitinib and Nivolumab slightly increased OR (52%) and PFS (12 months) compared to Sunitinib alone arm OR (47%) and PFS (9.5 to 11 months). This minimal survival advantage at a cost of significant toxicity over monotherapy will remain a challenge in bringing such combination therapies to clinical practice (Table 2).

In metastatic RCC at two different dose combinations of Nivolumab in combination with the anti-CTLA-4 antibody Ipilimumab was studied in a phase I/II clinical trial: Nivolumab dose of 3 mg/kg and Ipilimumab dose of 1 mg/kg versus Nivolumab dose of 1 mg/kg and Ipilimumab dose of 3 mg/kg in 44 patients with metastatic renal cell carcinoma [76]. The overall response rate was 39% and PFS ranging from 9 to 10 months with prolonged antitumor effects. CTCAE grades 3-4 gastrointestinal and liver toxicities were seen in 43% patients. Phase III clinical trials of Nivolumab in renal cell carcinoma and combination studies are ongoing.

In a phase I clinical trial of MPDL3280A (humanized IgG1 monoclonal antibody against PD-L1), 53 patients with metastatic renal cell carcinoma (RCC) were enrolled. More than 80% patients had prior systemic therapy; MPDL3280A was administered intravenous every 3 weeks at doses between 3 and 20 mg/kg [75]. CTCAE grades 3-4 adverse events were seen in 13% of patients. Responses per RECIST criteria were seen across all doses with prolonged interval of stable disease and at 24 month PFS was 50% [75].

A phase I/II trial of Pembrolizumab (MK-3475, formerly called Lambrolizumab) in combination with Pazopanib in advanced clear cell RCC patients is currently underway to assess safety, efficacy, and response. This trial analysis of patients with RCC treated with Pazopanib showed that patients' whose tumors have high expression of PD-L1 have shorter PFS (NCT02014636).

3.4. Bladder Cancer.
Phase I trial of MPDL3280A (humanized IgG1 monoclonal antibody blocking PD-L1) in 31 patients with heavily pretreated metastatic urothelial bladder cancer showed a 50% ORR [97]. The treatment was well tolerated and the responses were rapid and durable with median OS of 6-7 months. Responses were reported according to expression of PD-L1 by IHC on tumors. PD-L1 positive tumors, defined as immunohistochemistry score (IHC) of 2 or 3, had a 43% response rate by RECIST criteria, while tumors with (IHC score of 0 or 1) had 11% response rate. The study showed that expression of PD-L1 status changes over time and should not be used as a reliable marker for clinical applications. CTCAE adverse events grades 3-4 were seen in 3.2% of patients which showed a 50% ORR [97].

3.5. Prostate Cancer.
A phase I/II trial in 33 men with metastatic castrate-resistant prostate cancer (mCRPC) studied Ipilimumab alone or in combination with radiotherapy, given 24–48 h prior to Ipilimumab, either before or after chemotherapy [71]. At the highest dose level (10 mg/kg),

immune-related adverse events (irAEs) were manageable and included colitis (16%), diarrhea (8%), and hepatitis (10%). Of the 50 patients in the 10 mg/kg dose level cohort, 8 had a ≥50% decline in PSA. Of the 28 subjects in the 10 mg/kg cohort with evaluable tumors, one had a complete response and six had stable disease [71]. CTCAE adverse events were GI and skin related, with only 10% having grades 3-4 [71, 72]. Two phase III trials evaluating Ipilimumab in men with metastatic castrate-resistant prostate cancer are in progress.

A phase III trial conducted in this setting did not show any improved overall survival in the Ipilimumab treatment group but was positive for one of its secondary endpoints time to progression [72]. The subgroup analysis suggested that Ipilimumab was beneficial in mCRPC patients with no visceral metastases and a favorable performance status.

In phase I/II trials, the combinations were generally well tolerated and had an acceptable toxicity profile [98–101]. In spite of preclinical rationale for dual blockade of PD-1/PD-L1 in prostate cancer, no objective responses were seen in the prostate cancer cohorts in phase I PD-1 and PD-L1 trials [98–101] (Table 2).

Combination immunotherapy trials of Ipilimumab with GM-CSF or GVAX have been conducted. In phase I/II trials, the combinations were generally well tolerated and had an acceptable toxicity profile [98–101] (Table 2).

3.6. Ovarian Cancer. A phase I/II trial of 11 patients with FIGO stage IV ovarian cancers previously treated with either chemotherapy or GVAX (a vaccine product comprised of autologous, irradiated tumor cells engineered to secrete the immune stimulatory cytokine, granulocyte macrophage colony-stimulating factor) used Ipilimumab at a dose level of 3 mg/kg. Two patients had CTCAE grade 3 gastrointestinal inflammatory adverse events [77, 78]. Two patients had exceptional responses: one patient a dramatic fall of serum CA125 levels and a substantial regression of a large hepatic metastasis, mesenteric lymph nodes, and an omental caking; another patient had reduction in pain and ascites and stabilization of CA125 levels [78]. Four other patients had stable disease as assessed by blood CA125 levels and imaging that lasted longer than 10 months [77, 78].

3.7. Squamous Cell Carcinoma of Head and Neck. Recurrent squamous cell carcinoma of head and neck (SCCHN) is incurable with palliative chemotherapy resulting in a median survival of 8–10 months. SCCHN tumors express high levels of PD-L1 expression in 46–100% in the primary, recurrent, and metastatic settings [83, 102–106].

Human papilloma virus (HPV) has prognostic significance in oropharyngeal SCCHN and there is higher expression of PD-L1 in the HPV positive patients [32, 83, 103]. HPV infection of oropharyngeal epithelium is accompanied by PD-L1 expression creating a pseudo-immuno-privileged site for the developing malignancy. While PD-1 expression on effector T-cells is seen in both HPV positive and negative SCCHN tumors, the degree of expression seems to be increased in those patients with HPV positive disease [32, 83]. Regulatory T-cells which mediate peripheral tolerance, suppress effector T-cells, and inhibit immune mediated destruction are increased in the blood and tumor microenvironment

in patients with SCCHN [107]. In SCCHN, a higher frequency of intratumoral regulatory T-cells expressing PD-1 and CTLA-4 have higher suppressive effects on immunity when compared to peripheral blood regulatory T-cells [108]. These data suggest that blocking the interaction between PD-L1 and PD-1 may trigger cellular antitumor immune response, in recurrent and metastatic SCCHN patients. Two ongoing phase I trials, with anti-PD-L1mAb MEDI4736 (IgG1 isotype) (NCT01693562) and MK-3475 anti-PD-1 monoclonal Ab (IgG4 isotype) (NCT01848834), include cohorts of recurrent/metastatic SCCHN patients.

4. Discussion

Cancer immunotherapy showed promising results in several solid tumors. The benefits of such therapies in metastatic incurable solid tumors exceed those seen with conventional cytotoxic chemotherapy. Harnessing the immune system to eliminate tumors has limitations most of them being off-target autoimmune side effects. Immunotherapy has the potential for durable response and significantly improved long-term survival, potentially even on treatment breaks. There are no biomarkers to predicting exceptional responders or the patients at risk for immune-related toxicity. Choueiri et al in a prospective randomized clinical trial of Nivolumab in previously treated and untreated metastatic RCC showed that responses correlated to expression of PD-L1 by immunohistochemistry (IHC) in tumors [73]. Responses were higher in tumors staining positive (IHC 2 or 3) for PD-L1 of 22% versus 8% in IHC 0-1 tumors [73]. Changing in tumor heterogeneity in time secondary to mutation accumulation and tumor immune editing will result in changes in PD-L1 expression over time. Additionally CD3 and CD8 T-cell infiltration in tumor environment appeared to correlate with clinical responses. Prognostic implications of PD-1 and PD-L1 in staining in SCCHN combined with data from phase 1 anti-PD-1 and anti-PD-L1 trials supports that immune staining of tumors for PD-1 and PD-L1 will help guide immune therapy [63, 109, 110].

PD-L1 and PD-L2 status by immunohistochemistry was independent predictor of prognostic factor in postoperative esophageal cancer patients [22]. Of the 41 patients evaluated, 18 were positive for PD-L1 or PD-L2 expression and 23 were negative. PD-L positive patients had a significantly poorer prognosis with worse OS than the negative patients. The OS was worse with tumor positive for both PD-L1 and PD-L2, than those with tumor negative for both 50% versus 100% 1-year survival [22]. Significant differences were also noted in 1-year survival rate after surgery between positive and negative patients of PD-L1 and PD-L2 with T2, T3 disease, and stage III cancer [22]. The effect of PD-L status on postoperative prognosis was more pronounced in the advanced stage of tumor than in the early stage. PD-L2 expression was inversely correlated with tumor-infiltrating CD8+ T-cells but not PD-L1 expression [22].

5. Conclusion

Therapies that limit immune suppression in malignancy are effective in prolonging survival in cancer patients. The effect of immune check point inhibitors appears limited in patients with advanced bulky tumors likely due to highly suppressive effect of the tumor microenvironment and established tolerance mechanisms. As a consequence, immune based therapies may be more effective in patients with low volume disease such as earlier stage cancers immediately after bulk cytoreduction or chemotherapy use and may be more effective in treatment of minimal residual disease. Tumors characterized by epithelial-mesenchymal transition [EMT] have high expression for immune inhibitory molecules like PD-1, PD-L1, PD-L2, and CTLA-4 and may be more amenable to treatment with immune of checkpoint inhibitors [111]. A major limitation of immune checkpoint inhibitors is lack of information on binding affinities to antigens on human immune cells and cancer cells to control for the unforeseen variation in protein function from individual to individual. Such variation in protein function amongst individuals may explain the off-target immune and adverse effects seen.

Disclosure

Please find enclosed our paper entitled "Evolving concepts: Immunity in oncology from targets to treatments" for your consideration. This material is original research and has been seen and approved by all authors. The paper has not been previously published and has not been submitted for publication elsewhere. The authors reviewed available literature looking for the clinical efficacy and safety of currently available immune checkpoint blockade therapies in malignancies. Human antibodies directed against immune checkpoint proteins cytotoxic T lymphocytes antigen-4 (CTLA-4) and programmed death-1 (PD-1), programmed death-ligand 1 (PD-L1), have shown therapeutic efficacy in cancer. Side effects are related to immune dysregulation and diminished tolerance to self.

Conflict of Interests

The authors declare that there is no conflict of interests regarding the publication of this paper.

Acknowledgments

The authors gratefully acknowledge Mrs. Linda and Dr. Myron Teitelbaum, Mrs. Susan and Henry Gabbay and the Manhasset Women's Coalition against Breast Cancer for supporting in part this work.

References

[1] H. Nakagomi, M. Petersson, I. Magnusson et al., "Decreased expression of the signal-transducing zeta chains in tumor-infiltrating T-cells and NK cells of patients with colorectal carcinoma," *Cancer Research*, vol. 53, no. 23, pp. 5610–5612, 1993.

[2] C. Renner, S. Ohnesorge, G. Held et al., "T cells from patients with hodgkin's disease have a defective T-cell receptor ζ chain expression that is reversible by T-cell stimulation with CD3 and CD28," *Blood*, vol. 88, no. 1, pp. 236–241, 1996.

[3] J. H. Finke, A. H. Zea, J. Stanley et al., "Loss of T-cell receptor ζ chain and p56lck in T-cells infiltrating human renal cell carcinoma," *Cancer Research*, vol. 53, no. 23, pp. 5613–5616, 1993.

[4] E. Tartour, S. Latour, C. Mathiot et al., "Variable expression of CD3-ζ chain in tumor-infiltrating lymphocytes (TIL) derived from renal-cell carcinoma: relationship with TIL phenotype and function," *International Journal of Cancer*, vol. 63, no. 2, pp. 205–212, 1995.

[5] H. Mizoguchi, J. J. O'Shea, D. L. Longo, C. M. Loeffler, D. W. McVicar, and A. C. Ochoa, "Alterations in signal transduction molecules in T lymphocytes from tumor-bearing mice," *Science*, vol. 258, no. 5089, pp. 1795–1798, 1992.

[6] S. J. Cotton, J. Belcher, P. Rose, S. K Jagadeesan, and R. D. Neal, "The risk of a subsequent cancer diagnosis after herpes zoster infection: primary care database study," *British Journal of Cancer*, vol. 108, no. 3, pp. 721–726, 2013.

[7] F. Buntinx, R. Wachana, S. Bartholomeeusen, K. Sweldens, and H. Geys, "Is herpes zoster a marker for occult or subsequent malignancy?" *British Journal of General Practice*, vol. 55, no. 511, pp. 102–107, 2005.

[8] A. M. Arvin, J. F. Moffat, and R. Redman, "Varicella-zoster virus: aspects of pathogenesis and host respone to natural infection and varicella vaccine," *Advances in Virus Research*, vol. 46, pp. 263–309, 1996.

[9] D. H. Munn and A. L. Mellor, "IDO and tolerance to tumors," *Trends in Molecular Medicine*, vol. 10, no. 1, pp. 15–18, 2004.

[10] A. J. Muller and G. C. Prendergast, "Marrying immunotherapy with chemotherapy: why say IDO?" *Cancer Research*, vol. 65, no. 18, pp. 8065–8068, 2005.

[11] D. H. Munn and A. L. Mellor, "Macrophages and the regulation of self-reactive T cells," *Current Pharmaceutical Design*, vol. 9, no. 3, pp. 257–264, 2003.

[12] C. D. Mills, "Macrophage arginine metabolism to ornithine/urea or nitric oxide/citrulline: a life or death issue," *Critical Reviews in Immunology*, vol. 21, no. 5, pp. 399–425, 2001.

[13] B. A. Irving and A. Weiss, "The cytoplasmic domain of the T cell receptor ζ chain is sufficient to couple to receptor-associated signal transduction pathways," *Cell*, vol. 64, no. 5, pp. 891–901, 1991.

[14] P. C. Rodriguez, A. H. Zea, J. DeSalvo et al., "L-arginine consumption by macrophages modulates the expression of CD3 zeta chain in T lymphocytes," *Journal of Immunology*, vol. 171, no. 3, pp. 1232–1239, 2003.

[15] W. Zou, "Immunosuppressive networks in the tumour environment and their therapeutic relevance," *Nature Reviews Cancer*, vol. 5, no. 4, pp. 263–274, 2005.

[16] L. Chen, "Co-inhibitory molecules of the B7-CD28 family in the control of T-cell immunity," *Nature Reviews Immunology*, vol. 4, no. 5, pp. 336–347, 2004.

[17] J. M. Chemnitz, R. V. Parry, K. E. Nichols, C. H. June, and J. L. Riley, "SHP-1 and SHP-2 associate with immunoreceptor tyrosine-based switch motif of programmed death 1 upon primary human T cell stimulation, but only receptor ligation prevents T cell activation," *The Journal of Immunology*, vol. 173, no. 2, pp. 945–954, 2004.

[18] J.-J. Park, R. Omiya, Y. Matsumura et al., "B7-H1/CD80 interaction is required for the induction and maintenance of peripheral T-cell tolerance," *Blood*, vol. 116, no. 8, pp. 1291–1298, 2010.

[19] H. Dong, S. E. Strome, D. R. Salomao et al., "Tumor-associated B7-H1 promotes T-cell apoptosis: a potential mechanism of immune evasion," *Nature Medicine*, vol. 8, no. 8, pp. 793–800, 2002.

[20] M. E. Keir, M. J. Butte, G. J. Freeman, and A. H. Sharpe, "PD-1 and its ligands in tolerance and immunity," *Annual Review of Immunology*, vol. 26, pp. 677–704, 2008.

[21] J. Konishi, K. Yamazaki, M. Azuma, I. Kinoshita, H. Dosaka-Akita, and M. Nishimura, "B7-H1 expression on non-small cell lung cancer cells and its relationship with tumor-infiltrating lymphocytes and their PD-1 expression," *Clinical Cancer Research*, vol. 10, no. 15, pp. 5094–5100, 2004.

[22] Y. Ohigashi, M. Sho, Y. Yamada et al., "Clinical significance of programmed death-1 ligand-1 and programmed death-1 ligand-2 expression in human esophageal cancer," *Clinical Cancer Research*, vol. 11, no. 8, pp. 2947–2953, 2005.

[23] B. Seliger and D. Quandt, "The expression, function, and clinical relevance of B7 family members in cancer," *Cancer Immunology, Immunotherapy*, vol. 61, no. 8, pp. 1327–1341, 2012.

[24] C. Wu, Y. Zhu, J. Jiang, J. Zhao, X.-G. Zhang, and N. Xu, "Immunohistochemical localization of programmed death-1 ligand-1 (PD-L1) in gastric carcinoma and its clinical significance," *Acta Histochemica*, vol. 108, no. 1, pp. 19–24, 2006.

[25] C. S. Brandt, M. Baratin, E. C. Yi et al., "The B7 family member B7-H6 is a tumor cell ligand for the activating natural killer cell receptor NKp30 in humans," *Journal of Experimental Medicine*, vol. 206, no. 7, pp. 1495–1503, 2009.

[26] H. Dong, G. Zhu, K. Tamada, and L. Chen, "B7-H1, a third member of the B7 family, co-stimulates T-cell proliferation and interleukin-10 secretion," *Nature Medicine*, vol. 5, no. 12, pp. 1365–1369, 1999.

[27] H. Ghebeh, A. Tulbah, S. Mohammed et al., "Expression of B7-H1 in breast cancer patients is strongly associated with high proliferative Ki-67-expressing tumor cells," *International Journal of Cancer*, vol. 121, no. 4, pp. 751–758, 2007.

[28] J. Nakanishi, Y. Wada, K. Matsumoto, M. Azuma, K. Kikuchi, and S. Ueda, "Overexpression of B7-H1 (PD-L1) significantly associates with tumor grade and postoperative prognosis in human urothelial cancers," *Cancer Immunology, Immunotherapy*, vol. 56, no. 8, pp. 1173–1182, 2007.

[29] C. Berthon, V. Driss, J. Liu et al., "In acute myeloid leukemia, B7-H1 (PD-L1) protection of blasts from cytotoxic T cells is induced by TLR ligands and interferon-gamma and can be reversed using MEK inhibitors," *Cancer Immunology, Immunotherapy*, vol. 59, no. 12, pp. 1839–1849, 2010.

[30] C. M. Wilke, S. Wei, L. Wang, I. Kryczek, J. Kao, and W. Zou, "Dual biological effects of the cytokines interleukin-10 and interferon-γ," *Cancer Immunology, Immunotherapy*, vol. 60, no. 11, pp. 1529–1541, 2011.

[31] B. T. Fife and J. A. Bluestone, "Control of peripheral T-cell tolerance and autoimmunity via the CTLA-4 and PD-1 pathways," *Immunological Reviews*, vol. 224, no. 1, pp. 166–182, 2008.

[32] C. Badoual, S. Hans, N. Merillon et al., "PD-1-expressing tumor-infiltrating T cells are a favorable prognostic biomarker in HPV-Associated head and neck cancer," *Cancer Research*, vol. 73, no. 1, pp. 128–138, 2013.

[33] D. L. Barber, E. J. Wherry, D. Masopust et al., "Restoring function in exhausted CD8 T cells during chronic viral infection," *Nature*, vol. 439, no. 7077, pp. 682–687, 2006.

[34] S. L. Topalian, C. G. Drake, and D. M. Pardoll, "Targeting the PD-1/B7-H1(PD-L1) pathway to activate anti-tumor immunity," *Current Opinion in Immunology*, vol. 24, no. 2, pp. 207–212, 2012.

[35] J. Duraiswamy, K. M. Kaluza, G. J. Freeman, and G. Coukos, "Dual blockade of PD-1 and CTLA-4 combined with tumor vaccine effectively restores T-cell rejection function in tumors," *Cancer Research*, vol. 73, no. 12, pp. 3591–3603, 2013.

[36] L. Ni, C. J. Ma, Y. Zhang et al., "PD-1 modulates regulatory T cells and suppresses T-cell responses in HCV-associated lymphoma," *Immunology and Cell Biology*, vol. 89, no. 4, pp. 535–539, 2011.

[37] W. Wang, R. Lau, D. Yu, W. Zhu, A. Korman, and J. Weber, "PD1 blockade reverses the suppression of melanoma antigen-specific CTL by CD4+CD25Hi regulatory T cells," *International Immunology*, vol. 21, no. 9, pp. 1065–1077, 2009.

[38] F. S. Hodi, S. J. O'Day, D. F. McDermott et al., "Improved survival with ipilimumab in patients with metastatic melanoma," *The New England Journal of Medicine*, vol. 363, no. 8, pp. 711–723, 2010.

[39] G. Q. Phan, J. C. Yang, R. M. Sherry et al., "Cancer regression and autoimmunity induced by cytotoxic T lymphocyte-associated antigen 4 blockade in patients with metastatic melanoma," *Proceedings of the National Academy of Sciences of the United States of America*, vol. 100, no. 14, pp. 8372–8377, 2003.

[40] R. H. Thompson, H. Dong, C. M. Lohse et al., "PD-1 is expressed by tumor-infiltrating immune cells and is associated with poor outcome for patients with renal cell carcinoma," *Clinical Cancer Research*, vol. 13, no. 6, pp. 1757–1761, 2007.

[41] P. Yu, Y. Lee, W. Liu et al., "Priming of naive T cells inside tumors leads to eradication of established tumors," *Nature Immunology*, vol. 5, no. 2, pp. 141–149, 2004.

[42] S. Valastyan and R. A. Weinberg, "Tumor metastasis: molecular insights and evolving paradigms," *Cell*, vol. 147, no. 2, pp. 275–292, 2011.

[43] T. Bakacs, J. N. Mehrishi, and R. W. Moss, "Ipilimumab (Yervoy) and the TGN1412 catastrophe," *Immunobiology*, vol. 217, no. 6, pp. 583–589, 2012.

[44] R. J. Motzer, B. I. Rini, D. F. McDermott et al., "Nivolumab for metastatic renal cell carcinoma (mRCC): results of a randomized, dose-ranging phase II trial," *Journal of Cinical Oncology*, vol. 32, abstract 5009, 2014.

[45] M. A. Curran, W. Montalvo, H. Yagita, and J. P. Allison, "PD-1 and CTLA-4 combination blockade expands infiltrating T cells and reduces regulatory T and myeloid cells within B16 melanoma tumors," *Proceedings of the National Academy of Sciences of the United States of America*, vol. 107, no. 9, pp. 4275–4280, 2010.

[46] M. Huemer, S. Rebhandl, N. Zaborsky et al., " AID induces intraclonal diversity and genomic damage in CD86 ," *European Journal of Immunology*, vol. 44, no. 12, pp. 3747–3757, 2014.

[47] K. Waki, T. Yamada, K. Yoshiyama et al., "PD-1 expression on peripheral blood T-cell subsets correlates with prognosis in non-small cell lung cancer," *Cancer Science*, vol. 105, no. 10, pp. 1229–1235, 2014.

[48] J. Faget, N. Bendriss-Vermare, M. Gobert et al., "ICOS-ligand expression on plasmacytoid dendritic cells supports breast cancer progression by promoting the accumulation of immuno-suppressive CD4+ T cells," *Cancer Research*, vol. 72, no. 23, pp. 6130–6141, 2012.

[49] M. Shi, M. G. Roemer, B. Chapuy et al., "Expression of programmed cell death 1 ligand 2 (PD-L2) is a distinguishing feature of primary mediastinal (thymic) large B-cell lymphoma and associated with PDCD1LG2 copy gain," *The American Journal of Surgical Pathology*, vol. 38, no. 12, pp. 1715–1723, 2014.

[50] J. S. Weber, S. O'Day, W. Urba et al., "Phase I/II study of ipilimumab for patients with metastatic melanoma," *Journal of Clinical Oncology*, vol. 26, no. 36, pp. 5950–5956, 2008.

[51] C. Robert, L. Thomas, I. Bondarenko et al., "Ipilimumab plus dacarbazine for previously untreated metastatic melanoma," *The New England Journal of Medicine*, vol. 364, no. 26, pp. 2517–2526, 2011.

[52] E. M. Hersh, S. J. O'Day, J. Powderly et al., "A phase II multicenter study of ipilimumab with or without dacarbazine in chemotherapy-naïve patients with advanced melanoma," *Investigational New Drugs*, vol. 29, no. 3, pp. 489–498, 2011.

[53] L. H. Camacho, S. Antonia, J. Sosman et al., "Phase I/II trial of tremelimumab in patients with metastatic melanoma," *Journal of Clinical Oncology*, vol. 27, no. 7, pp. 1075–1081, 2009.

[54] A. Ribas, R. Kefford, M. A. Marshall et al., "Phase III randomized clinical trial comparing tremelimumab with standard-of-care chemotherapy in patients with advanced melanoma," *Journal of Clinical Oncology*, vol. 31, no. 5, pp. 616–622, 2013.

[55] J. R. Brahmer, C. G. Drake, I. Wollner et al., "Phase I study of single-agent anti-programmed death-1 (MDX-1106) in refractory solid tumors: Safety, clinical activity, pharmacodynamics, and immunologic correlates," *Journal of Clinical Oncology*, vol. 28, no. 19, pp. 3167–3175, 2010.

[56] S. L. Topalian, M. Sznol, D. F. McDermott et al., "Survival, durable tumor remission, and long-term safety in patients with advanced melanoma receiving nivolumab," *Journal of Clinical Oncology*, vol. 32, no. 10, pp. 1020–1030, 2014.

[57] O. Hamid, C. Robert, A. Daud et al., "Safety and tumor responses with lambrolizumab (anti-PD-1) in melanoma," *The New England Journal of Medicine*, vol. 369, no. 2, pp. 134–144, 2013.

[58] R. Kefford, A. Ribas, O. Hamid et al., "Clinical efficacy and correlation with tumor PD-L1 expression in patients (pts) with melanoma (MEL) treated with the anti-PD-1 monoclonal antibody MK-3475," *Journal of Clinical Oncology*, vol. 32, abstract 3005, 2014.

[59] C. Robert, A. Ribas, J. D. Wolchok et al., "Anti-programmed-death-receptor-1 treatment with pembrolizumab in ipilimumab-refractory advanced melanoma: a randomised dose-comparison cohort of a phase 1 trial," *The Lancet*, vol. 384, no. 9948, pp. 1109–1117, 2014.

[60] O. Hamid, J. A. Sosman, D. P. Lawrence et al., "Clinical activity, safety, and biomarkers of MPDL3280A, an engineered PD-L1 antibody in patients with locally advanced or metastatic melanoma (mM)," *Journal of Clinical Oncology*, vol. 31, abstract 9010, 2013.

[61] J. R. Brahmer, S. S. Tykodi, L. Q. M. Chow et al., "Safety and activity of anti-PD-L1 antibody in patients with advanced cancer," *The New England Journal of Medicine*, vol. 366, no. 26, pp. 2455–2465, 2012.

[62] T. J. Lynch, I. Bondarenko, A. Luft et al., "Ipilimumab in combination with paclitaxel and carboplatin as first-line treatment in stage IIIB/IV non-small-cell lung cancer: results from a randomized, double-blind, multicenter phase II study," *Journal of Clinical Oncology*, vol. 30, no. 17, pp. 2046–2054, 2012.

[63] S. L. Topalian, F. S. Hodi, J. R. Brahmer et al., "Safety, activity, and immune correlates of anti-PD-1 antibody in cancer," *The New England Journal of Medicine*, vol. 366, no. 26, pp. 2443–2454, 2012.

[64] J. R. Brahmer, L. Horn, S. J. Antonia et al., "Survival and long-term follow-up of the phase I trial of nivolumab (Anti-PD-1; BMS-936558; ONO-4538) in patients (pts) with previously treated advanced non-small cell lung cancer (NSCLC)," *Journal of Clinical Oncology*, vol. 31, abstract 8030, 2013, Proceedings of the ASCO Annual Meeting.

[65] J. R. Brahmer, L. Horn, S. J. Antonia et al., "Nivolumab (anti-PD-1; BMS-936558; ONO-4538) in patients with non-small cell lung cancer (NSCLC): overall survival and long-term safety in a phase 1 trial," in *Proceedings of the 15th International Association for the Study of Lung Cancer World Conference on Lung Cancer*, Sydney, Australia, October 2013.

[66] E. Garon, A. Balmanoukian, O. Hamid et al., "Preliminary clinical safety and activity of MK-3475 monotherapy for the treatment of previously treated patients with non-small cell lung cancer," in *Proceedings of the 15th World Conference on Lung Cancer (IASLC '13)*, Sydney, Australia, October 2013.

[67] J. Soria, C. Cruz, R. Bahleda et al., "Clinical activity, safety and biomarkers of PD-L1 blockade in non-small cell lung cancer (NSCLC): additional analyses from a clinical study of the engineered antibody MPDL3280A (anti-PDL1)," in *Proceedings of the European Cancer Conference (ECC '13)*, Amsterdam, The Netherlands, October 2013.

[68] L. Horn, R. S. Herbst, D. R. Spigel et al., "An analysis of the relationship of clinical activity to baseline EGFR status, PD-L1 expression and prior treatment history in patients with non-small cell lung cancer (NSCLC) following PD-L1 blockade with MPDL3280A (anti-PDL1)," in *Proceedings of the 15th International Association for the Study of Lung Cancer World Conference on Lung Cancer*, Sydney, Australia, 2013.

[69] J. R. Brahmer, N. A. Rizvi, J. Lutzky et al., "Clinical activity and biomarkers of MEDI4736, an anti-PD-L1 antibody, in patients with NSCLC," *Journal of Clinical Oncology*, vol. 32, abstract 8021, 2014, Proceedings of the ASCO Annual Meeting.

[70] P. Zatloukal, D. S. Heo, K. Park et al., "Randomized phase II clinical trial comparing tremelimumab (CP-675,206) with best supportive care (BSC) following first-line platinum-based therapy in patients (pts) with advanced non-small cell lung cancer (NSCLC)," *Journal of Clinical Oncology*, vol. 27, abstract 8071, 2009, Proceedings of the ASCO Annual Meeting.

[71] S. F. Slovin, C. S. Higano, O. Hamid et al., "Ipilimumab alone or in combination with radiotherapy in metastatic castration-resistant prostate cancer: results from an open-label, multicenter phase I/II study," *Annals of Oncology*, vol. 24, no. 7, pp. 1813–1821, 2013.

[72] W. R. Gerritsen, E. D. Kwon, K. Fizazi et al., "CA184-043: a randomized, multicenter, double-blind phase 3 trial comparing overall survival (OS) in patients (pts) with post-docetaxel castrationresistant prostate cancer (CRPC) and bone metastases treated with ipilimumab (ipi) vs placebo (pbo), each following single-dose radiotherapy (RT)," in *Proceedings of the European Cancer Congress*, 2013.

[73] T. K. Choueiri, M. N. Fishman, B. J. Escudier et al., "Immunomodulatory activity of nivolumab in previously treated and untreated metastatic renal cell carcinoma (mRCC): biomarker-based results from a randomized clinical trial," *Journal of Clinical Oncology*, vol. 32, no. 5, abstract 5012, 2014.

[74] A. Amin, E. R. Plimack, J. R. Infante et al., "Nivolumab (anti-PD-1; BMS-936558, ONO-4538) in combination with sunitinib or pazopanib in patients (pts) with metastatic renal cell carcinoma (mRCC)," *Journal of Clinical Oncology*, vol. 32, abstract 5010, 2014, Proceedings of the ASCO Annual Meeting.

[75] D. C. Cho, J. A. Sosman, M. Sznol et al., "Clinical activity, safety, and biomarkers of MPDL3280A, an engineered PD-L1 antibody in patients with metastatic renal cell carcinoma (mRCC)," *Journal of Clinical Oncology*, vol. 31, abstract 4505, 2013.

[76] H. J. Hammers, E. R. Plimack, J. R. Infante et al., "Phase I study of nivolumab in combination with ipilimumab in metastatic renal cell carcinoma (mRCC)," *Journal of Clinical Oncology*, vol. 32, abstract 4504, 2014, Proceedings of the ASCO Annual Meeting.

[77] F. S. Hodi, M. C. Mihm, R. J. Soiffer et al., "Biologic activity of cytotoxic T lymphocyte-associated antigen 4 antibody blockade in previously vaccinated metastatic melanoma and ovarian carcinoma patients," *Proceedings of the National Academy of Sciences of the United States of America*, vol. 100, no. 8, pp. 4712–4717, 2003.

[78] F. S. Hodi, M. Butler, D. A. Oble et al., "Immunologic and clinical effects of antibody blockade of cytotoxic T lymphocyte-associated antigen 4 in previously vaccinated cancer patients," *Proceedings of the National Academy of Sciences of the United States of America*, vol. 105, no. 8, pp. 3005–3010, 2008.

[79] R. S. Herbst, M. S. Gordon, G. D. Fine et al., "A study of MPDL3280A, an engineered PD-L1 antibody in patients with locally advanced or metastatic tumors," *Journal of Clinical Oncology*, vol. 31, abstract 3000, 2013.

[80] T. Y. Seiwert, B. Burtness, J. Weiss et al., "A phase Ib study of MK-3475 in patients with human papillomavirus (HPV)-associated and non-HPV–associated head and neck (H/N) cancer," *Journal of Clinical Oncology*, vol. 32, no. 5, abstract 6011, 2014.

[81] N. H. Segal, S. J. Antonia, J. R. Brahmer et al., "Preliminary data from a multi-arm expansion study of MEDI4736, an anti-PD-L1 antibody," *Journal of Clinical Oncology*, vol. 32, no. 5, abstract 3002, 2014.

[82] T. Azuma, S. Yao, G. Zhu, A. S. Flies, S. J. Flies, and L. Chen, "B7-H1 is a ubiquitous antiapoptotic receptor on cancer cells," *Blood*, vol. 111, no. 7, pp. 3635–3643, 2008.

[83] S. Lyford-Pike, S. Peng, G. D. Young et al., "Evidence for a role of the PD-1:PD-L1 pathway in immune resistance of HPV-associated head and neck squamous cell carcinoma," *Cancer Research*, vol. 73, no. 6, pp. 1733–1741, 2013.

[84] C. M. Balch, J. E. Gershenwald, S.-J. Soong et al., "Final version of 2009 AJCC melanoma staging and classification," *Journal of Clinical Oncology*, vol. 27, no. 36, pp. 6199–6206, 2009.

[85] C. Garbe, T. K. Eigentler, U. Keilholz, A. Hauschild, and J. M. Kirkwood, "Systematic review of medical treatment in melanoma: current status and future prospects," *Oncologist*, vol. 16, no. 1, pp. 5–24, 2011.

[86] T. Petrella, I. Quirt, S. Verma, A. E. Haynes, M. Charette, and K. Bak, "Single-agent interleukin-2 in the treatment of metastatic melanoma," *Current Oncology*, vol. 14, no. 1, pp. 21–26, 2007.

[87] J. M. Kirkwood, M. H. Strawderman, M. S. Ernstoff, T. J. Smith, E. C. Borden, and R. H. Blum, "Interferon alfa-2b adjuvant therapy of high-risk resected cutaneous melanoma: the Eastern Cooperative Oncology Group trial EST 1684," *Journal of Clinical Oncology*, vol. 14, no. 1, pp. 7–17, 1996.

[88] A. Ribas, L. H. Camacho, G. Lopez-Berestein et al., "Antitumor activity in melanoma and anti-self responses in a phase I trial with the anti-cytotoxic T lymphocyte-associated antigen 4 monoclonal antibody CP-675,206," *Journal of Clinical Oncology*, vol. 23, no. 35, pp. 8968–8977, 2005.

[89] E. J. Lipson, W. H. Sharfman, C. G. Drake et al., "Durable cancer regression off-treatment and effective reinduction therapy with an anti-PD-1 antibody," *Clinical Cancer Research*, vol. 19, no. 2, pp. 462–468, 2013.

[90] R. W. Joseph, J. Elassaiss-Schaap, J. D. Wolchok et al., "Baseline tumor size as an independent prognostic factor for overall survival in patients with metastatic melanoma treated with the anti-PD-1 monoclonal antibody MK-3475," *Journal of Clinical Oncology*, vol. 32, abstract 3015, 2014, Proceedings of the ASCO Annual Meeting.

[91] J. D. Wolchok, H. Kluger, M. K. Callahan et al., "Nivolumab plus Ipilimumab in advanced melanoma," *The New England Journal of Medicine*, vol. 369, no. 2, pp. 122–133, 2013.

[92] R. J. Kelly and G. Giaccone, "Lung cancer vaccines," *Cancer Journal*, vol. 17, no. 5, pp. 302–308, 2011.

[93] E. Ruffini, S. Asioli, P. L. Filosso et al., "Clinical significance of tumor-infiltrating lymphocytes in lung neoplasms," *Annals of Thoracic Surgery*, vol. 87, no. 2, pp. 365–372, 2009.

[94] K. Shimizu, M. Nakata, Y. Hirami, T. Yukawa, A. Maeda, and K. Tanemoto, "Tumor-infiltrating Foxp3+ regulatory T cells are correlated with cyclooxygenase-2 expression and are associated with recurrence in resected non-small cell lung cancer," *Journal of Thoracic Oncology*, vol. 5, no. 5, pp. 585–590, 2010.

[95] A. Belalcazar, L. E. Raez, and E. S. Santos, "Immunotherapy for nonsmall-cell lung cancer," *Magazine of European Medical Oncology*, vol. 5, no. 2, pp. 90–93, 2012.

[96] J. R. Brahmer, L. Horn, S. Antonia et al., "Clinical activity and safety of anti-PD1 (BMS-936558, MDX-1106) in patients with advanced non-small-cell lung cancer (NSCLC)," *Journal of Clinical Oncology*, vol. 30, abstract 7509, 2012, Proceedings of the ASCO Annual Meeting.

[97] T. Powles, N. J. Vogelzang, G. D. Fine et al., "Inhibition of PD-L1 by MPDL3280A and clinical activity in pts with metastatic urothelial bladder cancer (UBC)," *Journal of Clinical Oncology*, vol. 35, abstract 5011, 2014, Proceedings of the ASCO Annual Meeting.

[98] L. Fong, S. S. Kwek, S. O'Brien et al., "Potentiating endogenous antitumor immunity to prostate cancer through combination immunotherapy with CTLA4 blockade and GM-CSF," *Cancer Research*, vol. 69, no. 2, pp. 609–615, 2009.

[99] W. R. Gerritsen, A. J. van den Eertwegh, T. D. de Gruijl et al., "Biochemical and immunologic correlates of clinical response in a combination trial of the GM-CSF-gene transduced allogeneic prostate cancer immunotherapy and ipilimumab in patients with metastatic hormone-refractory prostate cancer (mHRPC)," *Journal of Clinical Oncology*, vol. 25, no. 18, abstract 5120, 2007.

[100] A. L. Harzstark, L. Fong, V. K. Weinberg et al., "Final results of a phase I study of CTLA-4 blockade in combination with GM-CSF for metastatic castration resistant prostate cancer (mCRPC)," *Journal of Clinical Oncology*, vol. 28, abstract 4689, 2010, Proceedings of the ASCO Annual Meeting.

[101] A. J. M. van den Eertwegh, J. Versluis, H. P. van den Berg et al., "Combined immunotherapy with granulocyte-macrophage colony-stimulating factor-transduced allogeneic prostate cancer cells and ipilimumab in patients with metastatic castration-resistant prostate cancer: a phase 1 dose-escalation trial," *The Lancet Oncology*, vol. 13, no. 5, pp. 509–517, 2012.

[102] S. E. Strome, H. Dong, H. Tamura et al., "B7-H1 blockade augments adoptive T-cell immunotherapy for squamous cell carcinoma," *Cancer Research*, vol. 63, no. 19, pp. 6501–6505, 2003.

[103] O. C. Ukpo, W. L. Thorstad, and J. S. Lewis Jr., "B7-H1 expression model for immune evasion in human papillomavirus-related oropharyngeal squamous cell carcinoma," *Head and Neck Pathology*, vol. 7, no. 2, pp. 113–121, 2013.

[104] Y.-A. Cho, H.-J. Yoon, J.-I. Lee, S.-P. Hong, and S.-D. Hong, "Relationship between the expressions of PD-L1 and tumor-infiltrating lymphocytes in oral squamous cell carcinoma," *Oral Oncology*, vol. 47, no. 12, pp. 1148–1153, 2011.

[105] M.-C. Hsu, J.-R. Hsiao, K.-C. Chang et al., "Increase of programmed death-1-expressing intratumoral CD8 T cells predicts a poor prognosis for nasopharyngeal carcinoma," *Modern Pathology*, vol. 23, no. 10, pp. 1393–1403, 2010.

[106] F. Zhang, Z. Liu, Y. Cui, G. Wang, and P. Cao, "The clinical significance of the expression of costimulatory molecule PD-L1 in nasopharyngeal carcinoma," *Lin Chung Er Bi Yan Hou Tou Jing Wai Ke Za Zhi*, vol. 22, no. 9, pp. 408–410, 2008.

[107] C. T. Allen, N. P. Judd, J. D. Bui, and R. Uppaluri, "The clinical implications of antitumor immunity in head and neck cancer," *Laryngoscope*, vol. 122, no. 1, pp. 144–157, 2012.

[108] H.-B. Jie, N. Gildener-Leapman, J. Li et al., "Intratumoral regulatory T cells upregulate immunosuppressive molecules in head and neck cancer patients," *British Journal of Cancer*, vol. 109, no. 10, pp. 2629–2635, 2013.

[109] J. Grosso, C. E. Horak, D. Inzunza et al., "Association of tumor PD-L1 expression and immune biomarkers with clinical activity in patients (pts) with advanced solid tumors treated with nivolumab (anti-PD-1; BMS-936558; ONO-4538)," *Journal of Clinical Oncology*, vol. 31, abstract 3016, 2013.

[110] J. D. Powderly, H. Koeppen, F. S. Hodi et al., "Biomarkers and associations with the clinical activity of PD-L1 blockade in a MPDL3280A study," *Journal of Clinical Oncology*, vol. 31, abstract 3001, 2013, Proceedings of the ASCO Annual Meeting.

[111] Y. Lou, L. Diao, L. A. Byers et al., "Association of epithelial-mesenchymal transition status with PD1/PDL1 expression and a distinct immunophenotype in non-small cell lung cancer: implications for immunotherapy biomarkers," *Journal of Clinical Oncology*, vol. 32, abstract 3018, 2014, Proceedings of the ASCO Annual Meeting.

16

Epithelial Plasticity in Cancer: Unmasking a MicroRNA Network for TGF-β-, Notch-, and Wnt-Mediated EMT

Eugenio Zoni,[1] **Gabri van der Pluijm,**[1] **Peter C. Gray,**[2] **and Marianna Kruithof-de Julio**[3,4]

[1] *Department of Urology, Leiden University Medical Center, Albinusdreef 2, 2333 ZA Leiden, The Netherlands*
[2] *Clayton Foundation Laboratories for Peptide Biology, The Salk Institute for Biological Studies, La Jolla, CA 92037, USA*
[3] *Department of Molecular Cell Biology, Cancer Genomics Centre and Centre for Biomedical Genetics, Einthovenweg 20, 2333 ZC Leiden, The Netherlands*
[4] *Department of Dermatology, Leiden University Medical Center, Einthovenweg 20, 2333 ZC Leiden, The Netherlands*

Correspondence should be addressed to Marianna Kruithof-de Julio; m.de_julio@lumc.nl

Academic Editor: George Lambrou

Epithelial-to-mesenchymal transition (EMT) is a reversible process by which cancer cells can switch from a sessile epithelial phenotype to an invasive mesenchymal state. EMT enables tumor cells to become invasive, intravasate, survive in the circulation, extravasate, and colonize distant sites. Paracrine heterotypic stroma-derived signals as well as paracrine homotypic or autocrine signals can mediate oncogenic EMT and contribute to the acquisition of stem/progenitor cell properties, expansion of cancer stem cells, development of therapy resistance, and often lethal metastatic disease. EMT is regulated by a variety of stimuli that trigger specific intracellular signalling pathways. Altered microRNA (miR) expression and perturbed signalling pathways have been associated with epithelial plasticity, including oncogenic EMT. In this review we analyse and describe the interaction between experimentally validated miRs and their target genes in TGF-β, Notch, and Wnt signalling pathways. Interestingly, in this process, we identified a "signature" of 30 experimentally validated miRs and a cluster of validated target genes that seem to mediate the cross talk between TGF-β, Notch, and Wnt signalling networks during EMT and reinforce their connection to the regulation of epithelial plasticity in health and disease.

1. Introduction

In the last decade the amount of data regarding microRNAs (miRs) and their target genes described in the literature has expanded tremendously. The volume of information on this new group of regulators (i.e., miRs) has complicated attempts to integrate this data within existing metabolic and signalling networks. As regulators of gene expression, miRs have indeed added a new level of interaction between different networks. In addition, a single miR can potentially regulate multiple different genes at the same time, leading to complex functional outcomes. However, from another perspective, the identification of groups of genes targeted by the same miR and the clustering of these genes within individual signalling pathways represents a means to understand the cross talk between multiple signalling networks and their role in a common biological process.

The focus of this review is to summarize the validated groups of miRs functionally linked to the cross talk between TGF-β, Notch, and Wnt signalling during the common biological process of epithelial-to-mesenchymal transition (EMT). In particular, this review will address whether the documented cross talk between these three important EMT-associated pathways could be further reinforced by the identification of a "signature" of miRs, already depicted in the literature but not yet "sharpened" or clearly defined in this role. In the past years, many studies have elegantly described the role of TGF-β, Notch, and Wnt pathways in promoting EMT and EMT-associated disorders including fibrosis and metastatic dissemination in cancer [1–6]. Here we identify published and validated interactions between miRs and genes involved in TGF-β, Notch, and Wnt signalling. This led to the discovery of a signature of 30 miRs each regulating all three pathways. We then searched for additional

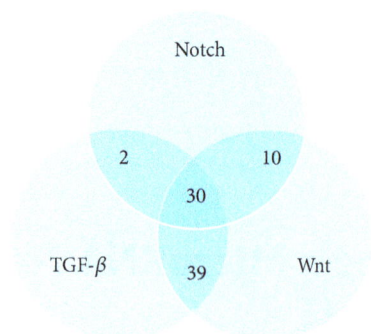

FIGURE 1: Venn diagram showing number of overlapping, experimentally validated miRs targeting KEGG pathway genes from the TGF-β, Wnt, and Notch pathways.

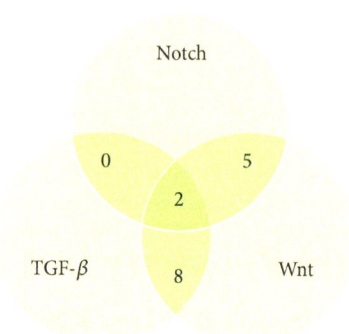

FIGURE 2: Venn diagram showing number of overlapping KEGG pathway genes from the TGF-β, Wnt, and Notch pathways.

validated genes targeted by these 30 miRs and then further clustered these into the TGF-β, Notch, and Wnt signalling pathways. Interestingly, in our attempt to identify miRs that were common to all three of these signalling pathways, we found that the 30-miR signature strongly reinforced existing evidence supporting cross talk between these three pathways during EMT.

2. Data Sources and Analysis

In this review we used TarBase v6.0, the largest currently available manually curated miR target gene database, which includes targets derived from specific and high throughput experiments [7]. Using TarBase v6.0 we searched the collection of manually curated, experimentally validated miR-gene interactions for TGF-β (hsa04350), Wnt (hsa04310), and Notch (hsa04330) signalling KEGG pathways in *Homo sapiens* [8].

Using DIANA-miRPath [9], a miR pathway analysis web-server, we clustered the validated miRs using experimentally validated miR interactions derived from DIANA-TarBase v6.0. Results were merged using a union of genes and analysed with a priori analysis methods (overrepresentation statistical analysis). This statistical analysis identified pathways significantly enriched with targets belonging to a union of genes. A P value threshold of 0.05 was applied with false discovery rate (FDR) correction to the resulting significance levels.

3. A Network of Experimentally Validated MicroRNA Highlights the Cross Talk between TGF-β, Wnt, and Notch Signalling in EMT

Using TarBase v6.0 we explored the collection of manually curated, experimentally validated miR interactions with genes in the TGF-β, Wnt, and Notch KEGG pathways. We identified 84 experimentally validated miRs interacting with genes involved in the TGF-β signalling pathway, 104 miRs in the Wnt pathway, and 48 miRs interacting with genes involved in Notch signalling. We clustered the miRs identified

in our search in order to obtain a list of experimentally validated miRs shared between all three pathways focusing first on clusters of two out of three pathways (i.e., experimentally validated miRs shared between only TGF-β and Notch, TGF-β and Wnt, or Notch and Wnt) (Figure 1). We identified 2 experimentally validated miRs shared between the TGF-β and Notch pathways (Figure 1 and Supplementary Table 1 available online at http://dx.doi.org/10.1155/2015/198967); 10 miRs shared between the Notch and Wnt pathways (Figure 1 and Supplementary Table 2); 39 miRs shared between the TGF-β and Wnt pathways (Figure 1 and Supplementary Table 3). We further identified a signature of 30 experimentally validated miRs targeting all three pathways (Figure 1 and Tables 1, 2, and 3). Within this 30-miR signature, 4 miRs (miR-103a, miR-132, miR-30a, and miR-10a) had validated target genes not ascribable to the manually annotated interactions within the KEGG pathways.

DIANA-miRPath was used to collect the complete list of manually annotated, experimentally validated, and published target genes for the 30 miRs identified. This was done in order to get better insight into the experimental data and understand the functional relevance of our analysis. Of all validated target genes 48 genes could be ascribed to the TGF-β pathway (P value = $6.9e - 09$), 30 to the Notch pathway (P value = $4.7e - 05$), and 88 to the Wnt signalling pathway (P value = $5.07e - 14$). Using the same approach as for the miRs, a cluster of genes was found to be shared between only two of the three pathways (i.e., experimentally validated miR-gene interactions from TGF-β and Notch, TGF-β and Wnt, or Notch and Wnt KEGG pathways). With this procedure, we identified 8 manually annotated and validated target genes shared by TGF-β and Wnt KEGG pathways (SMAD2, SMAD3, SMAD4, ROCK2, RHOA, MYC, PPP2R1A, and PPP2R1B) and 5 manually annotated and validated target genes shared by Notch and Wnt KEGG pathways (CTBP1, CTBP2, DVL2, DVL3, and PSEN1). Interestingly, no genes were shared between TGF-β and Notch KEGG pathways (Figure 2). Finally, we determined whether a new cluster of experimentally validated target genes coupled to our signature described above could be connected to a common biological process among TGF-β, Notch, and Wnt signalling pathways. Strikingly, only 2 validated target genes, the

TABLE 1: List of experimentally validated miRNA—gene interactions for TGF-β signalling pathway. Interactions with Notch and Wnt signalling are also indicated (genes among those in TGF-β pathway).

miRNA	Gene (TGF-β pathway)	Notch signalling	Wnt signalling
hsa-miR-335-5p	INHBB, **SMAD3**, ID4, ACVR1, ACVR2B, E2F5, **MYC**, BMP2, SP1, GDF5, AMHR2, TGFB2, THBS3, LTBP1, TGFBR2, INHBE	—	**SMAD3, MYC**
hsa-miR-34a-5p	E2F5, **MYC**	—	**MYC**
hsa-miR-1	E2F5, BMP7, THBS1	—	—
hsa-miR-124-3p	ID2, **ROCK2**, ID4, BMP6, **RHOA**, E2F5, SMAD5, ID1, SP1, BMPR1A, ID3, E2F4, **PPP2R1B**	—	**ROCK2, RHOA, PPP2R1B**
hsa-miR-26b-5p	SMAD6, BMP8B, RPS6KB2, ID1, BMP2, **EP300**, IFNG, SMAD7, BMPR2	**EP300**	**EP300**
hsa-miR-155-5p	**SMAD2**, THBS1, **SMAD3**, **RHOA**, SMAD5, SMAD1	—	**SMAD2, SMAD3, RHOA**
hsa-miR-375	CDKN2B, **RHOA**, TGFB2	—	**RHOA**
hsa-miR-21-5p	TGFBR1, THBS1, ZFVYE16, **MYC**, TGFB2, TGFBR2, BMPR2	—	**MYC**
hsa-miR-98	TGFBR1, THBS1, CDKN2B, RPS6KB2, **MYC**, SMAD7, INHBE, RPS6KB1	—	**MYC**
hsa-miR-122-5p	NODAL, SMURF2, **RHOA**	—	**RHOA**
hsa-miR-200c-3p	**EP300**	**EP300**	**EP300**
hsa-miR-9-5p	ID4, **EP300**	**EP300**	**EP300**
hsa-miR-324-3p	**CREBBP**	**CREBBP**	**CREBBP**
hsa-miR-24-3p	**MYC**	—	**MYC**
hsa-miR-194-5p	**EP300**	**EP300**	**EP300**
hsa-miR-92a-3p	THBS1, **SMAD4**, TGFBR2, BMPR2	—	**SMAD4**
hsa-miR-16-5p	SMURF2, **PPP2R1A**, SMAD5, ACVR2A, SP1, SMAD7, SMAD1, RPS6KB1	—	**PPP2R1A**
hsa-miR-93-5p	TGFBR2, BMPR2	—	—
hsa-miR-19a-3p	**SMAD4**, TGFBR2, BMPR2	—	**SMAD4**
hsa-miR-103a-3p	ACVR2B, SMAD7, RPS6KB1	—	—
hsa-miR-132-3p	THBS1	—	—
hsa-miR-30a-5p	THBS1, MAPK1	—	—
hsa-miR-200b-3p	**EP300**	**EP300**	**EP300**
hsa-miR-19b-3p	ACVR1, **SMAD4**, TGFBR2, BMPR2	—	**SMAD4**
hsa-miR-145-5p	**MYC**	—	**MYC**
hsa-miR-31-5p	**RHOA**	—	**RHOA**
hsa-miR-429	**EP300**	**EP300**	**EP300**
hsa-miR-10a-5p	ACVR2A	—	—
hsa-miR-182-5p	**EP300**	**EP300**	**EP300**
Hsa-miR-374a-5p	**EP300**	**EP300**	**EP300**

transcriptional coactivator cAMP-response element-binding protein- (CREB-) binding protein (CBP) and the adenovirus E1A-associated cellular p300 transcriptional coactivator protein p300 (EP300), were shared exclusively between the TGF-β, Notch, and Wnt signalling KEGG pathways (Figure 2). These results indicate the relevance of the 30-identified-miR signature thus suggesting a possible link between these miRs and cross talk between TGF-β, Notch, and Wnt pathways during EMT.

4. Identification of a Signature of miRs Targeting Genes Linked to TGF-β-, Notch-, and Wnt-Dependent EMT

4.1. Identification of miRs That Regulate Canonical and Noncanonical TGF-β Signalling during EMT. TGF-β signalling plays complex roles during tumor progression and can either inhibit or promote tumor growth depending on the cellular context. The complexity of TGF-β signalling derives in part

TABLE 2: List of experimentally validated miRNA—gene interactions for Wnt signalling pathway. Interactions with Notch and TGF-β signalling are also indicated (genes among those in Wnt pathway).

miRNA	Gene (Wnt pathway)	Notch signalling	TGF-β signalling
hsa-miR-335-5p	CTNNBIP1, LRP6, TBL1X, WNT10B, CCND2, DKK2, **SMAD3**, AXIN1, WNT3, FZD8, PPP2R5A, NFAT5, FZD10, **MYC**, VANGL2, PRKCG, DKK4, FZD1, PRICKLE2, SFRP1, WIF1, DAAM1, WNT7B, WNT9A, PPP3R2	—	**SMAD3, MYC**
hsa-miR-34a-5p	WNT1, CCND1, CTNNB1, AXIN2, **MYC**, PPP3R1, LEF1, MAP3K7, CCND3	—	**MYC**
hsa-miR-1	CSNK2A2, CAMK2G, **CTBP1, CTBP2**, PPP2R5A, PLCB3, CCND1, DKK1	**CTBP1, CTBP2**	—
hsa-miR-124-3p	VANGL1, PORCN, **ROCK2, RHOA**, WNT5B, CTNNB1, **PPP2R1B**, NFATC1, **DVL2**	**DVL2**	**ROCK2, PPP2R1B, RHOA**
hsa-miR-26b-5p	SFRP4, **DVL3**, FZD5, RUVBL1, VANGL1, GPC4, JUN, CCND1, VANGL2, PPP3R1, **EP300**, PLCB4, PLCB2	**EP300, DVL3**	**EP300**
hsa-miR-155-5p	**GSK3B, SMAD2**, APC, VANGL1, WNT5A, **SMAD3**, CSNK1A1L, **RHOA**, CTNNB1, CSNK1A1, RAC1, **PSEN1**	**PSEN1**	**SMAD2, SMAD3, RHOA,**
hsa-miR-375	PRKCA, **RHOA**, FZD4, PRKX	—	**RHOA**
hsa-miR-21-5p	TCF4, APC, WNT1, WNT5A, NFAT5, CSNK1A1, **MYC**, PRICKLE2, DAAM1, TBL1XR1	—	**MYC**
hsa-miR-98	VANGL1, WNT10B, SENP2, FZD10, **MYC**	—	**MYC**
hsa-miR-122-5p	**RHOA**, RAC1, TBL1XR1	**RHOA**	**RHOA**
hsa-miR-200c-3p	TCF7L1, **EP300**	**EP300**	**EP300**
hsa-miR-9-5p	WNT8A, WNT6, **EP300**, NFATC3, PLCB4	**EP300**	**EP300**
hsa-miR-324-3p	WNT9B, **CREBBP, DVL2**	**CREBBP, DVL2**	**CREBBP**
hsa-miR-24-3p	FZD5, CHD8, FZD4, NFAT5, NKD1, **MYC**, PPP3R1	—	**MYC**
hsa-miR-194-5p	**EP300**	**EP300**	**EP300**
hsa-miR-92a-3p	**SMAD4**	—	**SMAD4**
hsa-miR-16-5p	CAMK2G, WNT5A, CCND2, PPP2R5C, JUN, CCND1, AXIN2, **PPP2R1A**, WNT3A, CCND3	—	**PPP2R1A**
hsa-miR-93-5p	MAPK9, CCND1, PRKACB	—	—
hsa-miR-19a-3p	CCND1, **SMAD4**	—	**SMAD4**
hsa-miR-103a-3p	AXIN2, WNT3A, MAP3K7	—	—
hsa-miR-132-3p	WNT3A	—	—
hsa-miR-30a-5p	WNT5A, PPP2R5C, PPP3CA, JUN, CTNNB1, PPP3R1	—	—
hsa-miR-200b-3p	TCF7L1, **EP300**	**EP300**	**EP300**
hsa-miR-19b-3p	DAAM2, TCF4, CCND2, **SMAD4**, PRKACB	—	**SMAD4**
hsa-miR-145-5p	PPP3CA, **MYC**	—	**MYC**
hsa-miR-31-5p	**RHOA**, NFAT5	—	**RHOA**
hsa-miR-429	TCF7L1, **EP300**	**EP300**	**EP300**
hsa-miR-10a-5p	BTRC, MAPK8, MAP3K7	—	—
hsa-miR-182-5p	**EP300**	**EP300**	**EP300**
Hsa-miR-374a-5p	**EP300**	**EP300**	**EP300**

from the capability of its receptors to activate distinct canonical and noncanonical signalling pathways. In the SMAD-dependent canonical pathway, TGF-β ligands assemble their specific type II and type I transmembrane serine kinase receptors, allowing the constitutively active type II receptor kinase to phosphorylate the type I receptor, thereby activating its kinase. The active type I receptor then phosphorylates its cognate cytoplasmic SMAD proteins which then enter the nucleus to regulate the transcription of target genes. By contrast, the noncanonical pathway is SMAD-independent and includes TGF-β signalling via the Rho family of GTPases and MAPK/PI3K pathways. In this context, TGF-β has been shown to rapidly activate the Rho-GTPases and its activation of RHOA in epithelial cells leads to induction of stress fibers and acquisition of mesenchymal characteristics, thus promoting EMT [10]. Additionally, RHOA is a crucial regulator in

TABLE 3: List of experimentally validated miRNA—gene interactions for Notch signalling pathway. Interactions with Wnt and TGF-β signalling are also indicated (genes among those in Notch pathway).

miRNA	Gene (Notch pathway)	Wnt signalling	TGF-β signalling
hsa-miR-335-5p	NUMB, MFNG, LFNG, DLL1, NOTCH3, DTX1, MAML2, JAG2	—	—
hsa-miR-34a-5p	HDAC1, NOTCH2, NOTCH1, DLL1, JAG1	—	—
hsa-miR-1	**CTBP1, CTBP2**, NOTCH2, HDAC2, DTX1	**CTBP1, CTBP2**	—
hsa-miR-124-3p	RBPJ, **DVL2**, MAML1, JAG2	**DVL2**	—
hsa-miR-26b-5p	**DVL3**, KAT2B, **EP300**	**EP300, DVL3**	**EP300**
hsa-miR-155-5p	NOTCH2, PSEN1, RBPJ	—	—
hsa-miR-375	NUMB, JAG1, RBPJ	—	—
hsa-miR-21-5p	JAG1, NCSTN, DTX3L	—	—
hsa-miR-98	DTX4, JAG1	—	—
hsa-miR-122-5p	NUMBL, ADAM17	—	—
hsa-miR-200c-3p	JAG1, **EP300**	**EP300**	**EP300**
hsa-miR-9-5p	NCOR2, **EP300**	**EP300**	**EP300**
hsa-miR-324-3p	**CREBBP, DVL2**	**CREBBP, DVL2**	**CREBBP**
hsa-miR-24-3p	HDAC1, NOTCH1	—	—
hsa-miR-194-5p	**EP300**	**EP300**	**EP300**
hsa-miR-92a-3p	KAT2B	—	—
hsa-miR-16-5p	NOTCH2	—	—
hsa-miR-93-5p	KAT2B	—	—
hsa-miR-19a-3p	KAT2B	—	—
hsa-miR-103a-3p	NUMB	—	—
hsa-miR-132-3p	LFNG	—	—
hsa-miR-30a-5p	NOTCH1	—	—
hsa-miR-200b-3p	**EP300**	**EP300**	**EP300**
hsa-miR-19b-3p	KAT2B	—	—
hsa-miR-145-5p	APH1A	—	—
hsa-miR-31-5p	NUMB	—	—
hsa-miR-429	**EP300**	**EP300**	**EP300**
hsa-miR-10a-5p	NCOR2	—	—
hsa-miR-182-5p	**EP300**	**EP300**	**EP300**
Hsa-miR-374a-5p	**EP300**	**EP300**	**EP300**

the signal transduction events that link activation of latent TGF-β by plasma membrane receptors (e.g., integrins) to the assembly of focal adhesions and sites of F-actin fiber organization [11].

Interestingly, we have identified interactions between RHOA and a group of 5 validated miRs (miR-155, miR-124, miR-375, miR-122, and miR-31) [12–17] (Figure 3). More specifically, in endothelial cells, miR-155 was shown to block the acquisition of the mesenchymal phenotype induced by TGF-β by directly targeting RHOA [17]. Similar observations were made in osteoclast precursor cells, where overexpression of miR-124 decreased RHOA expression and reduced cell migration [18]. miR-375 also interferes with cytoskeletal organization by indirectly targeting RHOA during neuronal development [12]. Dramatic effects on migration and cytoskeleton disruption have also been reported for miR-122 in hepatocellular carcinoma (HCC). In this context, miR-122 and RHOA interact directly and overexpression of RHOA reverts miR-122-induced

mesenchymal-to-epithelial transition (MET) and inhibition of migration [16]. Finally, in breast cancer cells it was demonstrated that overexpression of miR-31 decreases invasion and metastasis via downregulation of RHOA [15] (Figure 3). Together, these findings highlight the relevance of these miRs in interfering with RHOA mediated EMT.

Modulation of stress fibers and cytoskeletal rearrangements are key events in the acquisition of a mesenchymal phenotype and in the modulation of cellular motility. Two key players in this process are the Rho-serine/threonine kinases ROCK1 and ROCK2 which regulate smooth muscle contraction, formation of stress fibers, and focal adhesions [19]. ROCK1 and ROCK2 are two major downstream effectors of RHOA that constitute additional important mediators of TGF-β-induced EMT. Interestingly, among the 30 miRs in our signature, we found 2 validated miRs (miR-335 and miR-124) that regulate expression of ROCK1 and ROCK2 [20, 21]. Low levels of miR-335 were correlated with poor overall patient survival in neuroblastoma while overexpression of

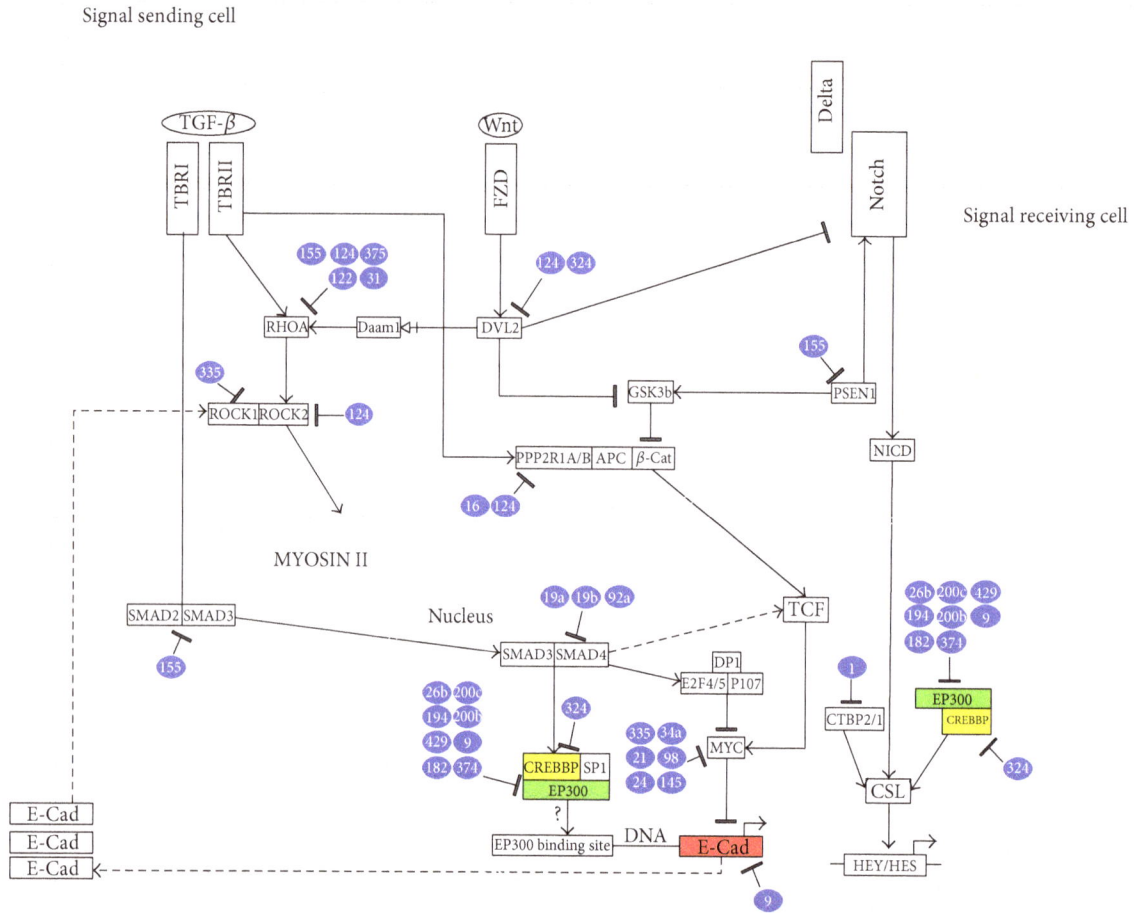

FIGURE 3: Interaction between miRs from the 30-miR signature and their predicted target genes overlaid on KEGG TGF-β, Notch, and Wnt pathways.

this miR strongly reduced cell migration and impaired F-actin organization [20]. Further analysis revealed that miR-335 directly targets ROCK1 providing an explanation for its ability to reduce cell invasion [20]. Low levels of miR-124 have been associated with poor prognosis in aggressive HCC while overexpression of miR-124 in HCC cell lines strongly decreased ROCK2 expression and inhibited EMT, formation of stress fibers, filopodia, and lamellipodia [21]. Taken together these experimental data highlight an important role for miR-335 and miR-124 in SMAD-independent, noncanonical TGF-β effects on cytoskeletal rearrangements via RHOA-dependent signalling pathways (Figure 3).

TGF-β also induces mesenchymal characteristics via canonical signalling, that is, via SMAD2 and SMAD3. In the previous paragraph we described the ability of miR-155 to directly decrease RHOA expression and thereby inhibit cell motility and EMT characteristics [17]. Interestingly, miR-155 has also been shown to interfere with the canonical TGF-β pathway by directly affecting the formation of the SMAD2/3 signalling complex. Louafi et al. have demonstrated that miR-155 directly targets SMAD2, leading to a reduction of TGF-β-induced SMAD2 phosphorylation and blocking

SMAD2-dependent activation of a TGF-β-inducible, SMAD-dependent CAGA reporter plasmid [22]. Additionally, miR-155 targets presenilin 1 (PSEN1), a catalytic subunit of the gamma-secretase complex which catalyzes the cleavage of membrane proteins including Notch receptors [23]. In this regard, Gudey et al. have shown that PSEN1 plays a crucial role in mediating the interaction between TGF-β and Notch signalling by promoting the association between the TGF-β type I receptor intracellular domain (TβRI-ICD) and the Notch intracellular domain (NICD) which in turn triggers cell-invasive behaviour in prostate cancer [24]. Altogether, these data suggest that miR-155 can disrupt both the canonical and noncanonical TGF-β pathways and might represent an interesting modulator of cross talk between TGF-β and Notch signalling pathways (Figure 3).

4.2. Identification of miRs Regulating the Cross Talk between TGF-β and Wnt Signalling during EMT. The observation that TGF-β alone can be sufficient to induce EMT in epithelial cells [10] while other cell types may not be sensitive to this effect of TGF-β [25] suggests that induction of EMT by TGF-β requires cooperation with other signalling pathways.

Indeed, several studies indicate that TGF-β acts together with the Notch and Wnt pathways to promote EMT [4, 6, 26, 27]. Remarkably, in our analysis we could not identify any validated miR target genes shared exclusively between the TGF-β and Notch pathways. However, Notch is able to antagonize TGF-β via sequestration of EP300, a factor that in turn acts as a transcriptional coactivator for NOTCH1 [28]. The interaction in the cluster of miR target genes ascribable to Notch signalling and their interactions with miR target genes associated with both TGF-β and Wnt signalling pathways are discussed below.

Concerning Wnt signalling, two interesting genes highlighted in our analysis are PPP2R1A and PPP2R1B. These are the catalytic subunits of the PP2A holoenzyme, a protein phosphatase that reverts the action of protein kinases in many signalling cascades, including Wnt signalling [29]. Several reports support the notion that PP2A plays a dual role in Wnt signalling and can act as either a positive or a negative regulator of the pathway [30]. On one hand, in the absence of Wnt, β-catenin forms a complex with APC, AXIN, and GSK3β. This allows GSK3β to phosphorylate β-catenin that is then ubiquitinated and targeted for proteasomal degradation. In this context, different PP2A subunits bind to AXIN and APC, decreasing β-catenin levels and thereby negatively regulating Wnt signalling. On the other hand, in the presence of Wnt, PP2A seems to exert a positive role in β-catenin stabilization [30]. In this situation, the complex of APC, AXIN, and GSK3β is degraded by Dishevelled (DSH) leading to nuclear β-catenin accumulation and activation of Wnt target genes. Stabilized β-catenin can subsequently localize at plasma membrane in complex with E-Cadherin and PP2A, thus reducing EMT.

Recently, we have demonstrated that activation of Wnt signalling via GSK3β inhibition in metastatic and androgen independent prostate cancer cells (PC3, DU145, and C4-2B) induces dramatic changes in their morphology, blocks their migration, reduces their metastatic growth, and strongly affects their mesenchymal phenotype [31]. This highlights the ability of Wnt signalling to stabilize E-Cadherin and interfere with EMT in prostate cancer suggesting that PP2A may act as a negative regulator of EMT. Consistent with this possibility, it has been shown that restoring expression of a catalytic subunit of PP2A can revert EMT and suppress tumor growth and metastasis in an orthotopic mouse model of human prostate cancer [32]. Interestingly, we identified two miRs in our signature (miR-16 and miR-124) that directly block the expression of catalytic subunits of PP2A (PPP2R1A and PPP2R1B) and that have been positively validated by proteomics and microarray, respectively [13, 23]. Strikingly, homozygous deletion (HD) of the miR-16 locus was observed in androgen independent prostate cancer in xenograft models [33]. The HD of miR-16 in a subset of androgen independent prostate cancer xenograft might suggest that, in this context, PP2A is present and stable. In turn, this might also suggest that activation of Wnt signalling in androgen independent prostate cancer cells could act synergistically with PP2A to promote stabilization of β-catenin and E-Cadherin leading to reduced EMT. Taken together, these data might identify a subset of androgen independent prostate cancers in which

restoration of Wnt signalling reduces the aggressiveness of tumor cells and abolishes their mesenchymal phenotype.

The involvement of miR-16 in EMT in the context of prostate cancer is further reinforced by an interesting observation regarding its role in the tumor-supportive capacity of stromal cells. Musumeci et al. have shown that miR-16 is downregulated in fibroblasts surrounding prostate tumors in patients [34]. Additionally, they have demonstrated that miR-16 restoration considerably impairs the tumor-supportive capability of stromal cells in vitro and in vivo [34]. From this perspective, it is important to note that the prostate tumor microenvironment is rich in TGF-β superfamily members including TGF-βs, bone morphogenetic proteins (BMPs), growth/differentiation factors (GDFs), activins, inhibins, Nodal, and anti-Müllerian hormone (AMH) [35]. Among them, miR-16 has been suggested to regulate activin/Nodal signalling via direct interaction with teratocarcinoma-derived growth factor 1 (Cripto, TDGF1). Chen et al. have indeed shown using luciferase reporter assays that miR-16 (together with miR-15a) directly interacts with the 3′UTR of Cripto [36].

Cripto is a small, GPI-anchored protein that functions as a secreted growth factor and as an obligatory cell surface coreceptor for a subset of TGF-β superfamily ligands including Nodal [37]. Cripto regulates both cell movement and EMT during embryonic development and cancer [38] and, strikingly, Nodal, which has been implicated in enhancing tumor cell plasticity and aggressiveness, is expressed in cancerous but not normal human prostate specimens [39]. Although it is required for Nodal signalling, Cripto suppresses TGF-β signalling in multiple cell types [40], reinforcing the inclusion of miR-16 in our signature. Therefore, the reduced expression of miR-16 in the tumor microenvironment in prostate cancer is predicted to facilitate Cripto-dependent Nodal signalling which together with Cripto's other tumor-promoting effects could trigger invasiveness, bone metastasis, and EMT.

Similar to miR-16, overexpression of miR-124 in androgen independent prostate cancer cell lines (DU145) strongly reduces aggressiveness and invasion [41]. This further supports the hypothesis that the increased PP2A stability caused by low levels of miR-16 and miR-124 in a subset of androgen independent prostate cancer cell lines could explain reduced cell migration and invasion, an effect that we also documented upon GSK3β inhibition [31]. miR-124 is also likely to be an important player in Wnt signal transduction since proteomics and microarray analyses have revealed that it interacts with DVL2 (a member of DSH protein family) [13, 42]. DVL2 binds the cytoplasmic C-terminus of the frizzled family of Wnt receptors and transduces the Wnt signal to downstream effectors. Interestingly, DVL2 also interacts with insulin receptor substrates (IRS1/2) and thereby promotes canonical Wnt signalling [43]. Moreover, IRS1/2 have been identified as key players in the regulation of E-Cadherin expression during EMT [44, 45]. IRS1/2 have also been implicated in the progression and etiology of prostate cancer. The IRS1/2 ratio has been shown to be significantly lower in malignant prostate tumors than in benign prostatic tissue and functional polymorphisms in IRS1 have been associated with a more advanced Gleason score [46, 47]. Also reduced migration was documented after miR-124 overexpression in androgen independent prostate cancer suggesting a mechanism in which low levels of miR-124 boost DVL2. This, in turn, would be predicted to lead to GSK3β blockade with subsequent β-catenin and E-Cadherin stabilization. Additionally, low levels of miR-124 strengthen PP2A, which further contribute to stabilization of β-catenin and E-Cadherin, therefore reducing EMT.

Another miR in our signature, miR-324, has also been shown to regulate expression of DVL2. Ragan et al. used a luciferase reporter plasmid to demonstrate that miR-324 directly targets DVL2 [48]. Interestingly, dysregulation of miR-324 has been linked to macrophage dysfunction in colorectal cancer, where altered Wnt signalling is known to play a pivotal role [49]. More specifically, miR-324 was found to be highly expressed in infiltrated macrophages in fresh colon cancer tissues isolated immediately after surgical removal [49]. Additionally, in the same work, the oncogene c-Myc was identified as a candidate transcription factor capable of regulating miR-324. This, combined with the identification of miR-324 in our analysis, suggests a fascinating role for miR-324 in the cross talk between TGF-β and Wnt signalling in EMT and colorectal cancer. The role of TGF-β as a "double edged sword" during colon cancer progression has been extensively documented in the literature. In its tumor suppressive role, TGF-β inhibits progression of the cell cycle by inducing the tumor suppressors p15 (INK4B) and p21 (CDKN1A) and inhibiting expression c-Myc [50]. At the same time, c-Myc is also a crucial downstream target of altered Wnt signalling in colon cancer [51] and has been shown to cause loss of E-Cadherin, which is a hallmark of EMT [52]. Therefore, miR-324 could be involved in a feedback loop between Wnt, TGF-β, and c-Myc. More specifically, altered Wnt signalling during colorectal cancer development could modulate c-Myc levels and therefore miR-324 expression. In turn, abnormal miR-324 levels can interfere with DVL2 expression leading to alteration in the Wnt signalling pathway that further alter c-Myc and E-Cadherin levels (Figure 3).

We have identified a group of 6 miRs (miR-335, miR-34a, miR-21, miR-98, miR-24, and miR-145) directly linked to c-Myc, reinforcing the role of c-Myc as a common downstream target between TGF-β- and Wnt-mediated EMT. Among them, we have already discussed the role of miR-335 in EMT induced by TGF-β, particularly its interaction with ROCK1 and ROCK2 [20]. Interestingly, Tavazoie et al. have shown by microarray that miR-335 also interacts with c-Myc [53], suggesting a more comprehensive role for miR-335 in TGF-β- and Wnt-mediated EMT. Additionally, Sampson et al. have suggested that miR-98 (from let-7/miR-98 family) might regulate c-Myc expression [54]. They have shown that administration of 10058-F4, a compound that inhibits MYC, strongly increases the expression of miR-98 and other let-7 family members [54]. Strikingly, treatment of melanoma cells with 10058-F4 efficiently diminished EMT mediated by TGF-β and S-phase kinase-associated protein 2 (SKP2) [55]. Taken together, these data suggest that miR-98 could represent an important mediator in the cross talk between TGF-β and Wnt and their effect in modulation of EMT.

Deregulated expression of c-Myc has been reported in a wide variety of human cancers and among several key regulators of c-Myc expression, an important role is exerted by p53. Interestingly miR-145 has been reported to repress c-Myc in response to the p53 pathway [56] reinforcing its identification in our EMT signature. Similarly, members of miR-34 family are known to be direct transcriptional targets of p53 and p53-binding sites are localized on the miR-34 gene promoter [57]. However, Christoffersen et al. demonstrated that miR-34a is capable of repressing c-Myc in a p53 independent manner [58]. This suggests that, beside the cross talk between p53 and c-Myc, there are additional mechanisms that contribute to fine tuning of the role of c-Myc in TGF-β- and Wnt-dependent EMT. From this perspective, a crucial outcome of deregulated MYC signalling is represented by E-Cadherin repression. Lal et al. have shown that miR-24 directly targets MYC, suggesting that this miR could potentially play an interesting role in EMT modulation [59]. To support this hypothesis, miR-24 has also been recently shown to regulate the EMT program in response to TGF-β in breast cancer cells. Papadimitriou et al. have demonstrated that miR-24 is capable of modulating TGF-β-induced breast cancer cell invasiveness through regulation of RHOA-specific guanine nucleotide exchange factor Net1 isoform2 (Net1A), a protein that is necessary for TGF-β-mediated RHOA activation [60]. Together, these findings reinforce the identification of miR-24 in our EMT signature.

The last miR included in the group of those targeting c-Myc is miR-21. Singh et al. have suggested that miR-21 regulates self-renewal in mouse embryonic stem (ES) cells and could potentially interact with MYC and other self-renewal markers (Oct4, Nanog, and Sox2) [61]. They have shown that enforced expression of miR-21 in ES cells downregulates renewal markers, including c-Myc [61]. This suggests that in specific contexts modulation of miR-21 could potentially affect c-Myc expression and therefore modulate E-Cadherin levels and affect EMT.

Finally, in the previous paragraphs we have described the role of miR-155 as an interesting player capable of disrupting the tumor-promoting effects of SMAD-dependent and SMAD-independent TGF-β signalling [22]. Interestingly, in our analysis we identified another group of 4 miRs linked to TGF-β signalling and belonging to the miR-17-92 cluster (i.e., miR-19a, miR-19b, and miR-92a) and to its paralog cluster miR-106b-25 (i.e., miR-93). Interestingly, c-Myc has been reported to upregulate the miR-17-92 cluster, providing further evidence of cross talk between Wnt and TGF-β signalling [62]. Dews et al. performed a detailed study to elucidate the mechanism of interaction between the miR-17-92 cluster and TGF-β signalling, particularly with SMAD4 [63]. Using qPCR and microarray analyses they provide evidence suggesting that miR-19a, miR-19b, and miR-92a regulate SMAD4 indirectly, that is, without interacting with the SMAD4 $3'$UTR [63].

4.3. A Group of miRs Targeting the CREBBP/EP300 Interaction Highlight the Cross Talk between TGF-β, Wnt, and Notch Signalling during EMT. As mentioned above, EP300 (p300) and CREBBP (CREB-binding protein, CBP) are the only two KEGG pathway genes shared among all three pathways (i.e., TGF-β, Wnt, and Notch). EP300 and CREBBP are functionally related transcriptional coactivator proteins that play many important roles in processes including cell proliferation, differentiation, and apoptosis. In the context of Wnt signalling, EP300 has been shown to act synergistically with β-catenin and T cell factor (TCF) during neoplastic transformation [64]. Similarly, in the context of TGF-β signalling, it has been reported that phosphorylated SMAD3 interacts with the CREBBP/EP300 complex to augment transcriptional activation [65]. Additionally, the Notch intracellular domain (NICD) can recruit the complex CREBBP/EP300 to interact with the transcription factor CSL (CBF1/Su(H)/Lag-1) which, in turn, activates the transcription of two known Notch related basic-helix-loop-helix transcription factor families, HEY and HES [66].

EP300 regulates transcription and remodels chromatin by acting as histone acetyltransferase. It regulates p53 dependent transcription and binds specifically to phosphorylated CREBBP [67]. EP300 and CREBBP were originally identified in protein interaction assays through their association with the transcription factor CREB and with the adenoviral-transforming protein E1A, respectively [68–70]. The roles of CREBBP and EP300 and their interaction during EMT have been extensively studied. However, the large degree of cellular heterogeneity within different organs and tissues makes the role of EP300 in EMT difficult to define with precision [71].

Strikingly, some reports have linked the expression of wild-type EP300 in colorectal and prostate cancer with the degree of intravascular dissemination of cancer cells (probably affected by ongoing EMT) and poor prognosis [72–74]. In this context, EP300 seems to promote cancer cells EMT. In support of this, elevated expression of EP300 in hepatocellular carcinomas (HCC) correlates with enhanced vascular invasion, intrahepatic metastasis, shortened survival, and, strikingly, low E-Cadherin expression [75]. EP300 knockdown strongly increased E-Cadherin expression and significantly decreased migration and invasion in a hepatoma cell line (HLE) that is otherwise highly invasive and poorly differentiated [75].

In the context of cancerous hepatocytes, TGF-β is one factor that plays a major role in the induction of EMT, causing type I collagen induction and formation of liver fibrosis. In this situation, EP300 interacts with SMAD3 and functions as signal integrator for mediating regulation of collagen synthesis by TGF-β [76]. Treatment with HDAC inhibitor strongly decreases EP300 levels and restores E-Cadherin distribution to the hepatocytes cell membrane therefore reducing TGF-β-induced EMT [77].

As outlined above, targeting the expression of EP300 and/or CREBBP can simultaneously affect TGF-β, Wnt, and Notch pathways. In this regard, miR-9, which is represented in our 30-miR signature, was shown to target EP300 as determined by microarray analysis [78] (Figure 3). Remarkably, miR-9 has also been shown to be involved in the modulation of E-Cadherin levels via c-Myc. More specifically, Ma et al. have shown that MYC acts as a transcriptional activator of miR-9 and that miR-9, in turn, directly targets E-Cadherin

[79]. Therefore, not only is miR-9 one of the common miRs linking TGF-β, Wnt, and Notch signalling but also it has the ability to target E-Cadherin which links it directly to EMT. Thus, it appears that miR-9 might represent an interesting regulator of the cross talk between TGF-β, Wnt, and Notch signalling pathways in both normal cells and cancer cells. On one hand, through its effect on E-Cadherin and EP300, miR-9 may maintain the balance between epithelial and mesenchymal cell state in normal cells. On the other hand, in cancer cells that have lost the tumor suppressive effect of TGF-β, the disruption of the TGF-β cytostatic program could cause c-Myc induced upregulation of miR-9 leading to loss of E-Cadherin and subsequent EMT. Bonev et al. have further shown that, in the context of Notch signalling, in addition to its connection with EP300, miR-9 also interacts directly with Hes1 [80]. This reinforces the hypothesis that miR-9 represents an interesting regulator of the Notch signalling pathway with a role in the cross talk between TGF-β, Wnt, and Notch.

Regulation of the CREBBP/EP300 complex by miR-9 represents an interesting mechanism of coregulation of TGF-β, Wnt, and Notch signalling pathways. In this regard, it is interesting to note that we identified another group of 5 miRs (miR-26b, miR-194, miR-182, miR-374, and miR-324) that also were shown to interact with EP300 and CREBBP by microarray [81]. Among these, notable observations have been reported for miR-26 and miR-324. Cai et al. have shown that miR-26 is strongly downregulated in HT-29 colon cancer cells undergoing TGF-β-induced EMT, whereas Ragan et al. have described an interaction between miR-324 and CREBBP by transcriptomic analysis [48, 82]. Moreover, interestingly in our analysis we have also identified miR-1, that has been shown to interact with CTBP1/2, two proteins that bind to the C-terminus of adenovirus E1A protein [13] and act as corepressors of Notch target genes [83] (Figure 3).

As discussed above, there is a connection between miR-324 and DVL2 in the context of Wnt signalling and colon cancer [48, 49]. Interactions between TGF-β and Wnt are important in many biological processes. In particular, in the context of colon cancer, the cascade of events that drives tumor progression is characterized by series of genetic modifications involving components of the Wnt and TGF-β signalling pathways. In colon cancer, the adenoma-carcinoma sequence is initiated by alteration in Wnt signalling (i.e., inactivation of APC). Subsequently, the late stage adenoma shows loss of 18q-arm, where it maps the best candidate tumor suppressor gene DPC4/MADH4, which encodes SMAD4, involved in the TGF-β pathway [84]. This event drives the progression from the intermediate adenoma stage to late adenoma, resulting in loss of the cytostatic effect of TGF-β. Strikingly, the interaction between β-catenin and the TGF-β pathway depends on the transcriptional coactivator CREBBP as demonstrated by Zhou et al. who used chromatin immune precipitation to show that a complex forms between SMAD3, β-catenin, and CREBBP [85]. These findings together with the identification of EP300 and CREBBP in our analysis suggest that miR-26 and miR-324 may link TGF-β and Wnt signalling with EMT in colon cancer progression.

4.4. Interaction between CREBBP/EP300 and miR-200 Family.
Recent studies have indicated that the switch in tumor
cells from a sessile, epithelial phenotype towards a motile,
mesenchymal phenotype is accompanied by the acquisition
of stem/progenitor cell characteristics [86]. In particular, cells
undergoing EMT acquire chemoresistance, a key property
attributed to cancer stem cells (CSCs) [86]. In this context,
the miR-200 family is particularly interesting. The miR-
200 family includes miR-200c-3p, miR-200b-3p, and miR-
429 (all identified in our analysis) and inhibits EMT and
cancer cell migration by directly targeting the E-Cadherin
transcriptional repressors ZEB1 and ZEB2 [87]. Additionally,
downregulation of miR-200 family has been described in
docetaxel resistant prostate cancer cells, reinforcing the link
between EMT and resistance to chemotherapy [88].

Interestingly, our analysis revealed a connection between
miR-200 family members and EP300 regulation. Mizuguchi
et al. have shown that acetyltransferase EP300 regulates
expression of miR-200c-3p overcoming its transcriptional
suppression by ZEB1 [89]. The same authors showed that
treatment with an HDAC inhibitor significantly increased
miR-200c-3p levels causing a decrease in Vimentine and
ZEB1 and upregulation of E-Cadherin. Strikingly, miR-200c-
3p, miR-200b-3p, and miR-429 have also been shown to
interact with EP300 by microarray and protein analysis [81].
These observations enhance the complexity of the regulatory
mechanisms governing the interplay between EP300 and E-
Cadherin and suggest a positive feedback loop between miR-
200 family and EP300. The inhibitory effect of ZEB1 on miR-
200 could be attenuated by EP300 which upregulates miR-
200 expression. Furthermore, higher levels of miR-200 could
decrease ZEB1, suggesting that the positive effect of EP300 on
E-Cadherin expression could also be mediated via miR-200
family (Figure 3).

5. Conclusion

In this review, we discussed and summarized the known
interactions between miRs and genes involved in TGF-
β, Notch, and Wnt signalling pathways and highlighted a
signature of 30 validated miRs linking these pathways to the
process of EMT. Our novel approach led to the identification
of a cluster of validated and known miRs involved in different
pathways in an attempt to reduce the extraordinary volume
of information related to the interaction between miRs and
different target genes. We believe that the identification of
groups of genes targeted by the same miR and the clustering
of these genes in different pathways could potentially represent an interesting strategy to better understand the cross
talk between multiple signalling networks, thus facilitating
the understanding of their connections and their role in a
common biological process.

Conflict of Interests

The authors disclose no potential conflict of interests.

Acknowledgments

The research leading to these results has received funding
from the FP7 Marie Curie ITN under Grant Agreement no.
264817-BONE-NET (EZ), Prostate Action UK (EZ, GP), and
Clayton Foundation (PG).

References

[1] J. P. Thiery and J. P. Sleeman, "Complex networks orchestrate
epithelial-mesenchymal transitions," *Nature Reviews Molecular
Cell Biology*, vol. 7, no. 2, pp. 131–142, 2006.

[2] R. Kalluri, "EMT: when epithelial cells decide to become
mesenchymal-like cells," *Journal of Clinical Investigation*, vol.
119, no. 6, pp. 1417–1419, 2009.

[3] J. Fuxe, T. Vincent, and A. G. de Herreros, "Transcriptional
crosstalk between TGFβ and stem cell pathways in tumor cell
invasion: role of EMT promoting Smad complexes," *Cell Cycle*,
vol. 9, no. 12, pp. 2363–2374, 2010.

[4] L. A. Timmerman, J. Grego-Bessa, A. Raya et al., "Notch
promotes epithelial-mesenchymal transition during cardiac
development and oncogenic transformation," *Genes and Development*, vol. 18, no. 1, pp. 99–115, 2004.

[5] J. Zavadil and E. P. Böttinger, "TGF-β and epithelial-to-
mesenchymal transitions," *Oncogene*, vol. 24, no. 37, pp. 5764–
5774, 2005.

[6] J. Zavadil, L. Cermak, N. Soto-Nieves, and E. P. Böttinger,
"Integration of TGF-β/Smad and Jagged1/Notch signalling in
epithelial-to-mesenchymal transition," *The EMBO Journal*, vol.
23, no. 5, pp. 1155–1165, 2004.

[7] T. Vergoulis, I. S. Vlachos, P. Alexiou et al., "TarBase 6.0: captur-
ing the exponential growth of miRNA targets with experimental
support," *Nucleic Acids Research*, vol. 40, no. 1, pp. D222–D229,
2012.

[8] M. Kanehisa and S. Goto, "KEGG: kyoto encyclopedia of genes
and genomes," *Nucleic Acids Research*, vol. 28, no. 1, pp. 27–30,
2000.

[9] I. S. Vlachos, N. Kostoulas, T. Vergoulis et al., "DIANA miRPath
v.2.0: investigating the combinatorial effect of microRNAs in
pathways," *Nucleic Acids Research*, vol. 40, no. 1, pp. W498–
W504, 2012.

[10] N. A. Bhowmick, M. Ghiassi, A. Bakin et al., "Transforming
growth factor-β1 mediates epithelial to mesenchymal transdifferentiation through a RhoA-dependent mechanism," *Molecular Biology of the Cell*, vol. 12, no. 1, pp. 27–36, 2001.

[11] C. Margadant and A. Sonnenberg, "Integrin-TGF-β crosstalk in
fibrosis, cancer and wound healing," *EMBO Reports*, vol. 11, no.
2, pp. 97–105, 2010.

[12] K. Abdelmohsen, E. R. Hutchison, E. K. Lee et al., "miR-375
inhibits differentiation of neurites by lowering HuD levels,"
Molecular and Cellular Biology, vol. 30, no. 17, pp. 4197–4210,
2010.

[13] D. Baek, J. Villén, C. Shin, F. D. Camargo, S. P. Gygi, and D. P.
Bartel, "The impact of microRNAs on protein output," *Nature*,
vol. 455, no. 7209, pp. 64–71, 2008.

[14] T. D. Schmittgen, "miR-31: a master regulator of metastasis?"
Future Oncology, vol. 6, no. 1, pp. 17–20, 2010.

[15] S. Valastyan, F. Reinhardt, N. Benaich et al., "A pleiotropically
acting microRNA, miR-31, inhibits breast cancer metastasis,"
Cell, vol. 137, no. 6, pp. 1032–1046, 2009.

[16] S.-C. Wang, X.-L. Lin, J. Li et al., "MicroRNA-122 triggers mesenchymal-epithelial transition and suppresses hepatocellular carcinoma cell motility and invasion by targeting RhoA," *PLoS ONE*, vol. 9, no. 7, Article ID e101330, 2014.

[17] R. Bijkerk, R. G. de Bruin, C. van Solingen et al., "MicroRNA-155 functions as a negative regulator of RhoA signaling in TGF-beta-induced endothelial to mesenchymal transition," *MicroRNA*, vol. 1, no. 1, pp. 2–10, 2012.

[18] Y. Lee, H. J. Kim, C. K. Park et al., "MicroRNA-124 regulates osteoclast differentiation," *Bone*, vol. 56, no. 2, pp. 383–389, 2013.

[19] F. E. Lock, K. R. Ryan, N. S. Poulter, M. Parsons, and N. A. Hotchin, "Differential regulation of adhesion complex turnover by ROCK1 and ROCK2," *PLoS ONE*, vol. 7, no. 2, Article ID e31423, 2012.

[20] J. Lynch, J. Fay, M. Meehan et al., "MiRNA-335 suppresses neuroblastoma cell invasiveness by direct targeting of multiple genes from the non-canonical TGF-β signalling pathway," *Carcinogenesis*, vol. 33, no. 5, pp. 976–985, 2012.

[21] F. Zheng, Y.-J. Liao, M.-Y. Cai et al., "The putative tumour suppressor microRNA-124 modulates hepatocellular carcinoma cell aggressiveness by repressing ROCK2 and EZH2," *Gut*, vol. 61, no. 2, pp. 278–289, 2012.

[22] F. Louafi, R. T. Martinez-Nunez, and T. Sanchez-Elsner, "MicroRNA-155 targets SMAD2 and modulates the response of macrophages to transforming growth factor-β," *Journal of Biological Chemistry*, vol. 285, no. 53, pp. 41328–41336, 2010.

[23] M. Selbach, B. Schwanhäusser, N. Thierfelder, Z. Fang, R. Khanin, and N. Rajewsky, "Widespread changes in protein synthesis induced by microRNAs," *Nature*, vol. 455, no. 7209, pp. 58–63, 2008.

[24] S. K. Gudey, R. Sundar, Y. Mu et al., "TRAF6 stimulates the tumor-promoting effects of TGFβ type I receptor through polyubiquitination and activation of presenilin," *Science Signaling*, vol. 7, no. 307, 2014.

[25] K. A. Brown, M. E. Aakre, A. E. Gorska et al., "Induction by transforming growth factor-beta1 of epithelial to mesenchymal transition is a rare event in vitro," *Breast Cancer Research*, vol. 6, no. 3, pp. R215–R231, 2004.

[26] A. Eger, A. Stockinger, J. Park et al., "β-Catenin and TGFβ signalling cooperate to maintain a mesenchymal phenotype after FosER-induced epithelial to mesenchymal transition," *Oncogene*, vol. 23, no. 15, pp. 2672–2680, 2004.

[27] W. J. Nelson and R. Nusse, "Convergence of wnt, β-catenin, and cadherin pathways," *Science*, vol. 303, no. 5663, pp. 1483–1487, 2004.

[28] S. Masuda, K. Kumano, K. Shimizu et al., "Notch 1 oncoprotein antagonizes TGF-β/Smad-mediated cell growth suppression via sequestration of coactivator p300," *Cancer Science*, vol. 96, no. 5, pp. 274–282, 2005.

[29] A. H. Schönthal, "Role of PP2A in intracellular signal transduction pathways," *Frontiers in Bioscience*, vol. 3, pp. D1262–D1273, 1998.

[30] P. J. A. Eichhorn, M. P. Creyghton, and R. Bernards, "Protein phosphatase 2A regulatory subunits and cancer," *Biochimica et Biophysica Acta: Reviews on Cancer*, vol. 1795, no. 1, pp. 1–15, 2009.

[31] J. Kroon, L. S. In't Veld, J. T. Buijs, H. Cheung, G. van der Horst, and G. van der Pluijm, "Glycogen synthase kinase-3β inhibition depletes the population of prostate cancer stem/progenitor-like cells and attenuates metastatic growth," *Oncotarget*, vol. 5, no. 19, pp. 8986–8994, 2014.

[32] A. Bhardwaj, S. Singh, S. K. Srivastava et al., "Restoration of PPP2CA expression reverses epithelial-to-mesenchymal transition and suppresses prostate tumour growth and metastasis in an orthotopic mouse model," *British Journal of Cancer*, vol. 110, no. 8, pp. 2000–2010, 2014.

[33] K. P. Porkka, E.-L. Ogg, O. R. Saramäki et al., "The miR-15a-miR-16-1 locus is homozygously deleted in a subset of prostate cancers," *Genes, Chromosomes and Cancer*, vol. 50, no. 7, pp. 499–509, 2011.

[34] M. Musumeci, V. Coppola, A. Addario et al., "Control of tumor and microenvironment cross-talk by miR-15a and miR-16 in prostate cancer," *Oncogene*, vol. 30, no. 41, pp. 4231–4242, 2011.

[35] M. Y. Wu and C. S. Hill, "TGF-β superfamily signaling in embryonic development and homeostasis," *Developmental Cell*, vol. 16, no. 3, pp. 329–343, 2009.

[36] F. Chen, S. K. Hou, H. J. Fan, and Y. F. Liu, "MiR-15a-16 represses Cripto and inhibits NSCLC cell progression," *Molecular and Cellular Biochemistry*, vol. 391, no. 1-2, pp. 11–19, 2014.

[37] P. C. Gray and W. Vale, "Cripto/GRP78 modulation of the TGF-β pathway in development and oncogenesis," *FEBS Letters*, vol. 586, no. 14, pp. 1836–1845, 2012.

[38] M. C. Rangel, H. Karasawa, N. P. Castro, T. Nagaoka, D. S. Salomon, and C. Bianco, "Role of Cripto-1 during epithelial-to-mesenchymal transition in development and cancer," *The American Journal of Pathology*, vol. 180, no. 6, pp. 2188–2200, 2012.

[39] M. G. Lawrence, N. V. Margaryan, D. Loessner et al., "Reactivation of embryonic nodal signaling is associated with tumor progression and promotes the growth of prostate cancer cells," *Prostate*, vol. 71, no. 11, pp. 1198–1209, 2011.

[40] P. C. Gray, G. Shani, K. Aung, J. Kelber, and W. Vale, "Cripto binds transforming growth factor β (TGF-β) and inhibits TGF-β signaling," *Molecular and Cellular Biology*, vol. 26, no. 24, pp. 9268–9278, 2006.

[41] S. Kang, Y. Zhao, K. Hu et al., "MiR-124 exhibits antiproliferative and antiaggressive effects on prostate cancer cells through PACE4 pathway," *Prostate*, vol. 74, pp. 1095–1106, 2014.

[42] L. P. Lim, N. C. Lau, P. Garrett-Engele et al., "Microarray analysis shows that some microRNAs downregulate large numbers of-target mRNAs," *Nature*, vol. 433, no. 7027, pp. 769–773, 2005.

[43] Y. Geng, Y. Ju, F. Ren et al., "Insulin receptor substrate 1/2 (IRS1/2) regulates Wnt/β-Catenin signaling through blocking autophagic degradation of dishevelled," *Journal of Biological Chemistry*, vol. 289, no. 16, pp. 11230–11241, 2014.

[44] R. M. Carew, M. B. Browne, F. B. Hickey, and D. P. Brazil, "Insulin receptor substrate 2 and FoxO3a signalling are involved in E-cadherin expression and transforming growth factor-β1-induced repression in kidney epithelial cells," *The FEBS Journal*, vol. 278, no. 18, pp. 3370–3380, 2011.

[45] A. V. Sorokin and J. Chen, "MEMO1, a new IRS1-interacting protein, induces epithelial-mesenchymal transition in mammary epithelial cells," *Oncogene*, vol. 32, no. 26, pp. 3130–3138, 2013.

[46] M. Heni, J. Hennenlotter, M. Scharpf et al., "Insulin receptor isoforms A and B as well as insulin receptor substrates-1 and -2 are differentially expressed in prostate cancer," *PLoS ONE*, vol. 7, no. 12, Article ID e50953, 2012.

[47] S. L. Neuhausen, M. L. Slattery, C. P. Garner, Y. C. Ding, M. Hoffman, and A. R. Brothman, "Prostate cancer risk and IRS1, IRS2, IGF1, and INS polymorphisms: strong association of IRS1 G972R variant and cancer risk," *Prostate*, vol. 64, no. 2, pp. 168–174, 2005.

[48] C. Ragan, N. Cloonan, S. M. Grimmond, M. Zuker, and M. A. Ragan, "Transcriptome-wide prediction of miRNA targets in human and mouse using FASTH," *PLoS ONE*, vol. 4, no. 5, Article ID e5745, 2009.

[49] Y. Chen, S. X. Wang, R. Mu et al., "Dysregulation of the MiR-324-5p-CUEDC2 axis leads to macrophage dysfunction and is associated with colon cancer," *Cell Reports*, pp. 1982–1993, 2014.

[50] K. Yagi, M. Furuhashi, H. Aoki et al., "c-myc is a downstream target of the Smad pathway," *Journal of Biological Chemistry*, vol. 277, no. 1, pp. 854–861, 2002.

[51] T.-C. He, A. B. Sparks, C. Rago et al., "Identification of c-MYC as a target of the APC pathway," *Science*, vol. 281, no. 5382, pp. 1509–1512, 1998.

[52] V. H. Cowling and M. D. Cole, "E-cadherin repression contributes to c-Myc-induced epithelial cell transformation," *Oncogene*, vol. 26, no. 24, pp. 3582–3586, 2007.

[53] S. F. Tavazoie, C. Alarcón, T. Oskarsson et al., "Endogenous human microRNAs that suppress breast cancer metastasis," *Nature*, vol. 451, no. 7175, pp. 147–152, 2008.

[54] V. B. Sampson, N. H. Rong, J. Han et al., "MicroRNA let-7a down-regulates MYC and reverts MYC-induced growth in Burkitt lymphoma cells," *Cancer Research*, vol. 67, no. 20, pp. 9762–9770, 2007.

[55] X. Qu, L. Shen, Y. Zheng et al., "A signal transduction pathway from TGF-β1 to SKP2 via Akt1 and c-Myc and its correlation with progression in human melanoma," *Journal of Investigative Dermatology*, vol. 134, no. 1, pp. 159–167, 2014.

[56] M. Sachdeva, S. Zhu, F. Wu et al., "p53 represses c-Myc through induction of the tumor suppressor miR-145," *Proceedings of the National Academy of Sciences of the United States of America*, vol. 106, no. 9, pp. 3207–3212, 2009.

[57] G. T. Bommer, I. Gerin, Y. Feng et al., "p53-mediated activation of miRNA34 candidate tumor-suppressor genes," *Current Biology*, vol. 17, no. 15, pp. 1298–1307, 2007.

[58] N. R. Christoffersen, R. Shalgi, L. B. Frankel et al., "P53-independent upregulation of miR-34a during oncogene-induced senescence represses MYC," *Cell Death and Differentiation*, vol. 17, no. 2, pp. 236–245, 2010.

[59] A. Lal, F. Navarro, C. A. Maher et al., "miR-24 Inhibits cell proliferation by targeting E2F2, MYC, and other cell-cycle genes via binding to "Seedless" 3′UTR microRNA recognition elements," *Molecular Cell*, vol. 35, no. 5, pp. 610–625, 2009.

[60] E. Papadimitriou, E. Vasilaki, C. Vorvis et al., "Differential regulation of the two RhoA-specific GEF isoforms Net1/Net1A by TGF-β and miR-24: role in epithelial-to-mesenchymal transition," *Oncogene*, vol. 31, no. 23, pp. 2862–2875, 2012.

[61] S. K. Singh, M. N. Kagalwala, J. Parker-Thornburg, H. Adams, and S. Majumder, "REST maintains self-renewal and pluripotency of embryonic stem cells," *Nature*, vol. 453, no. 7192, pp. 223–227, 2008.

[62] K. A. O'Donnell, E. A. Wentzel, K. I. Zeller, C. V. Dang, and J. T. Mendell, "c-Myc-regulated microRNAs modulate E2F1 expression," *Nature*, vol. 435, no. 7043, pp. 839–843, 2005.

[63] M. Dews, J. L. Fox, S. Hultine et al., "The Myc-miR-17 ∼ 92 axis blunts TGFβ signaling and production of multiple TGFβ-dependent antiangiogenic factors," *Cancer Research*, vol. 70, no. 20, pp. 8233–8246, 2010.

[64] Y. Sun, F. T. Kolligs, M. O. Hottiger, R. Mosavin, E. R. Fearon, and G. J. Nabel, "Regulation of β-catenin transformation by the p300 transcriptional coactivator," *Proceedings of the National Academy of Sciences of the United States of America*, vol. 97, no. 23, pp. 12613–12618, 2000.

[65] R. Janknecht, N. J. Wells, and T. Hunter, "TGF-β-stimulated cooperation of Smad proteins with the coactivators CBP/p300," *Genes and Development*, vol. 12, no. 14, pp. 2114–2119, 1998.

[66] S. E. Pursglove and J. P. Mackay, "CSL: a notch above the rest," *International Journal of Biochemistry and Cell Biology*, vol. 37, no. 12, pp. 2472–2477, 2005.

[67] N. Vo and R. H. Goodman, "CREB-binding protein and p300 in transcriptional regulation," *Journal of Biological Chemistry*, vol. 276, no. 17, pp. 13505–13508, 2001.

[68] J. C. Chrivia, R. P. S. Kwok, N. Lamb, M. Hagiwara, M. R. Montminy, and R. H. Goodman, "Phosphorylated CREB binds specifically to the nuclear protein CBP," *Nature*, vol. 365, no. 6449, pp. 855–859, 1993.

[69] R. W. Stein, M. Corrigan, P. Yaciuk, J. Whelan, and E. Moran, "Analysis of E1A-mediated growth regulation functions: binding of the 300-kilodalton cellular product correlates with E1A enhancer repression function and DNA synthesis-inducing activity," *Journal of Virology*, vol. 64, no. 9, pp. 4421–4427, 1990.

[70] R. Eckner, M. E. Ewen, D. Newsome et al., "Molecular cloning and functional analysis of the adenovirus E1A- associated 300-kD protein (p300) reveals a protein with properties of a transcriptional adaptor," *Genes and Development*, vol. 8, no. 8, pp. 869–884, 1994.

[71] D. C. Bedford, L. H. Kasper, T. Fukuyama, and P. K. Brindle, "Target gene context influences the transcriptional requirement for the KAT3 family of CBP and p300 histone acetyltransferases," *Epigenetics*, vol. 5, no. 1, pp. 9–15, 2010.

[72] K. Ishihama, M. Yamakawa, S. Semba et al., "Expression of HDAC1 and CBP/p300 in human colorectal carcinomas," *Journal of Clinical Pathology*, vol. 60, no. 11, pp. 1205–1210, 2007.

[73] H. V. Heemers, J. D. Debes, and D. J. Tindall, "The role of the transcriptional coactivator p300 in prostate cancer progression," *Advances in Experimental Medicine and Biology*, vol. 617, pp. 535–540, 2008.

[74] C. Peña, J. M. García, V. García et al., "The expression levels of the transcriptional regulators p300 and CtBP modulate the correlations between SNAIL, ZEB1, E-cadherin and vitamin D receptor in human colon carcinomas," *International Journal of Cancer*, vol. 119, no. 9, pp. 2098–2104, 2006.

[75] C. Yokomizo, K. Yamaguchi, Y. Itoh et al., "High expression of p300 in HCC predicts shortened overall survival in association with enhanced epithelial mesenchymal transition of HCC cells," *Cancer Letters*, vol. 310, no. 2, pp. 140–147, 2011.

[76] A. K. Ghosh and J. Varga, "The transcriptional coactivator and acetyltransferase p300 in fibroblast biology and fibrosis," *Journal of Cellular Physiology*, vol. 213, no. 3, pp. 663–671, 2007.

[77] A. Kaimori, J. J. Potter, M. Choti, Z. Ding, E. Mezey, and A. A. Koteish, "Histone deacetylase inhibition suppresses the transforming growth factor β1-induced epithelial-to-mesenchymal transition in hepatocytes," *Hepatology*, vol. 52, no. 3, pp. 1033–1045, 2010.

[78] A. Grimson, K. K.-H. Farh, W. K. Johnston, P. Garrett-Engele, L. P. Lim, and D. P. Bartel, "MicroRNA targeting specificity in mammals: determinants beyond seed pairing," *Molecular Cell*, vol. 27, no. 1, pp. 91–105, 2007.

[79] L. Ma, J. Young, H. Prabhala et al., "MiR-9, a MYC/MYCN-activated microRNA, regulates E-cadherin and cancer metastasis," *Nature Cell Biology*, vol. 12, no. 3, pp. 247–256, 2010.

[80] B. Bonev, P. Stanley, and N. Papalopulu, "MicroRNA-9 modulates hes1 ultradian oscillations by forming a double-negative feedback loop," *Cell Reports*, vol. 2, no. 1, pp. 10–18, 2012.

[81] S. T. Mees, W. A. Mardin, C. Wendel et al., "EP300—a miRNA-regulated metastasis suppressor gene in ductal adenocarcinomas of the pancreas," *International Journal of Cancer*, vol. 126, no. 1, pp. 114–124, 2010.

[82] Z. G. Cai, S. M. Zhang, H. Zhang, Y. Y. Zhou, H. B. Wu, and X. P. Xu, "Aberrant expression of microRNAs involved in epithelial-mesenchymal transition of HT-29 cell line," *Cell Biology International*, vol. 37, no. 7, pp. 669–674, 2013.

[83] F. Oswald, M. Winkler, Y. Cao et al., "RBP-Jκ/SHARP recruits CtIP/CtBP corepressors to silence notch target genes," *Molecular and Cellular Biology*, vol. 25, no. 23, pp. 10379–10390, 2005.

[84] S. A. Frank, *Dynamics of Cancer: Incidence, Inheritance, and Evolution*, Princeton University Press, Princeton, NJ, USA, 2007.

[85] B. Zhou, Y. Liu, M. Kahn et al., "Interactions between β-catenin and transforming growth factor-β signaling pathways mediate epithelial- mesenchymal transition and are dependent on the transcriptional co-activator cAMP-response element-binding protein (CREB)-binding protein (CBP)," *Journal of Biological Chemistry*, vol. 287, no. 10, pp. 7026–7038, 2012.

[86] G. van der Pluijm, "Epithelial plasticity, cancer stem cells and bone metastasis formation," *Bone*, vol. 48, no. 1, pp. 37–43, 2011.

[87] M. Korpal, E. S. Lee, G. Hu, and Y. Kang, "The miR-200 family inhibits epithelial-mesenchymal transition and cancer cell migration by direct targeting of E-cadherin transcriptional repressors ZEB1 and ZEB2," *Journal of Biological Chemistry*, vol. 283, no. 22, pp. 14910–14914, 2008.

[88] M. Puhr, J. Hoefer, G. Schäfer et al., "Epithelial-to-mesenchymal transition leads to docetaxel resistance in prostate cancer and is mediated by reduced expression of miR-200c and miR-205," *The American Journal of Pathology*, vol. 181, no. 6, pp. 2188–2201, 2012.

[89] Y. Mizuguchi, S. Specht, J. G. Lunz et al., "Cooperation of p300 and PCAF in the control of microRNA 200c/141 transcription and epithelial characteristics," *PLoS ONE*, vol. 7, no. 2, Article ID e32449, 2012.

17

Gallbladder Cancer in the 21st Century

Rani Kanthan,[1] Jenna-Lynn Senger,[2] Shahid Ahmed,[3] and Selliah Chandra Kanthan[4]

[1]*Department of Pathology & Laboratory Medicine, University of Saskatchewan, Saskatoon, SK, Canada S7N 0W8*
[2]*Department of Surgery, University of Alberta, Edmonton, AB, Canada T6G 2B7*
[3]*Division of Medical Oncology, Division of Medical Oncology, University of Saskatchewan, Saskatoon, SK, Canada S7N 0W8*
[4]*Department of Surgery, University of Saskatchewan, Saskatoon, SK, Canada S7N 0W8*

Correspondence should be addressed to Rani Kanthan; rani.kanthan@saskatoonhealthregion.ca

Academic Editor: Massimo Aglietta

Gallbladder cancer (GBC) is an uncommon disease in the majority of the world despite being the most common and aggressive malignancy of the biliary tree. Early diagnosis is essential for improved prognosis; however, indolent and nonspecific clinical presentations with a paucity of pathognomonic/predictive radiological features often preclude accurate identification of GBC at an early stage. As such, GBC remains a highly lethal disease, with only 10% of all patients presenting at a stage amenable to surgical resection. Among this select population, continued improvements in survival during the 21st century are attributable to aggressive radical surgery with improved surgical techniques. This paper reviews the current available literature of the 21st century on PubMed and Medline to provide a detailed summary of the epidemiology and risk factors, pathogenesis, clinical presentation, radiology, pathology, management, and prognosis of GBC.

1. Introduction

Gallbladder cancer is the most common malignant tumour of the biliary tract worldwide [1]. It is also the most aggressive cancer of the biliary tract with the shortest median survival from the time of diagnosis [2]. This poor prognosis is due, in part, to an aggressive biologic behavior and a lack of sensitive screening tests for early detection resulting in delayed diagnosis at advanced stage [3]. The only chance for a complete cure is by surgical resection; however, at initial presentation, only 10% of patients are candidates for surgery with a curative intent [2]. Even among those suitable for resection, the anatomical complexity of the portobiliary hepatic system, the morbidity/mortality associated with liver resection, and the risks of tumoural spread second to tumour manipulation portend a high mortality rate [4]. Additionally, among those that do undergo surgical resection, recurrence rates remain high [2].

This paper adds to the body of existing literature in gallbladder carcinomas to enhance awareness of this uncommon but otherwise potentially curable disease. In this paper, we review salient features of the epidemiology and risk factors, pathogenesis, clinical presentations, imaging findings, pathology, and prognosis of gallbladder cancer with special emphasis on advances in the management of gallbladder cancer through evidence-based reviews published in the 21st century (2000–present).

2. Methodology

A systematic review of the published medical literature using PubMed and Medline was carried out using the search terms "gallbladder" AND "cancer [OR] carcinoma" with a special emphasis on review articles. Secondary references obtained from these publications were identified by a manual search and reviewed as relevant. Case reports except for rare pathological entities were predominantly excluded. Manuscripts focusing on gallbladder cancer were included in this review, while those dedicated exclusively to biliary tract malignancies were excluded. Selected relevant abstracts from key oncology meetings (American Society of Clinical Oncology, European Cancer Congress, Gastrointestinal Cancer Symposium,

World Congress on Gastrointestinal Cancer, and Society of Surgical Oncology meeting) have also been reviewed. We have predominately limited our search to publications since 2000 to review concepts of gallbladder cancer in the 21st century.

3. Epidemiology and Risk Factors

Estimates by the American Cancer Society suggest 10,910 new cases of GBC will be diagnosed in the United States in 2015, with 3,700 deaths [5]. Gallbladder cancer is three times more common in females than in males [1, 6]. Among women, higher gravidity and parity increase the risk of developing this cancer [7]. The incidence of gallbladder cancer increases with age [1]. Within the United States, GBC is more prevalent among Mexican Americans and Native Americans, two populations who also have higher rates of gallstones. The average age at diagnosis is 72, with more than two out of three people with GBC over the age of 65 years [5].

The pathogenesis of gallbladder cancer is likely multifactorial, with no single causative factor being identified.

Risk factors for gallbladder cancer can be divided into four broad categories as annotated in the following list including (1) patient demographics, (2) gallbladder abnormalities, (3) patient exposures, and (4) infections [1, 8, 9].

Risk factors for the development of gallbladder cancer are listed as follows:

(1) Demographic factors:

  (a) advanced age,
  (b) female gender,
  (c) obesity,
  (d) geography: South American, Indian, Pakistani, Japanese, and Korean,
  (e) ethnicity: Caucasians, Southwestern Native American, Mexican, and American,
  (f) genetic predisposition.

(2) Gallbladder pathologies/abnormalities:

  (a) cholelithiasis,
  (b) porcelain gallbladder,
  (c) gallbladder polyps,
  (d) congenital biliary cysts,
  (e) pancreaticobiliary maljunction anomalies.

(3) Exposures:

  (a) heavy metals,
  (b) medications: methyldopa, OCP, isoniazid, and estrogen,
  (c) smoking.

(4) Infections:

  (a) *Salmonella*,
  (b) *Helicobacter*.

3.1. Demographic Factors. A striking geographical variability is observed in the prevalence of gallbladder carcinoma worldwide. Regions reporting a high incidence of gallbladder cancer include Delhi, India (21.5/100,000), La Paz, Bolivia (15.5/100,000), South Karachi, Pakistan (13.8/100,000), and Quito, Ecuador (12.9/100,000) [1]. High rates are reported in Chile (27/100,000), Poland (14/100,000), Japan (7/100,000), and Israel (5/100,000) [6]. Northern India, Korea, Japan, and central/eastern Europe including Slovakia, Czech Republic, and Slovenia have also reported a higher prevalence than the worldwide average [1]. By contrast, gallbladder cancer is rare in the western world (USA, UK, Canada, Australia, and New Zealand) with incidence rates of 0.4–0.8 in men and 0.6–1.4 in women per 100,000 [10]. In keeping with this, a retrospective review of the International Agency for Research on Cancer identified increasing rates of male gallbladder cancer mortality only in Iceland, Costa Rica, and Korea with declining rates in all other countries studied [11]. This geographic variability is most likely attributable to differences in environmental exposures and a regional intrinsic predisposition to carcinogenesis [7]. This genetic predisposition is proposed to originate from population migration patterns in Central Asia/Himalayas through Bering Strait during the last glacial era [12]. However, though such patterns of prevalence are observed, there is no true unifying factor that explains this unusual geographic distribution. Alternatively, this variability may be due to dietary factors, with diets high in calories, carbohydrates, red meats, oils, and red chili peppers conferring a higher risk. Intake of green leafy vegetables and fruits may be protective [9]. In keeping with this observation, obesity is a well-recognized risk factor for the development of gallbladder cancer. For each 5-point increase in BMI, the relative risk of developing gallbladder cancer increases by 1.59 for women and 1.09 for men [7, 13].

3.2. Gallbladder Pathologies

3.2.1. Cholelithiasis. The most important risk factor for the development of gallbladder cancer is gallstones, with an 8.3x higher risk than the general population [6]. Among patients with gallbladder cancer, 70–90% have a history of cholelithiasis [8, 9]. Larger stones portend a greater risk, with stones >3 cm being 9.2–10.1 times greater than stones <1 cm [1]. This increased risk is most likely attributable to greater local epithelial irritation. Gallstones and biliary duct stones are hypothesized to cause chronic inflammation leading to dysplasia. The exact mechanism whereby cholelithiasis causes/predisposes to gallbladder cancer remains debatable. Perhaps chronic mucosal damage due to mechanical forces exerted by the gallstone may be involved [8]. Between 0.5 to 1.5% of patients who undergo a simple cholecystectomy for presumed cholelithiasis are discovered incidentally to have gallbladder cancer [1]. Autopsy studies have revealed a 1-2% incidence of gallbladder carcinoma in patients with cholelithiasis [8].

3.2.2. Chronic Inflammation. Chronic inflammation is considered a major factor in carcinogenesis, causing DNA damage, tissue proliferation, and cytokine and growth factor release. Another result of chronic inflammation is deposition of calcium within the gallbladder wall, causing the gallbladder to develop a bluish hue and become fragile—the "porcelain gallbladder." While less than 1% of gallbladder specimens demonstrate this change, it is frequently (~25%) associated with gallbladder cancer. Only specimens with stippled calcification on imaging are considered potentially "premalignant" as transmural calcification is less likely to develop malignancy [7].

Chronic inflammatory diseases such as primary sclerosing cholangitis (PSC) are reported to be associated with a higher incidence of GBC. It is therefore recommended that patients with PSC should undergo annual gallbladder surveillance screening with ultrasound for the detection of any abnormal lesions [7].

Given the association between chronic cholecystitis and gallbladder cancer, it is questioned whether routine prophylactic cholecystectomy may be an effective way to prevent malignancy. Seretis et al. sought to answer this question by reviewing the prevalence of metaplasia in routine cholecystectomy specimens and found an increased prevalence of dysplastic changes, gallbladder wall thickening, and microlithiasis in specimens with metaplastic features. Microlithiasis is, however, more likely to be asymptomatic than macrolithiasis and therefore the practice of performing a cholecystectomy for all symptomatic cholecystitis patients may not be treating the population at the greatest risk as opposed to treating those with incidentally discovered microlithiasis on abdominal imaging [14].

3.2.3. Gallbladder Polyps.

While nearly 5% of all adults have gallbladder polyps, the majority are pseudopolyps with no neoplastic potential: cholesterolosis (60% gallbladder polyps), adenomyosis (25%), or inflammatory (10%) [7]. Other potential gallbladder polyps include nonneoplastic (hyperplastic and inflammatory) and neoplastic polyps (adenomas, leiomyomas, fibromas, and lipomas). Differentiating nonneoplastic from malignant/premalignant polyps is an important major preoperative diagnostic challenge [15]. Benign adenomas, constituting 4% of all gallbladder polyps, play an unclear role in neoplastic transformation; however, the absence of adenoma remnants in mucosa adjacent to adenocarcinoma suggests these tumours may not play a role in carcinogenesis in all cases [7].

Polyps at risk of malignant transformation are typically rapidly growing and >10 mm in size and solitary/sessile polyps in patients with gallstones of the age of 50+ years [7]. General consensus guidelines for removal of gallbladder polyps include polyps >10 mm in size, patients older than 60 years, increasing growth on serial imaging, and/or the presence of gallstones. These suggestions are, however, not firm evidence-based consensus guidelines. A recent study suggests that polyps larger than 2 cm are more likely to harbor high-grade dysplasia/malignancy and the authors concluded that all polyps >2 cm should be removed, whereas those <2 cm can be followed by serial ultrasound every 3–6 months [16]. By contrast, other authors point out that up to 40% of malignant gallbladder polyps may be <1 cm in size and thus patients with a polyp of 5–10 mm should not be excluded from investigation [17].

In summary, therefore, two treatment options are available for the treatment of polyps <10 mm: (i) cholecystectomy for symptomatic gallbladder polyps irrespective of size or (ii) serial ultrasounds until the polyp attains a size of ~10 mm [15].

3.2.4. Pancreaticobiliary Maljunction Anomalies.

Pancreaticobiliary maljunction (PBM) is an abnormal union of the biliary and pancreatic ducts located outside the duodenal wall in which a sphincter is not present. This congenital anatomic anomaly allows pancreatic fluids to reflux into the biliary system, causing chronic inflammation and genetic alterations, leading to increased cellular proliferation resulting in hyperplasia/dysplasia/carcinoma. This anomaly may be detected by cholangiography either with endoscopic retrograde cholangiopancreatography (ERCP) or magnetic resonance cholangiopancreatography (MRCP) or through endoscopic ultrasound (EUS) imaging [7]. EUS shows two thickened layers with epithelial hyperplasia and subserosal fibrosis, with or without a third layer containing a hypoechoic hypertrophic muscular layer [10]. Approximately 10% of patients with gallbladder cancer have this anomaly [7]. These patients also have a higher frequency of Kras mutations [18].

Among non-PBM patients, pancreaticobiliary reflux may occur secondary to a long common channel or high confluence of pancreaticobiliary ducts (HCPBD). A channel length greater than 8 mm is more frequent in patients with gallbladder cancer (38%) compared with normal gallbladders (3%) [10]. In these patients, it is thought that pancreaticobiliary reflux causes severe irritation of the gallbladder mucosa.

3.3. Exposures.

A number of substances have been hypothesized to increase the risk of gallbladder cancer, including heavy metals and radon. It has been shown that patients with gallbladder cancer have significantly lower levels of selenium and zinc and higher levels of copper, lead, cadmium, chromium, and nickel in serum and bile compared to patients with cholelithiasis. Whereas selenium and zinc are antioxidants, the remaining heavy metals are well-recognized carcinogens [9, 19].

Workers in oil, paper, chemical, shoe, textile, and cellulose acetate fiber manufacturing have an increased risk of developing gallbladder cancer. Tobacco is also well recognized to be a significant risk factor. Drugs including methyldopa and isoniazid may additionally increase the risk of GBC. The risk associated with taking oral contraceptives remains controversial [7, 9, 19].

3.4. Infection.

An association between Helicobacter infection of the bile and gallbladder carcinogenesis may be related to bacterial-induced degradation of bile acid; however, precise mechanisms remain poorly understood [6]. Liver flukes, particularly Clonorchis sinensis and Opisthorchis viverrini, have been implicated in cancer of the gallbladder [7].

Chronic bacterial cholangitis, usually due to Salmonella and Helicobacter, increases the risk of biliary tree malignancy. Colonization by bacteria may increase the risk of malignant transformation as the microorganisms degrade bile constituents by hydrolyzing bile salts and forming carcinogens. Chronic typhoid carrier status is thus a significant risk factor, with 6% of carriers developing this cancer (a 12x increased risk) [7].

4. Pathogenesis

Gallbladder cancer may arise in the gallbladder's fundus (60%), body (30%), or neck (10%) [20]. The development of gallbladder cancer is proposed to occur over a span of 5–15 years, with tissue alterations including metaplasia, dysplasia, carcinoma in situ, and invasive cancer [7].

The anatomy of the gallbladder is unique and predisposes the cancer to direct invasion as histologically the gallbladder wall is composed of a mucosa, lamina propria, smooth muscle layer, perimuscular connective tissue, and serosa: note the lack of submucosa in the gallbladder. Additionally, no serosa is present where the gallbladder attaches to the liver and, as such, direct infiltration of gallbladder cancer to the liver is the most common form of direct local spread [18, 21].

Patterns of Spread. Spread of gallbladder cancer occurs via four routes: (a) local invasion of the liver or other nearby structures, (b) lymphatic dissemination, (c) peritoneal spread, and (d) hematogenous spread. Direct extension of gallbladder cancer typically involves the liver (segments IV and V), bile duct, duodenum, colon, parietal wall, and/or abdominal viscera [1, 8]. Hepatic metastasis is most often the result of direct liver and portal tract invasion. Portal tract invasion can also be the result of lymphatic spread [22].

4.1. Molecular Pathogenesis

4.1.1. Biological Pathways. Two distinct independent biological pathways based on morphological, genetic, and molecular evidence leading to gallbladder cancer are hypothesized: (1) a dysplasia-carcinoma sequence arising from metaplastic epithelium and (2) an adenoma-carcinoma sequence [23, 24].

Theory #1. In the chronically inflamed gallbladder, metaplasia is common, being present in over 50%. Similar to metaplasia of the stomach, gallbladder metaplasia occurs in two forms: gastric type and intestinal type [24]. Chronically inflamed gallbladders (both fluke-infested and sporadic) may express both pyloric gland and intestinal metaplasia; however, fluke-infested gallbladders more commonly express intestinal metaplasia and p53 mutations than sporadic gallbladder cancers [25]. However, the precise relationship between metaplasia and dysplasia remains ill-established.

The first theory suggests that dysplasia progresses to carcinoma in situ (CIS) which becomes invasive. This theory is supported by the finding that over 80% of invasive gallbladder cancers have adjacent regions of CIS and epithelial dysplasia [26]. One study demonstrated the presence of metaplasia, dysplasia, and CIS adjacent to the cancer in 66%, 81.3%, and 69%, respectively. Dysplastic lesions have molecular genetic evidence that supports progression towards CIS. It is well recognized that gallbladder dysplasia progresses to invasive cancer typically over a course of 15 to 19 years [27].

Theory #2. By contrast, less than 3% of early carcinomas have adenomatous remnants, suggesting this mechanism has limited importance in the carcinogenic pathway. There remains no way to predict which of these will undergo malignant transformation. Unlike well-established carcinogenic pathways in colorectal cancer [28], it remains debated in the literature whether or not adenomas are true precursors of invasive gallbladder carcinomas. Only 1% of cholecystectomy specimens have adenomatous polyps as preneoplastic lesions [6].

4.1.2. Genetic Mutations. The precise genetic changes involved in the development of gallbladder cancer are poorly understood. A variety of genetic alterations are likely implicated in gallbladder cancer including oncogene activation, tumour suppressor gene inhibition, microsatellite instability, and methylation of gene promoter areas. Over 1281 genetic mutations have been identified in gallbladder cancer [23]. Specific genes implicated in carcinogenesis are summarized in Table 1 [23, 26, 29–37]. Early molecular changes are thought to include p53 mutation, cyclooxygenase-2 (COX2) overexpression, mitochondrial DNA mutations, and hypermethylation of promotors in tumour suppressor genes, with later events including inactivation of the fragile histidine triad (FHIT) and cyclin-dependent kinase inhibitor 2A (CDKN) tumour suppressor genes as well as loss of regions on chromosomes 9, 18, and 22. Dysplasia further leads to overexpression of p16 [23].

Like many malignancies, *Kras* and *TP53* are the best described genes implicated in gallbladder cancer. Carcinogenic pathways may include (1) inflammation secondary to gallstones leading to *p53* mutations and eventual carcinoma, (2) point mutation of *Kras* contributing to hyperplasia then carcinoma as seen in patients with an anomalous junction of pancreaticobiliary duct, and (3) neoplastic foci in gallbladder polyps secondary to *Kras* mutation [7].

Epigenetics may play a distinct role in gallbladder carcinogenesis. Methylation patterns of the tumour suppressor genes p16, APC, MGMT, hMLH1, RARbeta2, and p73 have been detected in 72% of GBCs and 28% of chronic cholecystitis, though rare in normal tissue [38, 39]. In keeping with the global prevalence variability, rates of methylation were compared in GBC patients from Chile versus the United States, and a significant difference in the methylation of APC (42% versus 13%) and p73 (14% versus 40%) was identified, suggesting a unique geographic-dependent biology. It is believed that the methylation level accumulates throughout the progression from chronic cholecystitis through the development of metaplasia [38].

The role of microsatellite instability (MSI) in the carcinogenesis of gallbladder cancer remains poorly described, with literature reporting MSI rates between 0 and 40% of cases; the largest and most recent study reported a prevalence of 7.8%. Moy et al. reported a strong correlation between global DNA methylation as measured by long interspersed

TABLE 1: Summary of the major genes implicated in gallbladder carcinogenesis as available in the published literature (2000–present).

	Gene	Expression in GBC	Tissues of comparison	Additional information	Reference(s)
Oncogene	KRAS	Higher (10–67%)	Adenoma (0%)	Marker of GBC in PBM No correlation with stage, histology, and survival	[23, 26, 29]
	EGFR	Higher (63.4%)	Dysplasia (71.4%) Hyperplasia (15.4%) Normal (0%)		[23]
	HER-2/neu (ERBB2)	Higher (16–64%)	Carcinoma in situ (0%) Gallstones (0%)	Marker of metastatic disease (70%) Marker of poor prognosis (10x mortality)	[23, 30, 31]
Tumor suppressor	TP53	Higher (58.3–100%)	Adenoma (10–20%) Normal (0%)	Unknown relation to prognosis More prominent with poor differentiation	[23, 32]
	P16	Lower (48.8%)	Adenoma (100%) Chronic cholecystitis (100%)	Related to poorer prognosis Negative correlation with cyclin D1	[33]
	Fragile histidine triad (FHIT)	Lower	Normal	Early change in carcinogenesis	[26]
	Retinoblastoma	Lower (58.5%)	Adenoma (100%) Cholecystitis (100%)	Causes cell proliferation, apoptosis, and developmental defects	[33]
	VHL	Lower (48.1%)	Peritumoral tissue (80.4%) Polyps (80%) Chronic cholecystitis (88.6%)	Marker progression, biological behavior, and prognosis	[34]
Adhesion molecules and mucins	Cadherins	Higher (N-cadherin 55%; P-cadherin 53%)	None	Associated with large tumor size, invasion, and node metastases	[35]
	MUC1	Higher (78%)	Normal tissue (absent)	Higher expression in more advanced tumours; poor survival	[36]
	Erythrocyte complement receptor 1 (CR1)	Lower	Chronic cholecystitis Cholelithiasis Normal	Role under investigation	[23]
Angiogenesis	Thrombospondin-1	Higher (74.5%)	Normal (0%) T1 cancer (0%)	Associated with venous involvement Predictor of vascular involvement and nodal metastases	[23]
	Cyclooxygenase-2	Higher (59.2–71.9%)	Normal (0–25%) Dysplasia (70.3%)	Associated with poor prognosis, mean survival, and tumor progression	[23, 26]
	VEGF-A	Higher (81%)	Chronic cholecystitis (5.1%)	Expression related to histologic grade, TNM stage, and prognosis	[37]
Cell cycle regulators	Cyclin E	Higher (33%)	Adenoma (12.5%)		[23]
	Cyclin D1	Higher (41–68.3%)	Adenoma (57.1–67%) Chronic cholecystitis (7.1%) Normal (0%)	Marker of lymphatic/venous involvement and lymph node metastases	[23, 33]
	P27Kip1	Lower (43–65%)	None		[23]
Apoptosis	Caspases	Higher (95%; caspase 3; 77%; caspases 6 and 8)	None	Higher extent apoptosis in grade II/III GBC compared with grade I/dysplasia	[23]
	Bcl-2	Higher (34.7%)			

element-1 (LINE-1) and loss of mismatch repair proteins suggesting that methylation causes silencing of these genes [40]. It is suggested that MSI may be more common in patients developing GBC secondary to abnormal anatomy and is not associated with Lynch syndrome. There is no reported significant difference in tumour grade, tumour stage, and overall survival in gallbladder cancer patients with or without MSI.

Loss of heterozygosity (LOH) has been described in a number of tumour suppressor genes in gallbladder cancer including chromosomes 1p34–36 (*p73*), 3p (*VHL, RAR-beta, RASSF1A,* and *FHIT*), 5q21 (*APC*), 8p21–23 (*PRLTS* and *FEZ1*), 9p21 (*p15, p16*), 9q (*DBCCR1*), 13q14 (*RB*), 16q24 (*WWOX* and *FRA16D*), and 17p13 (*p53*) [29].

Also associated with gallbladder cancers are sporadic reports that implicate lesser known genes. In gallbladder cancer, expression of ADAM-17 is increased in tumours with a high histological grade and pT stage as well as shorter overall survival [41, 42]. The ADAM gene family, of which the best known member is ADAM-17, has been implicated in regulation of ECM remodeling and cell migration. ADAM-17 (tumour necrosis factor-alpha converting enzyme, TACE) cleaves TNF-alpha from its precursor and releases EGFR ligands, amphiregulin, and heparin-binding epidermal growth factor (HB-EGF).

High mobility group protein A2 (HMGA2) is a nonhistone chromatin protein involved in tumorigenesis, invasion, and metastasis of tumours. Zou et al. showed statistically higher expression of HMGA2 in gallbladder cancer compared with normal tissue, polyps, and chronic cholecystitis. He also showed significantly decreased expression of CD9 in cancers compared to benign tissues [43]. Mobility related protein-1 (MRP1 aka CD9) is a glycoprotein that belongs to the transmembrane 4 superfamily and is related to tumour progression.

Thus, in summary, the pathogenesis of gallbladder cancer continues to be ill understood. As chronic inflammation is recognized as a key player in carcinogenesis causing DNA damage and tissue proliferation with cytokine and growth factor release, perhaps research may have to be undertaken in alternative pathways such as deciphering immune surveillance with special reference to intracellular and intercellular cell "chatter" which may be the earliest alteration that occurs in the carcinogenesis pathway. The field of cell signaling resulting in signal transduction in the immune system is yet to be explored in the pathogenesis of gallbladder cancers.

5. Staging

A number of staging systems have been described for gallbladder cancer including Nevin's staging system (Table 2) [44], the Japanese Biliary Surgical Society staging system (Table 3) [1, 45], and the TNM staging system of the American Joint Committee on Cancer (Table 4) [46].

6. Clinical Presentation

Gallbladder cancer typically presents in one of three ways: (a) malignancy suspected preoperatively, (b) malignancy

TABLE 2: Nevin's staging.

Stage	Definition
I	Tumour invades mucosa
II	Tumour invades mucosa + muscularis
III	Tumour invades mucosa + muscularis + subserosa
IV	Tumour invades all 3 layers of gallbladder + cystic lymph node
V	Tumour extends into liver bed or metastases

discovered accidentally at cholecystectomy performed for presumed benign disease, and (c) malignancy diagnosed incidentally at pathological examination following routine cholecystectomy [6]. Over two-thirds of patients with gallbladder cancer are only diagnosed during surgery or postoperatively [47]. Symptomatic patients most commonly present with advanced disease, a truth that has not greatly changed in the past 85 years [48]. At presentation, gallbladder cancer is often similar to biliary colic or chronic cholecystitis. Right upper quadrant or epigastric pain is the most common symptom (54–83%), followed by jaundice (10–46%), nausea and vomiting (15–43%), anorexia (4–41%), and weight loss (10–39%) [1]. Jaundice may result either from direct invasion of the biliary tree or from metastatic disease to the hepatoduodenal ligament [6]. Only 3–8% of patients have a palpable mass [1]. Among patients who present symptomatically, tumours are typically advanced with 75% being nonresectable [6]. Among patients with a preoperative diagnosis of Mirizzi syndrome, 6–27.8% of patients will have a final diagnosis of gallbladder cancer [1].

Unsuspected gallbladder cancer is most commonly diagnosed incidentally after routine cholecystectomy. Lack of preoperative clinical suspicion and the absence of specific clinical or serological markers on history and physical exam are likely contributing factors for advanced stage diagnosis.

7. Diagnostic Imaging

7.1. Ultrasound. Ultrasonography is most frequently the initial diagnostic study obtained when gallbladder disease is suspected. On ultrasonography, gallbladder carcinoma may have one of three appearances: (1) a mass replacing or invading the gallbladder, (2) an intraluminal gallbladder growth/polyp, or (3) an asymmetric gallbladder wall thickening. In advanced disease, sensitivity and specificity of ultrasound imaging is 85% and 80%, respectively; however, in early disease, ultrasound examination often fails to detect any abnormality, particularly when the tumour is flat or sessile and is associated with cholelithiasis [6]. High-resolution contrast-enhanced ultrasonography accurately identifies up to 70–90% of polypoid gallbladder lesions [49]. Cholesterol pseudopolyps are typically pedunculated with a thin stalk, <1 cm in maximal diameter, and multiple in number with ultrasound findings of echogenicity without posterior acoustic shadowing. In contrast, malignant polyps are usually sessile, solitary, and >1 cm [20]. Contrast-enhanced ultrasonography with perflubutane has been described in which

TABLE 3: Japanese Biliary Surgical Society staging system.

Stage	I	II	III	IV
Capsular invasion	No capsular invasion (S_0)	Suspected capsular invasion (S_1)	Marked capsular invasion (S_2)	Direct invasion of adjacent viscera (S_3)
Hepatic invasion	No hepatic invasion ($Hinf_0$)	Suspected hepatic invasion ($Hinf_1$)	Marked hepatic invasion around gallbladder ($Hinf_2$)	Extensive hepatic invasion ($Hinf_3$)
Bile duct invasion	No involvement of extrahepatic bile duct ($Binf_0$)	Suspected involvement of bile duct ($Binf_1$)	Marked biliary involvement ($Binf_2$)	Extensive involvement of bile duct ($Binf_3$)
Lymph node metastases	No lymph node metastasis (N_0)	Metastases to lymph nodes around extrahepatic bile duct (primary group, N_1)	Metastases in lymph nodes of hepatoduodenal ligament (secondary group, N_2) OR surrounding area (tertiary group, N_3)	Metastases more distant than in stage III (fourth group, N_4)
Liver metastasis	No liver metastases (H_0)	No liver metastases (H_0)	No liver metastases (H_0)	Liver metastases in 1 lobe (H_1) OR Small liver metastases in bilateral lobes (H_2) OR Multiple liver metastases in bilateral lobes (H_3)
Peritoneal dissemination	No peritoneal dissemination (P_0)	No peritoneal dissemination (P_0)	No peritoneal dissemination (P_0)	Peritoneal dissemination near tumour (P_1) OR Small number of peritoneal disseminations distant from tumour (P_2) OR Multiple peritoneal disseminations distant from tumour (P_3)

TABLE 4: TNM staging.

Stage	T-stage	N-stage	M-stage
0	T_{is}	N_0	M_0
I	T_1	N_0	M_0
II	T_2	N_0	M_0
IIIA	T_3	N_0	M_0
IIIB	T_1, T_2, T_3	N_1	M_0
IVA	T_4	N_0, N_1	M_0
IVB	Any T	Any N	M_1
	Any T	N_2	M_0

Primary Tumour (T): T_{is} Carcinoma in situ; T_1 Tumour invades lamina propria (a) or muscular layer (b); T_2 Tumour invades perimuscular connective tissue; T_3 Tumour perforates serosa and/or invades liver and/or other adjacent organs (stomach, duodenum, colon, pancreas, and extrahepatic bile ducts); T_4 Tumour invades main porta vein or hepatic artery or multiple extrahepatic organs.
Regional Lymph Nodes (N): N_0 No regional lymph node metastasis; N_1 Metastases to nodes along cystic duct, common bile duct, hepatic artery, and/or portal vein; N_2 Metastases to periaortic, pericaval, superior mesenteric artery, and/or celiac artery nodes.
Distant Metastasis (M): M_0 No distant metastasis; M_1 Distant metastasis.

gallbladder cancer shows continuous staining throughout the tumour and an "eruption sign" [10]. Aside from its diagnostic utility, ultrasonography may provide information for disease staging by defining the extent of biliary tree involvement and confirming the presence of hepatic, arterial, or portal vein invasion.

Endoscopic ultrasound (EUS) is currently the definitive imaging modality in the staging of gallbladder cancer, allowing for precise imaging and acquisition of a fine needle aspiration (FNA) biopsy. Ultrasound- or CT-guided biopsy of mass lesions has a diagnostic accuracy of 80–90% [8]. A scoring system was devised by Choi et al. to predict the risk of neoplastic polyps, based on layer structure, echo patterns, polyp margin, polyp stalk, presence of gallstones, gender, age, and number of polyps, with a cut-off score of 6 conferring a sensitivity and specificity of 81% and 86% [50].

Newer technologies include contrast-enhanced harmonic EUS (CEH-EUS) to characterize gallbladder polyps. This modality has a greater accuracy than EUS, with a sensitivity of 93.5% and specificity of 93.2% [51]. They also include real-time elastography using acoustic radiation force impulse (ARFI) that uses high intensity focused ultrasound to determine tissue stiffness in a variety of organs, differentiating malignant from benign [10].

7.2. CT Scan. The most common evaluative imaging in gallbladder cancer is the CT scan, the utilization of which has been increasing over time [52]. CT scan may be useful in the diagnosis and staging of gallbladder cancer. This imaging modality may detect liver or porta hepatis invasion, lymphadenopathy, and involvement of the adjacent organs. Four patterns of gallbladder cancer have been described on CT scan: (a) a polypoid mass within the gallbladder lumen (15–25%), (b) focal wall thickening, (c) diffuse wall thickening (20% gallbladder cancers), and (d) a mass replacing the gallbladder (40–65%). These findings are, however, also features of inflammatory conditions such as xanthogranulomatous cholecystitis and adenomyomatosis, benign lesions, and metastatic disease [53]. Multidetector row CT (MDCT) may be used to further distinguish between malignant gallbladder wall thickening and benign gallbladder wall thickening, with 75.9% specificity and 82.5% sensitivity [10].

7.3. ERCP. Endoscopic retrograde cholangiopancreatography (ERCP) may demonstrate anomalous junction of pancreaticobiliary ducts and allows for the collection of bile samples, brush cytology, and/or intralesional biopsy [8]. ERCP is a poor tool for diagnosing gallbladder cancer as, while it accurately demonstrates filling defects, it does not delineate the surface of polypoid lesions. As such, it is best used for identifying tumour extension into the bile ducts.

7.4. MRI, MRA, and MRCP. The combination of MRI (magnetic resonance imaging) with MRA (magnetic resonance angiography) and MRCP (magnetic resonance cholangiopancreatography) is useful in detecting vascular invasion (100% sensitivity and 87% specificity), biliary tract involvement (100% sensitivity and 89% specificity), liver invasion (67% sensitivity and 89% specificity), and lymph node involvement (56% sensitivity and 89% specificity) [6]. MRI has been shown to be superior to CT scan for differentiating T1a lesions from T1b or greater and as such may be useful in preoperative management planning [54].

The early and prolonged enhancement of malignant lesions differs from the early enhancement with subsequent washout of benign masses. Similar patterns of enhancement can assist in differentiating malignant wall thickening from benign wall thickening along with an irregular versus a smoothly delineated enhancement, respectively [55]. Differentiation of gallbladder cancer from adenomyomatosis may be challenging as the latter can also present with focal or diffuse wall thickening. Intramural cyst-like spaces due to dilated Rokitansky-Aschoff sinuses on MRI, the "pearl-necklace appearance," are indicative of adenomyomatosis, though they are not necessary to make this diagnosis [20, 56].

Addition of *diffusion-weighted imaging (DWI)* may aid in the differentiation of malignant from benign gallbladder disease as it provides a greater sensitivity [56]. Addition of DWI to standard T2WI improves the sensitivity, specificity, positive predictive value (PPV), and negative predictive value (NPV) from 97.2%, 86.7%, 74.5%, and 98.7% to 97.2%, 92.2%, 83.3%, and 98.8% [55].

7.5. FDG-PET Scan. PET scanning may be useful in diagnosing ambiguous primary lesions, detecting residual disease after cholecystectomy, and uncovering distant disease not otherwise appreciable by other imaging modalities. Given the high incidence of metastatic disease, PET scan is a useful

preoperative imaging modality. Indeed nearly 25% of patients with gallbladder cancer who underwent preoperative PET scanning had a change in their operative management in one study [52].

FDG-PET scanning with CT (PET/CT) combines metabolic and anatomical localizations of suspicious lesions. It has been shown to detect 95.9% of primary gallbladder cancers, 85.7% of lymph node involvement, and 95.9% of metastatic disease [4]. This combination of diagnostic imaging can be used (a) preoperatively to define the possibility of curative surgery and (b) in patients postoperatively for restaging. The authors reported a negative predictive value of 100%, indicating a negative study that excludes the presence of malignancy; false positives were due to inflammation secondary to cholecystitis, RAS, or adenomyomatosis [4]. Elevated CRP may negatively affect the accuracy of this imaging modality [57].

7.6. Percutaneous Approaches. Percutaneous transhepatic fine needle aspiration and percutaneous transhepatic cholecystoscopy may be used in the evaluation of gallbladder polyps. While these modalities portend an accurate diagnosis, they are time consuming, more invasive, and poorly tolerated by the patient [49]. Image-guided FNA including ultrasound-guided or CT-guided biopsy has the potential for a diagnostic accuracy of 80–90% [8]. False-negative results of 11–41% may be attributable to incorrect sampling, necrosis, or fibrosis. FNA can be used to detect the uncommon variants of gallbladder cancer [58].

8. Pathology

8.1. Gross Pathology. Gallbladder cancer may present as a mass lesion, localized wall thickening with induration of the wall, or polypoidal growth. Obstruction of the neck and/or cystic duct may cause distension or collapse of the gallbladder; neoplasms in the body may constrict the lateral wall resulting in an hour-glass deformity. These lesions are typically grey-white in colour; however, mucinous and signet ring lesions have a gelatinous cut surface.

8.2. Cytopathology. A recent study by Yadav et al. described the cytopathology of various subtypes of gallbladder cancer as follows:

(i) Papillary adenocarcinoma: papillae with vascular core and minimal pleomorphism.

(ii) Mucinous adenocarcinoma: single cells or clusters with >50% extracellular mucin.

(iii) Signet ring cell carcinoma: a predominance of signet ring cells.

(iv) Adenosqumous carcinoma: an admixture of glandular and squamous components.

(v) Squamous cell carcinoma: atypical keratinized cells and/or polliwog cells in a necrotic background.

(vi) Neuroendocrine carcinoma: rosettes, salt/pepper chromatin, anisonucleosis, and/or nuclear molding

(vii) Small cell carcinoma: smudge cells, scant cytoplasm, necrosis, salt/pepper chromatin, and/or nuclear molding

(viii) Undifferentiated carcinoma NOS: dispersed and highly pleomorphic cells with abundant necrosis [58].

8.3. Histopathology. Adenocarcinoma is the most common histologic type, accounting for 98% of all gallbladder tumours, two-thirds of which are moderately/poorly differentiated. The remaining common histopathological variants include papillary, mucinous, squamous, and adenosquamous subtypes [7]. Other rare types of gallbladder cancer include carcinosarcoma, small cell carcinoma, lymphoma, signet ring cell-type tumours, and metastases [59]. Tumours may contain more than one histological variant [60].

Though most traditional gastrointestinal adenocarcinomas are classified as either differentiated or undifferentiated, biliary tract cancer is predominately a well-differentiated adenocarcinoma with a minor component of poor differentiation, thus allowing venous, lymphatic, and perineural invasion in "advanced disease" that is not as readily apparent in "early" biliary cancers. Intramural invasion can be classified as either infiltrative growth-type or destructive growth-type, the latter conferring a worse overall prognosis [61].

As extensive tumour necrosis with minimal residual viable tumour can mimic acute gangrenous cholecystitis, adequate sampling is critical. Features of cholecystitis such as edema, vascular congestion, hemorrhage, and fibrin deposition to the adventitia/muscle may help in identifying a benign process [60].

Distinguishing between well-differentiated adenocarcinoma and Rokitansky-Aschoff sinuses (RAS) can be challenging as RAS can extend deep into the perimuscular adipose tissue and be located throughout the gallbladder. Desmoplasia does not rule out RAS as it may surround RAS particularly in the setting of chronic cholecystitis. Adenomyosis can mimic gallbladder adenocarcinoma as it is characterized by epithelial proliferation with deep diverticulae extending into the muscular layer; however, the glands are cytologically bland with cystic dilatations that communicate with the lumen of the gallbladder [60].

Immunohistochemistry of gallbladder adenocarcinoma is similar to that of bile duct and pancreatic carcinoma. These tumours are positive for cytokeratin 7 (CK7) with focal expression of carcinoembryonic monoclonal antibody (CEA-M), CA19-9, MUC1, B72.3, and MUC5AC [60].

The remaining 2% of gallbladder cancers include the following:

(i) *Papillary Adenocarcinoma.* It represents ~5% of gallbladder cancers. Two subtypes of papillary adenocarcinoma have been described: invasive and noninvasive [62]. On histologic examination, these tumours typically consist of fibrovascular stalks lined by malignant epithelial cells, often with the production of mucin in the gallbladder. Noninvasive papillary tumours have a tendency towards intraluminal growth, filling the gallbladder prior to locoregional invasion, and are therefore typically associated with a better prognosis than routine gallbladder cancers [59]. Regardless of size and degree of differentiation, these do not metastasize and are best treated with a simple cholecystectomy. In contrast, invasive papillary adenocarcinoma is associated with a 10-year relative survival rate for tumours confined to the gallbladder wall of 52% and <10% among those with lymph node metastases [62].

(ii) *Mucinous Adenocarcinoma.* Defined as a carcinoma with >50% stromal mucin deposition, it comprises 2.5% of all gallbladder cancers and is very poorly described in the literature. These tumours have less preponderance for females (1.1) and typically present with an initial diagnosis of acute cholecystitis. They are typically larger than adenocarcinoma (4.8 cm versus 2.9 cm). These tumours are usually mixed mucinous rather than pure colloid [63]. The presence of abundant mucin on radiographs (i.e., spotty and hyperechoic contents on sonography) is diagnostic [59]. Differentiation between mucinous carcinoma of the gallbladder and pseudomyxoma peritonei is challenging [60]. The tendency of mucinous adenocarcinoma towards invasive growth confers a poor prognosis.

(iii) *Signet Ring Cell Carcinoma.* It is identified by intracytoplasmic mucin displacing the nuclei to the periphery. These tumours characteristically have infiltrative submucosal growth patterns resembling *linitis plastica* of the stomach. On sonography and CT, these tumours show an echogenic polypoid mass with target-like wall thickening [59].

(iv) *Squamous/Adenosquamous Cell Carcinoma (SC/ASC).* Its incidence ranges from 1.4–12.7% [59]. There remains no consistent definition in the literature outlining the extent of squamous differentiation required to categorize a tumour as "adenosquamous" carcinoma rather than adenocarcinoma [64]. These tumours typically arise from the gallbladder fossa and present with rapid and aggressive growth. Adenosquamous carcinoma may show comedo-like necrosis with associated tumour giant cells. Pure squamous cell carcinoma often shows prominent keratinization. Due to the rarity of this lesion, exact treatment protocols and outcome data are controversial in the published literature. Residual disease is established as a significant independent prognostic factor for these tumours [65].

(v) *Cribriform Carcinoma.* It accounts for <1% of all gallbladder carcinomas and is thought to occur in younger patients. The histopathological characteristics are highly reminiscent of mammary gland cribriform carcinoma and as such this diagnosis must be excluded. The presence of bonafide "comedonecrosis" may help accurately distinguish primary gallbladder cribriform carcinoma from metastatic breast cancer. Lack of estrogen and progesterone receptor immunoreactivity may aid in differentiating primary gallbladder cribriform carcinoma from its counterpart metastatic breast lesion [66].

(vi) *Hepatoid Adenocarcinoma*. It is characterized by foci of both adenomatous differentiation and hepatocellular differentiation of the gallbladder with a natural history similar to hepatocellular carcinoma. On histopathology, these tumours are composed of large or polygonal cells with an abundant eosinophilic cytoplasm with or without medullary proliferation. On immunohistochemistry, hepatoid adenocarcinomas may express alpha-fetoprotein (AFP), albumin, transferrin, PIVKA, and alpha-1-antitrypsin. While AFP remains the most important marker of this lesion, not all hepatoid adenocarcinomas are positive for AFP. These tumours must be differentiated from hepatocellular carcinoma invasion into the gallbladder [67].

(vii) *Clear Cell Adenocarcinoma*. It is exceedingly rare and is often identified with other components such as adenocarcinoma, adenosquamous carcinoma, or mucinous carcinoma. On histopathology, clear cell adenocarcinoma (CCA) has an infiltrative growth pattern with or without glandular differentiation, composed of polygonal/cuboidal clear cells with minimal cytological atypia [68]. CCA of the gallbladder should be differentiated from a metastases most commonly from the kidneys [68, 69].

(viii) *Undifferentiated Carcinoma*. It can present as four histologic variants: (i) spindle and giant cell type, (ii) osteoclast-like giant cell type, (iii) small cell type, and (iv) nodular or lobular type. These tumours characteristically lack glandular structures [70]. Spindle cell carcinoma (SpCC) of the gallbladder is composed predominately of sarcomatous elements with areas of carcinomatous differentiation and demonstration of this biphasic appearance is essential for diagnosis. On immunohistochemistry, SpCC will usually demonstrate biphasic reactivity to cytokeratins (CK, EMA) and mesenchymal antibodies such as vimentin. This tumour confers a worse prognosis compared with gallbladder adenocarcinoma [71]. Giant cell type carcinomas are assumed to arise when there is dedifferentiation of a preexisting well-differentiated adenocarcinoma to anaplastic giant cell components [70].

(ix) *Gallbladder Sarcoma*. It is exceedingly rare and patients present similarly to gallbladder adenocarcinoma. Tumour types include leiomyosarcoma, rhabdomyosarcoma, angiosarcoma, Kaposi's sarcoma, malignant fibrous histiocytoma, synovial sarcoma, malignant GIST, and liposarcoma. Though the pathogenesis of these tumours remains unclear, gallbladder sarcomas are hypothesized to arise from totipotential stem cells or paramesonephric tissue [72]. Gallbladder carcinosarcoma is rare and very aggressive as it spreads by direct invasion, hematogenously, and via the lymph nodes [73]. The mean survival after diagnosis is measured in months.

(x) *Neuroendocrine Tumours*. Neuroendocrine Tumours of the gallbladder comprise only 0.5% of all neuroendocrine tumours and ~2% of gallbladder cancers. These tumours are thought to derive from multipotent stem cells, as normal gallbladder mucosa does not contain neuroendocrine cells, though mucosa undergoing gastric/intestinal metaplasia can express a variety of neuroendocrine hormones including serotonin, histamine, gastrin, somatostatin, and glucagon. Virtually all neuroendocrine tumours of the gallbladder reported have coexisting gallstones with chronic cholecystitis with less than 1% of patients presenting as functioning lesions such as carcinoid syndrome [74] and/or hyperglycemia [75]. Some authors suggest these lesions should be treated similarly to gallbladder adenocarcinoma, while others recommend a more aggressive approach. They are typically identified at an advanced stage, with a 5-year reported survival rate of ~20% [74]. Neuroendocrine tumours are classified according to their differentiation as carcinoid tumours (well differentiated) or small cell carcinoma (poorly differentiated).

Carcinoid tumours are rare with differentiation between them and carcinoma preoperatively being often impossible as imaging features are similar. Patients typically present with vague symptoms, and only 3.3–3.7% present with carcinoid syndrome [76, 77]. On histopathological examination, atypical variants may have cellular atypia and mitosis which are associated with a worse prognosis [77]. Immunohistochemistry is useful in the accurate identification of carcinoids, with positivity for neuroendocrine markers [76]. A SEER database review reported a 10-year survival of 36% [78].

Small cell carcinoma (SCC) of the gallbladder is extremely rare, comprising only 0.5% of all gallbladder cancers [79]. These patients may present with paraneoplastic syndromes including Cushing's syndrome and sensory neuropathy [80]. These tumours are most common in elderly females, particularly those with cholelithiasis [79]. Gallbladder SCC usually presents as a large mass containing extensive necrosis with a marked propensity for invasive submucosal growth. On histopathology, ~72% are pure SCC and the remaining 28% are mixed SCC + adenocarcinoma or squamous cell carcinoma [81]. Unlike adenocarcinoma, SCCs are bulky tumours with local invasion, paraneoplastic leukocytosis, and/or hypercalcemia and are associated with metastases and worse prognosis [82]. Based on the SEER database, gallbladder SCC has essentially no survivors at 10 years [78].

9. Surgical Treatment

Complete surgical tumour resection is the only curative treatment for GBC. A complete resection is often challenging as the gallbladder has anatomically neighboring vital structures such as the porta hepatica, and this malignancy has a propensity for hepatic invasion with early lymphatic metastases. The "radical cholecystectomy" was first proposed by Glenn and Hays in 1954 in which the gallbladder bed with a rim of liver tissue and lymphatic tissue within the hepatoduodenal ligament were excised en bloc [83]. An "extended radical cholecystectomy" that was proposed in 1982 differs in that the lymphatic tissue within the hepatoduodenal ligament, the posterosuperior head of the pancreas, with dissection around the portal vein, and common hepatic artery are removed en bloc with the gallbladder, a rim of liver tissue, and the extrahepatic bile duct [83]. During surgical resection, it is imperative to avoid incising the gallbladder or spilling its contents as this is associated with increased morbidity and mortality.

Prior to definitive management by laparotomy, staging laparoscopy is often helpful to assess for peritoneal spread or discontiguous liver disease. Weber et al. reported that unresectable disease was identified in 48% of their study patients by laparoscopy, thereby preventing unnecessary morbidity with open laparotomy [6]. While many recommend routine diagnostic laparoscopy for all gallbladder cancer-directed operations, there are authors that suggest staging laparoscopy is a waste of healthcare resources. However, when a gallbladder cancer is suspected preoperatively, laparoscopic cholecystectomy is contraindicated.

The extent of surgical intervention may range from simple cholecystectomy to being combined with partial hepatectomy, with or without regional lymph node dissection. At a minimum, definitive surgery includes removal of involved liver parenchyma as well as regional lymph nodes. While the appropriate surgical intervention may be estimated using TNM staging (Table 4) [84], there remains a paucity of randomized data to definitely guide management.

9.1. Incidental/Unsuspected Gallbladder Carcinoma. Incidental identification of gallbladder cancer occurs in 0.2–3% of all cholecystectomies for presumed benign disease [85]. In fact only 30% of patients with gallbladder cancer are suspected of harbouring a malignancy preoperatively [86]. Intraoperative findings that may indicate gallbladder cancer include ulcerations or small plaques on gross examination of the opened specimen or a firm mass in more advanced tumours. It has been proposed that ideally all cholecystectomy specimens should be opened and examined intraoperatively. If gallbladder cancer is suspected at routine laparoscopic cholecystectomy an intraoperative frozen section should be sent to the pathology laboratory for immediate tissue confirmation. Features indicating the need for intraoperative frozen section include (a) macroscopically contracted or sclerotic mucosa, (b) thickening of one part of the gallbladder wall, (c) normal tissue replaced by connective tissue in all wall layers, (d) macroscopic mucosal color change, and/or (e) presence of a polypoid lesion. Sensitivity and specificity of intraoperative frozen section are reported at 90% and 100%, respectively [84]. Though frozen section may be unable to differentiate carcinoma in situ from epithelial atypia, it has a 70–86% accuracy rate in determining the depth of invasion of the carcinoma [86].

The decision whether or not to convert to open laparotomy with a positive frozen section remains controversial, and no consensus guidelines have been established. Indications for conversion to open laparotomy include difficult dissection or a high risk of gallbladder rupture. Some surgeons advocate for immediate conversion to radical resection including port sites. As T1a lesions are treated with a simple laparoscopic cholecystectomy, and T3/T4 lesions should have been preoperatively diagnosed with imaging, it is the T1b and T2 lesions that are most commonly encountered unexpectedly intraoperatively and cause this management dilemma. An incomplete oncologic operation is undesirable, yet so is major resection for lesions that are ultimately benign or diffusely metastatic [84]. It is recently suggested that T1b tumours are best treated with a wedge resection of 2-3 cm of the gallbladder bed with lymph node dissection of the hepatoduodenal ligament with the initial cholecystectomy. Radical reresection of these tumours confers a survival benefit of 60–100% [86]. Other studies have, however, found no improved prognosis in patients with pT1b tumours treated with radical resection [87]. Tumours that invade the subserosal layer (T2+) require reoperating for radical surgery to improve survival. These patients require resection of liver segments IVb and V [86]. Evaluation of the initial cystic duct margin guides surgical management: a negative margin spares the biliary tree and a lymphadenectomy with IVb/V liver resection is performed. By contrast, a positive margin requires intraoperative identification of the cystic duct with resampling and resection of the common duct with portal nodes and liver bed [47].

After cholecystectomy, time to recurrence is generally rapid, with a mean of 4 months [8]. The ideal timeframe between cholecystectomy and radical surgery for incidentally discovered gallbladder cancer remains ill-defined; however, some authors suggest delayed referral to a tertiary center after cholecystectomy is not a risk factor for finding inoperable disease [88]. It is however suggested that reresection should be performed within 10 days of the initial surgery [86].

9.2. Port Site Recurrences. Port site recurrence is traditionally a major concern, reported in 14–29% of patients within 6–10 months. This risk is elevated in the event of gallbladder perforation at a rate of 40%. The precise mechanism responsible for port site recurrence remains ill understood. Theories include (a) direct mechanical contamination—tumour cells left at the site during tissue retrieval or removal of contaminated instruments, (b) indirect mechanical contamination due to leakage of gas along the trocars (chimney effect), (c) changes in the host immune response, (d) hematogenous dissemination, and (e) surgical technique [1]. Use of a retrieval bag in all laparoscopic cholecystectomies is recommended to prevent recurrences as it is not always possible to foresee problems with retraction and, should the gallbladder rupture, it is preferable to do so in a retrieval bag [47].

One-year survival rate among patients with port site recurrence is <30% [87]. Though port site seeding is associated with peritoneal carcinomatosis and is a poor prognostic factor, port site excision does not improve survival. A recent study by Fuks et al. retrospectively reviewed 218 incidentally discovered gallbladder cancers after laparoscopic cholecystectomy and concluded that port site excision did not improve survival and as such should not be routinely advocated during definitive surgical treatment. Poor prognosis in these patients may be due to several factors that include the following: these tumours are advanced stage, lymph node involvement is nearly exclusive (100% and 92% in two series), and concomitant peritoneal carcinomatosis is common [85].

9.3. Tis/T1a Disease. Tis/T1 gallbladder cancer is typically diagnosed after cholecystectomy. In those with Tis and T1a, simple cholecystectomy is sufficient therapy [84]. Specific attention to the cystic duct margin is, however, imperative as this remains the most important prognostic factor in these early cancers. Intraepithelial extension into Rokitansky-Aschoff sinuses (RAS) significantly shortens the survival and is an independent prognostic factor. Some authors suggest that RAS involvement may indicate the need for additional radical surgery [89]. In the absence of gallbladder perforation, port site excision is not indicated [84]. With a simple cholecystectomy, the 5-year survival rate is reported at 100% with no possible benefit of more aggressive surgical management; however, unfortunately few cases of gallbladder cancer are identified at this early stage [2].

9.4. T1b Disease. Management of T1b tumours that invade the muscular layer of the gallbladder remains controversial. While some authors maintain simple cholecystectomy is adequate in this population with 5-year survival up to 100%, locoregional recurrence has been well reported with 5-year survival rates as low as 37.5–68% [1]. Up to 30–60% of patients treated with simple cholecystectomy will have recurrence [84]. A 21-year analysis of stage I GBC recommends review of extensive resection (cholecystectomy + lymph node dissection or radical cholecystectomy) as it allegedly improved disease-specific survival when compared with a simple cholecystectomy [90]. As such, some authors recommend extended cholecystectomy including wedge resection of the gallbladder bed with segment IVb and V resection and/or N1 lymph node dissection. Other authors have failed to show any survival improvement with the addition of liver wedge resection/common bile duct resection/pancreaticoduodenectomy compared with a cholecystectomy and hepatoduodenal lymph node dissection [91]. Lymphatic metastases are more common than in T1a, with 20% of patients having nodal and 28% lymphovascular disease [84].

9.5. T2 Disease. Simple cholecystectomy is insufficient in the treatment of T2 disease as it confers a 5-year survival rate of only 20–40% [6]. One large study found a nearly threefold increase in median survival among patients with T2 disease who underwent radical resection compared with simple cholecystectomy [52]. Radical cholecystectomy with wedge resection of the gallbladder bed (or segments IVb and V) and regional lymph node dissection are therefore necessary in the treatment of T2 disease. The use of en bloc resection increases five-year survival to over 80–90% [2, 6]. The extent of hepatic resection depends on involvement of the major hepatic arterial or portal venous structures. Involvement of the right portal pedicle necessitates a right

hepatectomy; however, in its absence, resection of segments IVb and V is adequate [6]. In many centers, bile duct resection and reconstruction are standard for T2 gallbladder cancers; however, there remains a paucity of literature to support this practice [6]. In T2 disease, the rate of lymph node metastases is 19–62% [1]. The optimal extent of lymph node resection remains undetermined.

9.6. T3/T4 Disease. The best management of advanced gallbladder cancer remains a challenge for tumours that invade the serosa and/or adjacent organs (T3) and those that invade the main portal vein or hepatic artery or two or more extrahepatic organs/structures (T4). The morbidity and mortality of aggressive surgical management compared with the potential survival benefits remain unclear. Factors that may preclude extensive surgery in patients with advanced disease include poor physiologic status, the extent of the disease, and the presence of comorbidities. As such, surgical resection is only recommended when there is potential for a curative R0 resection.

In T3 tumours with direct invasion to adjacent duodenum, stomach, or colon, surgical resection is indicated. These tumours are usually amenable to a radical resection; however, such intervention is associated with a high degree of morbidity. Five-year survival rates for T3 gallbladder cancer range from 30–50% [6].

Management of hepatic invasion is inconclusive. No significant difference in survival was found between patients treated with gallbladder bed resection and those who underwent a formal segmental IVa + V hepatectomy [92].

The National Comprehensive Cancer Network (NCCN) recommends that tumours with T1b, T2, and T3 tumours should undergo radical reoperation including hepatic resection and lymph node dissection with or without common bile duct resection and reconstructive hepaticojejunostomy. Poor compliance, however, with these guidelines has been described, with only 13% and 6.9% of patients receiving radical repeat resections/hepatectomy and lymphadenectomy, respectively [52].

T4 tumours are typically unresectable, and palliation is indicated. Criteria for nonresectability include metastatic disease, involvement of main portal vein or hepatic artery, involvement of the portal vein or hepatic artery branches of both lobes of liver, simultaneous involvement of ipsilateral hepatic artery and contralateral portal vein, simultaneous involvement in both lobes of liver at the level of confluence of segmental bile ducts to form hepatic ducts, and contiguous involvement of more than 2 segments each in both lobes of liver. These criteria are, however, not binding. For example, two exceptions in the literature are the following: (a) if main portal vein invasion is present, then portal vein resection and reconstruction may be indicated rarely or (b) if there is extensive extrahepatic organ involvement this may be resected en bloc [6]. Traditionally, paraaortic lymph node metastasis was a contraindication to surgical resection; however, it is reported that resection in these patients confers a similar survival to those with isolated liver metastases and better survival than unresected tumours with other sites of metastatic spread. Contraindications to surgical resection in advanced tumours however remain poorly defined and as such each case should be evaluated on an individual basis [93].

The combination of hepatectomy and pancreaticoduodenectomy is commonly indicated when there is direct duodenal or pancreatic invasion and peripancreatic lymph node involvement. The presence of peripancreatic nodal involvement is not a contraindication for pancreaticoduodenectomy for gallbladder cancers provided an R0 resection is feasible. This procedure provides the greatest number of dissected lymph nodes [83]. The survival benefits of these procedures remain ill defined and geographically dependent. As such, aggressive surgery is not currently recommended routinely in this particular scenario.

9.7. Liver and Bile Duct Resection. Typically hepatic invasion occurs initially to segments IV and V. The extent of hepatectomy is dictated by the T-stage, the anatomical location, and size of the tumour. A surgical tumour-free margin of 2 cm is required; however, the extent of liver resection for T1b or higher tumours remains controversial. Some authors maintain that hepatic wedge excision is not appropriate for T1b/T2 disease as significant bleeds and bile leaks may result from an inconsistent thickness of tissue around the gallbladder. If there is invasion of the liver hilum, right hepatectomy with or without bile duct resection or portal vein resection is necessary for a curative intent. The operative mortality rate for extended radical surgery is <5% [1].

In the instance of a prior cholecystectomy with indications for a second operation, the status of the cystic duct margin is of utmost importance. If negative for malignant cells, the biliary tree may be preserved and a lymphadenectomy with IVB and V gallbladder bed liver resection is indicated. In contrast, a positive margin necessitates intraoperative identification of the cystic duct with resampling. If this sampling is positive, or the cystic duct stump cannot be identified, resection of the common duct, portal nodes, and liver bed to optimize surgically negative margins with Roux-en-Y hepaticojejunostomy is recommended. While some surgeons advocate for elective bile duct resection to improve node clearance, no survival benefit has been identified with this additional surgery [2].

9.8. Lymph Node Dissection. Regional lymph nodes of gallbladder cancer are classified based on the nodes involved: N1 (cystic, pericholedochal, and hilar lymph nodes, hepatoduodenal ligament), and N2 (peripancreatic (head only), peridutal, periportal, common hepatic artery, coeliac, and superior mesenteric artery lymph node). For T2–T4 disease, N1 and N2 regional lymph node dissection is indicated [1]. The most commonly involved initial nodes are the cystic and pericholedochal. It is strongly recommended that formal portal lymphadenectomy includes the nodal tissue of the hepatoduodenal ligament and portacaval and retroduodenal regions [2]. There remain no randomized control trials comparing survival with the extent of lymph node dissection [1]. It has been shown, however, that radical lymph node dissection is effective in up to three positive lymph nodes provided a R0 resection is attainable [83].

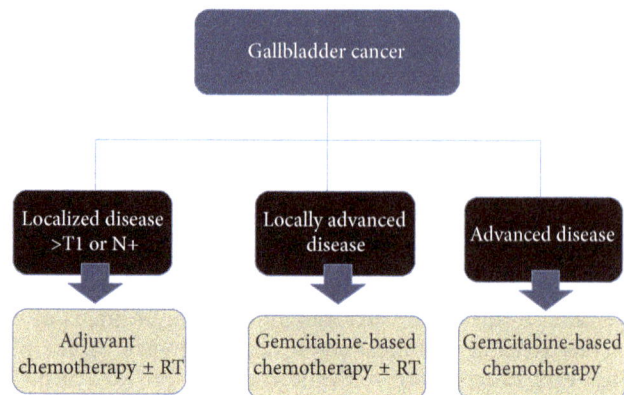

N+: node-positive
RT: radiation theraby

FIGURE 1: Role of systemic therapy in the management of gallbladder cancer.

As the most powerful predicting factor for survival is nodal status, effective lymph node dissection is reported to be the most valuable procedure for improving survival. Adequate assessment of lymph node involvement, per the American Joint Committee on Cancer (AJCC) guidelines, recommends resection and pathologic examination of a minimum of three regional lymph nodes (cystic, pericholedochal, retroportal, periduodenal, peripancreatic, coeliac, and superior mesenteric nodes) [90]. A survival advantage is reported when three or more nodes are removed compared with 2 or less, with overall median survival in one study of 18 versus 5 months, respectively [52]. Significant differences in survival are reported between node-negative and node-positive disease, with 5-year survivals of 58–77% versus 0–45%, respectively. Regional lymph node involvement in T2 and T3/T4 tumours occurs in 19–62% and 75–85% and N2 lymph node involvement occurs in 18–36% and 42–71% [1].

10. Medical Treatment

Systemic therapy is used in curative and palliative setting in the management of gallbladder cancer in 3 situations: (1) in adjuvant therapy alone or in combination with radiation following surgical resection, (2) in locally advanced nonmetastatic unresectable disease alone or in combination with radiation therapy, and (3) in advanced metastatic disease (Figure 1).

There is a paucity of randomized controlled studies in the management of gallbladder cancer in relationship with systemic therapy due to the rarity of gallbladder and other biliary tract cancers. Most studies are inclusive of all biliary tract cancers and there are very few gallbladder cancer-specific studies.

10.1. Resectable Gallbladder Cancer

10.1.1. Adjuvant Therapy. Evidence regarding adjuvant therapy in gallbladder cancer with few exceptions is mostly limited to retrospective studies. Most studies were comprised of small, heterogeneous groups of patients seen at a single institution. Several retrospective series and small phase II studies suggest better survival in patients who receive post-operative adjuvant treatment. The only phase III randomized trial regarding benefit of adjuvant therapy in gallbladder and biliary tract cancer is reported by the Japanese group. In this phase III multicenter randomized trial, 508 patients with resected pancreaticobiliary cancer were randomly assigned two cycles of intravenous mitomycin and 5-FU (MF) followed by maintenance oral 5-FU until disease recurrence versus observation. In a subgroup of 140 patients with gallbladder cancer, 5-year disease-free survival (DFS) rates of patients treated with adjuvant MF was 20.3% compared with 11.6% with observation ($P = 0.02$). The 5-year survival rate was significantly better in the adjuvant therapy group (26.0%) compared with the control group (14.4%) ($P = 0.03$) [94].

A meta-analysis which included 20 studies involving 6712 patients assessed the impact of chemotherapy, radiation therapy, or both therapies as an adjuvant to curative-intent surgery for the management of biliary tract cancers comprising extrahepatic and gallbladder cancers. Of 6712 patients 4915 were treated with surgery alone, and 1797 received adjuvant therapy. The meta-analysis reported a nonsignificant improvement in overall survival with any adjuvant therapy compared with surgery alone (odds ratio (OR), 0.74; $P = 0.06$). The association was significant when the two registry analyses were excluded. A nonsignificant benefit was also observed when disease sites were analyzed independently (gallbladder: OR, 0.81; 95% CI, 0.49 to 1.35; $P = 0.41$). The benefit of adjuvant therapy was dependent on treatment modality. Patients who received chemotherapy (OR, 0.39; 95% CI, 0.23 to 0.66; $P < 0.001$) or chemoradiotherapy (OR, 0.61; 95% CI, 0.38 to 0.99; $P = 0.049$) derived greater benefit than patients who were treated with radiation therapy alone (OR, 0.98; 95% CI, 0.67 to 1.43; $P = 0.90$). Nine studies reported nodal or margin positivity. Pooled data revealed a significant benefit for adjuvant chemotherapy or chemoradiation treatment ($n = 230$) in node-positive disease (OR, 0.49; 95% CI, 0.30–0.80; $P = 0.004$) or in cancers with R1 disease (OR, 0.36; 95% CI, 0.19 to 0.68; $P = 0.002$) [95]. An exploratory analysis that demonstrated greater magnitude of benefit from adjuvant therapy in studies included patients with node-positive disease, R1 disease, or both diseases compared to studies that did not include patients with node-positive or R1 disease. Similar findings were also seen in Surveillance, Epidemiology, and End Results- (SEER-) based study that was not included in this meta-analysis. This study demonstrated that, with the exception of T1N0 patients, 6 months of chemotherapy or radiation after surgery was associated with a better survival [96].

Even though the meta-analysis favors adjuvant therapy in patients with high risk, that is, node-positive gallbladder cancer, it does not resolve the question of the benefit of adjuvant therapy in patients with low risk disease. Moreover, the best treatment strategy, for instance, chemoradiotherapy versus chemotherapy alone, in adjuvant setting is not known.

The National Comprehensive Cancer Network (NCCN) guidelines for gallbladder cancer support adjuvant fluoropyrimidine chemoradiation or fluoropyrimidine or gemcitabine chemotherapy in patients with >T1N0 gallbladder cancer following curative surgery (National Comprehensive Cancer Network). Furthermore, the European Society of Medical Oncology (ESMO) guidelines also suggest consideration of postoperative chemoradiotherapy in patients with high risk gallbladder cancer [97].

The results of several phase III, randomized controlled trials evaluating the benefit of adjuvant chemotherapy are awaited. These trials included patients with completely resected biliary tract and gallbladder cancers. The United Kingdom trial [98] randomly assigned patients to eight cycles of capecitabine versus observation. The accrual for this study is completed. The French trial [99] that randomly assigns patients to 12 biweekly cycles of gemcitabine plus oxaliplatin versus observation is currently recruiting patients. ACTICCA-1 is a multicentre German phase III trial which is evaluating 24 weeks of gemcitabine and cisplatin after curative resection of biliary tract and muscle invasive gallbladder cancers (adjuvant chemotherapy with gemcitabine and cisplatin compared to observation after curative intent resection of biliary tract cancer [100]).

Given the poor prognosis of patients with gallbladder cancer with T ≥ 2 and/or node-positive disease, we recommend adjuvant therapy for such patients. As higher stage gallbladder cancers have a high incidence of both local failure and distant failure after surgical resection, despite limited evidence, a locoregional adjuvant treatment can be considered similar to other extrahepatic biliary cancers. The optimal adjuvant therapy is unknown though six months of gemcitabine or fluoropyrimidine-based chemotherapy with or without fluorouracil-based chemoradiation can be considered.

10.1.2. Neoadjuvant Therapy. Currently outside the setting of a clinical trial neoadjuvant therapy is not recommended for surgically resectable gallbladder cancer. Trials with a neoadjuvant strategy may provide opportunities for the development of predictive markers to guide personalized treatment in patients with gallbladder and biliary tract cancer.

10.1.3. Follow-Up after Curative Therapy. There is lack of level 1 evidence with respect to optimal follow-up of patients with gallbladder cancer who are treated with curative intention. Routine imaging studies and endoscopic examination are not recommended and can be performed as clinically indicated. Follow-up investigations should be individualized based on the stage of the cancer, adjuvant treatment provided, performance status, and clinical signs and symptoms.

10.2. Locally Advanced Unresectable Gallbladder Cancer. The optimal management of patients with locally advanced and unresectable gallbladder cancer is controversial, and there is no internationally embraced standard approach. The options for patients with locally advanced gallbladder cancers include fluoropyrimidine chemoradiation or gemcitabine-based chemotherapy (such as gemcitabine/cisplatin combination) or fluoropyrimidine-based chemotherapy. The available data suggest that tumour control is rarely achieved with external beam radiation alone [101, 102]. Most patients with locally advanced unresectable disease are treated with combination of chemotherapy and radiation rather than radiation alone. However, it is not known if chemoradiation therapy is superior to chemotherapy alone in this setting and there is a lack of level 1 evidence validating this approach. There is limited evidence that chemoradiation therapy with or without surgery (trimodality therapy) in selected patients with locally advanced gallbladder cancers may result in prolonged survival [103]. If restaging in patients with locally advanced disease shows potentially resectable tumours (conversion therapy), resection should be considered. The NCCN clinical practice guidelines and the ESMO Guidelines Working Group in biliary cancer support concomitant fluoropyrimidine-based chemoradiotherapy as a treatment option to palliative chemotherapy for patients with locally advanced, unresectable gallbladder cancer [97, 104].

10.3. Metastatic Gallbladder Cancer

10.3.1. Chemotherapy in Gallbladder Cancer. Systemic chemotherapy has shown significant but modest survival benefit in the management of advanced gallbladder cancer. A randomized trial compared systemic chemotherapy of gemcitabine plus oxaliplatin or 5-FU plus leucovorin versus best supportive care alone in 81 patients with unresectable gallbladder cancer [105]. Median overall survival in best supportive care and 5-FU/leucovorin groups was 4.5 and 4.6 months, respectively, versus 9.5 months in gemcitabine plus oxaliplatin group.

Of note, most published trials are small and have included patients with all biliary tract cancers. Only few clinical trials were performed exclusively in patients with gallbladder cancer [106–108]. There are three phase 2 trials that exclusively evaluated patients with gallbladder cancer. One study evaluated gemcitabine monotherapy and two trials assessed gemcitabine and cisplatin combination therapy (Table 5). In these trials, responses varied from 36 to 48% and median overall survival varied from 20 to 30 weeks. A pooled analysis of 104 chemotherapy trials involving 1,368 patients with biliary tract and gallbladder cancers that was conducted in 1985–2006 suggested differences in clinical behavior and responsiveness to chemotherapy between gallbladder and other biliary tract cancers. Pooled response rates and tumour control rates were 22.6 and 57.3%, respectively. Subgroup analysis showed superior response rate for gallbladder cancer compared with cholangiocarcinoma (36 versus 18%) but shorter overall survival for gallbladder cancer (7.2 versus 9.3 months) [109].

Most studies reported here are performed in patients with adenocarcinoma, the most common histology of gallbladder cancer. There is paucity of data regarding treatment of advanced adenosquamous or squamous cell gallbladder cancers, and in clinical practice these patients are treated similarly.

(1) Fluoropyrimidine-Based Regimens. 5-FU and 5-FU-based regimens were among the first reported in gallbladder cancers. In old trials, 5-FU alone or 5-FU-based combination therapies demonstrated objective response rates from 0 to 34% and median survival of four to six months in patients with advanced gallbladder and biliary tract cancers [110–112]. In contrast, most recent studies using infusional 5-FU combination therapy reported higher response rates and better overall survival [113–116]. In one study infusional 5-FU in combination with cisplatin resulted in partial response in six patients (24%). Median survival for patients with gallbladder cancer was 11.5 months [114].

Capecitabine is an orally active fluoropyrimidine derivative that has demonstrated efficacy in gallbladder cancer both as a single agent and in combination with cisplatin, gemcitabine, and oxaliplatin [117–121]. For instance, in a study involving 63 patients with hepatobiliary malignancies, which included eight patients with gallbladder cancer, capecitabine produced an objective response in four patients with gallbladder cancer, two of which were complete response [119]. In another trial involving 65 patients with biliary tract tumours, capecitabine was used in combination with oxaliplatin. Of 65 patients, 27 had gallbladder cancer. The patients with gallbladder cancer had a total disease control rate of 63% (one complete response, seven partial responses, and nine patients with stable disease) and a median survival of 8.2 months [120].

(2) Gemcitabine-Based Regimens. Gemcitabine is an active agent both as monotherapy and in combination regimens [107, 117, 118, 122, 123]. It has been extensively evaluated in patients with metastatic gallbladder and biliary tract cancer. The clinical benefit rates (partial response plus stable disease) with single agent gemcitabine are varied from 15 to 60% with overall response rates being as low as 7% [107, 122, 124–127]. Most studies reported median survival of 10 months or less. In contrast, reported response rates with gemcitabine combination therapies are varied from 17% to 50%, with median overall survival of up to 14 months (Table 6) [117, 118, 128–136]. At least four studies of gemcitabine plus cisplatin in patients with advanced gallbladder and biliary tract cancers have been reported. The reported response rates ranged from 21% to 34.5% and median survival times varied from 9.3 to 11 months [128–131]. The substitution of carboplatin for cisplatin decreases the severity of nonhematologic toxicity such as nausea, vomiting, nephropathy, and neuropathy; however, myelosuppression is sometimes worse. In a small trial, combination of gemcitabine and carboplatin was associated with response rate of 37% and median overall survival of about 11 months [137]. Several trials have demonstrated efficacy and good tolerability with a combination of gemcitabine and oxaliplatin [132–134]. The Groupe Coopérateur Multidisciplinaire en Oncologie study evaluated 56 patients with gallbladder and biliary tract cancers [133]. These patients were treated with gemcitabine and oxaliplatin combination and were stratified based on Eastern Cooperative Oncology Group performance status score (0–2 versus >2) and bilirubin. The median overall survival of patients with good performance status was almost double that of patients with

TABLE 5: Results of three phase 2 trials which exclusively evaluated efficacy of chemotherapy in patients with advanced gall bladder cancer.

Regimen	Number of patients	Response rate (%)	Median overall survival
Gemcitabine monotherapy [107]	26	36	30 weeks
Gemcitabine and cisplatin [106]	30	37	20 weeks
Gemcitabine and cisplatin [108]	42	48	7 months

Modified from [2].

TABLE 6: Efficacy of gemcitabine combination therapy in patients with advanced gallbladder and biliary tract cancer.

Regimens	Number of patients	Response rate (%)	Median overall survival (months)
Gemcitabine and cisplatin			
Meyerhardt et al. [128]	33	21	9.7
Thongprasert et al. [129]	40	26	8.4
Lee et al. [130]	24	21	9.3
Kim et al. [131]	29	35	11
Gemcitabine and oxaliplatin			
Harder et al. [132]	31	26	11
André et al. [133]	33[*]; 23[**]	36[*]; 22[**]	15.4[*]; 7.6[**]
Gebbia et al. [134]	24	50	14
Gemcitabine an capecitabine			
Knox et al. [118]	45	31	14
Cho et al. [117]	44	32	14
Riechelmann et al. [135]	75	29	12.7
Iyer et al. [136]	12	17	14

[*]Patients with good performance status; [**]patients with poor performance status. Modified from [2].

poor performance status (15.4 months versus 7.6 months). Of note, even patients with poor performance status tolerated this regimen fairly well. Others report a far lower objective response rate with this regimen in advanced gallbladder cancer (1 of 23 patients, 4%) as compared to nongallbladder biliary tract carcinomas (9 of 44, 21%). Similar to gemcitabine and platinum compounds combination, gemcitabine and the oral 5-FU prodrug capecitabine combination has been associated with higher response rates than gemcitabine plus 5-FU for advanced biliary and gallbladder tumours. At least four phase II trials report response rates up to 32% and a median survival of approximately 13 to 14 months [117, 118, 135, 136].

The result of a randomized phase III trial that reported improvement in outcomes of patients with locally advanced or metastatic biliary tract and gallbladder cancers who were treated with combination therapy was a major breakthrough in management of advanced gallbladder and biliary tract cancers [126]. In this trial, 410 patients with locally advanced (25%) or metastatic bile duct ($n = 242$), gallbladder, ($n = 149$) or ampullary ($n = 20$) cancer were randomly assigned to eight courses of cisplatin (25 mg/m^2) followed by gemcitabine (1000 mg/m^2) on days 1 and 8, every 21 days, or gemcitabine alone (1000 mg/m^2 on days 1, 8, and 15, every 28 days). At a median follow-up of 8.2 months, median progression-free survival (8 versus 5 months) and median overall survival (11.7 versus 8.1 months) were better with combination therapy.

(3) Taxanes and Other Chemotherapeutic Agents. Other chemotherapeutic agents have demonstrated limited benefit in gallbladder and biliary tract cancers. For instance, when paclitaxel was given every 21 days it demonstrated minimal efficacy in gallbladder cancer [138]. Likewise, the addition of pemetrexed to fixed-dose-rate gemcitabine, in a biweekly schedule, did not enhance the activity of gemcitabine in patients with biliary tract or gallbladder carcinoma [139]. Whereas docetaxel has shown a response rate of 20% in patients with advanced gallbladder and biliary tract cancers [140], single agent irinotecan demonstrated partial response rate of 8% and clinical benefit rate (partial response and stable disease) in 48% [141]. Based on the trial by Valle et al. [126] for patients with metastatic gallbladder cancer and good performance status, combination of cisplatin and gemcitabine is standard first line systemic therapy. In patients with borderline performance status, single agent gemcitabine or capecitabine is a reasonable alternative option.

10.3.2. Second-Line Therapy in Gallbladder Cancer. Currently there is no "standard" second-line therapy after failure of first-line gemcitabine and cisplatin in patients with gallbladder cancer. In a preliminary report of 18 patients with advanced gemcitabine-refractory pancreaticobiliary cancer who received CAPOX, one had a partial response, and 8 patients had stable disease with the median progression-free survival of about 16 weeks in all patients [142]. Several

TABLE 7: Targeted therapy alone or in combination with chemotherapy in gallbladder and biliary tract cancer.

Targeted agent	Disease site	Number GBC/total	Line of therapy	Response rate	Comments
Single agent targeting VGF					
Sorafenib [145]	BTC	12/31	First	6%	
Sunitinib [146]	BTC	NA/56	Second	9%	
Single agent targeting HER2					
Lapatinib [147]	HCC or BTC	17 BTC/57	First & second	0% in BTC	
Lapatinib [148]	HCC or BTC	NA/9	Any	0%	Trial was stopped early due to futility
Other single agents					
Bortezomib [149]	BTC	6/20	First, second, third	5%	Trial was stopped early due to futility
Selumetinib [150]	BTC	7/28	Second	10%	
Doublet of targeted agents					
Bevacizumab + erlotinib [151]	BTC	10/53	First	17%	
Bevacizumab + erlotinib [152]	Upper GI cancer	16 BTC/102	Second or later	6%	
Targeted agents with chemotherapy					
GEMOX ± cetuximab [153]	BTC	NA/50	First	23%	Response rate in control group: 29%
GEMOX + cetuximab [154]	BTC	NA/30	First	63%	9 patients underwent resection after response
GEMOX ± cetuximab [155]	BTC	50/122	First	27.3%	Response rate in control group: 15%
GEMOX + bevacizumab [156]	BTC	NA/35	First & second	40%	
Gem + triapine [157]	BTC	18/33	First	9%	
5FU/LV + imatinib [158]	BTC	19/41	First	8%	
GEMOX + erlotinib [159]	BTC	82/268	First	30%	16% in chemotherapy arm alone. No difference in OS

BTC, biliary tract cancer; GEMOX, gemcitabine and oxaliplatin; HCC, hepatocellular cancer; NA, not applicable; OS, overall survival. Modified from [143].

targeted therapies in combination with chemotherapy have shown modest clinical benefit (see below). In patients with good performance status oxaliplatin-based regimen, 5-FU/capecitabine, taxanes, or irinotecan based therapy may be considered following progression on cisplatin/gemcitabine.

10.3.3. Targeted Therapies in Gallbladder Cancer. Common mutations reported in gallbladder cancer are KRAS (10%–67%), EGFR (63%), BRAF (0% to 33%), and erbB2/HER2 (16%–64%) [23, 143, 144]. Early data suggest possible benefit from blockade of the epidermal growth factor receptor by the oral tyrosine kinase inhibitor erlotinib or anti-EGFR monoclonal antibody cetuximab (Table 7). [145–159]. A phase III Korean trial evaluated the efficacy of first-line treatment with gemcitabine and oxaliplatin with or without erlotinib in patients with advanced biliary tract cancer that included 31% of patients with gallbladder cancer. The median progression-free survival (PFS) was 5.8 months in the chemotherapy plus erlotinib group compared with 4.2 months in the chemotherapy alone group (HR, 0.80; 95% CI, 0.61–1.03; $P = 0.087$). Median OS was 9.5 months for both groups. However,

in a subgroup of patients with gallbladder cancer, no benefit of erlotinib was noted (HR, 0.9; 95% CI, 0.63 to 1.58) [159]. A randomized phase II study comparing gemcitabine plus oxaliplatin alone with the same chemotherapy regimen in combination with cetuximab demonstrated a higher 4-month PFS rate with the addition of cetuximab (44% versus 61%, resp.) [153].

Vascular endothelial growth factor (VEGF) is overexpressed in biliary tract cancers and has been proposed as a therapeutic target [145, 146, 151, 152, 156]. The efficacy of bevacizumab, a monoclonal antibody targeting VEGF, in combination with erlotinib was assessed in a phase II trial. Nine patients had partial response to double targeted therapy that was sustained beyond four weeks in six patients, with median response duration of 8.4 months. Overall stable disease was observed in about half of the treated patients [151]. Sunitinib and sorafenib have shown modest benefit in biliary tract and gallbladder cancers [145, 146]. Likewise, selumetinib, a BRAF inhibitor, triapine, a ribonucleotide reductase inhibitor, and imatinib, a tyrosine kinase inhibitor, have shown some efficacy in gallbladder and biliary tract cancers

[150, 157, 158]. In contrast, lapatinib targeting erB2/HER2 and bortezomib, a proteasome inhibitor, failed to demonstrate benefit in gallbladder and biliary tract cancers [147–149].

11. Radiation

While GBC's propensity for locoregional spread and recurrence suggest it is a rational target for intraoperative and postoperative radiotherapy, the role of adjuvant radiotherapy is poorly described in the literature with conflicting and largely disappointing results obtained in a small number of patients. The combination of external beam radiotherapy with fluorouracil has shown encouraging results, but further investigation is required. External radiation may be considered in palliative patients; however, tumour radioresistance typically precludes it from achieving tumour control as an independent therapeutic modality. Transhepatic percutaneous intraluminal brachytherapy using Ir-192 has been used as a palliative therapy for obstructive jaundice due to bile duct obstruction [160].

12. Palliation

Many patients who present symptomatically have advanced disease in whom palliation is the primary goal of treatment. Palliative bypass surgery may alleviate some of the symptoms commonly associated with incurable gallbladder cancer including jaundice, pruritus, cholangitis, pain, and biliary tract/gastrointestinal obstruction.

Biliary obstruction may be relieved by a number of procedures including Roux-en-Y or jejunal loop anastomosis with common hepatic duct or left duct or segment II or Longmire bilioenteric anastomosis. Segment III cholangiojejunostomy remains the most popular, with an associated high morbidity approaching 50% and mortality of 3.17%. Common complications include anastomotic leak and wound infection. As radiological and endoscopic stenting continues to evolve and improve, the future role of palliative surgery remains undetermined. No distinct advantage has been shown for one approach versus the other; however, it is suggested that the quality of life may be improved when treated surgically as postoperatively patients do not have the tubes and stents that would be present when treated by interventional radiological techniques [8].

Obstruction is a potential complication of late stage gallbladder cancer. Gastric outlet obstruction occurs in up to 30% of patients with advanced gallbladder cancer and may benefit from palliative gastrojejunostomy. The mortality and morbidity rates are high at 7.2% and 42%, respectively [8]. Palliative patients with bowel obstruction may be candidates for intestinal bypass procedures; however, morbidity is high in those with extensive peritoneal disease.

13. Prognosis

Gallbladder cancer is generally considered to confer a poor prognosis as this tumour typically remains silent until an advanced and often noncurative stage. Historically gallbladder cancer had an overall 5-year survival less than 5%. The recent advent of aggressive surgical resection with advances in perioperative care has markedly improved outcomes [1]. Other studies, however, have shown no significant improvement in OS in the past 20 years [52]. A retrospective review of gallbladder cancer throughout the 20th century found the overall survival has increased from 3.6 months in 1915–1932 to 10 months at the beginning of the 21st century [48]. Ongoing improvements in surgical techniques have resulted in a decline of both morbidity and mortality. In patients who undergo R0 curative resection, 5-year survival, by contrast, is 21–69%. Nevertheless, the French Surgical Association has demonstrated that 85% of T3/T4 tumours have an overall survival of only 2–8 months [18].

A recent (2012) multivariant Cox proportional hazard survival model by Hari et al. identified independent predictors of disease-specific survival to include age, T1 subtype, tumour grade, tumour histology, radiation, and surgery type, while independent predictors of overall survival were age, T1 subtype, tumour grade, tumour histology, race, and surgical procedure [90]. Prognostic factors specific for stage III/IV disease include adjuvant chemotherapy, tumour differentiation, hepatic invasion, and surgical margin status [92]. A recent (2013) study by D'Hondt et al. showed that patients with incidentally discovered gallbladder cancer have a significantly greater curability rate compared with nonincidentally discovered gallbladder cancer [88].

13.1. Patient Factors. Patient age is a well-recognized predictive factor. On multivariate analysis, treatment at a younger age is predictive of improved disease-specific survival [90]. On clinical exam, jaundice is a negative predictive finding, as it commonly indicates obstruction distal to the common hepatic duct or proximal common bile duct, therefore indicating advanced disease. The presence of a palpable mass, indicative of advanced disease, similarly confers a worse prognosis.

13.2. Tumour Factors. T-stage is an important prognostic feature. While the overall 5-year survival for T2 tumours is 70%, it falls dramatically to 0% for T3 tumours. Similarly, the rate of distant metastases increases from 16% in T2 to 79% in T4 disease, and the risk of nodal involvement increases from 33 to 69% [7]. Incidentally discovered gallbladder cancer has a better prognosis compared with patients with preoperative suspicion likely because of an earlier stage at incidental discovery [161, 162].

Among pT2–4 tumours, two patterns of intramural invasion are described: infiltrative (infiltration into the muscle without muscle destruction) and destructive (infiltration and destruction of muscle layer). Destructive growth confers a significantly lower overall survival than infiltrative, with higher rates of lymphovascular invasion, nodal positivity, and scirrhous growth pattern [162].

The extent of nodal involvement is an important prognostic factor. Whereas both the location and number of nodes were significant on univariate analysis, only the number of positive nodes is significant on multivariate analysis [83]. Other studies have shown a marked improvement in 5-year survival between node-negative (58–77%) and node-positive (0–45%) diseases [47]. It has been suggested that involvement of the peripancreatic nodes is indicative of a worse outcome. In patients with positive nodes, regional lymph node dissection may improve patient survival provided R0 resection is feasible [92]. Five-year survival rates following cholecystectomy alone are 5% and 13% with cholecystectomy and liver resection [8]. In patients who present with advanced disease, median survival is 2–4 months [6]. In all stages of GBC, R0 resection is an independent positive prognostic factor [88].

Hepatic involvement is well recognized as an independent prognostic factor in several series. In fact, on cox proportional regression, the importance of liver involvement is so dominant that no other covariants remained significant. While many of the other prognostic factors described in this section have been found on univariate analysis to be significant, hepatic involvement is consistently significant on both univariate and multivariate analyses [88].

13.3. Histology. The histological subtype of gallbladder cancer is another important prognostic factor. Papillary carcinoma confers the best prognosis, whereas squamous and adenosquamous carcinomas are more aggressive with a poorer prognosis. Small cell carcinoma, though very rare, metastasizes early and death often occurs shortly after diagnosis. The presence of perineural invasion is additionally significant for a worse outcome [88].

13.4. Miscellaneous

(i) *Lysosomal protein transmembrane 4 beta allele *2 (LAPTM4B)* is one of the two alleles of LAPTM4B, a cancer-related gene, that contains two 19-base pair sequences in the $5'$ untranslated region of exon 1. It is associated with poor histopathological differentiation, higher TNM stage, and the presence of lymph node metastases, with a shorter overall and disease-free survival. This allele is present in 37.9% of gallbladder cancers compared with 24.8% of controls [163]. The LAPTM4B status is suggested to be used to preoperatively evaluate patients for operability [163, 164].

(ii) Expressions of *Nectin-2, DDX3, integrin-linked kinase,* and *peroxiredoxin-1* have been shown to be independent poor prognostic factors in squamous/adenosquamous carcinomas of the gallbladder; however, these have not been studied in the more common gallbladder adenocarcinomas [164].

(iii) The prognostic role of *mucin* (MUC) expression in gallbladder remains disputed with MUC1 and MUC4 overexpression correlating with progression in some studies but not in others [164].

(iv) Overexpression of *histone-lysine N-methyltransferase* EZH2 or loss of phosphatase and tensin homolog expression may be implicated in the carcinogenesis of gallbladder cancer and convey a poorer prognosis [164]. Similarly, p53, bcl-2, bax, and COX-2 are all implicated in the pathogenesis of gallbladder carcinomas [164, 165].

(v) In contrast, *CDX2* and hepatocyte antigen expression increases the overall survival [164].

(vi) Expression of the *L1 cell adhesion molecule* is reported at the invasive front of 63.8% of gallbladder carcinomas and is associated with high histologic grade, advanced pathologic T-stage, clinical stage, and positive lymphovascular invasion. L1 cell adhesion molecule is reported to be an independent risk factor for disease-free survival [166].

(vii) Overexpression of *Skp2*, a SKP1-CUL1-F-box protein, has been shown to confer a shorter overall survival [166].

(viii) Expressions of *N(neural)-cadherin and P(placental)-cadherin* are associated with increased tumour size, invasion, and lymph node metastases in both adenocarcinoma and squamous cell/adenosquamous carcinomas of the gallbladder and with higher TNM staging in adenocarcinomas. N-cadherin is expressed in 52% of squamous cell/adenosquamous carcinomas and 55% of adenocarcinomas of the gallbladder; P-cadherin is expressed in 50% and 52.5%, respectively. Expressions of both N-cadherin and P-cadherin are both independent poor prognostic factors on multivariate Cox regression analysis [35].

(ix) Overexpression of CD54 is identified in gallbladder carcinoma, particularly in advanced disease [166].

(x) Intratumoural FoxP3 (transcriptional factor forkhead P3) is involved in the development and function of regulatory T cells and has been reported to be elevated in gallbladder cancers. FoxP3 and IL-17 positivity is correlated with nodal metastases and TNM stage. Additionally, FoxP3 positivity is associated with a poor disease-free survival on multivariate analysis [167].

(xi) Epithelial cell adhesion molecule (EpCAM) overexpression is reported to predict a decreased survival; however, its expression is not correlated with tumour grade or disease stage. Approximately 60% of patients with gallbladder cancer express EpCAM [168].

(xii) Frizzled (FZD1) is a member of a family of transmembrane receptors to which Wnt genes bind; these genes are well recognized to play a key role in controlling proliferation, specification, polarity, and cell migration. Expression of FZD1 is significantly associated with a large tumour size, high TMN staging, and lymph node involvement, with increased propensity for invasion, and thereby it is associated with a decreased overall survival in patients with gallbladder squamous cell and adenocarcinomas [169].

Prevention, Screening, and Future Directions. Eradication of gallstones remains the ideal target for the prevention of gallbladder cancer given their well-described association with carcinogenesis and given the fact that they are easily detected by ultrasound examination with a prolonged lead time of 20 years [3]. In this context, the role of prophylactic cholecystectomy in asymptomatic patients remains poorly defined. Patients at high risk (stones >2-3 cm, associated polyps, nonfunctioning gallbladder, porcelain gallbladder, pancreaticobiliary reflux, segmental adenomyomatosis, and xanthogranulomatous cholecystitis) may significantly benefit from prophylactic cholecystectomy, particularly those in a high risk geographical location [3, 12]. It is also recommended that gastrectomy patients undergo a concomitant cholecystectomy as these patients are predisposed to delayed gastric emptying with increased incidence of gallstones and rarely gallbladder cancers [12]. Potentially, unnecessary patient morbidity and the increased cost however remain barriers to this practice.

The future therefore should be directed towards research to promote early accurate diagnosis and improve management strategies which is dependent on global collaboration between general surgeons, gastroenterologists, radiologists, pathologists, and molecular biologists. Proposed areas for such research may include improved understanding of the molecular carcinogenesis with subsequent innovation of targeted chemotherapeutics, higher detection rates on imaging at an early T-stage, and the development of consensus-based guidelines for the management of T1b tumours. The creation of a sensitive and specific screening modality is perhaps of utmost importance to promote early detection of GBC at a resectable, low T-stage.

14. Conclusions

Gallbladder cancer is uncommon with a high case fatality occurring over a wide geographical distribution. Risk factors include advanced age, female gender, cholelithiasis, porcelain gallbladder, gallbladder polyps, congenital biliary cysts, chronic infection, and smoking. Most gallbladder cancers, unfortunately, are discovered incidentally at routine cholecystectomy or present as advanced stage disease. The role of radiological imaging, therefore, is limited to the use of ultrasound, CT scans, and endoscopic/FNA procedures for diagnostic and staging purposes. Adenocarcinoma accounts for the majority of gallbladder cancers. Surgery is the only curative therapy for gallbladder cancer. However, at diagnosis, less than ~20% of patients are candidates for curative surgery. The extent of surgical intervention is dependent on the TNM stage of the disease and may range from simple cholecystectomy in T1a tumour to partial hepatectomy and regional lymph node dissection in ≥T2 tumours. This may require reexcision of the tumor bed following the definitive pathological report.

Regional nodal status and the depth of tumor invasion (T status) are the two most important prognostic factors. The role of adjuvant therapy in GBC is not well defined. Nevertheless, in ≥T2 or node-positive disease, due to the high risk of recurrence, six months of gemcitabine or fluoropyrimidine-based chemotherapy can be considered. Such systemic chemotherapy has shown modest survival benefit in the management of advanced gallbladder cancer and is recommended in patients with good performance status along with best supportive care.

Currently, targeted therapy has limited role in the management of gallbladder cancer. Thus, the status of gallbladder cancers over the last century has not shown any definitive improvement in overall survival and continues to be plagued by the presence of advanced disease at diagnosis. This is directly related to the continued lack of sensitive screening modalities for the detection of early disease. The future, therefore, for improved success in the management of this disease may have to be directed towards the development of sensitive and specific screening strategies with relevant improved molecular understanding of the underlying pathogenesis of this "orphan disease."

Conflict of Interests

The authors declare that there is no conflict of interests regarding the publication of this paper.

References

[1] C. H. E. Lai and W. Y. Lau, "Gallbladder cancer—a comprehensive review," *Surgeon*, vol. 6, no. 2, pp. 101–110, 2008.

[2] A. X. Zhu, T. S. Hong, A. F. Hezel, and D. A. Kooby, "Current management of gallbladder carcinoma," *The Oncologist*, vol. 15, no. 2, pp. 168–181, 2010.

[3] U. Dutta, "Gallbladder cancer: can newer insights improve the outcome?" *Journal of Gastroenterology and Hepatology*, vol. 27, no. 4, pp. 642–653, 2012.

[4] C. Ramos-Font, M. Gómez-Rio, A. Rodríguez-Fernández, A. Jiménez-Heffernan, R. S. Sánchez, and J. M. Llamas-Elvira, "Ability of FDG-PET/CT in the detection of gallbladder cancer," *Journal of Surgical Oncology*, vol. 109, no. 3, pp. 218–224, 2014.

[5] Gallbladder Cancer, American Cancer Society, 2015, http://www.cancer.org/acs/groups/cid/documents/webcontent/003101-pdf.pdf.

[6] G. Miller and W. R. Jarnagin, "Gallbladder carcinoma," *European Journal of Surgical Oncology*, vol. 34, no. 3, pp. 306–312, 2008.

[7] R. Hundal and E. A. Shaffer, "Gallbladder cancer: epidemiology and outcome," *Clinical Epidemiology*, vol. 6, no. 1, pp. 99–109, 2014.

[8] S. P. Kaushik, "Current perspectives in gallbladder carcinoma," *Journal of Gastroenterology and Hepatology*, vol. 16, no. 8, pp. 848–854, 2001.

[9] T. Rustagi and C. A. Dasanu, "Risk factors for gallbladder cancer and cholangiocarcinoma: similarities, differences and updates," *Journal of Gastrointestinal Cancer*, vol. 43, no. 2, pp. 137–147, 2012.

[10] A. Vijayakumar, A. Vijayakumar, V. Patil, M. N. Mallikarjuna, and B. S. Shivaswamy, "Early diagnosis of gallbladder carcinoma: an algorithm approach," *ISRN Radiology*, vol. 2013, Article ID 239424, 6 pages, 2013.

[11] D. Hariharan, A. Saied, and H. M. Kocher, "Analysis of mortality rates for gallbladder cancer across the world," *HPB*, vol. 10, no. 5, pp. 327–331, 2008.

[12] A. Cariati, E. Piromalli, and F. Cetta, "Gallbladder cancers: associated conditions, histological types, prognosis, and prevention," *European Journal of Gastroenterology and Hepatology*, vol. 26, no. 5, pp. 562–569, 2014.

[13] K. Y. Wolin, K. Carson, and G. A. Colditz, "Obesity and cancer," *The Oncologist*, vol. 15, no. 6, pp. 556–565, 2010.

[14] C. Seretis, E. Lagoudianakis, G. Gemenetzis, F. Seretis, A. Pappas, and S. Gourgiotis, "Metaplastic changes in chronic cholecystitis: implications for early diagnosis and surgical intervention to prevent the gallbladder metaplasia-dysplasia-carcinoma sequence," *Journal of Clinical Medicine Research*, vol. 6, no. 1, pp. 26–29, 2014.

[15] R. Wiles, M. Varadpande, S. Muly, and J. Webb, "Growth rate and malignant potential of small gallbladder polyps—systematic review of evidence," *Surgeon*, vol. 12, no. 4, pp. 221–226, 2014.

[16] G. Donald, D. Sunjaya, T. Donahue, and O. Joe Hines, "Polyp on ultrasound: now what? the association between gallbladder polyps and cancer," *The American Surgeon*, vol. 79, no. 10, pp. 1005–1008, 2013.

[17] A. Maydeo and V. Dhir, "The gallbladder polyp conundrum: a riddler on the wall," *Gastrointestinal Endoscopy*, vol. 78, no. 3, pp. 494–495, 2013.

[18] Å. Andrén-Sandberg and Y. Deng, "Aspects on gallbladder cancer in 2014," *Current Opinion in Gastroenterology*, vol. 30, no. 3, pp. 326–331, 2014.

[19] S. Basu, M. K. Singh, T. B. Singh, S. K. Bhartiya, S. P. Singh, and V. K. Shukla, "Heavy and trace metals in carcinoma of the gallbladder," *World Journal of Surgery*, vol. 37, no. 11, pp. 2641–2646, 2013.

[20] K. S. Lim, C. C. Peters, A. Kow, and C. H. Tan, "The varying faces of gall bladder carcinoma: pictorial essay," *Acta Radiologica*, vol. 53, no. 5, pp. 494–500, 2012.

[21] K. Yoshimitsu, Y. Nishihara, D. Okamoto et al., "Magnetic resonance differentiation between T2 and T1 gallbladder carcinoma: significance of subserosal enhancement on the delayed phase dynamic study," *Magnetic Resonance Imaging*, vol. 30, no. 6, pp. 854–859, 2012.

[22] T. Wakai, Y. Shirai, J. Sakata, M. Nagahashi, Y. Ajioka, and K. Hatakeyama, "Mode of hepatic spread from gallbladder carcinoma: an immunohistochemical analysis of 42 hepatectomized specimens," *The American Journal of Surgical Pathology*, vol. 34, no. 1, pp. 65–74, 2010.

[23] S. K. Maurya, M. Tewari, R. R. Mishra, and H. S. Shukla, "Genetic aberrations in gallbladder cancer," *Surgical Oncology*, vol. 21, no. 1, pp. 37–43, 2012.

[24] I. Roa, X. de Aretxabala, J. C. Araya, and J. Roa, "Preneoplastic lesions in gallbladder cancer," *Journal of Surgical Oncology*, vol. 93, no. 8, pp. 615–623, 2006.

[25] N. R. Hughes and P. S. Bhathal, "Adenocarcinoma of gallbladder: an immunohistochemical profile and comparison with cholangiocarcinoma," *Journal of Clinical Pathology*, vol. 66, no. 3, pp. 212–217, 2013.

[26] R. D. Goldin and J. C. Roa, "Gallbladder cancer: a morphological and molecular update," *Histopathology*, vol. 55, no. 2, pp. 218–229, 2009.

[27] L. Solaini, A. Sharma, J. Watt, S. Iosifidou, J.-A. Chin Aleong, and H. M. Kocher, "Predictive factors for incidental gallbladder dysplasia and carcinoma," *Journal of Surgical Research*, vol. 189, no. 1, pp. 17–21, 2014.

[28] R. Kanthan, J.-L. Senger, and S. C. Kanthan, "Molecular events in primary and metastatic colorectal carcinoma: a review," *Pathology Research International*, vol. 2012, Article ID 597497, 14 pages, 2012.

[29] T. Kuroki, Y. Tajima, K. Matsuo, and T. Kanematsu, "Genetic alterations in gallbladder carcinoma," *Surgery Today*, vol. 35, no. 2, pp. 101–105, 2005.

[30] M. Li, Z. Zhang, X. Li et al., "Whole-exome and targeted gene sequencing of gallbladder carcinoma identifies recurrent mutations in the ErbB pathway," *Nature Genetics*, vol. 46, no. 8, pp. 872–876, 2014.

[31] N. Kumari, V. K. Kapoor, N. Krishnani, K. Kumar, and D. K. Baitha, "Role of c-erbB2 expression in gallbladder cancer," *Indian Journal of Pathology and Microbiology*, vol. 55, no. 1, pp. 75–79, 2012.

[32] S.-N. Wang, S.-C. Chung, K.-B. Tsai et al., "Aberrant p53 expression and the development of gallbladder carcinoma and adenoma," *Kaohsiung Journal of Medical Sciences*, vol. 22, no. 2, pp. 53–59, 2006.

[33] H.-B. Ma, H.-T. Hu, Z.-L. Di et al., "Association of cyclin D1, p16 and retinoblastoma protein expressions with prognosis and metastasis of gallbladder carcinoma," *World Journal of Gastroenterology*, vol. 11, no. 5, pp. 744–747, 2005.

[34] Z. Yang, Z. Yang, L. Xiong et al., "Expression of VHL and HIF-1α and their clinicopathologic significance in benign and malignant lesions of the gallbladder," *Applied Immunohistochemistry and Molecular Morphology*, vol. 19, no. 6, pp. 534–539, 2011.

[35] S. Yi, Z.-L. Yang, X. Miao et al., "N-cadherin and P-cadherin are biomarkers for invasion, metastasis, and poor prognosis of gallbladder carcinomas," *Pathology Research and Practice*, vol. 210, no. 6, pp. 363–368, 2014.

[36] M. Ghosh, H. Kamma, T. Kawamoto et al., "MUC1 core protein as a marker of gallbladder malignancy," *European Journal of Surgical Oncology*, vol. 31, no. 8, pp. 891–896, 2005.

[37] P. Letelier, P. Garcia, P. Leal et al., "Immunohistochemical expression of vascular endothelial growth factor a in advanced gallbladder carcinoma," *Applied Immunohistochemistry and Molecular Morphology*, vol. 22, no. 7, pp. 530–536, 2014.

[38] M. Tewari, A. Agarwal, R. R. Mishra, R. N. Meena, and H. S. Shukla, "Epigenetic changes in carcinogenesis of gallbladder," *Indian Journal of Surgical Oncology*, vol. 4, no. 4, pp. 356–361, 2013.

[39] M. G. House, I. I. Wistuba, P. Argani et al., "Progression of gene hypermethylation in gallstone disease leading to gallbladder cancer," *Annals of Surgical Oncology*, vol. 10, no. 8, pp. 882–889, 2003.

[40] A. P. Moy, M. Shahid, C. R. Ferrone et al., "Microsatellite instability in gallbladder carcinoma," *Virchows Archiv*, vol. 466, pp. 393–402, 2015.

[41] K. Wu, M. Liao, B. Liu, and Z. Deng, "ADAM-17 over-expression in gallbladder carcinoma correlates with poor prognosis of patients," *Medical Oncology*, vol. 28, no. 2, pp. 475–480, 2011.

[42] Å. Andrén-Sandberg, "Molecular biology of gallbladder cancer: potential clinical implications," *North American Journal of Medical Sciences*, vol. 4, no. 10, pp. 435–441, 2012.

[43] Q. Zou, L. Xiong, Z. Yang, F. Lv, L. Yang, and X. Miao, "Expression levels of HMGA2 and CD9 and its clinicopathological significances in the benign and malignant lesions of the gallbladder," *World Journal of Surgical Oncology*, vol. 10, article 92, 2012.

[44] J. E. Nevin, T. H. Moran, S. Kay, and R. King, "Carcinoma of gallbladder," *Cancer*, vol. 37, no. 1, pp. 141–148, 1976.

[45] H. Onoyama, M. Yamamoto, A. Tseng, T. Ajiki, and Y. Saitoh, "Extended cholecystectomy for carcinoma of the gallbladder," *World Journal of Surgery*, vol. 19, no. 5, pp. 758–763, 1995.

[46] AJCC, "Gallbladder," in *AJCC Cancer Staging Manual*, S. B. Edge, D. R. Byrd, C. C. Compton et al., Eds., pp. 211–217, Springer, New York, NY, USA, 7th edition, 2010.

[47] K. Jin, H. Lan, T. Zhu, K. He, and L. Teng, "Gallbladder carcinoma incidentally encountered during laparoscopic cholecystectomy: how to deal with it," *Clinical and Translational Oncology*, vol. 13, no. 1, pp. 25–33, 2011.

[48] S. R. Grobmyer, M. D. Lieberman, and J. M. Daly, "Gallbladder cancer in the twentieth century: single institution's experience," *World Journal of Surgery*, vol. 28, no. 1, pp. 47–49, 2004.

[49] K. Inui, J. Yoshino, and H. Miyoshi, "Diagnosis of gallbladder tumors," *Internal Medicine*, vol. 50, no. 11, pp. 1133–1136, 2011.

[50] W.-B. Choi, S.-K. Lee, M.-H. Kim et al., "A new strategy to predict the neoplastic polyps of the gallbladder based on a scoring system using EUS," *Gastrointestinal Endoscopy*, vol. 52, no. 3, pp. 372–379, 2000.

[51] J.-H. Choi, D.-W. Seo, J. H. Choi et al., "Utility of contrast-enhanced harmonic EUS in the diagnosis of malignant gallbladder polyps (with videos)," *Gastrointestinal Endoscopy*, vol. 78, no. 3, pp. 484–493, 2013.

[52] S. C. Mayo, A. D. Shore, H. Nathan et al., "National trends in the management and survival of surgically managed gallbladder adenocarcinoma over 15 years: a population-based analysis," *Journal of Gastrointestinal Surgery*, vol. 14, no. 10, pp. 1578–1591, 2010.

[53] S. D. Deshmukh, P. T. Johnson, S. Sheth, R. Hruban, and E. K. Fishman, "CT of gallbladder cancer and its mimics: a pattern-based approach," *Abdominal Imaging*, vol. 38, no. 3, pp. 527–536, 2013.

[54] S. J. Kim, J. M. Lee, E. S. Lee, J. K. Han, and B. I. Choi, "Preoperative staging of gallbladder carcinoma using biliary MR imaging," *Journal of Magnetic Resonance Imaging*, vol. 41, no. 2, pp. 314–321, 2015.

[55] N. K. Lee, S. Kim, T. U. Kim, D. U. Kim, H. I. Seo, and T. Y. Jeon, "Diffusion-weighted MRI for differentiation of benign from malignant lesions in the gallbladder," *Clinical Radiology*, vol. 69, no. 2, pp. e78–e85, 2014.

[56] S. J. Kim, J. M. Lee, H. Kim, J. H. Yoon, J. K. Han, and B. I. Choi, "Role of diffusion-weighted magnetic resonance imaging in the diagnosis of gallbladder cancer," *Journal of Magnetic Resonance Imaging*, vol. 38, no. 1, pp. 127–137, 2013.

[57] Q. Ke, Z. L. He, X. Duan, and S. S. Zheng, "Chronic cholecystitis with hilar bile duct stricture mimicking gallbladder carcinoma on positron emission tomography: a case report," *Molecular and Clinical Oncology*, vol. 1, no. 3, pp. 517–520, 2013.

[58] R. Yadav, D. Jain, S. R. Mathur, A. Sharma, and V. K. Iyer, "Gallbladder carcinoma: an attempt of WHO histological classification on fine needle aspiration material," *CytoJournal*, vol. 10, article 12, 2013.

[59] M.-J. Kim, K. W. Kim, H.-C. Kim et al., "Unusual malignant tumors of the gallbladder," *American Journal of Roentgenology*, vol. 187, no. 2, pp. 473–480, 2006.

[60] T. H. Giang, T. T. B. Ngoc, and L. A. Hassell, "Carcinoma involving the gallbladder: a retrospective review of 23 cases—pitfalls in diagnosis of gallbladder carcinoma," *Diagnostic Pathology*, vol. 7, article 10, 2012.

[61] H. Kijima, Y. Wu, T. Yosizawa et al., "Pathological characteristics of early to advanced gallbladder carcinoma and extrahepatic cholangiocarcinoma," *Journal of Hepato-Biliary-Pancreatic Sciences*, vol. 21, no. 7, pp. 453–458, 2014.

[62] J. Albores-Saavedra, M. Tuck, B. K. McLaren, K. S. Carrick, and D. E. Henson, "Papillary carcinomas of the gallbladder: analysis of noninvasive and invasive types," *Archives of Pathology and Laboratory Medicine*, vol. 129, no. 7, pp. 905–909, 2005.

[63] N. Dursun, O. T. Escalona, J. C. Roa et al., "Mucinous carcinomas of the gallbladder. Clinicopathologic analysis of 15 cases identified in 606 carcinomas," *Archives of Pathology and Laboratory Medicine*, vol. 136, no. 11, pp. 1347–1358, 2012.

[64] J. C. Roa, O. Tapia, A. Cakir et al., "Squamous cell and adenosquamous carcinomas of the gallbladder: clinicopathological analysis of 34 cases identified in 606 carcinomas," *Modern Pathology*, vol. 24, no. 8, pp. 1069–1078, 2011.

[65] Y. Oohashi, Y. Shirai, T. Wakai, S. Nagakura, H. Watanabe, and K. Hatakeyama, "Adenosquamous carcinoma of the gallbladder warrants resection only if curative resection is feasible," *Cancer*, vol. 94, no. 11, pp. 3000–3005, 2002.

[66] J. Albores-Saavedra, D. E. Henson, D. Moran-Portela, and S. Lino-Silva, "Cribriform carcinoma of the gallbladder: a clinicopathologic study of 7 cases," *American Journal of Surgical Pathology*, vol. 32, no. 11, pp. 1694–1698, 2008.

[67] S. Ellouze, C. Slim, G. Ahmad et al., "Hepatoid adenocarcinoma of the gallbladder," *World Journal of Surgical Oncology*, vol. 9, article 103, 2011.

[68] A. Bittinger, I. Altekruger, P. Barth, and L. A. Murakata, "Clear cell carcinoma of the gallbladder. A histological and immunohistochemical study," *Pathology Research and Practice*, vol. 191, no. 12, pp. 1259–1266, 1995.

[69] H. Eken, M. G. Balci, S. Buyukakincak, A. Isik, D. Firat, and O. Cimen, "Rare tumors of the gallbladder: clear cell carcinoma," *International Journal of Surgery Case Reports*, vol. 9, pp. 65–68, 2015.

[70] A. Manouras, M. Genetzakis, E. E. Lagoudianakis et al., "Undifferentiated giant cell type carcinoma of the gallbladder with sarcomatoid dedifferentiation: a case report and review of the literature," *Journal of Medical Case Reports*, vol. 3, article 6496, 2009.

[71] K. B. Badmos, L. Salah Seada, F. Fahad Al Rashid, and H. A. Oreiby, "Undifferentiated spindle-cell carcinoma of the gallbladder: a report of a case, an immunohistochemistry profile, and a review of the literature," *Case Reports in Pathology*, vol. 2013, Article ID 267194, 3 pages, 2013.

[72] E. A. Husain, R. J. Prescott, S. A. Haider et al., "Gallbladder sarcoma: a clinicopathological study of seven cases from the UK and Austria with emphasis on morphological subtypes," *Digestive Diseases and Sciences*, vol. 54, no. 2, pp. 395–400, 2009.

[73] H.-H. Kim, Y.-H. Hur, E.-H. Jeong et al., "Carcinosarcoma of the gallbladder: report of two cases," *Surgery Today*, vol. 42, no. 7, pp. 670–675, 2012.

[74] K. M. Eltawil, B. I. Gustafsson, M. Kidd, and I. M. Modlin, "Neuroendocrine tumors of the gallbladder: an evaluation and reassessment of management strategy," *Journal of Clinical Gastroenterology*, vol. 44, no. 10, pp. 687–695, 2010.

[75] S. Iype, T. A. Mirza, D. J. Propper, S. Bhattacharya, R. M. Feakins, and H. M. Kocher, "Neuroendocrine tumours of the gallbladder: three cases and a review of the literature," *Postgraduate Medical Journal*, vol. 85, no. 1002, pp. 213–218, 2009.

[76] V. Anjaneyulu, G. Shankar-Swarnalatha, and S. C.-S. Rao, "Carcinoid tumor of the gall bladder," *Annals of Diagnostic Pathology*, vol. 11, no. 2, pp. 113–116, 2007.

[77] Y.-P. Zou, W.-M. Li, H.-R. Liu, and N. Li, "Primary carcinoid tumor of the gallbladder: a case report and brief review of the

literature," *World Journal of Surgical Oncology*, vol. 8, article 12, 2010.

[78] J. Albores-Saavedra, K. Batich, S. Hossain, D. E. Henson, and A. M. Schwartz, "Carcinoid tumors and small-cell carcinomas of the gallbladder and extrahepatic bile ducts: a comparative study based on 221 cases from the Surveillance, Epidemiology, and End Results Program," *Annals of Diagnostic Pathology*, vol. 13, no. 6, pp. 378–383, 2009.

[79] D.-M. Kim, S.-O. Yang, H. Y. Han, K. S. Kim, and H. J. Son, "Small cell carcinoma of the gallbladder: 18F-FDG PET/CT imaging features—a case report," *Nuclear Medicine and Molecular Imaging*, vol. 44, no. 3, pp. 213–216, 2010.

[80] N. O. Uribe-Uribe, A. M. Jimenez-Garduño, D. E. Henson, and J. Albores-Saavedra, "Paraneoplastic sensory neuropathy associated with small cell carcinoma of the gallbladder," *Annals of Diagnostic Pathology*, vol. 13, no. 2, pp. 124–126, 2009.

[81] A. Mahipal and S. Gupta, "Small-cell carcinoma of the gallbladder: report of a case and literature review," *Case Reports in GI Oncology*, vol. 4, no. 4, pp. 135–136, 2011.

[82] H. Taniguchi, J. Sakagami, N. Suzuki et al., "Adenoendocrine cell carcinoma of the gallbladder clinically mimicking squamous cell carcinoma," *International Journal of Clinical Oncology*, vol. 14, no. 2, pp. 167–170, 2009.

[83] J. Sakata, Y. Shirai, T. Wakai, Y. Ajioka, and K. Hatakeyama, "Number of positive lymph nodes independently determines the prognosis after resection in patients with gallbladder carcinoma," *Annals of Surgical Oncology*, vol. 17, no. 7, pp. 1831–1840, 2010.

[84] C. Pilgrim, V. Usatoff, and P. M. Evans, "A review of the surgical strategies for the management of gallbladder carcinoma based on T stage and growth type of the tumour," *European Journal of Surgical Oncology*, vol. 35, no. 9, pp. 903–907, 2009.

[85] D. Fuks, J.-M. Regimbeau, P. Pessaux et al., "Is port-site resection necessary in the surgical management of gallbladder cancer?" *Journal of Visceral Surgery*, vol. 150, no. 4, pp. 277–284, 2013.

[86] X. Yi, X. Long, H. Zai, D. Xiao, W. Li, and Y. Li, "Unsuspected gallbladder carcinoma discovered during or after cholecystectomy: focus on appropriate radical re-resection according to the T-stage," *Clinical and Translational Oncology*, vol. 15, no. 8, pp. 652–658, 2013.

[87] L. Hu, B. Wang, X. Liu, and Y. Lv, "Unsuspected gallbladder cancer: a clinical retrospective study," *Archives of Iranian Medicine*, vol. 16, no. 11, pp. 631–635, 2013.

[88] M. D'Hondt, R. Lapointe, Z. Benamira et al., "Carcinoma of the gallbladder: patterns of presentation, prognostic factors and survival rate. An 11-year single centre experience," *European Journal of Surgical Oncology*, vol. 39, no. 6, pp. 548–553, 2013.

[89] J. C. Roa, O. Tapia, C. Manterola et al., "Early gallbladder carcinoma has a favorable outcome but Rokitansky-Aschoff sinus involvement is an adverse prognostic factor," *Virchows Archiv*, vol. 463, pp. 651–661, 2013.

[90] D. M. Hari, J. H. Howard, A. M. Leung, C. G. Chui, M.-S. Sim, and A. J. Bilchik, "A 21-year analysis of stage I gallbladder carcinoma: is cholecystectomy alone adequate?" *HPB*, vol. 15, no. 1, pp. 40–48, 2013.

[91] D. D. You, H. G. Lee, K. Y. Paik, J. S. Heo, S. H. Choi, and D. W. Choi, "What is an adequate extent of resection for T1 gallbladder cancers?" *Annals of Surgery*, vol. 247, no. 5, pp. 835–838, 2008.

[92] Y. Murakami, K. Uemura, T. Sudo et al., "Prognostic factors of patients with advanced gallbladder carcinoma following aggressive surgical resection," *Journal of Gastrointestinal Surgery*, vol. 15, no. 6, pp. 1007–1016, 2011.

[93] H. Nishio, M. Nagino, T. Ebata, Y. Yokoyama, T. Igami, and Y. Nimura, "Aggressive surgery for stage IV gallbladder carcinoma; what are the contraindications?" *Journal of Hepato-Biliary-Pancreatic Surgery*, vol. 14, no. 4, pp. 351–357, 2007.

[94] T. Takada, H. Amano, H. Yasuda et al., "Is postoperative adjuvant chemotherapy useful for gallbladder carcinoma? A phase III multicenter prospective randomized controlled trial in patients with resected pancreaticobiliary carcinoma," *Cancer*, vol. 95, no. 8, pp. 1685–1695, 2002.

[95] A. M. Horgan, E. Amir, T. Walter, and J. J. Knox, "Adjuvant therapy in the treatment of biliary tract cancer: a systematic review and meta-analysis," *Journal of Clinical Oncology*, vol. 30, no. 16, pp. 1934–1940, 2012.

[96] S. J. Wang, A. Lemieux, J. Kalpathy-Cramer et al., "Nomogram for predicting the benefit of adjuvant chemoradiotherapy for resected gallbladder cancer," *Journal of Clinical Oncology*, vol. 29, no. 35, pp. 4627–4632, 2011.

[97] F. Eckel, T. Brunner, and S. Jelic, "Biliary cancer: ESMO clinical practice guidelines for diagnosis, treatment and follow-up," *Annals of Oncology*, vol. 22, supplement 6, pp. vi40–vi44, 2011.

[98] Capecitabine or Observation after Surgery in Treating Patients with Biliary Tract Cancer, 2015, http://clinicaltrials.gov/show/NCT00363584.

[99] Gemcitabine Hydrochloride and Oxaliplatin or Observation in Treating Patients With Biliary Tract Cancer That Has Been Removed by Surgery, 2015, http://clinicaltrials.gov/ct2/show/NCT01313377?term=NCT01313377&rank=1.

[100] Adjuvant Chemotherapy With Gemcitabine and Cisplatin Compared to Observation After Curative Intent Resection of Biliary Tract Cancer (ACTICCA-1), 2015, https://clinicaltrials.gov/ct2/show/NCT02170090?term=ACTICCA&rank=1.

[101] M. A. Ben-David, K. A. Griffith, E. Abu-Isa et al., "External-beam radiotherapy for localized extrahepatic cholangiocarcinoma," *International Journal of Radiation Oncology Biology Physics*, vol. 66, no. 3, pp. 772–779, 2006.

[102] M. L. Foo, L. L. Gunderson, C. E. Bender, and S. J. Buskirk, "External radiation therapy and transcatheter iridium in the treatment of extrahepatic bile duct carcinoma," *International Journal of Radiation Oncology Biology Physics*, vol. 39, no. 4, pp. 929–935, 1997.

[103] A. R. Sasson, J. P. Hoffman, E. Ross et al., "Trimodality therapy for advanced gallbladder cancer," *American Surgeon*, vol. 67, no. 3, pp. 277–283, 2001.

[104] National Comprehensive Cancer Network (NCCN), "NCCN clinical practice guidelines in oncology," 2014, http://www.nccn.org/professionals/physician_gls/f_guidelines.asp.

[105] A. Sharma, A. D. Dwary, B. K. Mohanti et al., "Best supportive care compared with chemotherapy for unresectable gall bladder cancer: a randomized controlled study," *Journal of Clinical Oncology*, vol. 28, no. 30, pp. 4581–4586, 2010.

[106] D. C. Doval, J. S. Sekhon, S. K. Gupta et al., "A phase II study of gemcitabine and cisplatin in chemotherapy-naive, unresectable gall bladder cancer," *British Journal of Cancer*, vol. 90, no. 8, pp. 1516–1520, 2004.

[107] J. O. Gallardo, B. Rubio, M. Fodor et al., "A phase II study of gemcitabine in gallbladder carcinoma," *Annals of Oncology*, vol. 12, no. 10, pp. 1403–1406, 2001.

[108] J. Reyes-Vidal, J. Gallardo, E. Yáñez et al., "Gemcitabine: gemcitabine and cisplatin in the treatment of patients with unresectable or metastatic gallbladder cancer: results of the phase II GOCCHI study 2000-13," *Journal of Clinical Oncology*, vol. 22, abstract 1095, p. 273, 2003.

[109] F. Eckel and R. M. Schmid, "Chemotherapy in advanced biliary tract carcinoma: a pooled analysis of clinical trials," *British Journal of Cancer*, vol. 96, no. 6, pp. 896–902, 2007.

[110] M. Kajanti and S. Pyrhönen, "Epirubicin-sequential methotrexate-5-fluorouracil-leucovorin treatment in advanced cancer of the extrahepatic biliary system. A phase II study," *American Journal of Clinical Oncology*, vol. 17, article 223, 1994.

[111] J. H. Harvey, F. P. Smith, and P. S. Schein, "5-fluorouracil, mitomycin, and doxorubicin (FAM) in carcinoma of the biliary tract," *Journal of Clinical Oncology*, vol. 2, no. 11, pp. 1245–1248, 1984.

[112] G. Falkson, J. M. MacIntyre, and C. G. Moertel, "Eastern Cooperative Oncology Group experience with chemotherapy for inoperable gallbladder and bile duct cancer," *Cancer*, vol. 54, no. 6, pp. 965–969, 1984.

[113] S. R. Alberts, H. Al-Khatib, M. R. Mahoney et al., "Gemcitabine, 5-fluorouracil, and leucovorin in advanced biliary tract and gallbladder carcinoma: a north central cancer treatment group phase II trial," *Cancer*, vol. 103, no. 1, pp. 111–118, 2005.

[114] M. Ducreux, P. Rougier, A. Fandi et al., "Effective treatment of advanced biliary tract carcinoma using 5-fluorouracil continuous infusion with cisplatin," *Annals of Oncology*, vol. 9, no. 6, pp. 653–656, 1998.

[115] J.-S. Chen, Y.-Y. Jan, Y.-C. Lin, H.-M. Wang, W.-C. Chang, and C.-T. Liau, "Weekly 24 h infusion of high-dose 5-fluorouracil and leucovorin in patients with biliary tract carcinomas," *Anti-Cancer Drugs*, vol. 9, no. 5, pp. 393–397, 1998.

[116] P. A. Ellis, A. Norman, A. Hill et al., "Epirubicin, cisplatin and infusional 5-fluorouracil (5-FU) (ECF) in hepatobiliary tumours," *European Journal of Cancer*, vol. 31, no. 10, pp. 1594–1598, 1995.

[117] J. Y. Cho, Y. H. Paik, Y. S. Chang et al., "Capecitabine combined with gemcitabine (CapGem) as first-line treatment in patients with advanced/metastatic biliary tract carcinoma," *Cancer*, vol. 104, no. 12, pp. 2753–2758, 2005.

[118] J. J. Knox, D. Hedley, A. Oza et al., "Combining gemcitabine and capecitabine in patients with advanced biliary cancer: a phase II trial," *Journal of Clinical Oncology*, vol. 23, no. 10, pp. 2332–2338, 2005.

[119] Y. Z. Patt, M. M. Hassan, A. Aguayo et al., "Oral capecitabine for the treatment of hepatocellular carcinoma, cholangiocarcinoma, and gallbladder carcinoma," *Cancer*, vol. 101, no. 3, pp. 578–586, 2004.

[120] O. Nehls, H. Oettle, J. T. Hartmann et al., "Capecitabine plus oxaliplatin as first-line treatment in patients with advanced biliary system adenocarcinoma: a prospective multicentre phase II trial," *British Journal of Cancer*, vol. 98, no. 2, pp. 309–315, 2008.

[121] T. W. Kim, H. M. Chang, H. J. Kang et al., "Phase II study of capecitabine plus cisplatin as first-line chemotherapy in advanced biliary cancer," *Annals of Oncology*, vol. 14, no. 7, pp. 1115–1120, 2003.

[122] M. Penz, G. V. Kornek, M. Raderer et al., "Phase II trial of two-weekly gemcitabine in patients with advanced biliary tract cancer," *Annals of Oncology*, vol. 12, no. 2, pp. 183–186, 2001.

[123] A. D. Wagner, P. Buechner-Steudel, M. Moehler et al., "Gemcitabine, oxaliplatin and 5-FU in advanced bile duct and gallbladder carcinoma: two parallel, multicentre phase-II trials," *British Journal of Cancer*, vol. 101, no. 11, pp. 1846–1852, 2009.

[124] B. Mehrotra, S. Ahmed, and A. Bhargava, "Efficacy of gemcitabine in advanced unresectable biliary tract cancer," *Journal of Clinical Oncology*, vol. 22, no. 14, supplement, abstract 4259, p. 376, 2004.

[125] N. Tsavaris, C. Kosmas, P. Gouveris et al., "Weekly gemcitabine for the treatment of biliary tract and gallbladder cancer," *Investigational New Drugs*, vol. 22, no. 2, pp. 193–198, 2004.

[126] J. W. Valle, H. S. Wasan, D. H. Palmer et al., "Cisplatin plus gemcitabine versus gemcitabine for biliary tract cancer," *The New England Journal of Medicine*, vol. 362, no. 14, pp. 1273–1281, 2010.

[127] E. Suzuki, J. Furuse, M. Ikeda et al., "Treatment efficacy/safety and prognostic factors in patients with advanced biliary tract cancer receiving gemcitabine monotherapy: an analysis of 100 cases," *Oncology*, vol. 79, no. 1-2, pp. 39–45, 2010.

[128] J. A. Meyerhardt, A. X. Zhu, K. Stuart et al., "Phase-II study of gemcitabine and cisplatin in patients with metastatic biliary and gallbladder cancer," *Digestive Diseases and Sciences*, vol. 53, no. 2, pp. 564–570, 2008.

[129] S. Thongprasert, S. Napapan, C. Charoentum, and S. Moonprakan, "Phase II study of gemcitabine and cisplatin as first-line chemotherapy in inoperable biliary tract carcinoma," *Annals of Oncology*, vol. 16, no. 2, pp. 279–281, 2005.

[130] G.-W. Lee, J. H. Kang, H.-G. Kim, J.-S. Lee, J.-S. Lee, and J.-S. Jang, "Combination chemotherapy with gemcitabine and cisplatin as first-line treatment for immunohistochemically proven cholangiocarcinoma," *American Journal of Clinical Oncology: Cancer Clinical Trials*, vol. 29, no. 2, pp. 127–131, 2006.

[131] S. T. Kim, J. O. Park, J. Lee et al., "A Phase II study of gemcitabine and cisplatin in advanced biliary tract cancer," *Cancer*, vol. 106, no. 6, pp. 1339–1346, 2006.

[132] J. Harder, B. Riecken, O. Kummer et al., "Outpatient chemotherapy with gemcitabine and oxaliplatin in patients with biliary tract cancer," *British Journal of Cancer*, vol. 95, no. 7, pp. 848–852, 2006.

[133] T. André, C. Tournigand, O. Rosmorduc et al., "Gemcitabine combined with oxaliplatin (GEMOX) in advanced biliary tract adenocarcinoma: a GERCOR study," *Annals of Oncology*, vol. 15, no. 9, pp. 1339–1343, 2004.

[134] N. Gebbia, F. Verderame, R. Di Leo et al., "A phase II study of oxaliplatin (O) and gemcitabine (G) first line chemotherapy in patients with advanced biliary tract cancers," *Proceedings of the American Society of Clinical Oncology*, vol. 23, p. 4132, 2005.

[135] R. P. Riechelmann, C. A. Townsley, S. N. Chin, G. R. Pond, and J. J. Knox, "Expanded phase II trial of gemcitabine and capecitabine for advanced biliary cancer," *Cancer*, vol. 110, no. 6, pp. 1307–1312, 2007.

[136] R. V. Iyer, J. Gibbs, B. Kuvshinoff et al., "A phase II study of gemcitabine and capecitabine in advanced cholangiocarcinoma and carcinoma of the gallbladder: a single-institution prospective study," *Annals of Surgical Oncology*, vol. 14, no. 11, pp. 3202–3209, 2007.

[137] P. K. Julka, T. Puri, and G. K. Rath, "A phase II study of gemcitabine and carboplatin combination chemotherapy in gallbladder carcinoma," *Hepatobiliary & Pancreatic Diseases International*, vol. 5, no. 1, pp. 110–114, 2006.

[138] D. V. Jones Jr., R. Lozano, A. Hoque, A. Markowitz, and Y. Z. Patt, "Phase II study of paclitaxel therapy for unresectable biliary tree carcinomas," *Journal of Clinical Oncology*, vol. 14, no. 8, pp. 2306–2310, 1996.

[139] S. R. Alberts, J. R. Sande, N. R. Foster et al., "Pemetrexed and gemcitabine for biliary tract and gallbladder carcinomas: a North Central Cancer Treatment Group (NCCTG) phase I and II Trial, N9943," *Journal of Gastrointestinal Cancer*, vol. 38, no. 2–4, pp. 87–94, 2007.

[140] P. Papakostas, C. Kouroussis, N. Androulakis et al., "First-line chemotherapy with docetaxel for unresectable or metastatic carcinoma of the biliary tract. A multicentre phase II study," *European Journal of Cancer*, vol. 37, no. 15, pp. 1833–1838, 2001.

[141] P. M. Sanz-Altamira, E. O'Reilly, K. E. Stuart et al., "A phase II trial of irinotecan (CPT-11) for unresectable biliary tree carcinoma," *Annals of Oncology*, vol. 12, no. 4, pp. 501–504, 2001.

[142] A. Sancho, G. Lopez-Vivanco, I. D. de Concuera et al., "Oxaliplatin and capecitabine after gemcitabine failure in patients with advanced, pancreatic, biliary, and gallbladder adenocarcinoma," *Journal of Clinical Oncology*, vol. 26, no. 15, p. 665s, 2008.

[143] B. G. Müller, X. De Aretxabala, and M. G. Domingo, "A review of recent data in the treatment of gallbladder cancer: what we know, what we do, and what should be done," in *American Society of Clinical Oncology Educational Book*, vol. 34, pp. e165–e170, American Society of Clinical Oncology, Alexandria, Va, USA, 2014.

[144] A. F. Hezel, V. Deshpande, and A. X. Zhu, "Genetics of biliary tract cancers and emerging targeted therapies," *Journal of Clinical Oncology*, vol. 28, no. 21, pp. 3531–3540, 2010.

[145] A. B. El-Khoueiry, C. J. Rankin, E. Ben-Josef et al., "SWOG 0514: a phase II study of sorafenib in patients with unresectable or metastatic gallbladder carcinoma and cholangiocarcinoma," *Investigational New Drugs*, vol. 30, no. 4, pp. 1646–1651, 2012.

[146] J. H. Yi, S. Thongprasert, J. Lee et al., "A phase II study of sunitinib as a second-line treatment in advanced biliary tract carcinoma: a multicentre, multinational study," *European Journal of Cancer*, vol. 48, no. 2, pp. 196–201, 2012.

[147] R. K. Ramanathan, C. P. Belani, D. A. Singh et al., "A phase II study of lapatinib in patients with advanced biliary tree and hepatocellular cancer," *Cancer Chemotherapy and Pharmacology*, vol. 64, no. 4, pp. 777–783, 2009.

[148] J. Peck, L. Wei, M. Zalupski, B. O'Neil, M. Villalona Calero, and T. Bekaii-Saab, "HER2/neu may not be an interesting target in biliary cancers: results of an early phase II Study with Lapatinib," *Oncology*, vol. 82, no. 3, pp. 175–179, 2012.

[149] M. R. Costello, N. J. Meropol, C. S. Denlinger et al., "A phase II trial of the proteasome inhibitor bortezomib in patients with recurrent or metastatic adenocarcinoma of the bile duct or gallbladder (NCI #6135)," *Journal of Clinical Oncology*, vol. 27, supplement, abstract e15605, 2009, ASCO Annual Meeting.

[150] T. Bekaii-Saab, M. A. Phelps, X. Li et al., "Multi-institutional phase II study of selumetinib in patients with metastatic biliary cancers," *Journal of Clinical Oncology*, vol. 29, no. 17, pp. 2357–2363, 2011.

[151] S. J. Lubner, M. R. Mahoney, J. L. Kolesar et al., "Report of a multicenter phase II trial testing a combination of biweekly bevacizumab and daily erlotinib in patients with unresectable biliary cancer: a phase II consortium study," *Journal of Clinical Oncology*, vol. 28, no. 21, pp. 3491–3497, 2010.

[152] K. S. Rohrberg, R. K. Olesen, P. Pfeiffer et al., "Phase II trial of erlotinib and bevacizumab in patients with advanced upper gastrointestinal cancers," *Acta Oncologica*, vol. 51, no. 2, pp. 234–242, 2012.

[153] D. Malka, T. Trarbach, L. Fartoux et al., "A multicenter, randomized phase II trial of gemcitabine and oxaliplatin (GEMOX) alone or in combination with biweekly cetuximab in the first-line treatment of advanced biliary cancer: interim analysis of the BINGO trial," *Journal of Clinical Oncology*, vol. 27, no. 15, supplement, abstract 4520, 2009.

[154] B. Gruenberger, J. Schueller, U. Heubrandtner et al., "Cetuximab, gemcitabine, and oxaliplatin in patients with unresectable advanced or metastatic biliary tract cancer: a phase 2 study," *The Lancet Oncology*, vol. 11, no. 12, pp. 1142–1148, 2010.

[155] L. T. Chen, J. S. Chen, Y. Chao et al., "KRAS mutation status-stratified randomized phase II trial of GEMOX with and without cetuximab in advanced biliary tract cancer (ABTC): the TCOG T1210 trial," *Journal of Clinical Oncology*, vol. 31, supplement, abstract 4018, 2013.

[156] A. X. Zhu, J. A. Meyerhardt, L. S. Blaszkowsky et al., "Efficacy and safety of gemcitabine, oxaliplatin, and bevacizumab in advanced biliary-tract cancer and correlation of changes in 18-fluorodeoxyglucose PET with clinical outcome: a phase 2 study," *The Lancet Oncology*, vol. 11, no. 1, pp. 48–54, 2010.

[157] A. J. Ocean, P. Christos, J. A. Sparano et al., "Phase II trial of the ribonucleotide reductase inhibitor 3-aminopyridine-2-carboxaldehydethiosemicarbazone plus gemcitabine in patients with advanced biliary tract cancer," *Cancer Chemotherapy and Pharmacology*, vol. 68, no. 2, pp. 379–388, 2011.

[158] K. Schuette, E. Kettner, S. Al-Batran et al., "Preliminary results of a multicenter phase II study of imatinib and fluorourcail/leucovorin (FU/LV) in patients with unresectable or metastatic gallbladder or biliary tract cancer," *Journal of Clinical Oncology*, vol. 27, supplement, abstract e15622, 2009.

[159] J. Lee, S. H. Park, H.-M. Chang et al., "Gemcitabine and oxaliplatin with or without erlotinib in advanced biliary-tract cancer: a multicentre, open-label, randomised, phase 3 study," *The Lancet Oncology*, vol. 13, no. 2, pp. 181–188, 2012.

[160] S. Misra, A. Chaturvedi, N. C. Misra, and I. D. Sharma, "Carcinoma of the gallbladder," *The Lancet Oncology*, vol. 4, no. 3, pp. 167–176, 2003.

[161] L. M. Mazer, H. F. Losada, R. M. Chaudhry et al., "Tumour characteristics and survival analysis of incidental versus suspected gallbladder carcinoma," *Journal of Gastrointestinal Surgery*, vol. 16, no. 7, pp. 1311–1317, 2012.

[162] K.-I. Okada, H. Kijima, T. Imaizumi et al., "Wall-invasion pattern correlates with survival of patients with gallbladder adenocarcinoma," *Anticancer Research*, vol. 29, no. 2, pp. 685–692, 2009.

[163] G. Zhai, K. Yan, X. Ji et al., "LAPTM4B Allele *2 Is a Marker of Poor Prognosis for Gallbladder Carcinoma," *PLoS ONE*, vol. 7, no. 9, Article ID e45290, 2012.

[164] M. G. McNamara, C. Metran-Nascente, and J. J. Knox, "State-of-the-art in the management of locally advanced and metastatic gallbladder cancer," *Current Opinion in Oncology*, vol. 25, no. 4, pp. 425–431, 2013.

[165] R. Kanthan, J. M. Radhi, and S. C. Kanthan, "Gallbladder carcinomas: an immunoprognostic evaluation of P53, Bcl-2, CEA and alpha-fetoprotein," *Canadian Journal of Gastroenterology*, vol. 14, no. 3, pp. 181–184, 2000.

[166] S.-Y. Choi, Y. S. Jo, S.-M. Huang et al., "L1 cell adhesion molecule as a novel independent poor prognostic factor in gallbladder carcinoma," *Human Pathology*, vol. 42, no. 10, pp. 1476–1483, 2011.

[167] Y. Zhang, Y. Huang, and M. Qin, "Tumour-infiltrating FoxP3+ and IL-17-producing T cells affect the progression and prognosis of gallbladder carcinoma after surgery," *Scandinavian Journal of Immunology*, vol. 78, no. 6, pp. 516–522, 2013.

[168] S. Prince, A. Zeidman, Y. Dekel, E. Ram, and R. Koren, "Expression of epithelial cell adhesion molecule in gallbladder carcinoma and its correlation with clinicopathologic variables," *American Journal of Clinical Pathology*, vol. 129, no. 3, pp. 424–429, 2008.

[169] J. Li, Z.-L. Yang, X. Ren et al., "ACE2 and FZD1 are prognosis markers in squamous cell/adenosquamous carcinoma and adenocarcinoma of gallbladder," *Journal of Molecular Histology*, vol. 45, no. 1, pp. 47–57, 2014.

18

Does the Degree of Hepatocellular Carcinoma Tumor Necrosis following Transarterial Chemoembolization Impact Patient Survival?

Nathan Haywood,[1] **Kyle Gennaro,**[1] **John Obert,**[1] **Paul F. Sauer Jr.,**[1]
David T. Redden,[2] **Jessica Zarzour,**[3] **J. Kevin Smith,**[3] **David Bolus,**[3]
Souheil Saddekni,[3] **Ahmed Kamel Abdel Aal,**[3] **Stephen Gray,**[4] **Jared White,**[4]
Devin E. Eckhoff,[4] **and Derek A. DuBay**[4]

[1]*University of Alabama at Birmingham School of Medicine, Birmingham, AL 35233, USA*
[2]*Biostatistics Division, School of Public Health, University of Alabama at Birmingham, Birmingham, AL 35233, USA*
[3]*Department of Radiology, University of Alabama at Birmingham, Birmingham, AL 35233, USA*
[4]*Liver Transplant and Hepatobiliary Surgery, University of Alabama at Birmingham, Birmingham, AL 35233, USA*

Correspondence should be addressed to Derek A. DuBay; ddubay@uabmc.edu

Academic Editor: Kalpesh Jani

Purpose. The association between transarterial chemoembolization- (TACE-) induced HCC tumor necrosis measured by the modified Response Evaluation Criteria In Solid Tumors (mRECIST) and patient survival is poorly defined. We hypothesize that survival will be superior in HCC patients with increased TACE-induced tumor necrosis. *Materials and Methods*. TACE interventions were retrospectively reviewed. Tumor response was quantified via dichotomized (responders and nonresponders) and the four defined mRECIST categories. *Results*. Median survival following TACE was significantly greater in responders compared to nonresponders (20.8 months versus 14.9 months, $p = 0.011$). Survival outcomes also significantly varied among the four mRECIST categories ($p = 0.0003$): complete, 21.4 months; partial, 20.8; stable, 16.8; and progressive, 7.73. Only progressive disease demonstrated significantly worse survival when compared to complete response. Multivariable analysis showed that progressive disease, increasing total tumor diameter, and non-Child-Pugh class A were independent predictors of post-TACE mortality. *Conclusions*. Both dichotomized (responders and nonresponders) and the four defined mRECIST responses to TACE in patients with HCC were predictive of survival. The main driver of the survival analysis was poor survival in the progressive disease group. Surprisingly, there was small nonsignificant survival benefit between complete, partial, and stable disease groups. These findings may inform HCC treatment decisions following first TACE.

1. Introduction

Transarterial chemoembolization (TACE) is indicated for patients with hepatocellular carcinoma (HCC) who are not candidates for transplantation, resection, or ablation [1, 2]. TACE is the most common oncologic treatment for HCC patients with Medicare in the United States [3]. The Scientific Registry of Transplant Recipients (SRTR) shows that TACE is the most common bridging therapy for waitlisted liver transplant patients with HCC [3, 4]. The American Association for the Study of Liver Disease (AASLD) current HCC treatment recommendations state that "TACE is recommended as first line non-curative therapy for non-surgical patients with large/multifocal HCC who do not have vascular invasion or extrahepatic spread" [5, 6].

The goal of TACE is to induce HCC tumor necrosis via occlusion of tumor arterial blood flow along with local administration of cytotoxic chemotherapy [1]. Tumor necrosis is estimated via changes in HCC tumor arterial enhancement on post-TACE imaging, as quantified by the modified Response Evaluation Criteria In Solid Tumors (mRECIST) [7–9]. There are four categories of tumor response according to mRECIST: complete response, partial response, stable disease, or progressive disease [6, 8–10]. Studies have examined the correlation between post-TACE radiologic assessment and actual tumor necrosis on explant pathology [11–16]. However, relatively few studies have examined the correlation between radiologic evaluation of tumor necrosis and post-TACE survival [7, 8, 17].

A study by Memon et al. showed a correlation between radiologic evaluation of HCC tumor necrosis following locoregional therapies (including TACE and Y90) and overall survival in Child-Pugh classes A and B7 patients [17]. This study estimated HCC tumor necrosis via the European Association for the Study of Liver (EASL) response criteria [17]. A study by Kim et al. demonstrated that tumor response grading by mRECIST was predictive of overall survival in Child-Pugh classes A and B patients who underwent TACE for HCC [7]. Studies by Prajapati et al. and Gillmore et al. have also demonstrated that mRECIST response criteria are predictive of overall survival in HCC patients following TACE [18, 19]. However, in each of these analyses, patients were dichotomized into responders (complete and partial response mRECIST categories) or nonresponders (stable and progressive disease mRECIST categories) [7, 18, 19]. Few studies have shown that the 4 mRECIST categories are predictive of overall survival and in each case, the patient population was limited to only Child-Pugh class A or B patients [20–22]. Accordingly, there are two identified knowledge gaps in the literature regarding the impact of TACE-induced HCC necrosis and survival: the first is assessing patients with compromised liver disease (Child-Pugh class B8 or worse) and the second is to measure the difference between survival outcomes between each of the four mRECIST categories.

The purpose of this study was to measure the association between TACE-induced HCC tumor necrosis and survival in HCC patients with Child-Pugh class A, B, or C, measured by dichotomized (responder and nonresponder) and distinct (complete, partial, stable, and progressive) mRECIST categories. It is hypothesized that survival will be superior in HCC patients with increased TACE-induced tumor necrosis.

2. Methods

The research protocol for this study was approved by the UAB institutional review board. A retrospective chart review was performed for all patients receiving a TACE at UAB between January 2008 and April 2014. Methods presented here were adapted from previous studies [23].

2.1. Patient Population. Patients were diagnosed with HCC according to the AASLD criteria. The decision to offer TACE to patients with HCC was made by a multidisciplinary liver tumor board at UAB including medical oncologists, surgeons, hepatologists, and interventional radiologists. Patient candidacy for TACE was guided by established AASLD practice guidelines [5, 6]. One exception was the inclusion of highly selected Child-Pugh C candidates with single enhancing

peripheral HCC tumors felt to be "easy" TACE procedures by the interventional radiologists.

A list of consecutive patients treated with a first TACE was generated from the UAB Interventional Radiology procedures electronic database. TACE patients were excluded if they had non-HCC tumor type. Recurrent HCC following liver resection or transplantation also were excluded. In addition, HCC tumors that had previously been treated with another locoregional therapy such as radiofrequency ablation or external beam radiotherapy were excluded. Patients who received liver transplantation following TACE were censored at the time of transplant. Those who received multiple TACE procedures prior to assessing tumor response were excluded.

2.2. HCC Tumor Assessment and Post-TACE Tumor Necrosis Quantification

2.2.1. HCC Diagnosis. HCC is diagnosed according to AASLD criteria: when there is an arterially enhancing lesion with portal venous washout and/or pseudocapsule formation on delayed phase seen on multiphase contrast enhanced Computed Tomography (CT) or dynamic contrast enhanced Magnetic Resonance Imaging (MRI) of the liver [24, 25].

2.2.2. HCC Tumor Necrosis (Figure 1). Tumor response was assessed via the modified Response Evaluation Criteria in Solid Tumors (mRECIST). In 2008, the AASLD modified the National Cancer Institute RECIST criteria to unify assessment of radiographic response for hepatocellular carcinoma [8]. The modified RECIST criteria for tumor response are based on measurement of reduction in viable enhancing tumor in the arterial phase of dynamic CT or MRI imaging, rather than purely tumor shrinkage measured by the greatest diameter of the lesion. There are four categories of tumor response according to mRECIST: complete response, partial response, stable disease, or progressive disease [8]. Complete response is defined as the disappearance of tumor arterial enhancement. Partial response is defined as at least 30% decrease in the longest diameter of arterial enhancement. Stable disease is defined as a response that did not fall into the partial response or progressive disease category. Progressive disease is defined as growth of at least 20% of the sum of the longest diameter of the lesions. Electronic calipers were used to measure the longest diameter of arterial enhancement of the index lesion in the axial plane. Both MRI and CT imaging modalities were used to quantify HCC tumor necrosis. The tumor response used for statistical analysis was measured one month following initial TACE procedure for all patients included in this study.

2.3. TACE Protocol. The decision to offer TACE as locoregional oncologic therapy for patients with HCC was made at the UAB multidisciplinary liver tumor board. Over the course of this study, Lipiodol-based TACE was the most common approach initially, whereas most TACE procedures currently are performed with drug eluting beads (DEBS). Lipiodol-based TACE consisted of HCC embolization with a mixture of Lipiodol, 50 mg Doxorubicin, and 400 μm Embozene®

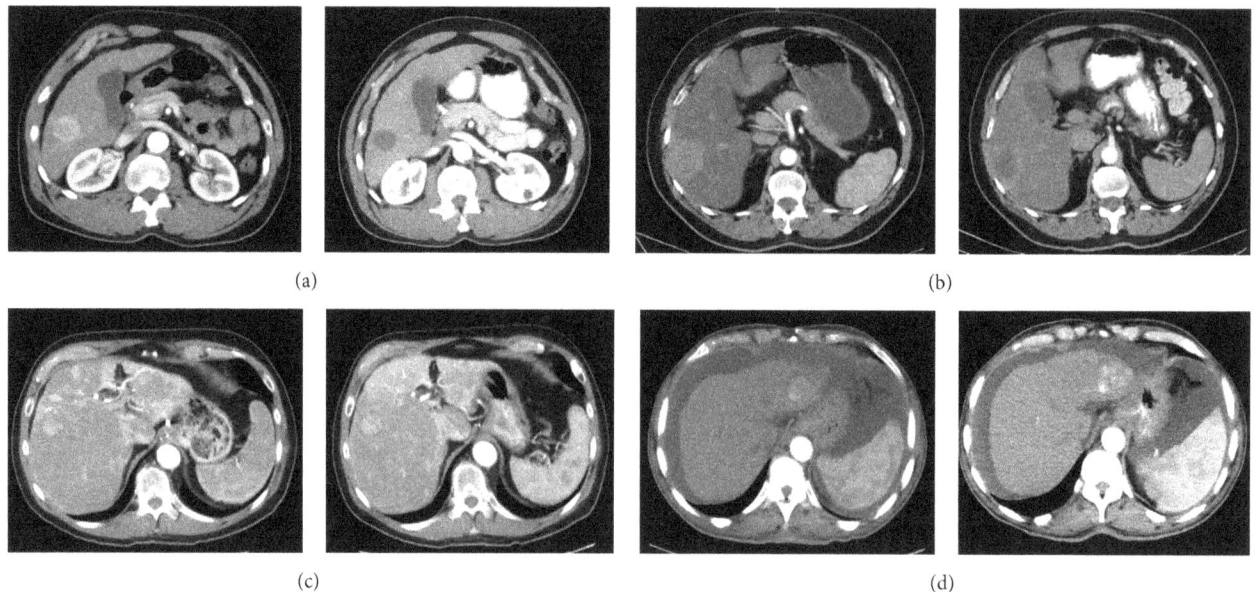

FIGURE 1: Axial CT images demonstrating the four mRECIST categories. (a) Complete: 100% HCC tumor necrosis. (b) Partial: 30%–99% HCC tumor necrosis. (c) Stable: between 29% HCC tumor necrosis and 20% HCC tumor growth. (d) Progressive: >20% HCC tumor growth.

microspheres (Celonova, USA). DEBS TACE consisted of either LC beads (Biocompatibles, UK) or QuadraSpheres® expanding microspheres (BioSphere Medical, France). These beads were eluted with 50 mg Doxorubicin. As a general strategy, selective targeted embolization was routinely done for focal lesions. In cases of multifocal disease, lesions larger than >2-3 cm were selectively targeted followed by lobar embolization if necessary.

2.4. Data Analysis. Patient demographics, clinical history, laboratory data, and cross sectional imaging characteristics were collected. Pre-TACE imaging CT and MRI variables include number of lesions, size of tumors, and sum of axial diameters of the 3 largest tumors in the case of multifocal HCC. Data collected from post-TACE CT and MRI imaging included HCC tumor necrosis measured according to mRECIST criteria [8]. To allow common statistical procedures, the analysis was restricted to examination of the index HCC tumor that was defined as the largest tumor (if more than one tumor per patient had been used in the analysis, the common assumption of independent data observations would have been violated). Analysis of Variance was used to compare means among mRECIST groups. The primary analytic approach for testing association between mRECIST and categorical variables utilized Chi-square analyses. Kaplan-Meier curves were constructed to evaluate patient survival. Survival probabilities were analyzed with the Wilcoxon test since it is more sensitive to detect differences at shorter survival times. Cox Proportional Hazard Regression was used for a multivariable adjusted analysis and to estimate survival curves adjusting for demographic and clinical baseline characteristics. For all inferences, the probability of a Type I error (α) was set to 0.05. All analyses were conducted using the SAS 9.4 (Cary, NC).

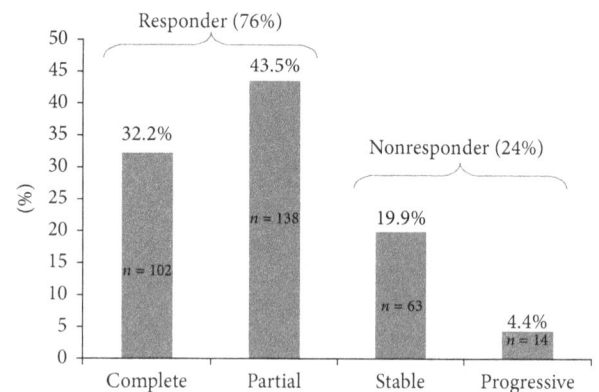

FIGURE 2: Distribution of HCC tumor necrosis following TACE as quantified by the mRECIST criteria.

3. Results

3.1. Patient Demographics. Between January 2008 and April 2014, 317 consecutive patients received a first TACE at UAB and were included in this study. The study population included Child-Pugh class A (39%), Child-Pugh class B (51%), and Child-Pugh class C (10%) patients. The most common etiologies of liver disease were hepatitis C virus (49%) alcohol (25%) and nonalcoholic steatohepatitis (19%). Tumor response was evaluated via MRI for 75 patients and CT for 242 patients. In total, 33 patients were treated with Sorafenib prior to TACE and 53 patients were treated with Sorafenib following TACE.

3.2. HCC Tumor Necrosis. HCC tumor necrosis distribution is shown in Figure 2. Patients were more likely to be responders (76%) than nonresponders (24%). Individual mRECIST

TABLE 1: Baseline characteristics of patients with hepatocellular carcinoma treated with transarterial chemoembolization.

	mRECIST categories				
	Complete (N = 102)	Partial (N = 138)	Stable (N = 63)	Progressive (N = 14)	p value
Age (mean ± SD)	61.5 ± 8.7	61.5 ± 10.1	63.1 ± 9.5	61.9 ± 8.3	0.697
Gender					
Female	73 (71.6%)	110 (79.7%)	40 (71.4%)	10 (63.5%)	0.102
Male	29 (28.4%)	28 (20.3%)	23 (28.6%)	4 (36.5%)	
Race					
White	78 (76.5%)	105 (76.1%)	43 (68.3%)	7 (50.0%)	0.064
Black	18 (17.7%)	30 (21.7%)	13 (20.6%)	6 (42.9%)	
Other	6 (5.8%)	3 (2.2%)	7 (11.1%)	1 (7.1%)	
Etiology					
Alcohol	29 (28.4%)	35 (25.4%)	13 (21.0%)	2 (14.3%)	0.563
HBV	7 (6.9%)	6 (4.4%)	5 (7.9%)	2 (14.3%)	0.434
HCV	57 (55.9%)	73 (52.9%)	21 (33.9%)	5 (35.7%)	0.024
NASH	22 (21.6%)	28 (20.3%)	10 (15.9%)	1 (7.1%)	0.402
Child-Pugh class					0.525
A	35 (34.3%)	53 (38.4%)	28 (44.4%)	7 (50.0%)	
B	54 (52.9%)	74 (53.6%)	28 (44.4%)	7 (50.0%)	
C	13 (12.8%)	11 (8.0%)	7 (11.2%)	0 (0.0%)	
AFP*	12.3 ± 100.8	22.0 ± 158.9	27.0 ± 132.6	132.0 ± 3601.0	0.179**
Diameter of largest tumor	3.6 ± 1.8	4.6 ± 2.5	5.6 ± 4.4	6.1 ± 3.7	<0.0001
Number of tumors	1.6 ± 0.8	1.5 ± 1.0	2.1 ± 1.4	1.9 ± 1.6	0.003

*Medians and interquartile range reported.
**Kruskal-Wallis procedure used.
TACE: transarterial chemoembolization; mRECIST: modified Response Evaluation Criteria In Solid Tumors, p value: probability, SD: standard deviation, HBV: hepatitis B virus, HCV: hepatitis C virus, NASH: nonalcoholic steatohepatitis, and AFP: alpha fetoprotein.

category analysis revealed that the most common response to TACE was partial (43.5%), followed by complete (32.2%) and stable (19.9%). The least frequent mRECIST response was progressive disease (4.4%).

Population basic demographics, stratified by mRECIST category, are presented in Table 1. There were no significant differences in the distribution of age, gender, race, or Child-Pugh class and mRECIST response. The prevalence of hepatitis C virus varies among the different mRECIST groups, with a higher prevalence in the complete and partial response groups. There was a significant association between worse mRECIST response and both increasing HCC tumor number ($p = 0.003$) and increasing max tumor diameter ($p < 0.0001$). A similar association was observed between total axial diameter of the 3 largest HCC tumors and worse mRECIST response ($p < 0.0001$). The mRECIST response was predictive of repeat TACE ($p = 0.025$). Patients with stable disease were the most likely to undergo repeat TACE (55.2%) while patients in the complete response were the least likely to undergo TACE (35.6%).

3.3. *Survival Outcomes.* Univariate and subsequent multi-variable analyses were carried out to examine post-TACE survival as a function of mRECIST response. Kaplan-Meier

curves were constructed for both the dichotomized, responders and nonresponders (Figure 3), and the 4 individual mRECIST groups (Figure 4(a)).

The survival analysis investigating mRECIST categories dichotomized into responders (complete and partial response) and nonresponders (stable and progressive disease) shows patient survival significantly varied according to the dichotomized mRECIST response (Figure 3). Median survival was significantly longer in responders than in nonresponders (20.8 months versus 14.9 months, $p = 0.011$).

Additional analyses were then carried out to examine survival in the four defined mRECIST categories. Crude, unadjusted survival analysis shows that patient survival following TACE varied according to mRECIST category ($p = 0.0003$, Figure 4(a)). Patients with a complete response had the longest median survival (21.44 months), followed by partial response (20.78 months) and stable response (16.82 months), while patients with progressive disease showed the shortest median survival (7.73 months).

A multivariate analysis of patient and HCC tumor predictors of post-TACE survival was performed (Table 2). There was no significant association between post-TACE survival and age, gender, or race. Child-Pugh class was significantly associated with post-TACE survival ($p < 0.001$). Compared to Child-Pugh A patients, Child-Pugh B [HR 2.67, 95% CI

TABLE 2: Multivariable analyses of post-TACE survival.

	Univariate			Multivariable		
	Hazard ratio	95% CI	p value	Hazard ratio	95% CI	p value
Age	0.99	(0.98, 1.01)	0.500	1.00	(0.98, 1.02)	0.721
Gender			0.295**			0.167**
Male	1.00 (reference)	(—, —)		1.00 (reference)	(—, —)	
Female	1.23	(0.84, 1.79)	0.295	1.35	(0.88, 2.06)	0.167
Race			0.108**			0.132**
White	1.00 (reference)	(—, —)		1.00 (reference)	(—, —)	
Black	0.88	(0.58, 1.36)		0.75	(0.47, 1.19)	0.222
Other	1.91	(0.99, 3.68)		1.57	(0.80, 3.08)	0.194
Child-Pugh			<0.001**			<0.001**
A	1.00 (reference)	(—, —)		1.00 (reference)	(—, —)	
B	2.17	(1.50, 3.15)	<0.001	2.67	(1.80, 3.94)	<0.001
C	2.09	(1.05, 4.16)	0.037	2.26	(1.09, 4.65)	0.028
Total tumor diameter*	1.04	(1.01, 1.07)	0.009	1.04	(1.01, 1.08)	0.009
mRECIST			0.034**			0.003**
Complete	1.00 (reference)	(—, —)		1.00 (reference)	(—, —)	
Partial	1.15	(0.77, 1.72)	0.499	1.18	(0.85, 2.14)	0.436
Stable	1.39	(0.83, 2.33)	0.209	1.28	(0.55, 2.03)	0.379
Progressive	3.21	(1.42, 7.24)	0.005	4.99	(1.19, 11.09)	<0.001

*Sum axial diameter of three largest hepatocellular carcinoma tumors.
**Multiple degree of freedom test to determine if any of the levels within the categorical variables differs from the reference group within that variable.
TACE: transarterial chemoembolization; mRECIST: modified Response Evaluation Criteria In Solid Tumors, p value: probability, and 95% CI: 95% confidence interval.

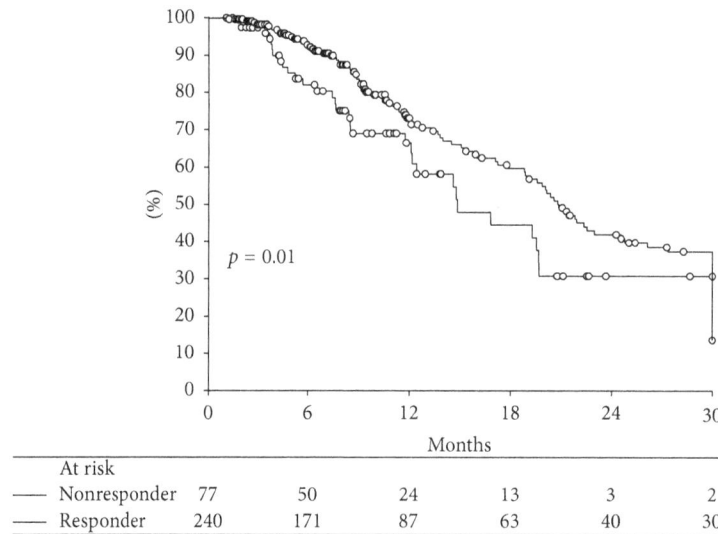

FIGURE 3: Unadjusted post-TACE survival as a function of mRECIST dichotomized into responders (complete and partial response) and nonresponders (stable and progressive disease).

(1.8, 3.94), $p < 0.001$] and Child-Pugh C [HR 2.26, 95% CI (1.09, 4.65), $p = 0.028$] have significantly increased mortality risk. Increased total tumor diameter was also significantly associated with decreased post-TACE survival [HR 1.04/cm of increasing tumor diameter, 95% CI (1.01, 1.08), $p = 0.009$]. The mRECIST response was also significantly associated with post-TACE survival ($p = 0.003$). However, when using complete response as a reference, there was no significant survival difference in partial and stable disease categories. Only the progressive disease category was significantly associated with decreased post-TACE survival (HR 4.99, 95% CI (1.19, 11.09), $p < 0.001$).

Adjusted survival curves were constructed adjusting for statistically significant covariates. Again, post-TACE survival was significantly associated with the four defined mRECIST categories ($p = 0.003$, Figure 4(b)). Adjusted median survival

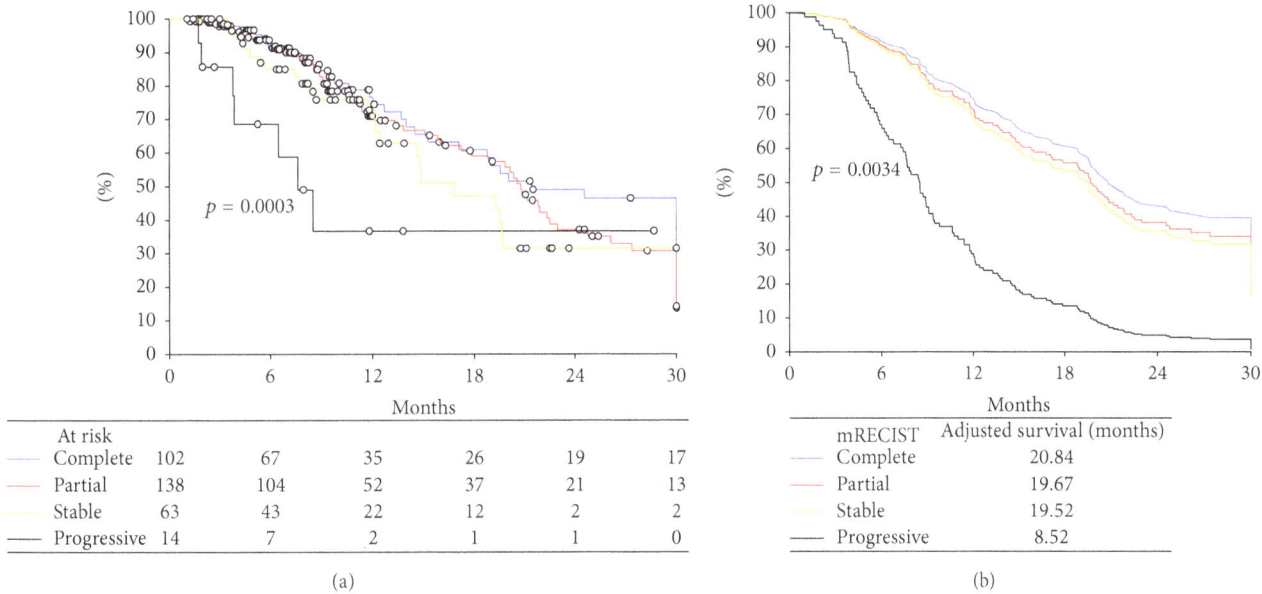

	At risk					
——	Complete	102	67	35	26	19	17
——	Partial	138	104	52	37	21	13
——	Stable	63	43	22	12	2	2
——	Progressive	14	7	2	1	1	0

(a)

	mRECIST	Adjusted survival (months)
——	Complete	20.84
——	Partial	19.67
——	Stable	19.52
——	Progressive	8.52

(b)

FIGURE 4: (a) Crude, unadjusted post-TACE survival as a function of mRECIST category. (b) Adjusted post-TACE survival as a function of mRECIST category.

estimates were greatest in patients with a complete response (20.84 months), followed by partial response (19.67 months) and stable response (19.52 months), while patients with progressive disease showed the shortest median survival (8.52 months).

4. Discussion

Similar to published reports [7, 17–22], this study demonstrates a significant survival advantage in responders compared to nonresponders following TACE for HCC. In isolation, this finding suggests that patients who exhibit a complete or partial response to TACE will experience approximately 6 months increased survival compared to patients with stable or progressive disease. To further investigate the association between TACE-induced HCC tumor necrosis and patient survival, we conducted survival analyses of the four defined mRECIST categories.

Patients with complete response experienced the longest median survival followed by patients with partial response and stable disease. Much to our surprise, there was only a small, nonstatistical difference in survival outcomes between patients with complete, partial, and stable disease mRECIST responses. Compared to complete response, the only statistically different survival outcome following TACE was observed in the progressive disease category. Patients with progressive disease experienced greatly decreased survival when compared to those in other mRECIST categories. The most important finding from this study is that the poor survival in the progressive disease group is the main statistical driver of the dichotomous (responder and nonresponder) and the four defined mRECIST group survival benefit analysis.

Findings presented here are congruent with previous works that have shown association between radiologic evaluation of tumor necrosis and survival [7, 17–22]. In the setting of HCC, disease progression following locoregional therapy is often associated with poor prognosis [26–28]. For example, studies have shown that HCC tumor progression measured by mRECIST following locoregional therapy is an independent risk factor of tumor recurrence and decreased survival following liver transplantation [26, 29]. Similarly, a study by De Carlis et al. demonstrated high recurrence rates and worse outcomes in patients with HCC progression while on the transplant wait list [27]. Recently the ART score was developed to aid in the decision making process for repeat TACE [28]. This scoring system predicts a poor prognosis following repeat TACE in patients with features of progressive HCC following initial TACE [28]. Predictive variables include a lack of radiologic response to initial TACE [28].

While this study does not address which HCC patients may benefit from an initial TACE, the data may inform treatment recommendations for patients after their first TACE procedure. Current HCC treatment goals focus on tumor eradication. However, the findings presented here suggest only a modest increase in median survival going from stable disease to partial and complete response. Perhaps the future paradigm should focus more on avoiding the progressive disease category, more of a "HCC treatment as a chronic disease" mindset instead of the (often unrealistic) goal of tumor eradication. Patients in the stable disease or partial response categories are the most common patients to undergo repeat TACE. These findings question the utility in giving these patients repeat TACE since only modest increases in median survival are seen with additional tumor necrosis. At the very least, it may be prudent not to rush to repeat TACE when a patient may require aggressive (nonselective) lobar embolization, in the setting of post-TACE liver dysfunction, or if a patient is on the liver transplant waitlist. In contrast, progressive disease as defined by mRECIST seems to carry an especially poor prognosis. The best approach for these patients may be alternative HCC treatments or even best supportive care.

This study has limitations to consider when interpreting the data. The retrospective design and practice patterns at UAB may bias the data. Well over half of the patients in this study (60%) were Child-Pugh B/C patients, which may not be representative of many patients receiving TACE. For example, studies included in a commonly referenced meta-analysis had patient populations with Child-Pugh A making up 70–100% [30]. Another practice pattern at UAB that may bias the data is that selective TACE procedures are commonly performed whereas nonselective lobar approaches are most common nationwide [31].

In conclusion, both the dichotomized (responders and nonresponders) and the four defined mRECIST responses to TACE in patients with HCC were predictive of survival. The main driver of this survival benefit analysis was the poor survival in the progressive disease group. Surprisingly, there was small nonsignificant survival benefit between complete response, partial response, and stable disease. Progressive disease, increasing total tumor diameter, and non-Child-Pugh class A were independent predictors of post-TACE mortality. These findings may inform HCC treatment decisions following first TACE procedures.

Disclosure

The data from this paper was presented at the 2015 AHPBA Conference.

Conflict of Interests

The authors declare that there is no conflict of interests regarding the publication of this paper.

Acknowledgment

This research was funded by National Institute of Health Grants nos. T35 HL007473 (Haywood) and 1 K23 DK091514-01A1 (DuBay).

References

[1] A. Forner, J. M. Llovet, and J. Bruix, "Hepatocellular carcinoma," The Lancet, vol. 379, no. 9822, pp. 1245–1255, 2012.

[2] R. Lencioni, "Loco-regional treatment of hepatocellular carcinoma," Hepatology, vol. 52, no. 2, pp. 762–773, 2010.

[3] S. A. Shah, J. K. Smith, Y. Li, S. C. Ng, J. E. Carroll, and J. F. Tseng, "Underutilization of therapy for hepatocellular carcinoma in the medicare population," Cancer, vol. 117, no. 5, pp. 1019–1026, 2011.

[4] P. J. Thuluvath, M. K. Guidinger, J. J. Fung, L. B. Johnson, S. C. Rayhill, and S. J. Pelletier, "Liver transplantation in the United States, 1999–2008: special feature," American Journal of Transplantation, vol. 10, no. 4, part 2, pp. 1003–1019, 2010.

[5] J. Bruix and M. Sherman, "Practice Guidelines Committee AAftSoLD. Management of hepatocellular carcinoma," Hepatology, vol. 42, no. 5, pp. 1208–1236, 2005.

[6] J. Bruix and M. Sherman, "Management of hepatocellular carcinoma: an update," Hepatology, vol. 53, no. 3, pp. 1020–1022, 2011.

[7] C. J. Kim, H. J. Kim, J. H. Park et al., "Radiologic response to transcatheter hepatic arterial chemoembolization and clinical outcomes in patients with hepatocellular carcinoma," Liver International, vol. 34, no. 2, pp. 305–312, 2014.

[8] R. Lencioni and J. M. Llovet, "Modified recist (mRECIST) assessment for hepatocellular carcinoma," Seminars in Liver Disease, vol. 30, no. 1, pp. 52–60, 2010.

[9] R. Lencioni, "New data supporting modified RECIST (mRECIST) for hepatocellular carcinoma," Clinical Cancer Research, vol. 19, no. 6, pp. 1312–1314, 2013.

[10] A. Arora and A. Kumar, "Treatment response evaluation and follow-up in hepatocellular carcinoma," Journal of Clinical and Experimental Hepatology, vol. 4, supplement 3, pp. S126–S129, 2014.

[11] B. C. Odisio, F. Galastri, R. Avritscher et al., "Hepatocellular carcinomas within the Milan criteria: predictors of histologic necrosis after drug-eluting beads transarterial chemoembolization," CardioVascular and Interventional Radiology, vol. 37, no. 4, pp. 1018–1026, 2014.

[12] X. Pauwels, M. Azahaf, G. Lassailly et al., "Drug-Eluting Beads Loaded with Doxorubicin (DEBDOX) chemoembolisation before liver transplantation for hepatocellular carcinoma: an imaging/histologic correlation study," CardioVascular and Interventional Radiology, vol. 38, no. 3, pp. 685–692, 2015.

[13] A. Riaz, L. Kulik, R. J. Lewandowski et al., "Radiologic-pathologic correlation of hepatocellular carcinoma treated with internal radiation using Yttrium-90 microspheres," Hepatology, vol. 49, no. 4, pp. 1185–1193, 2009.

[14] J. H. Shim, S. Han, Y. M. Shin et al., "Optimal measurement modality and method for evaluation of responses to transarterial chemoembolization of hepatocellular carcinoma based on enhancement criteria," Journal of Vascular and Interventional Radiology, vol. 24, no. 3, pp. 316–325, 2013.

[15] I. Bargellini, E. Bozzi, D. Campani et al., "Modified RECIST to assess tumor response after transarterial chemoembolization of hepatocellular carcinoma: CT-pathologic correlation in 178 liver explants," European Journal of Radiology, vol. 82, no. 5, pp. e212–e218, 2013.

[16] I. Bargellini, C. Vignali, R. Cioni et al., "Hepatocellular carcinoma: CT for tumor response after transarterial chemoembolization in patients exceeding Milan criteria—selection parameter for liver transplantation," Radiology, vol. 255, no. 1, pp. 289–300, 2010.

[17] K. Memon, L. Kulik, R. J. Lewandowski et al., "Radiographic response to locoregional therapy in hepatocellular carcinoma predicts patient survival times," Gastroenterology, vol. 141, no. 2, pp. 526.e2–535.e2, 2011.

[18] H. J. Prajapati, J. R. Spivey, S. I. Hanish et al., "mRECIST and EASL responses at early time point by contrast-enhanced dynamic MRI predict survival in patients with unresectable Hepatocellular Carcinoma (HCC) treated by Doxorubicin Drug-Eluting Beads Transarterial Chemoembolization (DEB TACE)," Annals of Oncology, vol. 24, no. 4, pp. 965–973, 2013.

[19] R. Gillmore, S. Stuart, A. Kirkwood et al., "EASL and mRECIST responses are independent prognostic factors for survival

in hepatocellular cancer patients treated with transarterial embolization," *Journal of Hepatology*, vol. 55, no. 6, pp. 1309–1316, 2011.

[20] B. K. Kim, S. U. Kim, K. A. Kim et al., "Complete response at first chemoembolization is still the most robust predictor for favorable outcome in hepatocellular carcinoma," *Journal of Hepatology*, vol. 62, no. 6, pp. 1304–1310, 2015.

[21] K. Han, J. H. Kim, H. M. Yoon et al., "Transcatheter arterial chemoembolization for infiltrative hepatocellular carcinoma: clinical safety and efficacy and factors influencing patient survival," *Korean Journal of Radiology*, vol. 15, no. 4, pp. 464–471, 2014.

[22] J. H. Shim, H. C. Lee, S.-O. Kim et al., "Which response criteria best help predict survival of patients with hepatocellular carcinoma following chemoembolization? A validation study of old and new models," *Radiology*, vol. 262, no. 2, pp. 708–718, 2012.

[23] J. A. White, D. T. Redden, M. K. Bryant et al., "Predictors of repeat transarterial chemoembolization in the treatment of hepatocellular carcinoma," *HPB*, vol. 16, no. 12, pp. 1095–1101, 2014.

[24] C. Wald, M. W. Russo, J. K. Heimbach, H. K. Hussain, E. A. Pomfret, and J. Bruix, "New OPTN/UNOS policy for liver transplant allocation: standardization of liver imaging, diagnosis, classification, and reporting of hepatocellular carcinoma," *Radiology*, vol. 266, no. 2, pp. 376–382, 2013.

[25] J. Bruix, M. Sherman, J. M. Llovet et al., "Clinical management of hepatocellular carcinoma. Conclusions of the barcelona-2000 EASL conference," *Journal of Hepatology*, vol. 35, no. 3, pp. 421–430, 2001.

[26] Q. Lai, A. W. Avolio, I. Graziadei et al., "Alpha-fetoprotein and modified response evaluation criteria in solid tumors progression after locoregional therapy as predictors of hepatocellular cancer recurrence and death after transplantation," *Liver Transplantation*, vol. 19, no. 10, pp. 1108–1118, 2013.

[27] L. De Carlis, S. D. Sandro, A. Giacomoni et al., "Beyond the Milan criteria: what risks for patients with hepatocellular carcinoma progression before liver transplantation?" *Journal of Clinical Gastroenterology*, vol. 46, no. 1, pp. 78–86, 2012.

[28] F. Hucke, W. Sieghart, M. Pinter et al., "The ART-strategy: sequential assessment of the ART score predicts outcome of patients with hepatocellular carcinoma re-treated with TACE," *Journal of Hepatology*, vol. 60, no. 1, pp. 118–126, 2014.

[29] D. J. Kim, P. J. Clark, J. Heimbach et al., "Recurrence of hepatocellular carcinoma: importance of mRECIST response to chemoembolization and tumor size," *American Journal of Transplantation*, vol. 14, no. 6, pp. 1383–1390, 2014.

[30] J. M. Llovet and J. Bruix, "Systematic review of randomized trials for unresectable hepatocellular carcinoma: chemoembolization improves survival," *Hepatology*, vol. 37, no. 2, pp. 429–442, 2003.

[31] R. C. Gaba, "Chemoembolization practice patterns and technical methods among interventional radiologists: results of an online survey," *American Journal of Roentgenology*, vol. 198, no. 3, pp. 692–699, 2012.

19

TIMP-1 as well as Microvessel Invasion and High Nuclear Grade Is a Significant Determinant Factor for Extension of Tumor Diameter in Localized RCC

Nozomu Kawata, Kenya Yamaguchi, Tomohiro Igarashi, and Satoru Takahashi

Department of Urology, Nihon University School of Medicine, 1-6 Kanda-Surugadai, Chiyoda-ku, Tokyo, Japan

Correspondence should be addressed to Nozomu Kawata; kawata.nozomu@nihon-u.ac.jp

Academic Editor: James L. Mulshine

Objectives. To clarify what kind of pathological factor is necessary for the extension of tumor diameter in localized RCC, we studied localized RCC patients. *Methods*. We retrospectively reviewed medical records of 237 RCC patients in our institute who underwent nephrectomy. We performed immune histological analysis of MMP-2, MMP-9, TIMP-1, TIMP-2, and MT-MMP-1 for all samples. *Results*. Among the clinicopathological factors, multivariate analysis revealed nuclear grade; TIMP-2 and MT-MMP-1 were independent prognostic factors of localized RCC (risk ratio 1.50, $p = 0.037$, risk ratio 1.12, $p = 0.008$, and risk ratio 1.84, $p = 0.045$, resp.). By the multiple logistic regression analysis among pT1a versus pT1b, TIMP-1 was an independent factor (risk ratio 3.30, $p = 0.010$) whereas all pT1 versus pT2a and all pT1 + pT2a versus pT2b high nuclear grade (risk ratio 5.15, $p = 0.0015$) and Micro vessel invasion (MVI, risk ratio 3.08, $p = 0.002$) were independent factors. For all pT1 + pT2a versus pT2b, nuclear grade (risk ratio 3.39, $p = 0.020$) and MVI (risk ratio 2.91, $p = 0.018$) were independent factors. *Conclusion*. Higher expression of TIMP-1 is necessary for advancement tumor diameter from pT1a to pT1b, and a process of tumor diameter extension beyond pT1 and pT2a category needs presence of MVI and high nuclear grade.

1. Introduction

Recently, Frank et al. [1] and Klatte et al. [2] proposed a subclassification of T2 RCC into pT2a and pT2b according to tumor diameter with a cutoff of 10 cm.

Based on their reports, the 7th edition of TNM classification [3], threshold value between T1 and T2 RCC was divided into T2a (up to 10 cm) and T2b (more than 10 cm) [3]. Lee et al. [4] reported that local control may be achieved in surgical management of contemporary patients with RCC of 4 cm or less either by radical or nephron sparing surgery, and, in addition, local recurrence rate after nephron sparing surgery was 0–12%. The rate decreases to 0% to 3% for microscopically organ confined disease and 0% to 5% for small renal tumors [5]. It is well known that renal cell carcinoma with a diameter of more than 10 cm has high potential to cause distant metastasis and generally recommended surgical procedure is radical nephrectomy [1].

Previously, we reported that systemic symptoms of RCC have a strong significant relationship with the expression of matrix metalloproteinase 9 (MMP-9) [6]. It is well known that both MMPs (matrix metalloproteinases) and TIMPs (tissue inhibitors of metalloproteinases) play an important role in the progression of RCC. However, there are no reports examining the relationships among tumor diameter and MMPs and TIMPs. To clarify what kind of clinicopathological feature is necessary for extension of the tumor diameter, we studied localized RCC patients.

2. Material and Method

Between January 1988 and December 2003, a total of 237 patients had underwent radical nephrectomy for localized renal cell carcinoma at Nihon University Itabashi or Surugadai Hospital. Patients consisted of 176 males and 61 females, mean age of 60 (33–83) and 58 (25–82), respectively.

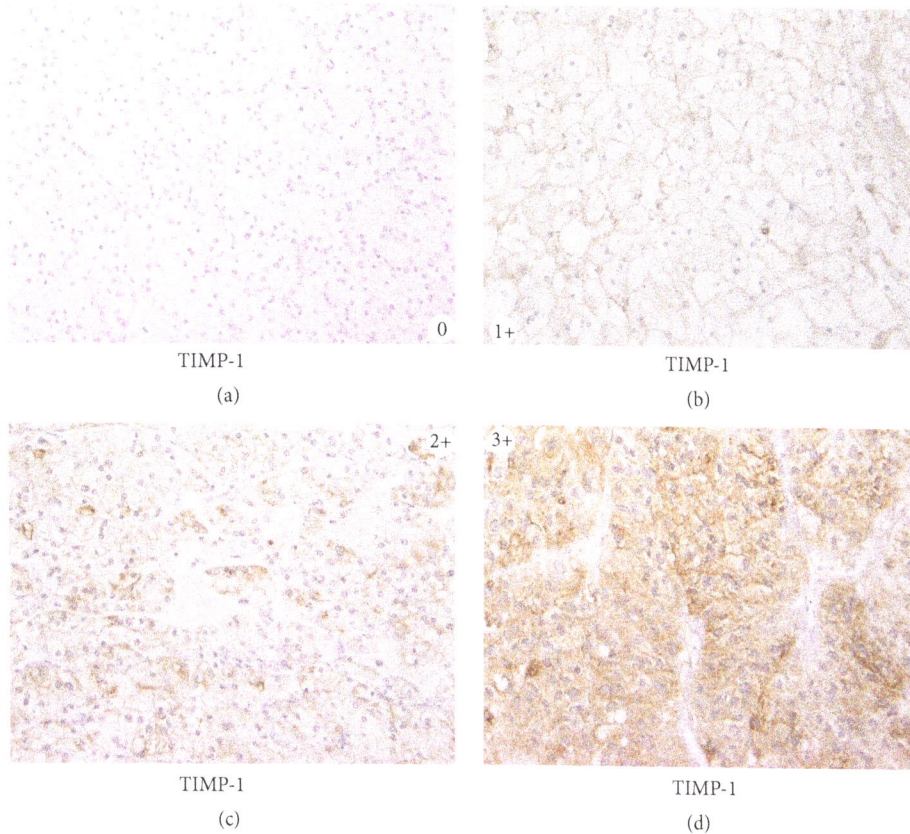

FIGURE 1: 0 indicates the absence of immune staining or faint membranous staining of rare tumor cells; 1+ indicates membranous staining in most tumor cells; 2+ indicates diffuse membranous and/or cytoplasmic staining in groups of tumor cells; and 3+ indicates significant cytoplasmic staining in most tumor cells. For the evaluation of immune histochemical staining, intensities of 2+ and 3+ were considered strong expressions of each protein.

The average postoperative follow-up period was 61 ± 3.6 months. All patients underwent preoperative chest and abdominal contrast enhanced CT, and bone scan if required. Pathological stages were determined according to the TNM classification of malignant tumors [3].

Tumors were classified as pT1a, pT1b, pT2a, and pT2b in 94 (40%), 74 (31%), 43(18%), and 26 (11%) cases, respectively.

The nuclear grade of RCC was determined using the criteria proposed by Fuhrman et al. [7]. Since several studies found no significant difference in survival results between patients with Grade 1 versus 2 tumors and those with Grade 3 versus 4 tumors [8], a total of 237 patients were divided into two groups according to nuclear grade: a low nuclear grade group (Grades 1 and 2, 190 patients) and a high nuclear grade group (Grades 3 and 4, 47 patients).

Microvessel invasion (MVI) was defined as a tumor infiltration locally through the intact vessel wall including the endothelium, leading to free extension of cancer cells into the lumen [9].

The maximum tumor diameter (MTD) was confirmed by pathological specimens. We applied immunohistochemistry on the cut surface of tumor with no necrosis nor intratumoral hemorrhage.

The immunohistochemical study for MMP-2, MMP-9, TIMP-1, TIMP-2, and MT-MMP-1 was performed by methods we previously reported [6]. For evaluation of immunohistochemical staining, staining intensities of 2+ and 3+ were considered strong expressions of each protein (Figure 1) [6].

Cancer-specific survival (CSS) was defined as the interval from initial surgery to death and was calculated by the method of Kaplan and Meier. Statistical significance was determined by the log-rank test. Cox multivariate analysis was performed to determine any independent predictive values.

To determine the relationships between T categories and 8 pathological features of RCC (histopathological type, nuclear grade, MVI, MMP-2, MMP-9, TIMP-1, TIMP-2, and MT-MMP-1), we compared the quantitative results using a multiple logistic regression analysis. Intergroup differences were considered statistically significant at $p < 0.05$. All analyses were performed using JMP4.0 (SAS Institute, Cory, NC, USA).

The study using these specimens was performed under the approval of Nihon University School of Medicine Ethics Board (IRB number 106-1).

TABLE 1: Predictors of localized 237 RCC cases postoperative specific mortality.

Categories	Univariate analysis		Multivariate analysis	
	Hazard ratio (95% CI)	p value	Hazard ratio (95% CI)	p value
pT1a versus pT1b 94 versus 74	2.38 (1.02–5.55)	0.046	1.35 (0.96–1.88)	0.086
pT1a versus pT2a 94 versus 43	1.40 (0.49–4.0)	0.53	1.07 (0.93–1.42)	0.74
pT1a versus pT2b 94 versus 26	4.0 (1.51–1.020)	0.005	1.09 (0.66–1.85)	0.71
Clear versus nonclear 190 versus 47	2.05 (1.00–4.019)	0.048	1.12 (0.77–1.65)	0.53
Nuclear Grades 1 and 2 versus 3 and 4 190 versus 47	1.79 (1.76–6.84)	<0.001	1.50 (1.03–2.22)	0.037
MVI (−) versus (+) 154 versus 83	1.95 (0.92–2.94)	0.025	1.04 (0.33–1.21)	0.94
MMP-2 weak versus strong 82 versus 155	3.69 (1.43–9.52)	0.0069	1.26 (0.30–5.23)	0.74
MMP-9 weak versus strong 181 versus 56	4.29 (2.17–8.16)	<0.0001	2.88 (0.92–2.94)	0.75
TIMP-1 weak versus strong 42 versus 195	2.52 (0.77–8.26)	0.12	1.014 (0.709–1.45)	0.34
TIMP-2 weak versus strong 201 versus 36	2.07 (0.99–4.31)	0.052	1.12 (1.36–3.29)	**0.020**
MT-MMP-1 weak versus strong 194 versus 43	3.44 (1.73–6.84)	0.005	1.84 (1.21–2.82)	**0.045**

3. Results

Among the tumors, 194 (82%) were conventional clear cell carcinomas, 42 (17%) were papillary carcinomas, and 1 (0.3%) was a chromophobe carcinoma. Tumors were classified as pT1a, pT1b, pT2a, and pT2b in 94 (40%), 74 (31%), 43 (18%), and 26 (11%) cases, respectively. The median tumor diameter was 50 mm (15–250 mm). Among a total of 237 patients, 190 were classified as having a low nuclear grade (Grades 1 and 2), whereas 47 as having a high nuclear grade (Grades 3 and 4).

The cancer-specific 10-year survival rates were 88.8%, 69.5%, 80.3%, and 50.0% for pT1a, pT1b, pT2a, and pT2b, respectively (Figure 2, $p < 0.001$).

With respect to the cancer-specific mortality, the univariate analysis showed no significance for pT1a versus pT2a and TIMP-1 and TIMP-2 as a determinant factor, while the remaining 8 factors were significant factors of postoperative specific mortality of 247 patients (Table 1). By the multivariate analysis of clinicopathological factors, nuclear grade, TIMP-2, and MT-MMP-1 were independent prognostic factors (risk ratio 1.50, $p = 0.037$, risk ratio 1.12, $p = 0.02$, and risk ratio 1.84, $p = 0.045$, resp.) (Table 1).

We compared the clinicopathological factors in three categories: pT1a versus pT1b, all pT1 versus pT2a, and all pT1 + pT2a versus pT2b. By the Cox multivariate analysis (Table 2), among the pT1a versus pT1b group, TIMP-1 was an independent factor (risk ratio 3.30, $p = 0.010$). For pT1 versus pT2a, both nuclear grade (risk ratio 5.15, $p = 0.0015$) and MVI (risk ratio 3.08, $p = 0.002$) were independent factors. For the remaining pT1 + pT2a versus pT2b, both nuclear

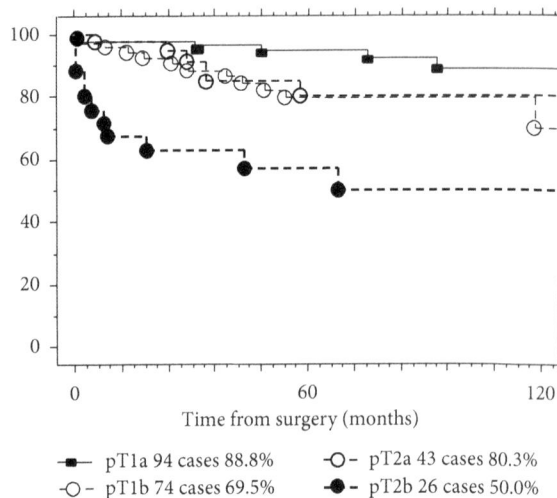

FIGURE 2: Cancer-specific survival rate according to the pT category.

grade (risk ratio 3.39, $p = 0.020$) and MVI (risk ratio 2.91, $p = 0.018$) were significant factors.

4. Discussion

Once MMPs are stimulated, they are susceptible to prohibition by the general serum proteinase inhibitor α2-macroglobulin and by a family of specific tissue inhibitors (TIMPs). On the other hand, TIMPs have been frequently

TABLE 2: Correlation between pT category and pathological features with localized 237 RCC cases.

	pT1a versus pT1b Odds ratio (95% CI) p value 94 versus 74 Cases of each category	pT1a and pT1b versus pT2a Odds ratio (95% CI) p value 168 versus 43 Cases of each category	pT1a, pT1b, and pT2a versus pT2b Odds ratio (95% CI) p value 211 versus 26 Cases of each category
Cell type	2.43 (0.85–6.89) 0.09	2.28 (0.76–6.82) 0.13	2.32 (0.84–6.36) 0.10
Clear versus others	139 versus 29	175 versus 36	190 versus 47
Nuclear grade	1.79 (0.57–5.56) 0.31	**5.15 (1.87–14.2) 0.0015**	**3.39 (1.20–9.58) 0.020**
Low versus high	147 versus 21	**176 versus 35**	**190 versus 47**
MVI	1.95 (0.92–4.16) 0.08	**3.08 (1.47–6.48) 0.002**	**2.91 (1.19–7.11) 0.018**
(−) versus (+)	123 versus 45	**144 versus 67**	**154 versus 83**
MMP-2	1.14 (0.55–2.36) 0.71	2.13 (0.90–5.0) 0.84	1.24 (0.41–3.70) 0.70
Weak versus strong	60 versus 108	76 versus 135	82 versus 156
MMP-9	1.79 (0.65–4.90) 0.205	1.47 (0.55–3.94) 0.43	1.31 (0.40–4.21) 0.64
Weak versus strong	134 versus 34	163 versus 48	181 versus 56
TIMP-1	**3.30 (1.32–8.26) 0.010**	1.18 (0.43–3.26) 0.74	1.59 (0.49–5.10) 0.42
Weak versus strong	**31 versus 137**	37 versus 174	42 versus 195
TIMP-2	1.41 (0.48–4.13) 0.53	2.14 (0.65–6.99) 0.84	3.03 (0.71–12.98) 0.13
Weak versus strong	142 versus 26	178 versus 33	201 versus 36
MT-MMP-1	1.93 (0.65–5.71) 0.096	2.28 (0.76–3.50) 0.15	1.98 (0.60–6.54) 0.26
Weak versus strong	144 versus 26	176 versus 35	194 versus 43

MVI: microvascular invasion.

reported that they may be multifunctional, because of additional effects on cell growth and apoptosis. These activities appear to be distinct from their MMP inhibitory capabilities in some cases [10].

Previously, we reported that high expression levels of MMP-9 were associated with poor prognosis of RCC [11]. Basically, TIMPs are known to inhibit MMP activity by forming a complex with active MMPs and are believed to be specific for enzymes of this family, such as TIMP-1 with MMP-9 and TIMP-2 with MMP-2 [12]. Members of the TIMP family have also been associated with cancer. In several cases, malignant tumors have elevated TIMP levels rather than decreased levels [12].

MMP-9 has a significant relationship with high nuclear grade RCC and was found to be an independent prognosticator by multivariate analysis. Furthermore, nuclear grade and TIMP-2 were independent prognostic factors among the incidental RCC patients [13].

With regard to MVI, Ishimura reported that MVI is not a significant prognostic factor in localized RCC patients; on the other hand, it is the only significant prognostic factor of disease free recurrence after radical operation for patients with pT1 and pT2 disease [14]. Additionally, Dall'Oglio et al. showed a significant relationship between MVI and clinical stage. In 95 tumors below 4 cm in diameter, MVI was detected in 11 (12%), while in 74 tumors of 4.1–7 cm, MVI was detected in 20 (27%), and in 61 of over 7 cm, 28 (48%) had MVI [15].

Previously we reported that cancer-specific 5-year survival was 45.0% for patients with high nuclear grade tumor (Grade 3.4) and 83.3% for patients with low nuclear grade tumor (Grade 1.2) ($p < 0.001$) [16]. Zhang et al. reported a significant correlation between tumor size and nuclear grade.

By their report, tumor diameters of G1, G2, and G3 tumors were significantly different (3.27 ± 1.46 cm, 4.87 ± 2.23 cm, and 7.39 ± 3.11 cm, $p < 0.05$). Tumors with larger diameter were prone to have higher nuclear grade. These results were consistent with ours [17].

5. Conclusion

In conclusion, higher expression of TIMP-1 is necessary for advancement of tumor diameter from pT1a to pT1b, and a process of tumor diameter extension beyond pT1 category needs the presence of MVI and high nuclear grade.

Conflict of Interests

The authors declare that there is no conflict of interests regarding the publication of this paper.

References

[1] I. Frank, M. L. Blute, B. C. Leibovich et al., "pT2 classification for renal cell carcinoma. Can its accuracy be improved?" *Journal of Urology*, vol. 173, no. 2, pp. 380–384, 2005.

[2] T. Klatte, J.-J. Patard, R. H. Goel et al., "Prognostic impact of tumor size on pT2 renal cell carcinoma: aninternational multicenter experience," *Journal of Urology*, vol. 178, no. 1, pp. 35–40, 2007.

[3] L. H. Sobin, M. K. Gospondarowics, and Ch. Wittekind, *TNM Classification of Malignant Tumours*, Wiley-Blackwell, New York, NY, USA, 7th edition, 2009.

[4] C. T. Lee, J. Katz, W. Shi, H. T. Thaler, V. E. Reuter, and P. Russo, "Surgical management of renal tumors 4 cm. Or less in

a contemporary cohort," *The Journal of Urology*, vol. 163, no. 3, pp. 730–736, 2000.

[5] S. E. Lerner, C. A. Hawkins, M. L. Blute et al., "Disease outcome in patients with low stage renal cell carcinoma treated with nephron sparing or radical surgery," *The Journal of Urology*, vol. 155, no. 6, pp. 1868–1873, 1996.

[6] N. Kawata, Y. Nagane, T. Igarashi et al., "Strong significant correlation between MMP-9 and systemic symptoms in patients with localized renal cell carcinoma," *Urology*, vol. 68, no. 3, pp. 523–527, 2006.

[7] S. A. Fuhrman, L. C. Lasky, and C. Limas, "Prognostic significance of morphologic parameters in renal cell carcinoma," *American Journal of Surgical Pathology*, vol. 6, no. 7, pp. 655–663, 1982.

[8] L. J. Medeiros, A. B. Gelb, and L. M. Weiss, "Renal cell carcinoma: prognostic significance of morphologic parameters in 121 cases," *Cancer*, vol. 61, no. 8, pp. 1639–1651, 1988.

[9] H. Lang, V. Lindner, C. Saussine, D. Havel, F. Faure, and D. Jacqmin, "Microscopic venous invasion: a prognostic factor in renal cell carcinoma," *European Urology*, vol. 38, no. 5, pp. 600–605, 2000.

[10] A. F. Chambers and L. M. Matrisian, "Changing views of the role of matrix metalloproteinases in metastasis," *Journal of the National Cancer Institute*, vol. 89, no. 17, pp. 1260–1270, 1997.

[11] A. Sato, H. Nagase, D. Obinata et al., "Inhibition of MMP-9 using a pyrrole-imidazole polyamide reduces cell invasion in renal cell carcinoma," *International Journal of Oncology*, vol. 43, no. 5, pp. 1441–1446, 2013.

[12] D. J. Grignon, W. Sakr, M. Toth et al., "High levels of tissue inhibitor of metalloproteinase-2 (TIMP-2) expression are associated with poor outcome in invasive bladder cancer," *Cancer Research*, vol. 56, no. 7, pp. 1654–1659, 1996.

[13] N. Kawata, Y. Nagane, H. Hirakata et al., "Significant relationship of matrix metalloproteinase 9 with nuclear grade and prognostic impact of tissue inhibitor of metalloproteinase 2 for incidental clear cell renal cell carcinoma," *Urology*, vol. 69, no. 6, pp. 1049–1053, 2007.

[14] T. Ishimura, I. Sakai, I. Hara, H. Eto, and H. Miyake, "Microscopic venous invasion in renal cell carcinoma as a predictor of recurrence after radical surgery," *International Journal of Urology*, vol. 11, no. 5, pp. 264–268, 2004.

[15] M. F. Dall'Oglio, A. A. Antunes, Á. S. Sarkis et al., "Microvascular tumour invasion in renal cell carcinoma: the most important prognostic factor," *BJU International*, vol. 100, no. 3, pp. 552–555, 2007.

[16] N. Kawata, K. Yamaguchi, H. Hirakata, T. Hachiya, T. Yoshida, and Y. Takimoto, "Immunosuppressive acidic protein detects high nuclear grade localized renal cell carcinoma," *Urology*, vol. 66, no. 4, pp. 736–740, 2005.

[17] C. Zhang, X. Li, H. Hao, W. Yu, Z. He, and L. Zhou, "The correlation between size of renal cell carcinoma and its histopathological characteristics: a single center study of 1867 renal cell carcinoma cases," *BJU International*, vol. 110, no. 11 B, pp. E481–E485, 2012.

20

The Regulatory Role of MicroRNAs in EMT and Cancer

Apostolos Zaravinos

Department of Laboratory Medicine, Karolinska Institutet Huddinge, 171 77 Stockholm, Sweden

Correspondence should be addressed to Apostolos Zaravinos; apostolos.zaravinos@ki.se

Academic Editor: Panos Papageorgis

The epithelial to mesenchymal transition (EMT) is a powerful process in tumor invasion, metastasis, and tumorigenesis and describes the molecular reprogramming and phenotypic changes that are characterized by a transition from polarized immotile epithelial cells to motile mesenchymal cells. It is now well known that miRNAs are important regulators of malignant transformation and metastasis. The aberrant expression of the miR-200 family in cancer and its involvement in the initiation and progression of malignant transformation has been well demonstrated. The metastasis suppressive role of the miR-200 members is strongly associated with a pathologic EMT. This review describes the most recent advances regarding the influence of miRNAs in EMT and the control they exert in major signaling pathways in various cancers. The ability of the autocrine TGF-β/ZEB/miR-200 signaling regulatory network to control cell plasticity between the epithelial and mesenchymal state is further discussed. Various miRNAs are reported to directly target EMT transcription factors and components of the cell architecture, as well as miRNAs that are able to reverse the EMT process by targeting the Notch and Wnt signaling pathways. The link between cancer stem cells and EMT is also reported and the most recent developments regarding clinical trials that are currently using anti-miRNA constructs are further discussed.

1. Epithelial to Mesenchymal Transition (EMT)

The epithelial to mesenchymal transition is a unique process that describes the molecular reprogramming and phenotypic changes characterized by a transition from polarized immotile epithelial cells to motile mesenchymal cells, thus leading to increased motility and invasion. This transition is characterized by a decrease in the expression of proteins that enhance cell-cell contact such as E-cadherin and γ-catenin, as well as an increase in the expression of mesenchymal markers such as vimentin, N-cadherin, and fibronectin, as well as the activity of some matrix metalloproteinases. EMT was initially identified during embryogenesis and was later shown to be involved in neural crest [1] and heart-valve formation [2] and palate fusion [3]. More recently, EMT was shown to play a critical role in tumor invasion and metastasis [4]. EMT is categorized into developmental (Type I), fibrosis and wound healing (Type II), and cancer (Type III) [5]. Mesenchymal to epithelial transition (MET) [6] is the reverse process and also plays an important role in the formation of the kidney nephron epithelium. It is now widely known that EMT constitutes an early metastatic step [7], where cells that have undergone EMT can detach from the primary tumor, invade through the basement membrane into the circulation, and converse back to an epithelial phenotype to form a metastasis at a distant secondary site [8].

2. Signaling Pathways Involved in EMT

Various signaling pathways can induce EMT and include key molecules such as transforming growth factor beta (TGF-β), growth factors that act through tyrosine kinase receptors (RTKs), like platelet-derived growth factor (PDGF) and fibroblast growth factor receptors (FGFRs) [4, 9], and the proteins nuclear factor kappa-light-chain-enhancer of activated B cells (NF-κB), Wnt (*wingless integrated*), and Notch and hedgehog (Hh) proteins [10] (Figure 1). These signaling pathways stimulate transcription factors like Snail, basic helix-loop-helix (bHLH), zinc finger E-box-binding homeobox1/2 (ZEB1/2), and NF-κB, among others, that repress epithelial gene expression and act as activators of EMT [11]. These proteins bind to the promoter of E-cadherin silencing its expression. E-cadherin is a central component of the adherens junction complex, responsible for the calcium-dependent cell-cell adhesion and the maintenance of the cytoskeletal

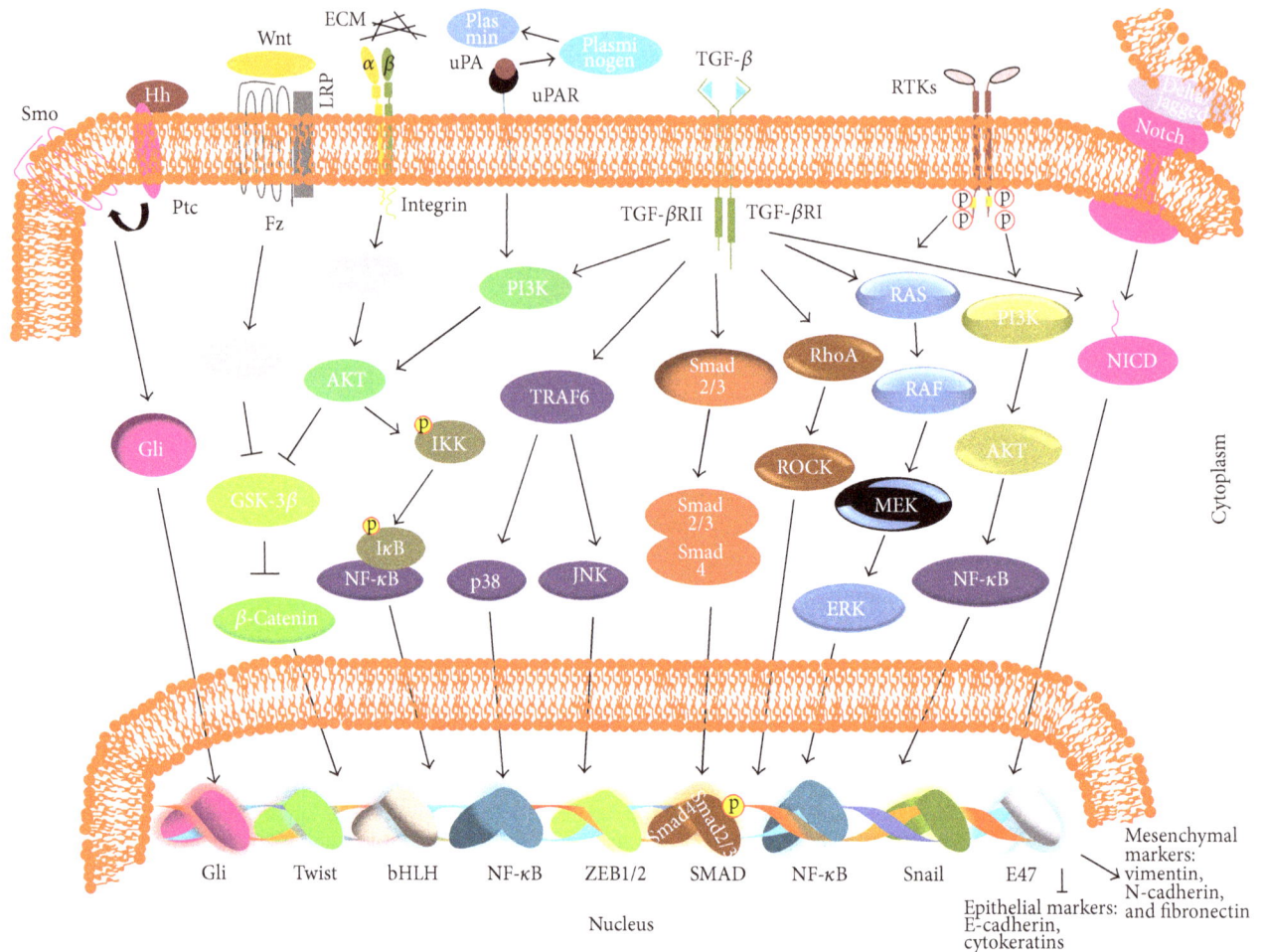

FIGURE 1: Major interconnected signaling pathways that regulate EMT. The Smad pathway for TGF-β signaling acts through the formation of a complex between Smad 2/3 and Smad 4. The complex then moves to the nucleus and stimulates the transcription of target genes. Sharp arrows denote activation/upregulation and blunt arrows denote inhibition/downregulation. Fz: frizzled receptors; Gli: glioma-associated oncogene family of transcription factors; GSK-3b: glycogen synthase kinase; Hh: hedgehog; PI3K: phosphatidylinositol-3-kinase; ILK: integrin-linked kinase; LRP: low-density lipoprotein receptor-related protein; p38 MAPK: mitogen-activated protein kinase; Ptc: patched receptor for Hh signaling; SMO: smoothened; TGF-β: transforming growth factor β; uPAR: urokinase plasminogen activator receptor.

organization. Its loss is a causal factor in cancer progression. Transcriptional repression of E-cadherin is an important emerging mechanism through which the gene is downregulated during tumor progression and several transcription factors, among them Snail, Slug/Snail2, ZEB1, ZEB2, and E47, directly bind to its promoter and repress its transcription. EMT is induced through various channels. Many of these E-cadherin repressors are induced by the stimulation of the TGF-β pathway and they can further repress the transcription of other cell polarity and adhesion genes [12] (Figure 1).

TGF-β is a major inducer of EMT [13–15]. It binds to its receptors (TGF-βRI, TGF-βRII, and TGF-βRIII) leading to the activation through phosphorylation of Smad 2 and Smad 3. These in turn form trimers with Smad 4 and the complex is translocated into the nucleus where it regulates the expression of TGF-β target genes along with other DNA binding factors, like Snail, ZEB, and Twist [16, 17]. The result is the downregulation of epithelial markers (E-cadherin and cytokeratins)

and the upregulation of mesenchymal markers (vimentin, N-cadherin, and fibronectin). The activation of RTKs and their downstream signaling effectors such as MAPK or PI3K is crucial for an increased rate of cell proliferation in epithelial cells. Signaling via either MAPK or PI3K along with TGF-β is also necessary and sufficient to regulate EMT [18]. Crosstalk of TGF-β with other signaling pathways like Notch, Wnt/β-catenin, NF-κB, and RTKs can also induce EMT which further helps in maintaining the mesenchymal phenotype of metastatic tumor cells [4, 9, 10, 19] (Figure 1).

Wnt signaling is also important for the regulation of EMT and diverse cell functions via canonical (β-catenin) or noncanonical pathways [20]. The formation of the Wnt-Fz-LRP complex through the binding of wnt1 and wnt3 ligands to their receptors, Frizzled (Fz) and LDL-receptor-related protein 5/6 (LRP 5/6), initiates the canonical pathway. Without the Wnt signaling pathway, cytoplasmic β-catenin forms a complex with Axin, adenomatous polyposis coli

(APC), glycogen synthase kinase-3b (GSK-3β), and casein kinase 1 (Ck1) [21]. When the cell receives Wnt signals, LRP5/6 and Fz form a complex. These structures affect the stabilization of β-catenin, its translocation to the nucleus, and its protein accumulation. In the nucleus, β-catenin forms a complex with T-cell factor/lymphoid enhancer factor (TCF/LEF) initiating the transcription of Wnt target genes, including Snail1 [21, 22]. During EMT, Smad 2 and Smad 4 influence Wnt signaling to repress E-cadherin expression in medial-edge epithelial cells (Figure 1).

Another important pathway in EMT is Hedgehog (Hh) signaling. Hh is a major regulator of cell proliferation, differentiation, and tissue polarity. The Hh family consists of three Hh proteins, including Sonic Hedgehog, Desert Hedgehog, and Indian Hedgehog [23]. Binding of Hh ligands to their receptors causes activation of a family of transcriptional factors through complex cascades. This leads to the upregulation of Wnt protein β-catenin and bone morphogenic protein accumulation in the cytoplasm. Wnt and Hh signaling are both mediated by the G-protein coupled Frizzled receptors, and both pathways prevent phosphorylation-dependent proteolysis of β-catenin. In addition, the molecules involved in Wnt signaling such as GSK-3β also regulate Hh signaling, suggesting crosstalk between the two potential pathways (Figure 1).

The Notch signaling pathway is also considered an important regulator for EMT induction, despite several reports that Notch signaling is insufficient to completely induce EMT and it requires crosstalk with other signaling molecules [20]. The Notch pathway is initiated through interactions between the Notch receptor and ligands on adjacent cells. Four Notch receptors (1–4) and five ligands (Dll-1, Dll-3, Dll-4, Jagged-1, and Jagged-2) have been shown to exist in mammals [24, 25]. Notch signaling is initiated through ligand binding to an adjacent receptor. Subsequently, the intramembrane Notch receptor (NICD) is cleaved by γ-secretase. The released NICD then translocates to the nucleus and interacts with C-protein binding factor 1/Suppressor of Hairless/Lag-1 (CBF1/Su (H)/Lag 1) [25, 26] and acts as an activator of target genes, including Hes and Hey (Figure 1). The Notch pathway maintains a balance between cell proliferation, differentiation, and apoptosis and plays an important role in determining cell fate and maintaining progenitor cell population. Notch signaling requires coordination with other signals to promote EMT. TGF-β increases Notch activity through Smad 3, subsequently promoting Slug expression which suppresses E-cadherin [27]. Slug-induced EMT is accompanied by the activation of β-catenin and resistance to anoikis. Wnt and Notch pathways have also been shown to cross-link between each other in order to induce a tumorigenic phenotype [19, 28].

E-cadherin is anchored to the cytoskeleton via β-catenin, a cytoplasmic plaque protein [29]. In loss of cell adhesion, during invasion, E-cadherin is endocytosed and β-catenin is released. In normal and noninvasive cells, β-catenin is usually localized to the cell membrane. In cells undergoing EMT, β-catenin is located in the cytoplasm. This cytosolic β-catenin translocates to the nucleus to promote transcription of genes that induce EMT (Figure 1).

The integrin-linked kinase (ILK) pathway has also been reported to induce EMT. Integrins are heterodimeric adhesion receptors composed of α and β subunits. There are 18 α and 8 β subunits that variously combine into 24 different integrins. Integrins bind to ligands, including collagens, laminins, and fibronectin in the ECM. Ligand-bound integrins induce several signaling cascades that control cell polarity, motility, survival, shape, proliferation, and differentiation [30] (Figure 1).

uPAR (urokinase-type plasminogen activator receptor) signaling also plays a role in EMT [31]. Urokinase was originally isolated from human urine but can also be present in several other locations including the ECM. The main physiological substrate for urokinase plasminogen activator (uPA) is plasminogen. When uPA, a serine protease, binds to uPAR, plasminogen is activated to form plasmin (Figure 1). Activation of plasmin triggers a proteolytic cascade that can participate in ECM remodeling, degrading components of the basement membrane, and hence allowing cells to move across and through these barriers [31, 32]. Binding of uPA to uPAR can induce EMT through activating a number of cell-signaling factors, including PI3K, Src family kinases, Akt, ERK/MAPK, and myosin light chain kinase [33, 34]. Among them, only the PI3K/AKT pathway has been studied in uPAR signaling in EMT. Activation of PI3K signaling catalyzes the formation of phosphatidylinositol 3,4,5-phosphate, which can influence cell morphology through its effect on actin cytoskeleton reorganization and migration [32]. Another mechanism by which PI3K may also be involved is through the activation of AKT, which can promote cell invasion [32] and regulate the activity of transcription factors like NF-κB that binds to the DNA sequence and induce EMT [35].

3. MicroRNAs (miRNAs)

miRNAs are small (19–25 nucleotides long) noncoding, single-stranded RNAs that control gene expression by targeting mRNA transcripts and leading to their translational repression or degradation, according to the level of complementarity with them [36, 37]. To date, over 2,500 potential human miRNAs have been recorded in miRBase v20 [36] and their number is increasing rapidly. Taking into account that one miRNA can target many mRNA transcripts and that one mRNA transcript can be targeted by many miRNAs, it can be roughly estimated that ~10–40% of the mRNA sequences are targeted by miRNAs in human [38]. Therefore, there is a great need to validate the targets of newly discovered miRNAs.

miRNAs can be both differentially and temporally expressed in a tissue- and developmental-specific mode [39–42]. Various miRNA signatures can accurately distinguish tumor from normal tissue, as well as various cancerous subtypes among them [39]. Furthermore, it is now well established that miRNAs can serve as candidate biomarkers for diagnostic and prognostic purposes [40, 43]. miRNA genes are usually intronic and clustered and are transcribed by RNA polymerase II producing a primary miRNA (pri-miRNA) of several kb in length. Pri-miRNAs are cleaved at specific sites in the nucleus (resulting in pre-miRNAs) and in the cytoplasm (resulting in mature miRNAs), by the RNases Drosha by Dicer, respectively [44]. Mature miRNAs are then activated by binding to the Argonaute 2 (AGO2) in the miRNA-induced silencing complex (miRISC) [45]. In particular, the "seed" sequence across nucleotides 2–8 at the $5'$ end of the mature miRNA binds its complementary sequence within the $3'$ UTRs of its target mRNA transcripts. Perfect complementarity between the miRNA and its mRNA target often leads to mRNA deadenylation and degradation, whereas imperfect complementarity leads to the inhibition of translation [46]. Mature miRNAs can also regulate gene expression by binding to the $5'$ UTR of their target genes or their coding regions (CDS) [47]. CDS-based sites are more effective at inhibiting translation, whereas sites in the $3'$ UTR are more specialized for promoting degradation [47]. Many miRNAs are now known to suppress various important cancer-related genes, therefore, acting as oncogenes or tumor suppressors [48]. Several miRNAs have been identified to regulate EMT.

4. The miR-200 Family and Its Metastasis Suppressive Role in Cancer

The miR-200 family is composed of 5 miRNA sequences: miR-200a, miR-200b, miR-200c, miR-141, and miR-429, clustered and expressed as two separate polycistronic pri-miRNA transcripts: miR-200a, miR-200b, and miR-429 (chromosome 1) and miR-200c and miR-141 (chromosome 12) [49]. The miR-200 family plays an essential role in EMT suppression mainly through targeting ZEB and its function was recently reviewed [50–52]. The role of miR-200 in EMT and tumor progression has been linked to several cancers [53–63]. Gregory et al. found markedly low miR-200 levels in cells that had undergone EMT, in response to TGF-β. The enforced miR-200 expression alone was also shown to be sufficient to prevent TGF-β-induced EMT and miR-200 inhibition was sufficient to induce EMT. Conversely, ectopic expression of the miR-200 members in mesenchymal cells initiated MET [64]. Moreover, in invasive breast cancer, the lack of miR-200 expression was positively correlated with absent E-cadherin [64]. Further supporting these results, both miR-200 clusters were shown to be clearly downregulated in a TGF-β inducible mouse model of mammary tumor with EMT. The overexpression of miR-200 members caused E-cadherin upregulation and inhibited EMT via targeting the transcription factors ZEB1 and ZEB2 [65].

The metastasis suppressive role of the miR-200 family was further studied in tumor cell lines derived from mice that develop metastatic lung adenocarcinoma owing to expression of mutant K-ras and p53. Following a TGF-β treatment, the cells entered EMT and this transition was entirely miR-200 dependent [63]. Furthermore, in non-small-cell lung cancer (NSCLC) cell lines, miR-200 was correlated with EMT markers, distinguishing between those lines that derived from primary lung tumors and the ones that originated from metastatic lesions [63]. In metastatic NSCLC cells, the reexpression of miR-200 downregulated genes that are involved in metastasis signaling and proliferation, such as DLC1, ATRX, HFE, HNRNPR3, HFE, and ATRX [66]. The miR-200 expression was also demonstrated to change the tumor microenvironment and inhibit EMT and metastasis,

in lung adenocarcinoma [67]. miR-200 was further reported to enhance macroscopic metastases in mouse breast cancer cell lines [56]. Dykxhoorn et al. [56] reported that, for some tumors, tumor colonization at metastatic sites might be enhanced by MET, which suggests that the epithelial nature of a tumor does not predict metastatic outcome.

5. The TGF-β/ZEB/miR-200 Regulatory Network

Gregory et al. recently demonstrated the existence of an autocrine TGF-β/ZEB/miR-200 signaling regulatory network that controls the plasticity between the epithelial and mesenchymal states of the cells. Strong correlation was reported between the ZEB1/2 and TGF-β and negative correlations were detected between miR-200 and TGF-β, as well as between miR-200 and ZEB1/2, in invasive ductal carcinomas [68]. ZEB1/2 can induce EMT by repressing various epithelial genes [69]. The TGF-β signaling pathway is a central activator of ZEB1/2, indicating that they are important intracellular mediators of the TGF-β-induced EMT. The crosstalk between the ZEB/miR-200 axis and several signal transduction pathways activated at different stages of tumor development was also reviewed recently [70]. ZEB1/2 and the miR-200 family are involved in a double-negative feedback loop, which controls EMT and MET programs both in development and tumorigenesis [70]. On one hand, the miR-200 members target and suppress ZEB1/2 and promote epithelial differentiation [64, 71, 72]. On the other hand, ZEB1 knockdown can enhance miR-200 [73] (Figure 2). This was supported when it was found that the common promoter region of the miR-200 members includes highly conserved ZEB-binding sites, through which ZEB factors control the transcription of the miR-200 family [73, 74]. ZEB downregulation leads to the enhancement of an epithelial pattern of gene expression through induction of the miR-200 members. On the contrary, ZEB expression induces a mesenchymal pattern of gene expression through miR-200 suppression. This feedback loop was shown to play important roles in the stabilization of cellular differentiation in response to prevalent extracellular cues [75]. In gastric cancer, miR-200b can control metastasis by regulating the expression of ZEB2 [76]. Cong et al. found inversely related expression levels between miR-200a and ZEB1/2 in gastric adenocarcinoma tissue arrays. The upregulated miR-200a expression was also found to increase E-cadherin and suppress the Wnt/β-catenin pathway by targeting ZEB1/2 in gastric adenocarcinoma, thus delaying tumor growth in vivo [77].

The permanence of the mesenchymal phenotype following EMT is sustained by TGF-β-containing autocrine loops (Figure 2) [78–80]. TGF-β can induce its own autocrine production, cooperating with the RAF-MAPK and the β-catenin signaling pathways that trigger EMT [81, 82]. TGF-β2 is a predominant target of the miR-200 family and the relief of miR-200-mediated inhibition of TGF-β2 increases the autocrine effect of TGF-β [73] (Figure 2). Therefore, the interconnection among TGF-β, miR-200, and ZEB can explain the reversibility of the mesenchymal phenotype. Nevertheless, the mechanism by which the

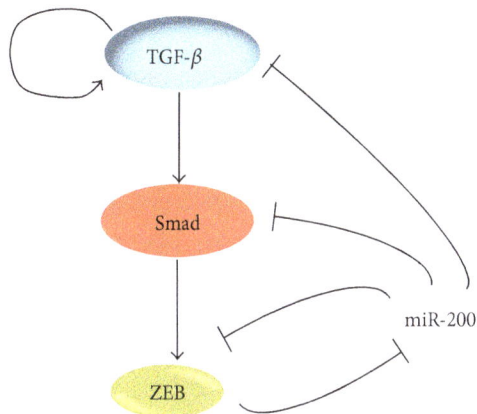

FIGURE 2: The TGF-β/ZEB/miR-200 regulatory network.

ZEB/miR-200 loop activates autocrine TGF-β signaling is not clear enough. One explanation is that Smads bind to the promoter of ZEB and induce its TGF-β-mediated transcription [68, 83] (Figure 2). On the other hand, the autocrine TGF-β signaling was shown to induce a reversible methylation of the miR-200 loci, through the recruitment of histone-modifying complexes by ZEB proteins. Smad and TGF-β were further shown to be direct targets of miR-200 [84] (Figure 2). Recently, microenvironment-dependent cues were suggested to trigger miRNA-regulated feedback loops facilitating the switch between EMT and MET [85]. Although many TGF-β-induced pathways are necessary for the induction and maintenance of EMT [86], it is not clear how they control the expression of ZEB.

6. Other EMT-Regulating miRNAs

6.1. miRNAs That Control EMT Transcription Factors. Many other miRNAs can directly target EMT transcription factors. miR-205 acts synergistically with miR-200 members in order to suppress ZEB and lead to MET [64]. In mammary gland cells, miR-205 maintains the epithelial differentiation [87–89]. In prostate cancer, miR-29b suppresses metastasis by regulating EMT signaling [90]. Also, miR-30a is downregulated during EMT in murine hepatocytes [91]. Furthermore, in NSCLC, Snail is posttranscriptionally targeted by miRNA-30a [92]. In hepatoma cells, miR-148a can negatively regulate Met/Snail signaling and prevent EMT and metastasis [93]. Snail and miR-34 form another double feedback loop, in which the first binds to E-boxes that are located within the promoter of the miR-34 gene, thereby leading to the transcriptional repression of the second [94]. In TGF-β-induced EMT, increased Snail expression can suppress miR-34. A novel miR-203/SNAI1 feedback loop was also reported in breast cancer [95]. These double-feedback loops can enhance the activation of EMT and control the balance between the two states of the cell (epithelial and mesenchymal). Recently, a novel EMT network integrating the negative feedback loops, miR-203/SNAI1 and miR-200/ZEB, was proposed to function as a switch that controls the plasticity of epithelial cells during their differentiation and the progression of cancer [95]. In

metastatic breast cancer cells, the expression of miR-10b was shown to be induced by the transcription factor Twist, which binds directly to the putative promoter of miR-10b [96]. The Twist-induced miR-10b thereby inhibits translation of the mRNA encoding homeobox D10, resulting in the increased expression of RHOC, a well-characterized prometastatic gene [96].

6.2. miRNAs Targeting Components of the Cell Architecture. Many miRNAs interfere with EMT by targeting components of the cell architecture [97–102]. A direct transcriptional target of the TGF-β/Smad 4 signaling is miR-155 [103]. Its knockdown can suppress TGF-β-induced EMT and the dissolution of tight junctions, as well as cell migration and invasion [99]. Furthermore, the ectopic expression of miR-155 can reduce the expression of RhoA (Ras homolog gene family, member A) protein, a small GTPase protein known to regulate the actin cytoskeleton in the formation of stress fibers and disrupt the formation of tight junctions [99].

In colon cancer cells upon treatment with TGF-β, miR-21 and miR-31 were induced and could lead to enhanced cellular motility and invasiveness. Their elevated expression was associated with lymph node positivity and the development of distant metastases in patients suffering from colorectal cancer [104]. In the progression of colorectal cancer, both miRNAs could promote TGF-β-induced EMT, by repressing the translation of TIAM1 (T-cell lymphoma invasion and metastasis 1), a guanidine exchange factor of the Rac GTPase [101]. In established metastases, the activation of miR-31 was shown to lead to regression of metastasis and prolongation of patient survival. Furthermore, its induction could reduce the metastatic potential of cancer cells, via targeting RhoA [105].

In human breast cancer cells, miR-9 is upregulated and directly represses cadherin-1 (CDH1), a calcium-dependent protein involved in mechanisms regulating cell-cell adhesions, mobility, and proliferation of epithelial cells. CDH1 repression leads to increased cell motility and invasiveness [106]. Furthermore, the loss of E-cadherin liberates β-catenin which translocates into the nucleus and activates prometastatic genes, such as VEGF [107], which in turn leads to increased tumor angiogenesis. During EMT, E-cadherin suppression is often accompanied by upregulation of N-cadherin. On the other hand, miR-194 negatively regulated the expression of N-cadherin. However, miR-194 expression is attenuated in advanced stage gastric cancer cells, whereas in mesenchymal hepatic cancer cells, miR-194 expression is enhanced and N-cadherin, cell migration, invasion, and metastasis are reduced [108].

In hepatocellular carcinoma cells (HCC), miR-490-3p enhances cell proliferation, migration, and invasion abilities and stimulates EMT, via targeting ERGIC3 (ER-Golgi intermediate compartment protein 3), also known as endoplasmic reticulum-localized protein/ERp43. ERGIC3 is a protein with a possible role in transport between ER and Golgi [109]. Overexpression of ERp43 was shown to accelerate cell growth and to inhibit ER stress-induced cell death, while its downregulation decreased the rate of cellular proliferation and enhanced cell death [110]. ERGIC3 was also shown to stimulate cell migration and their ability to invade [109].

The same authors found that, in HCC cells, miR-490-3p led to increased cell proliferation, migration, and invasion, thus contributing to EMT. ERGIC3 was shown to be directly targeted by miR-490-3p, which unexpectedly increased its mRNA and protein levels [109].

Furthermore, miR-29a was found to be the most highly upregulated miRNA during EMT in response to TGF-β in the murine mesenchymal, metastatic RasXT cells relative to epithelial EpRas cells. miR-29a can target tristetraproline (TTP), a protein involved in the degradation of messenger RNAs with AU-rich 3′-untranslated regions, and led to EMT and metastasis in cooperation with oncogenic Ras signaling [100]. All these results demonstrate the ability of miRNAs to regulate EMT in cancer progression, via the targeting of components of the cell architecture.

6.3. miRNAs Targeting Multiple EMT/MET Components.

Some miRNAs regulate EMT by targeting either the receptors that accept signals from EMT inducers or multiple EMT/MET components. TGF-βRII and Snail2 were demonstrated to be directly targeted by miR-204. A reduction in miR-204 expression led to reduced levels of claudins 10, 16, and 19 [111]. miR-204 has dual roles in maintaining the integrity of the epithelium, since it can also target Snail, which is rapidly induced by TGF-β signaling during EMT [111].

The Eph tyrosine kinase receptor A4 (EphA4) regulates MET of the paraxial mesoderm during somite morphogenesis [112]. It also promotes cell proliferation and migration through an EphA4-FGFR1 signaling pathway [113]. In HCC, miR-10a targets EphA4 and regulates the metastatic properties of the cancer cells [114]. EphA4 knockdown phenocopied the effect of miR-10a and its ectopic expression restored the effect of miR-10a on migration, invasion, and adhesion in HCC cells [114].

The induction of EMT in luminal breast cancer cells involves the downregulation of miR-200 members and the upregulation of the miR-221 family [115]. Luminal cells expressing miR-221/222 gained a more mesenchymal phenotype and increased cell motility and invasiveness [115], whereas the inhibition of miR-221/222 in basal-like cells promoted MET [116]. Providing a functional link between miR-221/222 expression and E-cadherin repression in breast cancer cells, miR-221/222 could directly target trichorhinophalangeal 1 (TRPS1), a transcriptional repressor of ZEB2 [115, 117]. miR-221/222 can also repress Dicer, a key protein in the maturation of miRNAs [118].

In squamous cells, miR-138 was shown to regulate EMT by targeting components of the EMT pathways, such as RhoC (Ras homolog gene family, member C) and ROCK2 (Rho-associated, coiled-coil containing protein kinase 2) [119]. Its enhanced expression could repress RhoC and ROCK2 in tongue squamous cell carcinoma, leading to diminished cellular migration and invasion [120]. Additionally, miR-138 regulates EMT either via direct targeting vimentin or via targeting ZEB2, which in turn regulates the transcription activity Cadherin-1. Furthermore, it can regulate EMT through targeting the epigenetic regulator enhancer of zeste homologue 2 (EZH2), which in turn modulates its gene silencing effects on downstream genes (e.g., E-cadherin)

[121]. miR-101 was recently reported to act as a crucial tumor suppressor which suppresses cell proliferation, invasiveness, and self-renewal in aggressive endometrial cancer cells via the modulation multiple critical oncogenes [122]. The axis miR-101-EZH2/MCL-1/FOS was proposed to be a potential therapeutic target for endometrial cancer [122].

6.4. miR-200 Members Regulate the Notch and Wnt Signaling Pathways.

Recently, a coupling between the ZEB/miR-200 axis and the Notch pathway was established in cancer [123–125]. ZEB1 was shown to trigger Notch signaling by stabilizing the expression of Jagged1, Maml2, and Maml3, through inhibition of the miR-200 members [124]. This suggests that the ZEB-dependent downregulation of miR-200 feeds back positively on ZEB expression and results in the stabilization of a mesenchymal cell phenotype [124].

Furthermore, a functional link was recently established between the canonical Wnt pathway and ZEB1, demonstrating that ZEB1 is a direct transcriptional target of β-catenin in colon cancer cells [126, 127]. However, the ZEB2/Wnt relationship in colon cancer yet remains unclear. Wnt signaling is also connected with the ZEB/miR-200 network in cancer. miR-200a was reported to downregulate β-catenin-mediated transcription via targeting either ZEB or β-catenin, thus downregulating the activation of Wnt/β-catenin signaling [128] (Figure 3). In contrast, miR-200b and miR-200c have no effect on β-catenin.

6.5. The ZEB/miR-200 Network and p53 Family Members.

The p53 transcription factor can induce or repress a large set of genes and miRNAs [129, 130]. The p53 and its homologs p63 and p73 are well involved in tumor metastasis and tumor progression [131–133]. The p63 and p73 members exist as full-size proteins (TAp63 and TAp73) or truncated forms (ΔNp63 and ΔNp73) that lack the transcriptional activation domain. In early studies, it was demonstrated that ΔNp63/73 expression is directly repressed by ZEB binding, establishing a link between the ZEB proteins and the p53 family. In addition, TAp73 isoforms were also found to be repressed to a lesser extent during myoblast differentiation and in mouse embryonic fibroblasts (MEFs) [134] (Figure 4).

In hepatocellular carcinoma (HCC), p53 upregulates the miR-200, miR-192, and other miRNAs [135]. The p53 protein inhibits EMT by downregulating the ZEB1/2 transcription factors. Furthermore, p53-regulated miR-200 and miR-192 family members were shown to be involved in a p53-adjusted EMT. Similarly, p53 knockdown could upregulate ZEB1 in epithelial cells, which in turn induced EMT and affected EMT-associated stem cell properties. On the other hand, p53 overexpression could reverse EMT and stem cell characteristics [136]. The work of Chang et al. reveals a role for p53 in regulating EMT-MET and stemness and implies a potential therapy of the suppression of cancer stem cells (CSCs), which is associated with EMT through the activation of the p53-miR-200 pathway. The above-mentioned findings elucidate a new function of p53 in which it ensures the epithelial properties. Although the p63/p73 genes are overexpressed as different isoforms, the p53 gene is usually mutated in a majority of carcinomas. Thus, in the absence of p53, p63

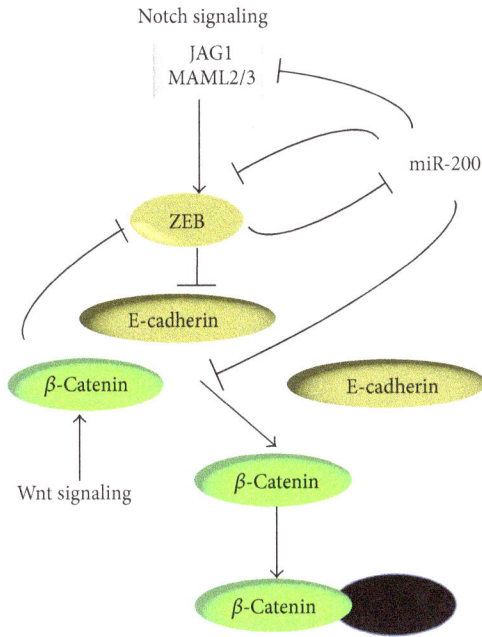

FIGURE 3: Regulation of the Notch and Wnt signaling pathways by miR-200.

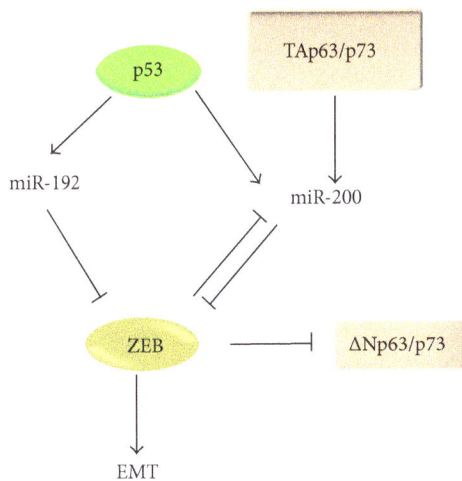

FIGURE 4: The ZEB/miR-200 network and the p53 family members.

and p73 may be involved in the control of the ZEB/miR-200 loop. In fact, both proteins have been identified as positive regulators of miR-200 in ovarian carcinoma cells by directly modulating its promoter activity [137].

7. EMT as a Characteristic of Cancer Stem Cells (CSCs)

The term cancer stem cell was adopted in 2006 [138] to define the population of cancer cells with the ability to self-renew and differentiate just like the stem cells. The name, cancer stem cell, was invented to represent its properties of self-renewal and multipotency. CSCs can self-renew but it is debatable whether they can differentiate into multiple types

of cells. Also, the term CSCs implies that these cells have originated from normal stem cells. The stem cells may be a source of origin of CSCs, but they are certainly not the only source [139]. For these reasons, many prefer to call them tumor initiating cells.

Many studies have recently linked the CSC phenotype to tumor cells undergoing EMT [140–148]. Morel et al. [141] recently showed that nontumorigenic mammary epithelial cells can give rise to a cell population that displays CD44+CD24– stem-like signatures through the activation of the RAS/MAPK pathway. This cell population displays an EMT phenotype that is characterized by the loss of E-cadherin and gain of vimentin expression [140, 141]. The linkage between EMT and stemness is further supported by the finding that Snail1 or Twist expression resulted in the loss of epithelial phenotype and the acquisition of mesenchymal phenotype in mammary epithelial cells and that the constitutive expression of either protein increased tumor initiating potential in transformed mammary epithelial cells [149, 150].

In prostate cancers, invasive cells exhibited CSC-like characteristics in an in vitro study of established and primary prostate cell lines. These cells were more tumorigenic than their counterparts and had a higher expression of the surface marker CD44, as well as of genes involved in the maintenance of a stem cell phenotype, including Nanog [151]. Although these authors did not investigate spontaneous metastasis by the invasive cells in vivo, Mulholland et al. [152] showed that EMT promotes the metastasis of cells with CSC characteristics. They engineered a mouse model of prostate cancer that better reflects the human situation, notably in terms of metastasis. The authors showed that RAS activation in PTEN-null cells resulted in EMT and that these EMT-induced cells had CSC characteristics and were responsible for micro- and macrometastases [152]. Similar results linking EMT and stemness were recently reported for putative CSCs from cervical cancer cell lines [153].

8. miRNA-Based Therapeutics and Clinical Trials

We have now entered the era that miRNAs are in trials to be used as a therapeutic tool against cancer. Depending on their pro- or antitumoral properties, different strategies based on blocking miRNA function or specific miRNA delivery to the tumor cells can be used. Several preclinical approaches have been developed in order to block miRNAs, including anti-miRNA oligonucleotides, miRNA sponges, miRNA masks (target protectors), and small molecule inhibitors [154].

Despite the challenges presented in delivering these molecules to the cells, there are currently two clinical trials for miRNA-based therapeutics [155]. Targeting miRNAs may be used directly to target tumor cells and also to enhance other therapies. For example, they could be used in reducing the drug resistance of tumors as has been shown by the chemoresistant properties of miR-100 in NSCLC [156] and the epigenetic silencing of miR-199b-5p in chemoresistant ovarian carcinoma [157].

The most advanced miRNA trial involves the use of anti-miR-122 (miravirsen) for hepatitis C therapy [158], which shows reduction in viral RNA with no evidence of resistance. Miravirsen is complementary to miR-122 but has also a modified locked-nucleic acid (LNA) structure which provides resistance to degradation and increased affinity for its target. Apart from targeting the mature miR-122, miravirsen was shown to target both the pri- and pre-miR-122 forms, thus leading to reduced processing and enhancement of its therapeutic effect [159].

The first miRNA-based therapy for cancer is MIRX34. It entered clinical testing in 2013 and is currently being studied in a multicenter, open-label Phase 1 clinical trial in patients with unresectable primary liver cancer or solid cancers with liver involvement. The trial also includes a separate cohort of patients with hematological malignancies. MRX34 was designed to deliver a mimic of the naturally occurring tumor suppressor, miR-34, which is lost or underexpressed in tumors of patients with a wide variety of cancers, including cervical cancer, ovarian cancer, glioblastoma, hepatocellular carcinoma (liver cancer), colon cancer, and non-small-cell lung cancer (NSCLC) and in cancer stem cells [160–162]. The miR-34 mimic is encapsulated using an innovative liposomal formulation called SMARTICLES.

The MRX34 Phase 1 clinical study in liver-based cancers is expected to be completed at the end of the first quarter of 2015, while the top-line results from the hematological malignancy cohort are expected in mid-2015. The primary objectives of the clinical trial are to establish the maximum tolerated dose and the recommended Phase 2 dose for future clinical trials. The secondary objectives are to assess the safety, tolerability, and pharmacokinetic profile of MRX34 as well as assess any biological activity and clinical outcomes. Nevertheless, miRNA-therapeutics is still in its infancy and the side effects of these therapies need to be carefully evaluated.

9. Conclusion

EMT plays a major role in cancer metastasis and is a complex, multifunctional, and tightly regulated developmental program. Understanding the different strategies employed by tumor cells to switch EMT on and off and the biological functions of the increasing number of the newly discovered miRNAs will lead to the development of new strategies in the diagnosis, prognosis, and treatment of human cancers. We have now entered a new exciting era, where clinical trials utilizing miRNA profiling for patient prognosis and clinical response are underway, and the first miRNA mimic has already entered the clinic for cancer therapy.

Abbreviations

TGF-β: Transforming growth factor-beta
RTKs: Receptor tyrosine kinases
PDGF: Platelet-derived growth factor
FGFRs: Fibroblast growth factor receptors
PI3K: Phosphatidylinositol-3-kinase
NF-κB: Nuclear factor kappa-light-chain-enhancer of activated B cells
JNK: c-Jun N-terminal kinase

ERK: Ras/Raf/Mitogen-activated protein kinase/ERK kinase (MEK)/extracellular-signal-regulated kinase
GEF: Guanine nucleotide exchange factor
EMT: Epithelial to mesenchymal transition
MET: Mesenchymal to epithelial transition
miRISC: miRNA-induced silencing complex.

Conflict of Interests

The author declares that there is no conflict of interests regarding the publication of this paper.

References

[1] J. L. Duband, F. Monier, M. Delannet, and D. Newgreen, "Epithelium-mesenchyme transition during neural crest development," *Acta Anatomica*, vol. 154, no. 1, pp. 63–78, 1995.

[2] D. L. Bolender and R. R. Markwald, "Epithelial-mesenchymal transformation in chick atrioventricular cushion morphogenesis," *Scanning Electron Microscopy*, vol. 3, pp. 313–321, 1979.

[3] C. M. Griffith and E. D. Hay, "Epithelial-mesenchymal transformation during palatal fusion: carboxyfluorescein traces cells at light and electron microscopic levels," *Development*, vol. 116, no. 4, pp. 1087–1099, 1992.

[4] M. Yilmaz and G. Christofori, "EMT, the cytoskeleton, and cancer cell invasion," *Cancer and Metastasis Reviews*, vol. 28, no. 1-2, pp. 15–33, 2009.

[5] R. Kalluri and R. A. Weinberg, "The basics of epithelial-mesenchymal transition," *Journal of Clinical Investigation*, vol. 119, no. 6, pp. 1420–1428, 2009.

[6] U. Soomets, M. Hällbrink, and U. Langel, "Antisense properties of peptide nucleic acids," *Frontiers in Bioscience*, vol. 4, pp. D782–D786, 1999.

[7] J. P. Thiery and J. P. Sleeman, "Complex networks orchestrate epithelial-mesenchymal transitions," *Nature Reviews Molecular Cell Biology*, vol. 7, no. 2, pp. 131–142, 2006.

[8] J. P. Their, "Epithelial-mesenchymal transitions in tumor progression," *Nature Reviews Cancer*, vol. 2, no. 6, pp. 442–454, 2002.

[9] S. M. Hansen, V. Berezin, and E. Bock, "Signaling mechanisms of neurite outgrowth induced by the cell adhesion molecules NCAM and N-Cadherin," *Cellular and Molecular Life Sciences*, vol. 65, no. 23, pp. 3809–3821, 2008.

[10] G. Ouyang, Z. Wang, X. Fang, J. Liu, and C. J. Yang, "Molecular signaling of the epithelial to mesenchymal transition in generating and maintaining cancer stem cells," *Cellular and Molecular Life Sciences*, vol. 67, no. 15, pp. 2605–2618, 2010.

[11] J. P. Thiery, H. Acloque, R. Y. J. Huang, and M. A. Nieto, "Epithelial-mesenchymal transitions in development and disease," *Cell*, vol. 139, no. 5, pp. 871–890, 2009.

[12] S. Spaderna, O. Schmalhofer, M. Wahlbuhl et al., "The transcriptional repressor ZEB1 promotes metastasis and loss of cell polarity in cancer," *Cancer Research*, vol. 68, no. 2, pp. 537–544, 2008.

[13] L. D. Wood, D. W. Parsons, S. Jones et al., "The genomic landscapes of human breast and colorectal cancers," *Science*, vol. 318, pp. 1108–1113, 2007.

[14] S. Jones, X. Zhang, D. W. Parsons et al., "Core signaling pathways in human pancreatic cancers revealed by global genomic analyses," *Science*, vol. 321, no. 5897, pp. 1801–1806, 2008.

[15] S. Lamouille, J. Xu, and R. Derynck, "Molecular mechanisms of epithelial-mesenchymal transition," *Nature Reviews Molecular Cell Biology*, vol. 15, no. 3, pp. 178–196, 2014.

[16] J. Fuxe, T. Vincent, and A. G. de Herreros, "Transcriptional crosstalk between TGFβ and stem cell pathways in tumor cell invasion: role of EMT promoting Smad complexes," *Cell Cycle*, vol. 9, no. 12, pp. 2363–2374, 2010.

[17] J. Zavadil and E. P. Böttinger, "TGF-β and epithelial-to-mesenchymal transitions," *Oncogene*, vol. 24, no. 37, pp. 5764–5774, 2005.

[18] J. Gotzmann, M. Mikula, A. Eger et al., "Molecular aspects of epithelial cell plasticity: implications for local tumor invasion and metastasis," *Mutation Research—Reviews in Mutation Research*, vol. 566, no. 1, pp. 9–20, 2004.

[19] Y. Wang and B. P. Zhou, "Epithelial-mesenchymal transition in breast cancer progression and metastasis," *Chinese Journal of Cancer*, vol. 30, no. 9, pp. 603–611, 2011.

[20] M. Garg, "Epithelial-mesenchymal transition-activating transcription factors-multifunctional regulators in cancer," *World Journal of Stem Cells*, vol. 5, no. 4, pp. 188–195, 2013.

[21] B. T. MacDonald, K. Tamai, and X. He, "Wnt/β-catenin signaling: components, mechanisms, and diseases," *Developmental Cell*, vol. 17, no. 1, pp. 9–26, 2009.

[22] T. P. Rao and M. Kühl, "An updated overview on wnt signaling pathways: a prelude for more," *Circulation Research*, vol. 106, no. 12, pp. 1798–1806, 2010.

[23] F. H. Sarkar, Y. Li, Z. Wang, and D. Kong, "The role of nutraceuticals in the regulation of Wnt and Hedgehog signaling in cancer," *Cancer and Metastasis Reviews*, vol. 29, no. 3, pp. 383–394, 2010.

[24] L. Miele, "Notch signaling," *Clinical Cancer Research*, vol. 12, no. 4, pp. 1074–1079, 2006.

[25] Z. Wang, Y. Li, D. Kong, and F. H. Sarkar, "The role of notch signaling pathway in Epithelial-Mesenchymal Transition (EMT) during development and tumor aggressiveness," *Current Drug Targets*, vol. 11, no. 6, pp. 745–751, 2010.

[26] S. J. Bray, "Notch signalling: a simple pathway becomes complex," *Nature Reviews Molecular Cell Biology*, vol. 7, no. 9, pp. 678–689, 2006.

[27] K. G. Leong, K. Niessen, I. Kulic et al., "Jagged1-mediated Notch activation induces epithelial-to-mesenchymal transition through Slug-induced repression of E-cadherin," *Journal of Experimental Medicine*, vol. 204, no. 12, pp. 2935–2948, 2007.

[28] G. M. Collu and K. Brennan, "Cooperation between Wnt and Notch signalling in human breast cancer," *Breast Cancer Research*, vol. 9, no. 3, article 105, 2007.

[29] M. J. Wheelock and K. R. Johnson, "Cadherin-mediated cellular signaling," *Current Opinion in Cell Biology*, vol. 15, no. 5, pp. 509–514, 2003.

[30] M. Zeisberg and E. G. Neilson, "Biomarkers for epithelial-mesenchymal transitions," *The Journal of Clinical Investigation*, vol. 119, no. 6, pp. 1429–1437, 2009.

[31] Q. Wang, Y. Wang, Y. Zhang, and W. Xiao, "The role of uPAR in epithelial-mesenchymal transition in small airway epithelium of patients with chronic obstructive pulmonary disease," *Respiratory Research*, vol. 14, no. 1, article 67, 2013.

[32] N. Chandrasekar, S. Mohanam, M. Gujrati, W. C. Olivero, D. H. Dinh, and J. S. Rao, "Downregulation of uPA inhibits migration and PI3k/Akt signaling in glioblastoma cells," *Oncogene*, vol. 22, no. 3, pp. 392–400, 2003.

[33] M. Jo, R. D. Lester, V. Montel, B. Eastman, S. Takimoto, and S. L. Gonias, "Reversibility of epithelial-mesenchymal transition (EMT) induced in breast cancer cells by activation of urokinase receptor-dependent cell signaling," *The Journal of Biological Chemistry*, vol. 284, no. 34, pp. 22825–22833, 2009.

[34] R. D. Lester, M. Jo, V. Montel, S. Takimoto, and S. L. Gonias, "uPAR induces epithelial-mesenchymal transition in hypoxic breast cancer cells," *Journal of Cell Biology*, vol. 178, no. 3, pp. 425–436, 2007.

[35] L. Larue and A. Bellacosa, "Epithelial-mesenchymal transition in development and cancer: role of phosphatidinositol 3′ kinase/AKT pathways," *Oncogene*, vol. 24, no. 50, pp. 7443–7454, 2005.

[36] A. Kozomara and S. Griffiths-Jones, "MiRBase: integrating microRNA annotation and deep-sequencing data," *Nucleic Acids Research*, vol. 39, no. 1, pp. D152–D157, 2011.

[37] J. Krol, I. Loedige, and W. Filipowicz, "The widespread regulation of microRNA biogenesis, function and decay," *Nature Reviews Genetics*, vol. 11, no. 9, pp. 597–610, 2010.

[38] T. Dalmay, "Mechanism of miRNA-mediated repression of mRNA translation," *Essays in Biochemistry*, vol. 54, no. 1, pp. 29–38, 2013.

[39] A. Zaravinos, G. I. Lambrou, N. Mourmouras et al., "New miRNA profiles accurately distinguish renal cell carcinomas and upper tract urothelial carcinomas from the normal kidney," *PLoS ONE*, vol. 9, no. 3, Article ID e91646, 2014.

[40] J. Radojicic, A. Zaravinos, T. Vrekoussis, M. Kafousi, D. A. Spandidos, and E. N. Stathopoulos, "MicroRNA expression analysis in triple-negative (ER, PR and Her2/neu) breast cancer," *Cell Cycle*, vol. 10, no. 3, pp. 507–517, 2011.

[41] I. Chaveles, A. Zaravinos, I. G. Habeos et al., "MicroRNA profiling in murine liver after partial hepatectomy," *International Journal of Molecular Medicine*, vol. 29, no. 5, pp. 747–755, 2012.

[42] D. V. Chartoumpekis, A. Zaravinos, P. G. Ziros et al., "Differential expression of microRNAs in adipose tissue after long-term high-fat diet-induced obesity in mice," *PLoS ONE*, vol. 7, no. 4, Article ID e34872, 2012.

[43] A. Zaravinos, J. Radojicic, G. I. Lambrou et al., "Expression of miRNAs involved in angiogenesis, tumor cell proliferation, tumor suppressor inhibition, epithelial-mesenchymal transition and activation of metastasis in bladder cancer," *Journal of Urology*, vol. 188, no. 2, pp. 615–623, 2012.

[44] T. M. Rana, "Illuminating the silence: understanding the structure and function of small RNAs," *Nature Reviews Molecular Cell Biology*, vol. 8, no. 1, pp. 23–36, 2007.

[45] B. Zhang, Q. Wang, and X. Pan, "MicroRNAs and their regulatory roles in animals and plants," *Journal of Cellular Physiology*, vol. 210, no. 2, pp. 279–289, 2007.

[46] W. Filipowicz, L. Jaskiewicz, F. A. Kolb, and R. S. Pillai, "Posttranscriptional gene silencing by siRNAs and miRNAs," *Current Opinion in Structural Biology*, vol. 15, no. 3, pp. 331–341, 2005.

[47] J. Hausser, A. P. Syed, B. Bilen, and M. Zavolan, "Analysis of CDS-located miRNA target sites suggests that they can effectively inhibit translation," *Genome Research*, vol. 23, no. 4, pp. 604–615, 2013.

[48] B. Zhang, X. Pan, G. P. Cobb, and T. A. Anderson, "microRNAs as oncogenes and tumor suppressors," *Developmental Biology*, vol. 302, no. 1, pp. 1–12, 2007.

[49] E. M. C. Ohlsson Teague, C. G. Print, and M. L. Hull, "The role of microRNAs in endometriosis and associated reproductive conditions," *Human Reproduction Update*, vol. 16, no. 2, pp. 142–165, 2009.

[50] M. Koutsaki, D. A. Spandidos, and A. Zaravinos, "Epithelial-mesenchymal transition-associated miRNAs in ovarian carcinoma, with highlight on the miR-200 family: prognostic value and prospective role in ovarian cancer therapeutics," *Cancer Letters*, vol. 351, pp. 173–181, 2014.

[51] X. Feng, Z. Wang, R. Fillmore, and Y. Xi, "MiR-200, a new star miRNA in human cancer," *Cancer Letters*, vol. 344, no. 2, pp. 166–173, 2014.

[52] A. Díaz-López, G. Moreno-Bueno, and A. Cano, "Role of microRNA in epithelial to mesenchymal transition and metastasis and clinical perspectives," *Cancer Management and Research*, vol. 6, no. 1, pp. 205–216, 2014.

[53] L. Adam, M. Zhong, W. Choi et al., "miR-200 expression regulates epithelial-to-mesenchymal transition in bladder cancer cells and reverses resistance to epidermal growth factor receptor therapy," *Clinical Cancer Research*, vol. 15, no. 16, pp. 5060–5072, 2009.

[54] V. P. Tryndyak, F. A. Beland, and I. P. Pogribny, "E-cadherin transcriptional down-regulation by epigenetic and microRNA-200 family alterations is related to mesenchymal and drug-resistant phenotypes in human breast cancer cells," *International Journal of Cancer*, vol. 126, no. 11, pp. 2575–2583, 2010.

[55] E. D. Wiklund, J. B. Bramsen, T. Hulf et al., "Coordinated epigenetic repression of the miR-200 family and miR-205 in invasive bladder cancer," *International Journal of Cancer*, vol. 128, no. 6, pp. 1327–1334, 2011.

[56] D. M. Dykxhoorn, Y. Wu, H. Xie et al., "miR-200 enhances mouse breast cancer cell colonization to form distant metastases," *PLoS ONE*, vol. 4, no. 9, Article ID e7181, 2009.

[57] I. Elson-Schwab, A. Lorentzen, and C. J. Marshall, "MicroRNA-200 family members differentially regulate morphological plasticity and mode of melanoma cell invasion," *PLoS ONE*, vol. 5, no. 10, Article ID e13176, 2010.

[58] X. Hu, D. M. Macdonald, P. C. Huettner et al., "A miR-200 microRNA cluster as prognostic marker in advanced ovarian cancer," *Gynecologic Oncology*, vol. 114, no. 3, pp. 457–464, 2009.

[59] S. Ali, A. Ahmad, S. Banerjee et al., "Gemcitabine sensitivity can be induced in pancreatic cancer cells through modulation of miR-200 and miR-21 expression by curcumin or its analogue CDF," *Cancer Research*, vol. 70, no. 9, pp. 3606–3617, 2010.

[60] Y. Li, T. G. Vandenboom II, D. Kong et al., "Up-regulation of miR-200 and let-7 by natural agents leads to the reversal of epithelial-to-mesenchymal transition in gemcitabine-resistant pancreatic cancer cells," *Cancer Research*, vol. 69, no. 16, pp. 6704–6712, 2009.

[61] D. Kong, Y. Li, Z. Wang et al., "miR-200 regulates PDGF-D-mediated epithelial-mesenchymal transition, adhesion, and invasion of prostate cancer cells," *Stem Cells*, vol. 27, no. 8, pp. 1712–1721, 2009.

[62] A. Shinozaki, T. Sakatani, T. Ushiku et al., "Downregulation of microRNA-200 in EBV-associated gastric carcinoma," *Cancer Research*, vol. 70, no. 11, pp. 4719–4727, 2010.

[63] D. L. Gibbons, W. Lin, C. J. Creighton et al., "Contextual extracellular cues promote tumor cell EMT and metastasis by regulating miR-200 family expression," *Genes and Development*, vol. 23, no. 18, pp. 2140–2151, 2009.

[64] P. A. Gregory, A. G. Bert, E. L. Paterson et al., "The miR-200 family and miR-205 regulate epithelial to mesenchymal transition by targeting ZEB1 and SIP1," *Nature Cell Biology*, vol. 10, no. 5, pp. 593–601, 2008.

[65] S.-M. Park, A. B. Gaur, E. Lengyel, and M. E. Peter, "The miR-200 family determines the epithelial phenotype of cancer cells by targeting the E-cadherin repressors ZEB1 and ZEB2," *Genes & Development*, vol. 22, no. 7, pp. 894–907, 2008.

[66] M. Pacurari, J. B. Addison, N. Bondalapati et al., "The microRNA-200 family targets multiple non-small cell lung cancer prognostic markers in H1299 cells and BEAS-2B cells," *International Journal of Oncology*, vol. 43, no. 2, pp. 548–560, 2013.

[67] M. J. Schliekelman, D. L. Gibbons, V. M. Faca et al., "Targets of the tumor suppressor miR-200 in regulation of the epithelial-mesenchymal transition in cancer," *Cancer Research*, vol. 71, no. 24, pp. 7670–7682, 2011.

[68] P. A. Gregory, C. P. Bracken, E. Smith et al., "An autocrine TGF-β/ZEB/miR-200 signaling network regulates establishment and maintenance of epithelial-mesenchymal transition," *Molecular Biology of the Cell*, vol. 22, no. 10, pp. 1686–1698, 2011.

[69] C. Vandewalle, F. Van Roy, and G. Berx, "The role of the ZEB family of transcription factors in development and disease," *Cellular and Molecular Life Sciences*, vol. 66, no. 5, pp. 773–787, 2009.

[70] L. Hill, G. Browne, and E. Tulchinsky, "ZEB/miR-200 feedback loop: at the crossroads of signal transduction in cancer," *International Journal of Cancer*, vol. 132, no. 4, pp. 745–754, 2012.

[71] G. J. Hurteau, J. A. Carlson, S. D. Spivack, and G. J. Brock, "Overexpression of the MicroRNA hsa-miR-200c leads to reduced expression of transcription factor 8 and increased expression of E-cadherin," *Cancer Research*, vol. 67, no. 17, pp. 7972–7976, 2007.

[72] M. Korpal, E. S. Lee, G. Hu, and Y. Kang, "The miR-200 family inhibits epithelial-mesenchymal transition and cancer cell migration by direct targeting of E-cadherin transcriptional repressors ZEB1 and ZEB2," *The Journal of Biological Chemistry*, vol. 283, no. 22, pp. 14910–14914, 2008.

[73] U. Burk, J. Schubert, U. Wellner et al., "A reciprocal repression between ZEB1 and members of the miR-200 family promotes EMT and invasion in cancer cells," *EMBO Reports*, vol. 9, no. 6, pp. 582–589, 2008.

[74] C. P. Bracken, P. A. Gregory, N. Kolesnikoff et al., "A double-negative feedback loop between ZEB1-SIP1 and the microRNA-200 family regulates epithelial-mesenchymal transition," *Cancer Research*, vol. 68, no. 19, pp. 7846–7854, 2008.

[75] S. Brabletz and T. Brabletz, "The ZEB/miR-200 feedback loop—a motor of cellular plasticity in development and cancer?" *EMBO Reports*, vol. 11, no. 9, pp. 670–677, 2010.

[76] J. Kurashige, H. Kamohara, M. Watanabe et al., "MicroRNA-200b regulates cell proliferation, invasion, and migration by directly targeting ZEB2 in gastric carcinoma," *Annals of Surgical Oncology*, vol. 19, supplement 3, pp. S656–S664, 2012.

[77] N. Cong, P. Du, A. Zhang et al., "Downregulated microRNA-200a promotes EMT and tumor growth through the Wnt/β-catenin pathway by targeting the E-cadherin repressors ZEB1/ZEB2 in gastric adenocarcinoma," *Oncology Reports*, vol. 29, no. 4, pp. 1579–1587, 2013.

[78] S. Grünert, M. Jechlinger, and H. Beug, "Diverse cellular and molecular mechanisms contribute to epithelial plasticity and metastasis," *Nature Reviews Molecular Cell Biology*, vol. 4, no. 8, pp. 657–665, 2003.

[79] M. Jechlinger, A. Sommer, R. Moriggl et al., "Autocrine PDGFR signaling promotes mammary cancer metastasis," *Journal of Clinical Investigation*, vol. 116, no. 6, pp. 1561–1570, 2006.

[80] J. Gotzmann, A. N. Fischer, M. Zojer et al., "A crucial function of PDGF in TGF-β-mediated cancer progression of hepatocytes," *Oncogene*, vol. 25, no. 22, pp. 3170–3185, 2006.

[81] K. Lehmann, E. Janda, C. E. Pierreux et al., "Raf induces TGFβ production while blocking its apoptotic but not invasive responses: a mechanism leading to increased malignancy in epithelial cells," *Genes and Development*, vol. 14, no. 20, pp. 2610–2622, 2000.

[82] A. Eger, A. Stockinger, B. Schaffhauser, H. Beug, and R. Foisner, "Epithelial mesenchymal transition by c-Fos estrogen receptor activation involves nuclear translocation of β-catenin and upregulation of β-catenin/lymphoid enhancer binding factor-1 transcriptional activity," *Journal of Cell Biology*, vol. 148, no. 1, pp. 173–187, 2000.

[83] J. Lu, H. Guo, W. Treekitkarnmongkol et al., "14-3-3ζ cooperates with ErbB2 to promote ductal carcinoma in situ progression to invasive breast cancer by inducing epithelial-mesenchymal transition," *Cancer Cell*, vol. 16, no. 3, pp. 195–207, 2009.

[84] J. Braun, C. Hoang-Vu, H. Dralle, and S. Hüttelmaier, "Down-regulation of microRNAs directs the EMT and invasive potential of anaplastic thyroid carcinomas," *Oncogene*, vol. 29, no. 29, pp. 4237–4244, 2010.

[85] J. L. Carstens, S. Lovisa, and R. Kalluri, "Microenvironment-dependent cues trigger miRNA-regulated feedback loop to facilitate the EMT/MET switch," *Journal of Clinical Investigation*, vol. 124, no. 4, pp. 1458–1460, 2014.

[86] G. Berx, E. Raspé, G. Christofori, J. P. Thiery, and J. P. Sleeman, "Pre-EMTing metastasis? Recapitulation of morphogenetic processes in cancer," *Clinical & Experimental Metastasis*, vol. 24, no. 8, pp. 587–597, 2007.

[87] L. F. Sempere, M. Christensen, A. Silahtaroglu et al., "Altered microRNA expression confined to specific epithelial cell sub-populations in breast cancer," *Cancer Research*, vol. 67, no. 24, pp. 11612–11620, 2007.

[88] P. A. Gregory, C. P. Bracken, A. G. Bert, and G. J. Goodall, "MicroRNAs as regulators of epithelial-mesenchymal transition," *Cell Cycle*, vol. 7, no. 20, pp. 3112–3118, 2008.

[89] M. Kato, J. Zhang, M. Wang et al., "MicroRNA-192 in diabetic kidney glomeruli and its function in TGF-β-induced collagen expression via inhibition of E-box repressors," *Proceedings of the National Academy of Sciences of the United States of America*, vol. 104, no. 9, pp. 3432–3437, 2007.

[90] P. Ru, R. Steele, P. Newhall, N. J. Phillips, K. Toth, and R. B. Ray, "miRNA-29b suppresses prostate cancer metastasis by regulating epithelial-mesenchymal transition signaling," *Molecular Cancer Therapeutics*, vol. 11, no. 5, pp. 1166–1173, 2012.

[91] J. Zhang, H. Zhang, J. Liu et al., "MiR-30 inhibits TGF-β1-induced epithelial-to-mesenchymal transition in hepatocyte by targeting Snail1," *Biochemical and Biophysical Research Communications*, vol. 417, no. 3, pp. 1100–1105, 2012.

[92] R. Kumarswamy, G. Mudduluru, P. Ceppi et al., "MicroRNA-30a inhibits epithelial-to-mesenchymal transition by targeting Snail and is downregulated in non-small cell lung cancer," *International Journal of Cancer*, vol. 130, no. 9, pp. 2044–2053, 2012.

[93] J. P. Zhang, C. Zeng, L. Xu, J. Gong, J. H. Fang, and S. M. Zhuang, "MicroRNA-148a suppresses the epithelial-mesenchymal transition and metastasis of hepatoma cells by targeting Met/Snail signaling," *Oncogene*, vol. 33, pp. 4069–4076, 2014.

[94] H. Siemens, R. Jackstadt, S. Hünten et al., "miR-34 and SNAIL form a double-negative feedback loop to regulate epithelial-mesenchymal transitions," *Cell Cycle*, vol. 10, no. 24, pp. 4256–4271, 2011.

[95] M. Moes, A. Le Béchec, I. Crespo et al., "A novel network integrating a mirna-203/snail feedback loop which regulates epithelial to mesenchymal transition," *PLoS ONE*, vol. 7, no. 4, Article ID e35440, 2012.

[96] L. Ma, J. Teruya-Feldstein, and R. A. Weinberg, "Tumour invasion and metastasis initiated by microRNA-10b in breast cancer," *Nature*, vol. 449, no. 7163, pp. 682–688, 2007.

[97] A. E. G. Lenferink, C. Cantin, A. Nantel et al., "Transcriptome profiling of a TGF-β-induced epithelial-to-mesenchymal transition reveals extracellular clusterin as a target for therapeutic antibodies," *Oncogene*, vol. 29, no. 6, pp. 831–844, 2010.

[98] G. Turcatel, N. Rubin, A. El-Hashash, and D. Warburton, "Mir-99a and mir-99b modulate TGF-β induced epithelial to mesenchymal plasticity in normal murine mammary gland cells," *PLoS ONE*, vol. 7, no. 1, Article ID e31032, 2012.

[99] W. Kong, H. Yang, L. He et al., "MicroRNA-155 is regulated by the transforming growth factor β/Smad pathway and contributes to epithelial cell plasticity by targeting RhoA," *Molecular and Cellular Biology*, vol. 28, no. 22, pp. 6773–6784, 2008.

[100] C. A. Gebeshuber, K. Zatloukal, and J. Martinez, "miR-29a suppresses tristetraprolin, which is a regulator of epithelial polarity and metastasis," *EMBO Reports*, vol. 10, no. 4, pp. 400–405, 2009.

[101] C. L. Cottonham, S. Kaneko, and L. Xu, "miR-21 and miR-31 converge on TIAM1 to regulate migration and invasion of colon carcinoma cells," *Journal of Biological Chemistry*, vol. 285, no. 46, pp. 35293–35302, 2010.

[102] G. Eades, Y. Yao, M. Yang, Y. Zhang, S. Chumsri, and Q. Zhou, "miR-200a regulates SIRT1 expression and epithelial to mesenchymal transition (EMT)-like transformation in mammary epithelial cells," *Journal of Biological Chemistry*, vol. 286, no. 29, pp. 25992–26002, 2011.

[103] P. S. Eis, W. Tam, L. Sun et al., "Accumulation of miR-155 and BIC RNA in human B cell lymphomas," *Proceedings of the National Academy of Sciences of the United States of America*, vol. 102, no. 10, pp. 3627–3632, 2005.

[104] O. Slaby, M. Svoboda, P. Fabian et al., "Altered expression of miR-21, miR-31, miR-143 and miR-145 is related to clinicopathologic features of colorectal cancer," *Oncology*, vol. 72, no. 5-6, pp. 397–402, 2008.

[105] S. Valastyan, A. Chang, N. Benaich, F. Reinhardt, and R. A. Weinberg, "Activation of miR-31 function in already-established metastases elicits metastatic regression," *Genes and Development*, vol. 25, no. 6, pp. 646–659, 2011.

[106] L. Ma, J. Young, H. Prabhala et al., "MiR-9, a MYC/MYCN-activated microRNA, regulates E-cadherin and cancer metastasis," *Nature Cell Biology*, vol. 12, no. 3, pp. 247–256, 2010.

[107] F. Ceteci, S. Ceteci, C. Karreman et al., "Disruption of tumor cell adhesion promotes angiogenic switch and progression to micrometastasis in RAF-driven murine lung cancer," *Cancer Cell*, vol. 12, no. 2, pp. 145–159, 2007.

[108] Z. Meng, X. Fu, X. Chen et al., "miR-194 is a marker of hepatic epithelial cells and suppresses metastasis of liver cancer cells in mice," *Hepatology*, vol. 52, no. 6, pp. 2148–2157, 2010.

[109] L.-Y. Zhang, M. Liu, X. Li, and H. Tang, "MiR-490-3p modulates cell growth and epithelial to mesenchymal transition of hepatocellular carcinoma cells by targeting endoplasmic reticulum-golgi intermediate compartment protein 3 (ERGIC3)," *Journal of Biological Chemistry*, vol. 288, no. 6, pp. 4035–4047, 2013.

[110] M. Nishikawa, Y. Kira, Y. Yabunaka, and M. Inoue, "Identification and characterization of endoplasmic reticulum-associated protein, ERp43," *Gene*, vol. 386, no. 1-2, pp. 42–51, 2007.

[111] F. E. Wang, C. Zhang, A. Maminishkis et al., "MicroRNA-204/211 alters epithelial physiology," *FASEB Journal*, vol. 24, no. 5, pp. 1552–1571, 2010.

[112] A. Barrios, R. J. Poole, L. Durbin, C. Brennan, N. Holder, and S. W. Wilson, "Eph/Ephrin signaling regulates the mesenchymal-to-epithelial transition of the paraxial mesoderm during somite morphogenesis," *Current Biology*, vol. 13, no. 18, pp. 1571–1582, 2003.

[113] J. Fukai, H. Yokote, R. Yamanaka, T. Arao, K. Nishio, and T. Itakura, "EphA4 promotes cell proliferation and migration through a novel EphA4-FGFR1 signaling pathway in the human glioma U251 cell line," *Molecular Cancer Therapeutics*, vol. 7, no. 9, pp. 2768–2778, 2008.

[114] Y. Yan, Y.-C. Luo, H.-Y. Wan et al., "MicroRNA-10a is involved in the metastatic process by regulating Eph tyrosine kinase receptor A4-mediated epithelial-mesenchymal transition and adhesion in hepatoma cells," *Hepatology*, vol. 57, no. 2, pp. 667–677, 2013.

[115] S. Stinson, M. R. Lackner, A. T. Adai et al., "TRPS1 targeting by miR-221/222 promotes the epithelial-to-mesenchymal transition in breast cancer," *Science Signaling*, vol. 4, no. 177, article ra41, 2011.

[116] Z. Gai, G. Zhou, S. Itoh et al., "Trps1 functions downstream of Bmp7 in kidney development," *Journal of the American Society of Nephrology*, vol. 20, no. 11, pp. 2403–2411, 2009.

[117] M. Y. Shah and G. A. Calin, "MicroRNAs miR-221 and miR-222: a new level of regulation in aggressive breast cancer," *Genome Medicine*, vol. 3, no. 8, article 56, 2011.

[118] I. K. Guttilla, K. N. Phoenix, X. Hong, J. S. Tirnauer, K. P. Claffey, and B. A. White, "Prolonged mammosphere culture of MCF-7 cells induces an EMT and repression of the estrogen receptor by microRNAs," *Breast Cancer Research and Treatment*, vol. 132, no. 1, pp. 75–85, 2012.

[119] U. Koch and F. Radtke, "Notch and cancer: a double-edged sword," *Cellular and Molecular Life Sciences*, vol. 64, no. 21, pp. 2746–2762, 2007.

[120] L. Jiang, X. Liu, A. Kolokythas et al., "Downregulation of the Rho GTPase signaling pathway is involved in the microRNA-138-mediated inhibition of cell migration and invasion in tongue squamous cell carcinoma," *International Journal of Cancer*, vol. 127, no. 3, pp. 505–512, 2010.

[121] X. Liu, C. Wang, Z. Chen et al., "MicroRNA-138 suppresses epithelial-mesenchymal transition in squamous cell carcinoma cell lines," *Biochemical Journal*, vol. 440, no. 1, pp. 23–31, 2011.

[122] Y. Konno, P. Dong, Y. Xiong et al., "MicroRNA-101 targets EZH2, MCL-1 and FOS to suppress proliferation, invasion and stem cell-like phenotype of aggressive endometrial cancer cells," *Oncotarget*, vol. 5, pp. 6049–6062, 2014.

[123] Z. Wang, Y. Li, D. Kong et al., "Acquisition of epithelial-mesenchymal transition phenotype of gemcitabine-resistant pancreatic cancer cells is linked with activation of the notch signaling pathway," *Cancer Research*, vol. 69, no. 6, pp. 2400–2407, 2009.

[124] S. Brabletz, K. Bajdak, S. Meidhof et al., "The ZEB1/miR-200 feedback loop controls Notch signalling in cancer cells," *The EMBO Journal*, vol. 30, no. 4, pp. 770–782, 2011.

[125] D. M. Vallejo, E. Caparros, and M. Dominguez, "Targeting Notch signalling by the conserved miR-8/200 microRNA family in development and cancer cells," *The EMBO Journal*, vol. 30, no. 4, pp. 756–769, 2011.

[126] S. Spaderna, O. Schmalhofer, F. Hlubek et al., "A transient, EMT-linked loss of basement membranes indicates metastasis and poor survival in colorectal cancer," *Gastroenterology*, vol. 131, no. 3, pp. 830–840, 2006.

[127] E. Sánchez-Tilló, O. de Barrios, L. Siles, M. Cuatrecasas, A. Castells, and A. Postigo, "β-catenin/TCF4 complex induces the epithelial-to-mesenchymal transition (EMT)-activator ZEB1 to regulate tumor invasiveness," *Proceedings of the National Academy of Sciences of the United States of America*, vol. 108, no. 48, pp. 19204–19209, 2011.

[128] Y. Shi and J. Massagué, "Mechanisms of TGF-β signaling from cell membrane to the nucleus," *Cell*, vol. 113, no. 6, pp. 685–700, 2003.

[129] H. Hermeking, "p53 enters the microRNA world," *Cancer Cell*, vol. 12, no. 5, pp. 414–418, 2007.

[130] N. S. Chari, N. L. Pinaire, L. Thorpe, L. J. Medeiros, M. J. Routbort, and T. J. McDonnell, "The p53 tumor suppressor network in cancer and the therapeutic modulation of cell death," *Apoptosis*, vol. 14, no. 4, pp. 336–347, 2009.

[131] B. C. Lewis, D. S. Klimstra, N. D. Socci, S. Xu, J. A. Koutcher, and H. E. Varmus, "The absence of *p53* promotes metastasis in a novel somatic mouse model for hepatocellular carcinoma," *Molecular and Cellular Biology*, vol. 25, no. 4, pp. 1228–1237, 2005.

[132] Y.-W. Chen, D. S. Klimstra, M. E. Mongeau, J. L. Tatem, V. Boyartchuk, and B. C. Lewis, "Loss of p53 and Ink4a/Arf cooperate in a cell autonomous fashion to induce metastasis of hepatocellular carcinoma cells," *Cancer Research*, vol. 67, no. 16, pp. 7589–7596, 2007.

[133] J. E. Hansen, L. K. Fischer, G. Chan et al., "Antibody-mediated p53 protein therapy prevents liver metastasis *in vivo*," *Cancer Research*, vol. 67, no. 4, pp. 1769–1774, 2007.

[134] G. Fontemaggi, A. Gurtner, S. Strano et al., "The transcriptional repressor ZEB regulates p73 expression at the crossroad between proliferation and differentiation," *Molecular and Cellular Biology*, vol. 21, no. 24, pp. 8461–8470, 2001.

[135] T. Kim, A. Veronese, F. Pichiorri et al., "p53 regulates epithelial-mesenchymal transition through microRNAs targeting ZEB1 and ZEB2," *Journal of Experimental Medicine*, vol. 208, no. 5, pp. 875–883, 2011.

[136] C.-J. Chang, C.-H. Chao, W. Xia et al., "p53 regulates epithelial-mesenchymal transition and stem cell properties through modulating miRNAs," *Nature Cell Biology*, vol. 13, no. 3, pp. 317–323, 2011.

[137] E. C. Knouf, K. Garg, J. D. Arroyo et al., "An integrative genomic approach identifies p73 and p63 as activators of miR-200 microRNA family transcription," *Nucleic Acids Research*, vol. 40, no. 2, pp. 499–510, 2012.

[138] M. F. Clarke, J. E. Dick, P. B. Dirks et al., "Cancer stem cells—perspectives on current status and future directions: AACR workshop on cancer stem cells," *Cancer Research*, vol. 66, no. 19, pp. 9339–9344, 2006.

[139] R. Chhabra and N. Saini, "MicroRNAs in cancer stem cells: current status and future directions," *Tumor Biology*, vol. 35, no. 9, pp. 8395–8405, 2014.

[140] S. A. Mani, W. Guo, M.-J. Liao et al., "The epithelial-mesenchymal transition generates cells with properties of stem cells," *Cell*, vol. 133, no. 4, pp. 704–715, 2008.

[141] A.-P. Morel, M. Lièvre, C. Thomas, G. Hinkal, S. Ansieau, and A. Puisieux, "Generation of breast cancer stem cells through epithelial-mesenchymal transition," *PLoS ONE*, vol. 3, no. 8, Article ID e2888, 2008.

[142] B. T. Hennessy, A. M. Gonzalez-Angulo, K. Stemke-Hale et al., "Characterization of a naturally occurring breast cancer subset enriched in epithelial-to-mesenchymal transition and stem cell characteristics," *Cancer Research*, vol. 69, no. 10, pp. 4116–4124, 2009.

[143] B. Aktas, M. Tewes, T. Fehm, S. Hauch, R. Kimmig, and S. Kasimir-Bauer, "Stem cell and epithelial-mesenchymal transition markers are frequently overexpressed in circulating tumor cells of metastatic breast cancer patients," *Breast Cancer Research*, vol. 11, no. 4, article R46, 2009.

[144] B. G. Hollier, K. Evans, and S. A. Mani, "The epithelial-to-mesenchymal transition and cancer stem cells: a coalition against cancer therapies," *Journal of Mammary Gland Biology and Neoplasia*, vol. 14, no. 1, pp. 29–43, 2009.

[145] M. Santisteban, J. M. Reiman, M. K. Asiedu et al., "Immune-induced epithelial to mesenchymal transition *in vivo* generates breast cancer stem cells," *Cancer Research*, vol. 69, no. 7, pp. 2887–2895, 2009.

[146] T. Blick, H. Hugo, E. Widodo et al., "Epithelial mesenchymal transition traits in human breast cancer cell lines parallel the CD44HI/CD24lO/-stem cell phenotype in human breast cancer," *Journal of Mammary Gland Biology and Neoplasia*, vol. 15, no. 2, pp. 235–252, 2010.

[147] D. Kong, S. Banerjee, A. Ahmad et al., "Epithelial to mesenchymal transition is mechanistically linked with stem cell signatures in prostate cancer cells," *PLoS ONE*, vol. 5, no. 8, Article ID e12445, 2010.

[148] J. Zavadil, "A spotlight on regulatory networks connecting EMT and cancer stem cells," *Cell Cycle*, vol. 9, no. 15, p. 2927, 2010.

[149] A. Martin and A. Cano, "Tumorigenesis: twist1 links EMT to self-renewal," *Nature Cell Biology*, vol. 12, no. 10, pp. 924–925, 2010.

[150] M.-H. Yang, D. S.-S. Hsu, H.-W. Wang et al., "Bmi1 is essential in Twist1-induced epithelial-mesenchymal transition," *Nature Cell Biology*, vol. 12, no. 10, pp. 982–992, 2010.

[151] G. J. Klarmann, E. M. Hurt, L. A. Mathews et al., "Invasive prostate cancer cells are tumor initiating cells that have a stem cell-like genomic signature," *Clinical and Experimental Metastasis*, vol. 26, no. 5, pp. 433–446, 2009.

[152] D. J. Mulholland, N. Kobayashi, M. Ruscetti et al., "Pten loss and RAS/MAPK activation cooperate to promote EMT and metastasis initiated from prostate cancer stem/progenitor cells," *Cancer Research*, vol. 72, no. 7, pp. 1878–1889, 2012.

[153] J. Lopez, A. Poitevin, V. Mendoza-Martinez, C. Perez-Plasencia, and A. Garcia-Carranca, "Cancer-initiating cells derived from established cervical cell lines exhibit stem-cell markers and increased radioresistance," *BMC Cancer*, vol. 12, article 48, 2012.

[154] R. Garzon, G. Marcucci, and C. M. Croce, "Targeting microRNAs in cancer: rationale, strategies and challenges," *Nature Reviews Drug Discovery*, vol. 9, no. 10, pp. 775–789, 2010.

[155] A. Bouchie, "First microRNA mimic enters clinic," *Nature Biotechnology*, vol. 31, no. 7, article 577, 2013.

[156] F. Xiao, Y. Bai, Z. Chen et al., "Downregulation of HOXA1 gene affects small cell lung cancer cell survival and chemoresistance under the regulation of miR-100," *European Journal of Cancer*, vol. 50, no. 8, pp. 1541–1554, 2014.

[157] M. X. Liu, M. K. Y. Siu, S. S. Liu, J. W. P. Yam, H. Y. S. Ngan, and D. W. Chan, "Epigenetic silencing of microRNA-199b-5p is associated with acquired chemoresistance via activation of JAG1-Notch1 signaling in ovarian cancer," *Oncotarget*, vol. 5, no. 4, pp. 944–958, 2014.

[158] H. L. A. Janssen, H. W. Reesink, E. J. Lawitz et al., "Treatment of HCV infection by targeting microRNA," *The New England Journal of Medicine*, vol. 368, no. 18, pp. 1685–1694, 2013.

[159] L. F. R. Gebert, M. A. E. Rebhan, S. E. M. Crivelli, R. Denzler, M. Stoffel, and J. Hall, "Miravirsen (SPC3649) can inhibit the biogenesis of miR-122," *Nucleic Acids Research*, vol. 42, no. 1, pp. 609–621, 2014.

[160] J. F. Wiggins, L. Ruffino, K. Kelnar et al., "Development of a lung cancer therapeutic based on the tumor suppressor microRNA-34," *Cancer Research*, vol. 70, no. 14, pp. 5923–5930, 2010.

[161] A. G. Bader, "MiR-34—a microRNA replacement therapy is headed to the clinic," *Frontiers in Genetics*, vol. 3, article 120, 2012.

[162] C. L. Daige, J. F. Wiggins, L. Priddy et al., "Systemic delivery of a miR34a mimic as a potential therapeutic for liver cancer," *Molecular Cancer Therapeutics*, vol. 13, no. 10, pp. 2352–2360, 2014.

21

Recombinant Human Thyroid Stimulating Hormone versus Thyroid Hormone Withdrawal for Radioactive Iodine Treatment of Differentiated Thyroid Cancer with Nodal Metastatic Disease

Robert M. Wolfson,[1] Irina Rachinsky,[1] Deric Morrison,[2] Al Driedger,[1] Tamara Spaic,[2] and Stan H. M. Van Uum[2]

[1]*Department of Diagnostic Imaging, Schulich School of Medicine and Dentistry, Western University, London, ON, Canada N6A 5W9*
[2]*Department of Medicine, Schulich School of Medicine and Dentistry, Western University, London, ON, Canada N6A 4V2*

Correspondence should be addressed to Stan H. M. Van Uum; stan.vanuum@sjhc.london.on.ca

Academic Editor: James L. Mulshine

Introduction. Recombinant human thyroid stimulating hormone (rhTSH) is approved for preparation of thyroid remnant ablation with radioactive iodine (RAI) in low risk patients with well differentiated thyroid cancer (DTC). We studied the safety and efficacy of rhTSH preparation for RAI treatment of thyroid cancer patients with nodal metastatic disease. *Methods.* A retrospective analysis was performed on 108 patients with histopathologically confirmed nodal metastatic DTC, treated with initial RAI between January 1, 2000, and December 31, 2007. Within this selected group, 31 and 42 patients were prepared for initial and all subsequent RAI treatments by either thyroid hormone withdrawal (THW) or rhTSH protocols and were followed up for at least 3 years. *Results.* The response to initial treatment, classified as excellent, acceptable, or incomplete, was not different between the rhTSH group (57%, 21%, and 21%, resp.) and the THW group (39%, 13%, and 48%, resp.; $P = 0.052$). There was no significant difference in the final clinical outcome between the groups. The rhTSH group received significantly fewer additional doses of RAI than the THW group ($P = 0.03$). *Conclusion.* In patients with nodal-positive DTC, preparation for RAI with rhTSH is a safe and efficacious alternative to THW protocol.

1. Introduction

Following initial surgery, the recurrence risk for differentiated thyroid cancer (DTC) is defined as low, intermediate, or high [1]. Treatment with radioactive iodine (RAI) is also used for remnant ablation and for patients with local and distant metastases [1]. Administration of RAI requires increased TSH to maximize RAI uptake in benign or malignant thyroid tissue. Traditionally, this has been achieved by thyroid hormone withdrawal (THW). Several studies, including one prospective study [2], demonstrated the effectiveness of recombinant human thyroid stimulating hormone (rhTSH) for thyroid remnant ablation. In 2007 this resulted in approval by the FDA for preparation of thyroid remnant ablation with radioactive iodine (RAI) in low risk patients with DTC and no evidence of metastatic disease. In Canada, rhTSH was

approved for this indication in 2009. In contrast, rhTSH has not been approved in the US or Canada for use in RAI treatment of recurrent disease or distant metastases [3]. Thus, THW, rather than rhTSH, is recommended for patients with intermediate or high recurrence risk. The use of rhTSH for these groups is considered off-label.

The conventional preparation method with THW causes hypothyroidism which is symptomatic in almost all patients. Luster et al. [4] reported that 92% of patients developed hypothyroid symptoms, and almost half of them sought medical attention because of this. These transient effects have not been described in relation to rhTSH administration, and it has no known long-term side effects. Recently Hugo et al. [5] reported that, compared to THW, rhTSH preparation for RAI treatment resulted in similar final clinical outcomes across a wide range of risks of recurrence and risks of thyroid cancer related death. In our centre, as early as 2000, we started offering rhTSH to patients who potentially could have higher incidence of hypothyroid complications, for example, patients with known depression and previous suicide attempts, professional drivers, and patients with heart or renal failure. Thus, we also prepared some patients with cervical lymph node metastases with rhTSH rather than with THW for RAI treatment. In the present retrospective study, we compare the effect of THW with that of rhTSH for preparation for RAI treatment in newly diagnosed thyroid cancer patients who had intermediate recurrence risk based on histological presence of cervical lymph node metastases at presentation. We analysed both initial response to treatment and clinical status after long-term follow-up.

2. Methods

Patients were recruited from the thyroid cancer clinics at the London Health Sciences Centre, the major referral centre for patients residing in Southwestern Ontario, Canada. Since 1998, all thyroid cancer patients attending our thyroid cancer clinics have been invited to participate in a thyroid cancer registry. More than 95% of invited patients provided written informed consent for inclusion in this registry. The study was approved by the Health Sciences Research Ethics Board of the University of Western Ontario.

For the present study, we searched the registry for all newly diagnosed thyroid cancer patients who were seen at our institution between January 1, 2000, and December 31, 2007. Patients were included if they had well DTC with nodal metastatic disease diagnosed on histopathology at the time of their thyroidectomy. They needed to have received RAI treatment at least once. In addition, we required that any subsequent RAI treatments were administered using the same protocol (THW or rhTSH administration) that was used for the initial therapy. The choice to use rhTSH was made jointly by the patient and the treating physician. For the treatment described in this study, the use of rhTSH was off-label. All patients were followed up for a minimum of 3 years or until death. Clinical follow-up occurred every 6–12 months for all patients and included baseline (suppressed) thyroglobulin (Tg), Tg antibody levels, and annual neck ultrasound. Stimulated thyroglobulin Tg test was performed within 2 years of initial RAI treatment.

For evaluation of the response to initial treatment and the clinical status at the time of final follow-up, we applied the criteria defined by Hugo et al. [5]. Briefly, the response to initial treatment was classified as *excellent* when both suppressed and stimulated Tg were <1 ng/mL, and there was no evidence of disease on neck ultrasound, whole body iodine scan, or CT scan. *Acceptable* response was defined as suppressed Tg <1 ng/mL, stimulated Tg 1–10 ng/mL, and/or equivocal findings on diagnostic imaging. *Incomplete* response was defined as suppressed Tg >1 ng/mL, stimulated Tg >10 ng/mL, and/or evidence of persistent disease on diagnostic imaging. For final outcome, patients were classified according to their status at last follow-up. *No evidence of disease* was defined as suppressed Tg <1 ng/mL, no detectable anti-Tg antibody,

and no structural evidence of disease on clinical examination or radiological studies. *Persistent disease* was defined as suppressed Tg values >1 ng/mL, stimulated Tg values >2 ng/mL, and/or evidence of persistent disease in structural or functional imaging.

Recurrent disease was defined as suppressed Tg >1 ng/mL and/or structural or functional evidence of disease identified following a period of no evidence of disease.

Patients who died from thyroid cancer were categorized as *death due to thyroid cancer*.

Results are described as mean ± SD or % as appropriate. The Student's *t*-test was used for group comparison of quantitative data. Categorical comparison of the groups was done using chi square testing and Fisher's exact test as appropriate (SPSS version 20.0). A *P* value <0.05 was considered statistically significant.

3. Results

We identified 108 patients with newly diagnosed well DTC with nodal metastatic disease diagnosed on histopathology at the time of thyroidectomy. All patients had received at least one RAI treatment, 56 patients were initially prepared with rhTSH, and 52 patients were prepared with THW for the first RAI treatment. Of the 56 patients in the rhTSH group, 7 were excluded because they underwent THW at one or more subsequent treatments, and 7 patients had insufficient follow-up. Of the 52 patients in the THW group, 8 were excluded because they received rhTSH at one or more subsequent treatments, and 13 patients had insufficient follow-up. Therefore we included 42 patients in the rhTSH group and 31 patients in the THW group. Clinical follow-up occurred every 6–12 months and laboratory and imaging studies were done as described above. In addition, at least one neck ultrasound and one stimulated Tg test were performed within the first 2 years following initial RAI. Patients were followed up clinically until they were deemed disease-free (undetectable or negative Tg, U/S) and discharged to a local endocrinologist or had succumbed to death.

Baseline parameters of both THW and rhTSH groups are presented in Table 1(a). Patients in the rhTSH group were older than those in the THW group (*P* = 0.039). However, there was no difference in the proportion of patients younger than 45 years between the two groups (*P* = 0.075). There were less male patients (19%) in the THW group than in the rhTSH group (40%), although this difference did not reach statistical significance (*P* = 0.08). There was no difference in histological subtype or thyroid cancer size at presentation between groups.

Information on staging and recurrence risk is presented in Table 1(b). There was no statistically significant difference in TNM staging, AJCC staging, or ATA risk between THW and rhTSH groups. The duration of follow-up was longer in the THW group than in the rhTSH group (*P* = 0.01), but there was no difference in total RAI activity that had been administered.

The response to initial treatment showed a trend towards superiority in the rhTSH group compared to the THW group

TABLE 1: (a) Baseline characteristics. (b) Thyroid cancer staging and initial RAI treatment.

(a)

Parameter	THW ($n = 31$)	rhTSH ($n = 42$)	P value
Age at ablation			
Mean ± SD (years)	38.2 ± 12.4	45.7 ± 16.2	0.039
<45	23 (74%)	22 (52%)	0.075
>45	8 (26%)	20 (48%)	
Male	6 (19%)	17 (40%)	
Female	25 (81%)	25 (60%)	0.08
Histology			0.92
Papillary thyroid cancer	29 (94%)	41 (98%)	
Classical variant	9 (29%)	10 (24%)	
Follicular variant	6 (19%)	9 (21%)	
Mixed classical/follicular variant	4 (13%)	6 (14%)	
Aggressive variant	3 (10%)	5 (12%)	
Cystic variant	1 (3%)	0 (0%)	
Variant not available	6 (19%)	11 (26%)	
Follicular thyroid cancer	0 (0%)	0 (0%)	
Hurthle cell thyroid cancer	0 (0%)	0 (0%)	
Poorly differentiated cancer	1 (3%)	1 (3%)	
Thyroid cancer not specified	1 (3%)	0 (0%)	
Size of primary thyroid cancer (cm)	2.9 ± 1.5	2.2 ± 1.5	0.09
Median	2.6	2.0	

(b)

Parameter	THW ($n = 31$)	rhTSH ($n = 42$)	P value
Tumor staging			0.59
1	7 (23%)	13 (31%)	
2	6 (19%)	4 (10%)	
3	15 (48%)	22 (52%)	
4a	3 (10%)	3 (7%)	
4b	0 (0%)	0 (0%)	
Nodal staging			0.73
1a	21 (68%)	30 (71%)	
1b	10 (32%)	12 (29%)	
Metastatic staging			0.24
0	30 (97%)	42 (100%)	
1	1 (3%)	0 (0%)	
AJCC staging			0.17
1	22 (71%)	22 (52%)	
2	1 (3%)	0 (0%)	
3	5 (16%)	13 (31%)	
4a	3 (10%)	7 (17%)	
4b	0 (0%)	0 (0%)	
4c	0 (0%)	0 (0%)	
ATA recurrence risk			0.33
Low	0 (0%)	0 (0%)	
Intermediate	23 (74%)	37 (88%)	
High	8 (26%)	5 (12%)	
Administered RAI activity (GBq)	4.58 ± 1.49	4.52 ± 0.92	0.48
Duration of follow-up (years)	8.6 ± 2.4	6.8 ± 2.1	0.01

TABLE 2: Response to initial treatment, additional treatments, and outcome.

Parameter	THW ($n = 31$)	rhTSH ($n = 42$)	P value
Response to initial treatment			0.052
Excellent	12 (39%)	24 (57%)	
Acceptable	4 (13%)	9 (21%)	
Incomplete	15 (48%)	9 (21%)	
Additional surgeries*			0.44
None	21 (68%)	33 (79%)	
1	6 (19%)	7 (17%)	
2	4 (13%)	2 (5%)	
Additional RAI treatments#			0.03
None	17 (55%)	28 (67%)	
1	9 (29%)	14 (33%)	
≥2	5 (16%)	0 (0%)	
Distant metastasis at any time			0.21
0	27 (87%)	40 (95%)	
1	4 (13%)	2 (5%)	
Clinical status at last visit			0.62
No evidence of disease	21 (68%)	30 (71%)	
Persistent disease	4 (13%)	8 (19%)	
Recurrent disease	3 (10%)	2 (5%)	
Death due to thyroid cancer	3 (10%)	2 (5%)	

*Additional surgery usually consisted of removal of one or more lymph nodes.
#The dose for each additional treatment, a fixed dose of 5.5 GBq (150 mCi) of 131-I.

($P = 0.052$). The majority of patients in the rhTSH group had an excellent response, while almost half of the patients in the THW group had an incomplete response (Figure 1). Table 2 presents further information on initial and additional treatments and clinical outcome at follow-up. Patients in the THW group received more additional RAI treatments than the rhTSH group. There was no difference between groups with respect to the outcome as assessed at the last visit (Figure 2). In both groups about 70% had no evidence of persistent disease, while 3 patients died of thyroid cancer in the THW group and 2 in the rhTSH group (Table 2).

The need for additional RAI treatments was higher in patients with N1b stage (41%) than in patients with N1a stage (31%; $P < 0.05$).

4. Discussion

In this study we compared THW with rhTSH for preparation of RAI treatment in DTC patients with intermediate recurrence risk and did not find any difference in clinical outcome after about seven years of follow-up between rhTSH and THW preparation. Over the last years several groups have compared rhTSH preparation with THW for

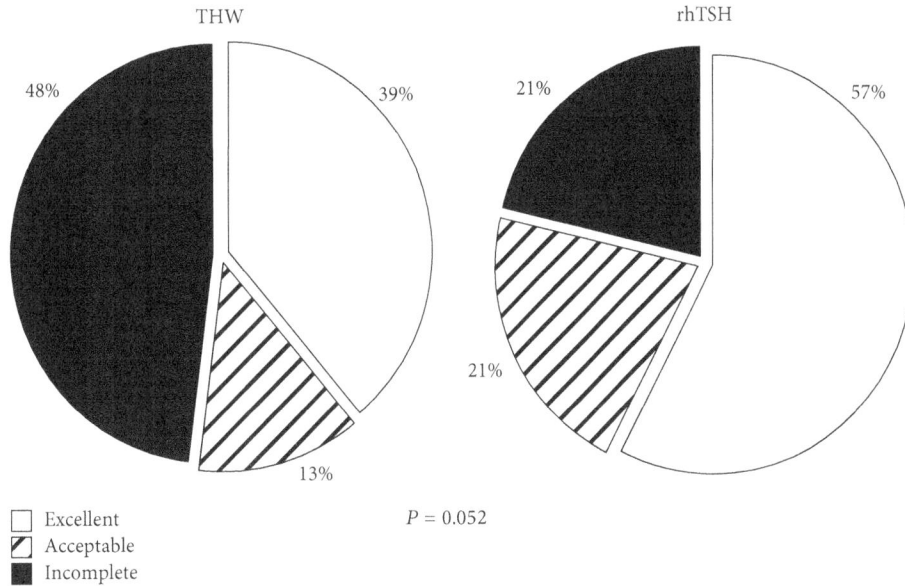

FIGURE 1: Response to initial treatment with radioactive iodine, specified according to preparation with thyroid hormone withdrawal (THW) versus preparation with recombinant human TSH (rhTSH).

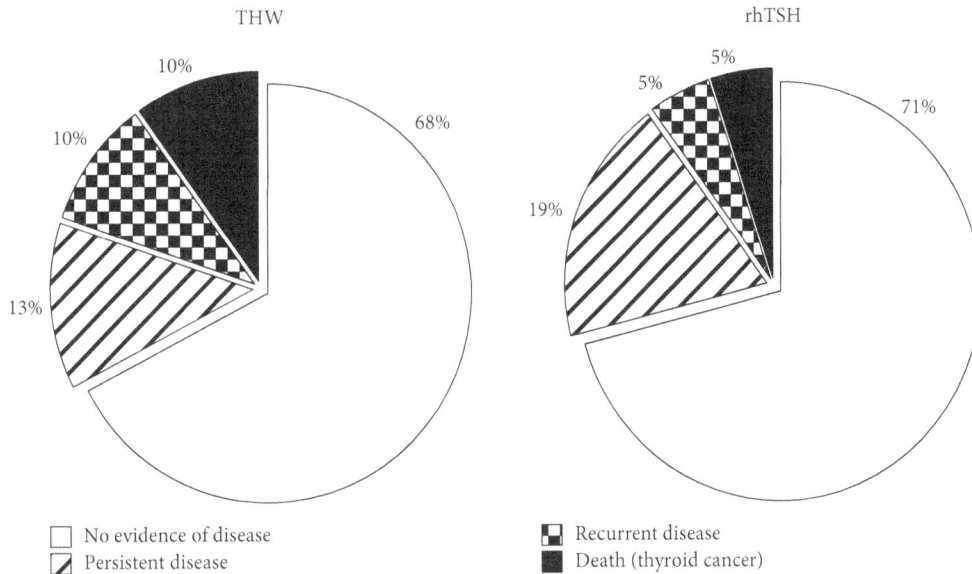

FIGURE 2: Final clinical outcome specified according to preparation with thyroid hormone withdrawal (THW) versus preparation with recombinant human TSH (rhTSH).

initial RAI. Sabra et al. [3] reviewed 9 studies that compared these two preparation modalities with respect to the effect of first adjuvant RAI treatment on the percentage of patients that achieved an undetectable stimulated thyroglobulin (<2 ng/mL). They found no difference between rhTSH and THW preparation; after 1-2 years, nearly 75% of patients were classified as having no evidence of disease. However, the stimulated thyroglobulin test is an intermediate endpoint and the follow-up duration was relatively short.

Focusing on clinical outcomes over longer follow-up time, Rosario et al. [6] reported clinical outcome after 5-year follow-up in a cohort of 276 patients with N1 disease and found no difference between rhTSH and THW prepared group.

For patients with ATA intermediate risk, Hugo et al. [5] also found no difference in final clinical outcome between 291 patients prepared with withdrawal and 141 patients prepared with rhTSH. A more recent study by Molinaro et al. [7]

prospectively evaluated 10-year follow-up in DTC patients. While the number of patients with ATA intermediate recurrence risk was relatively small, 11 in the rhTSH group and 9 in the THW group, they found no difference in final clinical outcome between preparation modalities. Similar results have also been reported for patients with RAI avid-metastatic disease by Klubo-Gwiezdzinska et al. [8], who found that rhTSH preparation and THW withdrawal resulted in similar clinical outcomes of RAI treatment.

In our patients the response to initial therapy showed a trend towards being more favorable in the rhTSH group than in the THW group. In addition, the rhTSH group required significantly fewer additional RAI treatments than the THW group, despite the increased prevalence of 2 risk factors for more aggressive disease (higher age and higher percentage of male patients) in the rhTSH group. Similar results have been found by other investigators. For patients with an intermediate ATA recurrence risk, Hugo et al. [5] reported an excellent response in 43.1 and 30.8%, an acceptable response for 26.6 and 24.8%, and an incomplete response for 30.3 and 44.4% for rhTSH and THW groups, respectively. They also found that patients in the THW group were more likely to require additional RAI treatments than patients treated with rhTSH. For patients with an intermediate ATA recurrence risk, Sabra et al. [3] reported an excellent response in 43% of rhTSH patients and 31% of THW patients ($P = 0.03$).

The 2015 ATA guidelines state in recommendation 34 that, for patients with ATA low and intermediate DTC, rhTSH stimulation is an acceptable alternative to THW for initial RAI treatment/remnant ablation [9]. The results of the present study support this. With respect to further RAI treatments, the 2015 ATA guideline suggests there is insufficient evidence to support use of rhTSH for RAI treatment. Our study suggests that in this situation use of rhTSH results in equal outcomes as compared to THW.

We are not sure why there was a trend towards higher incidence of male patients in the rhTSH group than in the THW group in our study. The age bias is most likely due to a higher prevalence of medical comorbidities in older patients, making the risks of hypothyroidism with the THW protocol higher, resulting in choosing rhTSH for more of these patients.

As these studies in patients with ATA intermediate recurrence risk suggest that there is no difference in longer-term clinical outcome between THW and rhTSH preparation and there is either no difference or improved response to initial treatment, it becomes important to compare side effects of the two preparation methods. THW is associated with hypothyroidism and a decrease in QOL. Luster et al. [4] reported that 92% of patients had symptomatic and 85% had multisymptomatic hypothyroidism. In 2006, Schroeder et al. [10] reported that THW is associated with significant decline in quality of life as assessed by SF-36 questionnaire, an effect that was not found after rhTSH administration. An important study was reported by Nygaard et al. [11] who performed a double blind, placebo-controlled randomized cross-over study comparing liothyronine L-T3 THW for 10 days with rhTSH in 56 patients with DTC receiving RAI treatment. Their primary outcome was QOL as assessed by SF-36

questionnaire, and THW was associated with a significantly worse QOL in 2 domains, social functioning and mental health. Indeed, severe hypothyroidism is associated with reversible depression, slowed reaction time, and decreased fine-motor performance and processing speed [12]. Thus, during severe hypothyroidism, patients should be cautioned against activities that could be affected by the effects of hypothyroidism, such as driving motor vehicles.

There are several limitations pertaining to the present study, including its retrospective, nonrandomized, non-blinded design. In addition, the number of patients was relatively small. Recent studies suggest that the outcome and treatment choice may be affected by the extent of node positivity (N1a versus N1b) and probably the lymph node size [9]. We also found that additional RAI treatment was required in more patients with N1b status than patients with N1a status. Regarding the size of lymph nodes, this was reported inconsistently during the study period, so that we are not able to perform this analysis.

Strengths of this study relate to its inclusion of patients from a well-defined regional area, reducing referral bias and the inclusion of a homogeneous group of patients all with pathologically proven cervical lymph node metastasis. In addition, all patients received only one method of preparation, either rhTSH or THW, for the initial and all subsequent RAI treatments. Finally, all patients were followed up on the long term in similar fashion in one single centre.

The 2015 ATA guideline definitions for assessment of clinical status during follow-up [9] vary slightly from the definitions in our study. The ATA guideline definition of excellent response is the same as that in our study. The ATA guideline differentiates between biochemical and structural incomplete response, while in our study these have been grouped together. The "indeterminate response" is defined in the 2015 ATA guideline as "non-specific, biochemical or structural findings which cannot be confidently classified as either benign or malignant" and is essentially the same as the "acceptable response" in our study. Based on the lower limit of detectable thyroglobulin in the assay used at the time of our study, we determined study-specific biochemical criteria to define clinical status, for example, "no evidence of disease" or "persistent" disease. In addition, we developed a specific definition for recurrent disease, which was important for the primary objective of our study.

The optimal management of regional lymph node metastases and ATA intermediate risk patients in thyroid cancer remains to be determined [13]. A recent study suggests that the presence of cervical lymph node metastasis increases the risk for recurrence of thyroid cancer and mortality [14], and another retrospective study suggests that treating these patients with RAI decreases mortality [15]. This indicates that it remains extremely important to determine how adjuvant RAI can be most effective with least side effects. The present study lends further support to the notion that use of rhTSH in thyroid cancer patients with nodal metastatic disease is associated with similar long-term outcomes while perhaps improving initial response to treatment. This suggests that it is time for a well-designed prospective randomized study comparing the effect of rhTSH and THW on the initial response, clinical outcomes, and short- and long-term side effects in patients with intermediate recurrence risk.

Disclosure

The funding body did not have any role in data analysis, interpretation, or paper preparation.

Conflict of Interests

The authors declare that there is no conflict of interests regarding the publication of this paper.

Acknowledgment

The authors' thyroid cancer registry was supported by unrestricted grants from Genzyme, a Sanofi Company. Up to the date of rhTSH approval by Health Canada, Genzyme generously provided free product for all cases.

References

[1] D. S. Cooper, G. M. Doherty, B. R. Haugen et al., "Revised American thyroid association management guidelines for patients with thyroid nodules and differentiated thyroid cancer," *Thyroid*, vol. 19, no. 11, pp. 1167–1214, 2009.

[2] F. Pacini, P. W. Ladenson, M. Schlumberger et al., "Radioiodine ablation of thyroid remnants after preparation with recombinant human thyrotropin in differentiated thyroid carcinoma: results of an international, randomized, controlled study," *Journal of Clinical Endocrinology and Metabolism*, vol. 91, no. 3, pp. 926–932, 2006.

[3] M. M. Sabra, R. K. Grewal, H. Tala, S. M. Larson, and R. M. Tuttle, "Clinical outcomes following empiric radioiodine therapy in patients with structurally identifiable metastatic follicular cell-derived thyroid carcinoma with negative diagnostic but positive post-therapy 131I whole-body scans," *Thyroid*, vol. 22, no. 9, pp. 877–883, 2012.

[4] M. Luster, R. Felbinger, M. Dietlein, and C. Reiners, "Thyroid hormone withdrawal in patients with differentiated thyroid carcinoma: a one hundred thirty-patient pilot survey on consequences of hypothyroidism and a pharmacoeconomic comparison to recombinant thyrotropin administration," *Thyroid*, vol. 15, no. 10, pp. 1147–1155, 2005.

[5] J. Hugo, E. Robenshtok, R. Grewal, S. Larson, and R. M. Tuttle, "Recombinant human thyroid stimulating hormone-assisted radioactive iodine remnant ablation in thyroid cancer patients at intermediate to high risk of recurrence," *Thyroid*, vol. 22, no. 10, pp. 1007–1015, 2012.

[6] P. W. Rosario, A. F. C. Mineiro Filho, R. X. Lacerda, and M. R. Calsolari, "Long-term follow-up of at least five years after recombinant human thyrotropin compared to levothyroxine withdrawal for thyroid remnant ablation with radioactive iodine," *Thyroid*, vol. 22, no. 3, pp. 332–333, 2012.

[7] E. Molinaro, C. Giani, L. Agate et al., "Patients with differentiated thyroid cancer who underwent radioiodine thyroid remnant ablation with low-activity (1)(3)(1)I after either recombinant human TSH or thyroid hormone therapy withdrawal showed the same outcome after a 10-year follow-up," *The Journal of Clinical Endocrinology & Metabolism*, vol. 98, pp. 2693–2700, 2013.

[8] J. Klubo-Gwiezdzinska, K. D. Burman, D. Van Nostrand, M. Mete, J. Jonklaas, and L. Wartofsky, "Radioiodine treatment of metastatic thyroid cancer: relative efficacy and side effect profile of preparation by thyroid hormone withdrawal versus recombinant human thyrotropin," *Thyroid*, vol. 22, no. 3, pp. 310–317, 2012.

[9] B. R. Haugen, E. K. Alexander, K. C. Bible et al., "2015 American Thyroid Association Management Guidelines for adult patients with thyroid nodules and differentiated thyroid cancer: The American Thyroid Association Guidelines Task Force on thyroid nodules and differentiated thyroid cancer," *Thyroid*, vol. 26, no. 1, pp. 1–133, 2016.

[10] P. R. Schroeder, B. R. Haugen, F. Pacini et al., "A comparison of short-term changes in health-related quality of life in thyroid carcinoma patients undergoing diagnostic evaluation with recombinant human thyrotropin compared with thyroid hormone withdrawal," *Journal of Clinical Endocrinology and Metabolism*, vol. 91, no. 3, pp. 878–884, 2006.

[11] B. Nygaard, L. Bastholt, F. N. Bennedbæk, T. W. Klausen, and J. Bentzen, "A placebo-controlled, blinded and randomised study on the effects of recombinant human thyrotropin on quality of life in the treatment of thyroid cancer," *European Thyroid Journal*, vol. 2, no. 3, pp. 195–202, 2013.

[12] C. D. Smith, R. Grondin, W. Lemaster, B. Martin, B. T. Gold, and K. B. Ain, "Reversible cognitive, motor, and driving impairments in severe hypothyroidism," *Thyroid*, vol. 25, no. 1, pp. 28–36, 2015.

[13] I. J. Nixon and A. R. Shaha, "Management of regional nodes in thyroid cancer," *Oral Oncology*, vol. 49, no. 7, pp. 671–675, 2013.

[14] A. Amin, G. Younis, K. Sayed, and Z. Saeed, "Cervical lymph node metastasis in differentiated thyroid carcinoma: does it have an impact on disease-related morbid events?" *Nuclear Medicine Communications*, vol. 36, no. 2, pp. 120–124, 2015.

[15] E. Ruel, S. Thomas, M. Dinan, J. M. Perkins, S. A. Roman, and J. A. Sosa, "Adjuvant radioactive iodine therapy is associated with improved survival for patients with intermediate-risk papillary thyroid cancer," *The Journal of Clinical Endocrinology & Metabolism*, vol. 100, no. 4, pp. 1529–1536, 2015.

22

Enchondroma versus Chondrosarcoma in Long Bones of Appendicular Skeleton: Clinical and Radiological Criteria—A Follow-Up

Eugenio M. Ferrer-Santacreu,[1] **Eduardo J. Ortiz-Cruz,**[2]
Mariana Díaz-Almirón,[3] **and Jose Juan Pozo Kreilinger**[4]

[1]Orthopaedic Surgery Department, Hospital Universitario de Móstoles, C/Río Júcar s/n, 28935 Móstoles, Spain
[2]Orthopaedic Oncology Unit, Orthopaedic Surgery Department, Hospital Universitario La Paz, Paseo de la Castellana 261, 28046 Madrid, Spain
[3]Hospital La Paz Research Institute (IdiPaz), Paseo de la Castellana 261, 28046 Madrid, Spain
[4]Pathology Department, Hospital Universitario La Paz, Paseo de la Castellana 261, 28046 Madrid, Spain

Correspondence should be addressed to Eduardo J. Ortiz-Cruz; eortiz@mdanderson.es

Academic Editor: Bruno Vincenzi

As of today two types of cartilage tumors remain a challenge even for the orthopedic oncologist: enchondroma (E), a benign tumor, and chondrosarcoma (LGC), a malignant and low aggressiveness tumor. A prospective study of 133 patients with a cartilaginous tumor of low aggressiveness in the long bones of the appendicular skeleton was done to prove this difficult differential diagnosis. Parameters including medical history and radiological and nuclear imaging were collected and compared to the result of the biopsy. A scale of aggressiveness was applied to each patient according to the number of aggressiveness episodes present. A comparison of the results of the biopsy with the initial diagnosis made by the orthopedic oncologist based solely on clinical data and imaging tests was also made. Finally, a management algorithm for these cases was proposed. A statistical significance for LGC resulted from the parameter as follows: pain on palpation, involvement of cortical in either the CT or MRI, and Tc99 bone scan uptake equal or superior to anterosuperior iliac crest. In our series, a tumor scoring 5 points or higher in the scale of aggressiveness can have 50% more chance of being LGC. When compared with the gold standard (the biopsy), surgeon's initial judgement showed a sensitivity of 73.5% and a specificity of 94.1%.

1. Introduction

Distinction between enchondroma (E) and low-grade chondrosarcoma (LGC) remains a challenge for any specialist on musculoskeletal sarcomas management including orthopaedic surgeons, pathologists, and radiologists (Table 1). Even in the most expert hands, these two entities can lead to a wrong diagnosis and, as a consequence, to an unsuitable treatment [1–3]. No previous published study has been able to show any distinctive feature between E and LGC in long bones of the appendicular skeleton [4–7]. An initial diagnosis based upon clinical, radiological, and metabolical data is capital, because the biopsy does not provide always an accurate result.

Firstly, our aim with this study was to find out if there was any feature enabling us to differentiate between E and LGC without performing any invasive procedure, as biopsy. On that purpose, we performed a prospective data collection of patients having a low aggressiveness chondral tumor in long bones of appendicular skeleton including information from their clinical stories and imaging. We also included the initial diagnosis based upon clinical and imaging data made by a single experienced sarcoma surgeon. Correlation between the biopsy and each radiological and clinical feature, as well

TABLE 1: Compared features of solitary enchondroma and low grade chondrosarcoma.

Features	Solitary enchondroma	Low grade chondrosarcoma
Clinical	(i) Younger patients (ii) Pain is rare (iii) Typical in appendicular skeleton (iv) In general <5 cm	(i) Patients > 25 years (ii) Inflammatory pain (iii) Axial skeleton (iv) Bigger size
Radiological	(i) Intramedullary (ii) No periosteal reaction (iii) No endosteal scalloping (iv) No changes over time (v) No soft tissue mass	(i) Intramedullary (ii) Periostealreaction and microfractures (iii) Endosteal scalloping (iv) Loss of calcification. Increasing size (v) Soft tissue mass in some cases
Pathology	(i) Encasement pattern (ii) No endosteal scalloping (iii) Multinodular (iv) Surrounded by lamellar bone (v) No bone marrow infiltration	(i) Haversian system invasion (ii) Periosteal reaction and endosteal scalloping (iii) Single mass (iv) Occasional sites of necrosis and haemorrhage (v) Bone marrow invasion

as surgeon's initial diagnosis, was performed. Secondly, we elaborated an aggressiveness score which could serve as a tool in decision-making based on clinical, radiological, and metabolical features. Finally, we have made a management algorithm proposal based on our findings for the management of these patients.

2. Patients and Methods

2.1. Data Collection. We have performed a prospective study in which 182 patients presenting a low aggressiveness cartilage-type lesion on plain radiographs in long bones of appendicular skeleton suggestive of E or LGC have been included. In the first visit to the clinic, personal and clinical data were collected. Further imaging (CT, MRI, and bone scan) including reports done by specialists were carefully collected to complete our database. We also included specialist's first diagnostic impression based upon clinical and imaging data and the final result of the biopsy. Patients under 18 years old, cartilage lesions in hands, feet, and axial skeleton, cases of enchondromatosis (including Ollier's disease and Maffucci's syndrome), osteochondromatosis, secondary chondrosarcomas or chondrosarcomas of intermediate or high grade according to Evans classification, and recurrences of previously operated tumors were excluded.

In each patient, a form was filled with personal data, physical examination, and symptoms (focusing on pain and its features: presence of pain with palpation, inflammatory or mechanic, evolution, etc.). Concerning age, patients were divided into two groups: up to 35 years of age and more than 35 years of age. The site of the tumor (bone, side, and bone area) was registered. In plain radiographs, we measured size, site, and appearance and changes in calcification over time. In CT, size, calcification (presence and changes over time) endosteal scalloping, and soft tissue mass (STM) were registered. In MRI, size, endosteal scalloping, and STM were also recorded. Concerning Tc99 bone scan, lesions were classified according to the presence of radionuclide uptake on whole-body image. The degree of uptake was compared to the physiological uptake of the iliac crest (similar to or lower or

higher than iliac crest uptake) focusing on the anterosuperior iliac crest (ASIC), as recorded by nuclear medicine specialists in their reports. In each case, an initial diagnosis (E or LGC) was made by a single specialist in musculoskeletal oncology surgery based upon clinical, radiological, and metabolic data. A decision of performing a biopsy or just doing a follow-up of the patient was made after this initial diagnosis. A record of the biopsy and final result was also included and all specimens were reviewed by the same department. The judgment made by the pathologist could confirm or reject surgeon's initial impression. In those cases in which an E was suspected, patients were followed periodically. If, after three years of follow-up, no changes in clinical or radiological features were registered, those cases were assumed hypothetically as E although diagnosis was made only based upon clinical and radiological criteria.

2.2. Aggressiveness Scale. As part of each patient's evaluation, an account of features indicating aggressiveness was performed (Table 2). One point was given to every feature of aggressiveness shown by the lesion in three categories: clinical (CA), radiological (RA), and metabolic (MA). As well, a final score was obtained with the sum of the score obtained in each category. Statistical significance between biopsy's result and the score obtained in each category as well as the final score was calculated.

2.3. Statistical Analysis. Statistical analysis of the collected data was performed by Hospital La Paz University Research Institute (IdIPaz). All statistical tests were bilateral and significance was considered when P values were under 0.05. Software employed was SAS 9.1 (SAS Institute Inc, Cary, NC, USA).

Quantitative data description of our series consisted of mean and standard deviation and median, minimal, and maximal values. To evaluate the accuracy of the first diagnosis made by the surgeon compared to the gold standard (biopsy's result) in each case, sensitivity and specificity, as well as false positive and false negative rates, were calculated. In order to establish statistical relationship between every feature

TABLE 2: Aggressiveness score employed in our study.

Aggressiveness categories	Features (1 point per each of the following features)
Clinical aggressiveness CA	Presence of inflammatory pain Presence of pain with palpation
Radiological aggressiveness RA	Size bigger than 5 cm Metaphyseal location Loss of calcification (calcification lysis) over time Cortical involvement in CT or MRI Presence of a soft tissue mass in CT or MRI
Metabolic aggressiveness MA	Presence of Tc99 uptake in bone scan Uptake equal to or higher than anterosuperior iliac crest (ASIC)
Total aggressiveness TA	=CA + RA + MA

TABLE 3: Tumor location distributed by diagnosis.

Bone	Enchondroma	LGC
Femur	48.1%	37.3%
Humerus	36.7%	41.2 %
Fibula	6.3%	11.3%
Tibia	7.6%	9.8%
Ulna	1.3%	

TABLE 4: Bone site affected.

Bone site affected	Enchondroma	LGC
Proximal metaphysis	35.4%	40.4%
Distal metaphyso-epiphyseal	30.4%	19.6%

included in the study and the possibility of being an E or a LGC, P values obtained by means of the Fisher's exact test and chi-square test were considered. This was also calculated between the scores obtained in every aggressiveness category.

As well, relationship between total score (TS) in the aggressiveness scale (AS) and biopsy's result was calculated. A statistical model was developed to show the risk increase of having a LGC with every additional point, that is, with every additional feature of aggressiveness shown by the lesion.

2.4. Literature Review. Previous peer-reviewed literature on the matter has been revised with the aid of Pubmed and Ovid databases using the following keywords: "enchondroma versus low grade chondrosarcoma" and "chondral tumors diagnosis". Papers older than 20 years were discarded unless they were considered as classics by experts.

2.5. Ethical Issues. According to our country legal requirements, patients were informed and gave a verbal consent to allow us to use their clinical data in this research. As well, we obtained a certificate of approval from the ethical committee for clinical research in our institution.

3. Results

3.1. Clinical, Radiological, and Metabolic Features. A prospective study has been performed in which 182 patients were included. Twenty-two variables were registered for analysis. At the end, only 133 patients completed the follow-up. Of these, 39 were diagnosed as E (29.3%) and 94 as LGC (70.7%).

A biopsy was performed in 90 patients (13 were percutaneous and CT-guided, 9 were incisional, and 68 were excisional). The remaining 43 patients were followed up because they had a chondral tumor without any sign of clinical or radiological aggressiveness. As explained above in the patients and methods section, they were considered as E.

Our series consisted of 33 men (24.8%) with a mean age of 49.8 years and 100 women with a mean age of 49.8 years. Global mean age in our series was 50.1 years. In patients finally diagnosed as E, 25.3% were male and 74.7% were female. In those having a LGC, 23.5% were male

and 76.5% female. Regardless of these differences in gender distribution, statistical analysis showed no relevance ($P = 0.494$). Concerning age groups, 14.3% of the patients were less than 35 years of age and 82.7% were of that age or older. Among those diagnosed as E, 16.7% were under 35 years of age and 83.3% were older. In the LGC group, 11.8% were less than 35 years of age and 88.2% were older. Analysis showed no relevance between final diagnosis and belonging to one specific age group ($P = 0.307$). Most common bone affected was the femur (44.1%) followed by the humerus (37.5%). Fibula (8.82%) and tibia (8.2%) were not so frequent in our study (Table 3). These differences turned out to be irrelevant when analyzed ($P = 0.575$). Among cases of E, 55.7% were on the right side and 44.3% on the left. In the LGC group, 39.2% of the lesions were on the right side while 60.8% were on the left. No relevance was found regarding this matter ($P = 0.116$).

Concerning the most frequent bone site affected, proximal metaphysis (36.09% of the cases) and distal metaphyso-epiphyseal zone (24.81%) followed by proximal epiphysometaphyseal zone (17.29%) were the three top sites in our study. Table 4 shows locations distribution by diagnosis. When analyzed, these data showed no statistical relationship with final diagnosis ($P = 0.575$).

Almost 60% of the cases were casual findings when the involved area was studied for other reasons, mostly pain or traumatism. In 61.2% of the patients pain had a mechanical pattern, while in 29.5% of the patients, pain was inflammatory. 9.3% of the patients had no pain at all. In the E group, 14.1% were asymptomatic whereas only 2% of the LGC showed no symptoms at all. Among those patients with E who had pain, in 74.6% pain was mechanic (58% in the LGC) and in 25.4% pain was inflammatory (42% in the LGC). Analyzing these data, P value was 0.111. No statistical significance was found for this feature. In the physical examination, 70.67% of the patients had pain with palpation. Among patients with E, 58.2% had pain with palpation and among patients with LGC, proportion reached 88.2%. Statistical analysis showed $P < 0.001$ establishing statistical relevance between the presence of pain during physical examination and the possibility of the lesion being a LGC.

TABLE 5: Size measured on plain radiographs.

Size	Enchondroma	LGC
>5 cm	31%	40%

TABLE 6: CT cortical involvement.

Involvement depth	Enchondroma	LGC
1/3	61.1%	63.63%
2/3	22.2%	15.15%
3/3	16.6%	21.21%

TABLE 7: MRI cortical involvement.

Involvement depth	Enchondroma	LGC
1/3	62.5%	63.3%
2/3	**18.75%**	**13.33%**
3/3	18.75%	23.33%

TABLE 8: Bone scan uptake.

Technetium 99 bone scan	Enchondroma	LGC
=Uptake to anterosuperior iliac crest	44.1%	54.3%
<Uptake to anterosuperior iliac crest	35.3%	10.9%
>Uptake to anterosuperior iliac crest	20.6%	34.8%

Size measured on plain radiographs was bigger than 5 cm in 40.61% of the cases. Analysis sowed $P = 0.326$ with no relevance for these differences (Table 5).

There were no cases of soft tissue mass in CT or MRI in our study. Cortex involvement in CT imaging was seen in 63.9% of the cases. As explained in the patients and methods section, involvement of the cortical bone was divided into three categories, according to the depth affected by the tumor: one-third, two-thirds, or total involvement (Table 6). Analysis showed $P < 0.01$ because most cases without cortical involvement (36.09%) were finally diagnosed as E. A relationship between E and lack of cortical involvement was present in our study.

In MRI, 31.7% of our series showed some cortical involvement, which represents half the cases detected with CT scan. Table 7 shows the MRI cortical involvement in each diagnosis. Statistical analysis showed $P < 0.001$ which is understandable after seeing that most E do not have cortical involvement and most LGC do. Because of this situation, patients were redistributed in two groups: cortical involvement in CT or MRI and no cortical involvement in CT and MRI.

Technetium 99 bone scan was positive in some degree in 97.5% of the patients in our study. 97.2% of the E and 97.5% of the LGC showed some uptake. As there was almost no difference between both groups, no significance was found after analysis ($P = 0.652$). Comparison between tumor's uptake and anterosuperior iliac crest (ASIC) physiological uptake is shown in Table 8. No statistical differences were detected between those cases having higher uptake and showing a similar uptake. But, if these two categories were considered as one and compared to those patients showing lower uptake than ASIC, then $P < 0.01$ which is statistically significant. Significance was also found in the fact that 82.8% of the cases showing lower uptake were finally diagnosed as E and 17.2% as LGC ($P < 0.01$).

To summarize our findings so far, pain with palpation, cortical involvement in any degree in CT or MRI, and a similar or higher Tc99 uptake than ASIC showed statistical relevance in the possibility of this lesion being a LGC.

3.2. Aggressiveness Score. As explained in the Patients and Methods, we employed an aggressiveness score in each patient giving one point for each feature of aggressiveness shown by the lesion in three fields: clinical (CA), radiological (RA), and metabolic (MA). Adding the points obtained in the three categories, we obtained a final score or total aggressiveness (TA). Considering CA, patients with E scored 0 points in 30.2% of the cases, 1 point in 57%, and 2 points in 12.7%. Among those having LGC, only 6% scored 0 points, 60% scored 1 point, and 34% scored two points. From another point of view, among patients having 0 points of CA, 88.9% were E and 11.1% were LGC. Among those patients scoring 1 point, 60% were E and 40% LGC. Finally, patients scoring 2 points turned out to be LGC in 63% of the cases and E in 37% of the cases. Analysis showed $P < 0.01$ for these differences, revealing a high possibility of E when CA is 0 and LGC when CA was 2.

Among patients having an E 3.8% scored 0 points (we had no cases among the LGC); 79.2% scored 1 point (20.8% of the LGC); 51.9% scored 2 points (48.1% of the LGC); 8.9% scored 3 points (28% of the LGC). Statistical analysis showed significance in the possibility of having an E when RA was 1 and having a LGC when RA was 3. Differences in the 0 points' group were not significant because only three patients were in that category (3 E and no LGC).

Finally, metabolic aggressiveness (MA) showed that 12.7% of the E had 0 points (8% of the LGC), 32.9% had 1 point (12% of the LGC), and 54.4% had 2 points (80% of the LGC). On the other hand, among those patients scoring 0 points, 71.4% were E and 28.6% LGC; among those scoring 1 point 81.2% were E and 18.8% LGC. Finally, among those scoring 2 points, 61.2% were E and 38.8% were LGC. These differences were statistically significant when analyzed ($P < 0.01$). When considering the final score or total aggressiveness, analysis showed that every new point increased the possibility of having a LGC rather than an E. Specifically, every new point in the score multiplies the risk of having a LGC by 2.3 ($P < 0.01$). Our model established that a patient scoring 5 points or more in the aggressiveness score had more than 50% of possibilities of having a LGC.

3.3. Expert's Initial Judgement. The surgeon in charge of the initial diagnosis classified 64 of the cases as LGC, of which 61 were confirmed by pathologists. On the other hand, 69 were classified as E but only 47 were confirmed as such and the other 22 patients were reclassified as LGC. Sensitivity in our series was 73.5% and specificity was 94.1% for diagnosis based exclusively on clinical and radiological features. Positive predictive value was 93.5% and negative predictive value was

68.1%. False positive rate was 5.9% while false negative rate was 26.5% (confidence interval of 95%).

4. Discussion

Distinction between clinical E and LGC remains a challenge for specialists in bone and soft tissue sarcomas. So far, we do not know a paper that has analyzed the relationship between specific clinical, radiological, and metabolic features and the possibility of that lesion to be an E or a LGC in long bones, except for the one published by this group in 2012 [4]. Our reference in the literature has been the study published by Murphey et al. [5, 6] in which this same idea was developed but taking into account chondrosarcomas of intermediate and high degree as well. They found relevant differences in the following features: gender, size, metaphyso-epiphyseal location for LGC and diaphyseal location for E, pain, STM, endosteal scalloping both in depth and in length, histological pattern, cortical remodeling, periosteal reaction, degree of mineralization, amount and homogeneity of Tc99 uptake in bone scan, pathologic fracture, and cortical thickening. In their study on the usefulness of radiographs and clinical data, Geirnaardt et al. [7] obtained relevant differences favoring LGC when the lesion was in axial skeleton and was bigger than 5 cm. Our previous paper in 2011 [4], also focused on long bones in appendicular skeleton and including 82 patients, showed no relevant differences between E and LGC when comparing the same clinical, radiological, and features analyzed in this paper. Our first hypothesis proposed the absence of any feature which had a statistical relationship with the final diagnosis of E or LGC in the biopsy. Statistical analysis in our series has shown that pain with palpation, cortical involvement in CT or MRI, and uptake in Tc99 bone scan similar or higher than ASIC had significant relationship with a final diagnosis of LGC. For that reason, we have rejected our initial hypothesis.

4.1. Clinical Findings and Plain Radiograph. In our study the only clinical feature showing statistical relationship with LGC has been pain with palpation. No differences were found concerning the type of pain or features found in the radiographs. Presence of pain, especially when having inflammatory pattern, has always been related to malignancy but in our series we did not find a relationship between this type of pain and LGC. Murphey et al. [5], in their study, found that tumor's size, pain of any kind, patient's age and gender, and tumor location (Metaphyso-epiphyseal for LGC and diaphyseal for E) were statistically significant to distinguish between E and LGC. We must remember that Murphey's study included chondrosarcomas of all grades. Geirnaardt et al. [7] reached the conclusion in their study that a tumor bigger than five cm in a plain radiograph was significant for LGC (including tumors in axial skeleton). Nevertheless, they found differences for clinical symptoms and stressed the scarce usefulness of these features to reach a correct diagnosis. Nevertheless, we consider that the presence of pain with palpation or inflammatory pain should make the clinician perform further imaging studies for a more accurate decision-making.

4.2. Imaging Studies. Imaging includes CT scan, MRI scan, and Tc99 bone scan. Some studies have tried to analyze medullary perilesional edema or contrast enhancement but we did not include these features because they were not part of the standard management of a low aggressiveness cartilage-like tumor [8–10]. In our series, no STM has been found. Concerning cortical involvement, our initial classification in one-third, two-thirds, or complete involvement did not show any differences. However when we redistributed our patients in two categories, that is, cortical involvement or no cortical involvement in CT or MRI, we detected an association between cortical involvement of any degree and final diagnosis of LGC in both CT or MRI. Moreover, these differences were especially significant in MRI images. This finding is of special interest considering that CT scan is supposed to provide a better detection of cortical involvement than MRI. Our conclusion was that the better sensitivity of CT scan in this matter makes it possible that involvement can be found even if it is of very small degree. This makes it possible that E and LGC show almost no differences between them in CT scan imaging. On the other hand, MRI only detects cortical involvement when it has certain degree and considering that LGC usually is more aggressive in its growth, it is easier to find differences between LGC and E in MRI images. This fact, as it will be discussed later, led us to avoid CT in the standard imaging protocol of these tumors and keep it only for patients in which an MRI is not available for some reason. In Tc99 bone scan, uptake presence and comparison with ASIC's physiological uptake were analyzed. Murphey et al. detected differences between E and chondrosarcomas of all grades. They found that a higher degree of uptake and its uniformity was an indication of malignancy. In our series, most patients showed some degree of uptake. When comparing with ASIC's uptake, analysis showed that patients with similar or higher uptake had more possibilities of having a LGC. This feature was not considered in other studies but has been included in the most recent management algorithms.

4.3. Aggressiveness Score. Another goal in our study was to elaborate an aggressiveness score (AS) as a tool to measure the likelihood of a low aggressiveness cartilage tumor to be a LGC. It was a support in doubtful cases to complement clinical and radiological data and in no way can be considered as an absolute indicator of malignancy. So far, we have no notice of any score of this kind being published in peer-reviewed literature. We must make it clear that the AS should be used with tumors in long bones of appendicular skeleton where differential diagnosis between E and LGC is complicated. As explained before, in the material and method section, this score includes three categories of evaluation: clinical aggressiveness (CA) with a top score of two points, radiological aggressiveness (RA) with a top score of four points, and metabolic aggressiveness (MA) with a top score of two points. Finally, the sum of the three categories provides a total aggressiveness (TA) score. Statistical analysis of the scores obtained in our patients showed significant differences for each category separately and for the final score indicating that the higher the score is, the higher the possibility of that

(a)   (b)   (c)

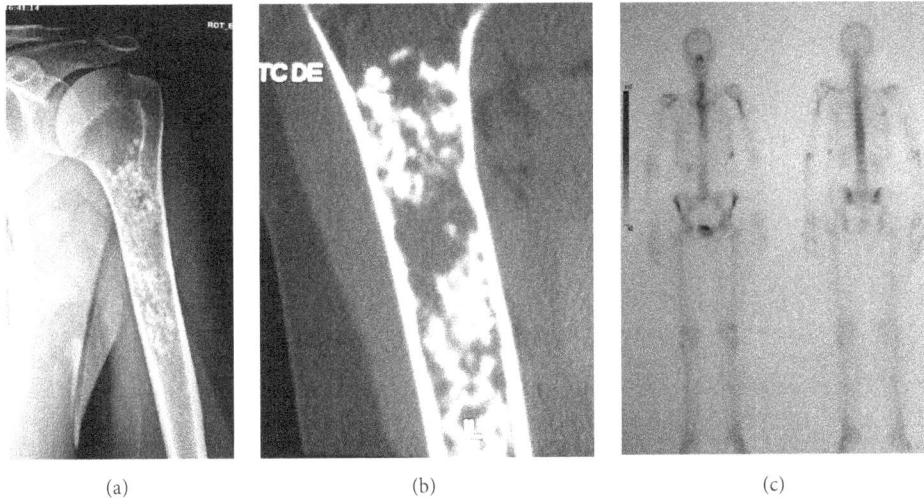

FIGURE 1: (a–c) A case of a big painless cartilage tumor with benign appearance in radiographs (a), endosteal scalloping in CT (b), and similar Tc99 uptake compared to ASIC. TA score was 5 and specimen analysis after intralesional resection with adjuvancies showed LGC.

tumor to be a LGC. It is remarkable that each feature showing significance in the first part of our study belongs to one of the three different categories of the score, that is, pain with palpation to CA, cortical involvement in CT or MRI to RA, and bone scan uptake similar or higher than ASIC to MA. A prediction model was established to appreciate the risk increase with every additional point obtained in the AS for each patient. A critical score was also established for the score in which the risk of having a LGC was higher than having an E. Our analysis established that those patients with a TA score of 5 or more had a risk of having LGC higher than 50%. We must consider that this model does not establish whether these points come from clinical, radiological, or metabolic features.

4.4. Specialist's Initial Diagnosis versus Final Diagnosis. The expert's opinion in the present study has shown a sensitivity of 73.5% and a specificity of 94.1% compared to biopsy. As mentioned at the beginning of this study, it is of key importance to have an algorithm to increase the sensitivity so no patient with a LGC is considered as an E. Specificity is also important but biopsying an E is not such a mistake compared to the opposite situation. False negative rate reaches 26.5%, showing that, even in the hands of a specialist, there is a certain risk of choosing the wrong option with these tumors.

4.5. Management Algorithm Proposal. The last of our goals in the present study was the elaboration of a management algorithm (Figure 4), trying to integrate previous conclusions in the literature and our results. Several authors such as Weiner et al. [11–14] have reviewed the management of these tumors. Our proposal is focused on tumors of long bones of appendicular skeleton and includes our aggressiveness score in the distinction of these two entities (Table 2). From our point of view, there are two key decisions when studying these tumors: when we have to perform a complete imaging study including CT/MRI and bone scan and when we have to make a surgical decision regarding these patients under the

suspicion of a LGC. The surgical technique preferred by the authors is an extensive intralesional resection associated with local adjuvant treatment (high-speed burr, phenolization, lavage with a high-pressure pulsatile system, and then packing the defect with cement). An additional internal fixation was indicated when needed (mainly distal femur) [15–23].

Those patients having a low aggressiveness cartilage tumor in long bones should be considered for further imaging studies if they have an inflammatory pain or pain with palpation is found. Even if many authors abandon the clinical signs as a reason to request more imaging studies, we think that clinical signs make the difference when a radiograph did not help with the diagnosis. Traditionally, CT scan, MRI scan, and Tc99 bone scan were included in the study. In our series, cortical involvement of any degree in both CT and MRI has shown significant relationship with those tumors that were finally considered as LGC in the biopsy. Moreover, MRI showed itself as the best tool to differentiate LGC from E according to cortical involvement. Geirnaardt et al. [7] concluded that a polilobular pattern, pop-corn calcification, absence of cortical involvement, and a nongeographical margin are indicative of an E. On the other hand, the presence of these features does not assure that the tumor is a LGC. In another paper, De Beuckeleer et al. [24] concluded that the use of contrast enhanced MRI can show features more typical of LGC such as arcs and rings enhancement, low signal septs, and lobulated tumors. Janzen et al. [9] found that peritumoral bone marrow contrast enhancement was more indicative of LGC in their series of 23 patients. Cortical involvement was not significant in their series. In our study, contrast was not employed because it is not a routine for cartilage tumors evaluation for our musculoskeletal radiologists. In addition, papers studying cartilage tumors have shorter series of patients compared to ours. Our proposal is to perform only an MRI and a Tc99 bone scan, leaving CT for those patients in which an MRI is not available (pacemakers, metal implants, etc.) or for doubtful cases, in which more information could be needed to complete the aggressiveness score.

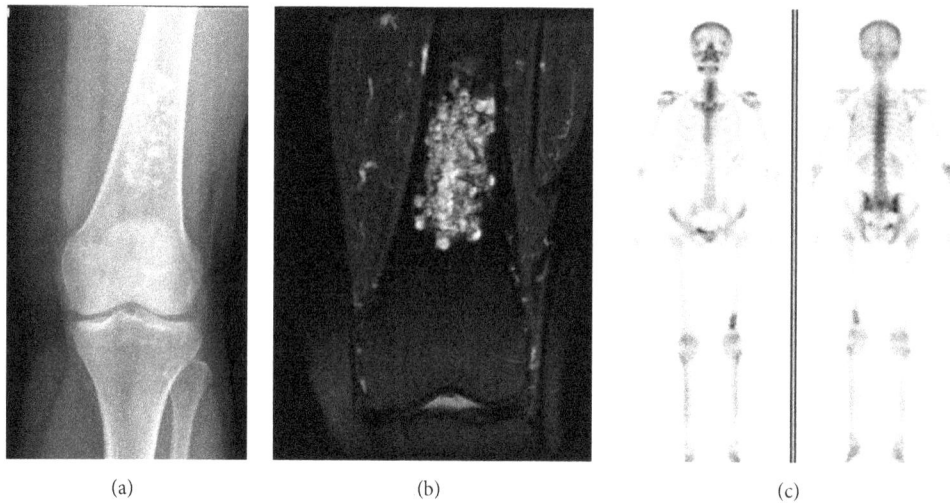

FIGURE 2: (a–c) Case of a tumor cartilage in distal femur (a) with cortical involvement in MRI (b) and increased Tc99 uptake compared to ASIC (c). TA was 5 and specimen showed LGC.

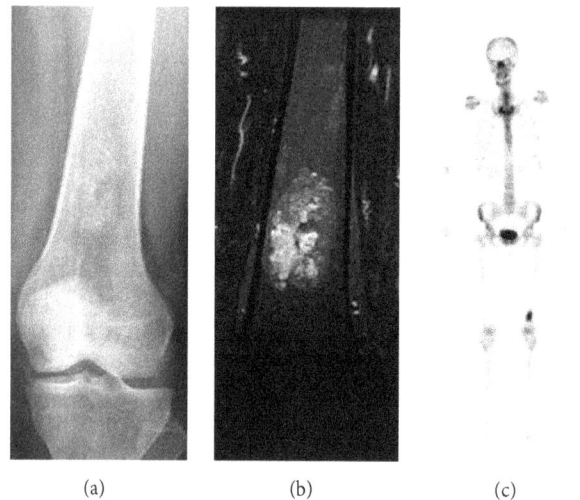

FIGURE 3: (a–c) Similar case of a tumor cartilage in distal femur (a) with cortical involvement in MRI (b) and increased Tc99 uptake compared to ASIC (c). TA was 5 and specimen showed enchondroma.

With the results of the imaging, four situations are possible:

  (i) With no cortical involvement in MRI:

    (a) No uptake or less than ASIC's in bone scan: clinical and radiological follow-up is our recommendation in these cases.

    (b) Uptake similar or higher than ASIC's. Doubts with these patients are logical with a clean MRI but strong metabolic activity. We recommend the use of the aggressiveness score and if 5 or more points are obtained, an intralesional resection with adjuvancies should be performed.

  (ii) With cortical involvement in MRI:

    (a) No uptake or uptake less than ASIC's in bone scan: doubts with these patients are logical with an MRI showing local damage but weak metabolic activity. We recommend the use of the aggressiveness score and if 5 or more points are obtained, an intralesional resection with adjuvancies should be performed.

    (b) Uptake similar or higher than ASIC's. In this situation in which signs of potential malignancy are present, an intralesional resection with adjuvancies is recommended.

We think that the AS can also be used in those cases where not all the images are available as we mentioned above in the discussion; the final score is taken into account regardless

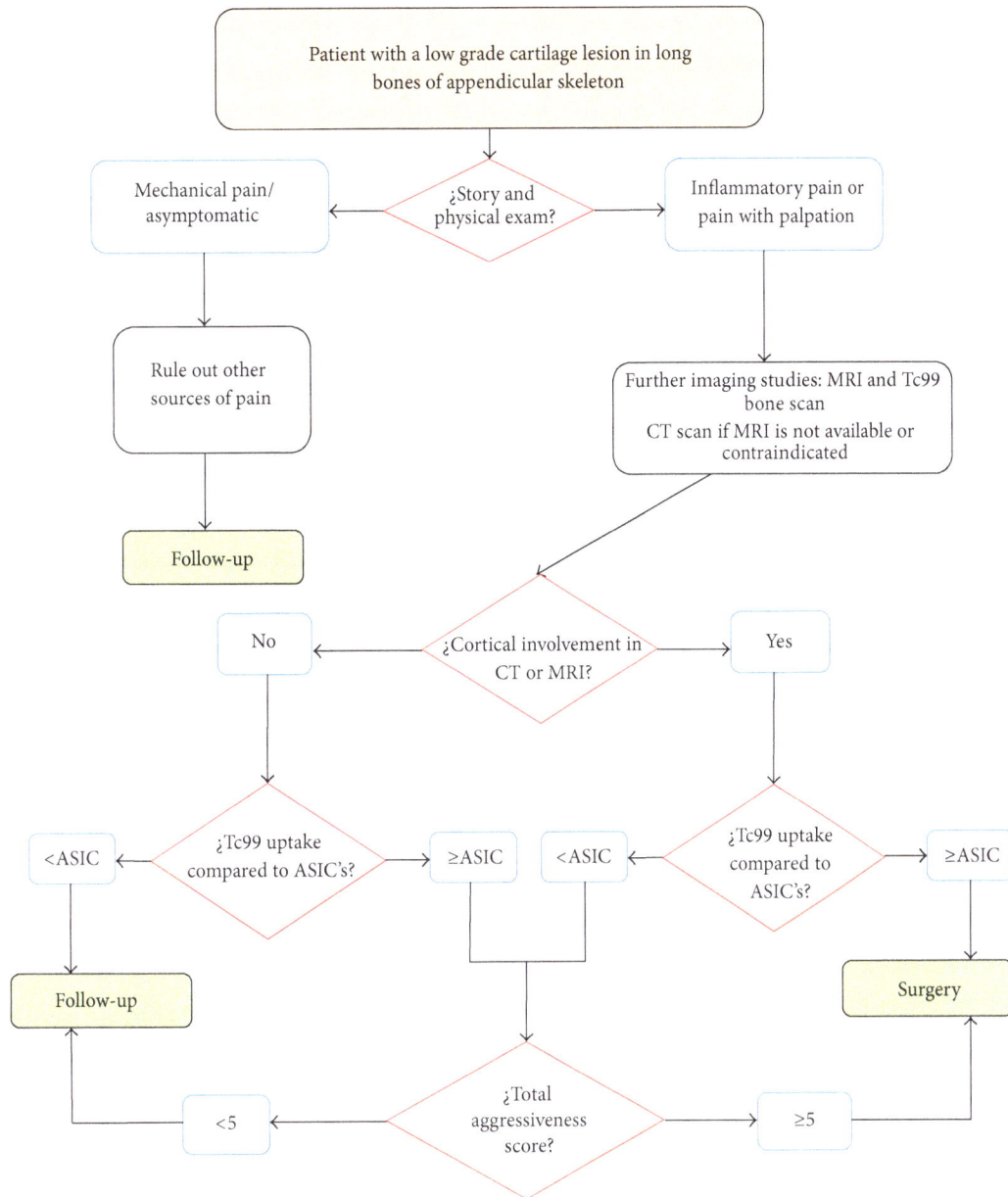

FIGURE 4: Management algorithm for low aggressiveness cartilage tumors in long bones of appendicular skeleton.

of which categories the points are obtained in (see cases in Figures 1, 2, and 3).

5. Strengths and Weaknesses of the Study

The strong points of this study include the fact that we focused our analysis on tumors located in long bones where the diagnosis is more difficult. Moreover, we have excluded the chondrosarcomas of grade II according to the Evans classification. Prospective data collection and patients being interrogated and examined by the same surgeon, who is a widely experienced specialist in bone sarcomas, enabled us to have a uniform database to analyze. Weaknesses of the study include the fact that imaging reports have been made by different radiologists and nuclear medicine specialists, although the same surgeon evaluated all the images and the most borderline cases were presented at the weekly multidisciplinary meeting of sarcomas. Not all the imaging studies were available for every patient which is the reason why only 133 patients were finally included in the study. The fact that not all the patients have been biopsied is a major limitation of the study. Authors found it ethically unsuitable to perform a biopsy in a patient whose tumor has been an incidental finding, with no signs of aggressiveness and a very small size, just to confirm it is an E which does not require further treatment.

6. Conclusions

Distinction between E and LGC remains a challenge even for experts in bone sarcomas as shown in the results obtained when comparing an expert's first opinion and the final diagnosis in the biopsy. In our study, three features showed statistical relationship with LGC: pain on palpation, cortical involvement in CT/MRI, and Tc99 uptake similar to or higher than ASIC. These three features belong to the three categories in which we have divided our aggressiveness score. This score orientates the risk for a cartilage tumor in long bones of the appendicular skeleton to be a LGC rather than an E. This happens when the patient obtains 5 points or more. In view of all these facts, we have proposed a management algorithm which stresses the use of MRI, instead of CT, and Tc99 bone scan to complete the information provided by physical examination and plain radiographs. In case of strong suspicion of LGC, an intralesional resection with adjuvancies should be performed to obtain a suitable specimen for final diagnosis.

Disclosure

The present study has been supervised by the ethical committee of Hospital Universitario La Paz. The present study was performed in Hospital Universitario La Paz.

Conflict of Interests

The authors declare that they do not have any competing interest regarding the preparation of the present study.

Authors' Contribution

Eugenio M. Ferrer-Santacreu carried out data collection, discussion, conclusions preparation, and paper preparation. Eduardo J. Ortiz-Cruz carried out study design and supervision, database design, data collection, discussion, and conclusions preparation. Mariana Díaz carried out statistical analysis. Jose Juan Pozo Kreilinger carried out pathology assessment and paper revision.

Acknowledgments

The authors would like to thank the contributing members of the Pathology Department and Musculoskeletal Radiology Section of Hospital Universitario La Paz. Their professional and technical support has been of a great value to them in the preparation of the present study.

References

[1] K. K. Unni, "Cartilaginous lesions of bone," *Journal of Orthopaedic Science*, vol. 6, no. 5, pp. 457–472, 2001.

[2] D. Eefting, Y. M. Schrage, M. J. A. Geirnaerdt et al., "Assessment of interobserver variability and histologic parameters to improve reliability in classification and grading of central cartilaginous tumors," *The American Journal of Surgical Pathology*, vol. 33, no. 1, pp. 50–57, 2009.

[3] Skeletal Lesions Interobserver Correlation among Expert Diagnosticians (SLICED) Study Group, "Reliability of histopathologic and radiologic grading of cartilaginous neoplasms in long bones," *The Journal of Bone & Joint Surgery—American Volume*, vol. 89, no. 10, pp. 2113–2123, 2007.

[4] E. M. Ferrer-Santacreu, E. J. Ortiz-Cruz, J. M. González-López, and E. P. Fernández, "Enchondroma versus low-grade chondrosarcoma in appendicular skeleton: clinical and radiological criteria," *Journal of Oncology*, vol. 2012, Article ID 437958, 6 pages, 2012.

[5] M. D. Murphey, D. J. Flemming, S. R. Boyea, J. A. Bojescul, D. E. Sweet, and H. T. Temple, "Enchondroma versus chondrosarcoma in the appendicular skeleton: differentiating features," *Radiographics*, vol. 18, no. 5, pp. 1213–1237, 1998.

[6] M. D. Murphey, E. A. Walker, A. J. Wilson, M. J. Kransdorf, H. T. Temple, and F. H. Gannon, "From the archives of the AFIP: imaging of primary chondrosarcoma: radiologic-pathologic correlation," *RadioGraphics*, vol. 23, no. 5, pp. 1245–1278, 2003.

[7] M. U. A. Geirnaardt, J. Hermans, J. L. Bloem et al., "Usefulness of radiography in differentiating enchondroma from central grade 1 chondrosarcoma," *American Journal of Roentgenology*, vol. 169, no. 4, pp. 1097–1104, 1997.

[8] D. G. Varma, A. G. Ayala, C. H. Carrasco, S. Q. Guo, R. Kumar, and J. Edeiken, "Chondrosarcoma: MR imaging with pathologic correlation," *Radiographics*, vol. 12, no. 4, pp. 687–704, 1992.

[9] L. Janzen, P. M. Logan, J. X. O'Connell, D. G. Connell, and P. L. Munk, "Intramedullary chondroid tumors of bone: correlation of abnormal peritumoral marrow and soft-tissue MRI signal with tumor type," *Skeletal Radiology*, vol. 26, no. 2, pp. 100–106, 1997.

[10] M. J. A. Geirnaerdt, P. C. W. Hogendoorn, J. L. Bloem, A. H. M. Taminiau, and H.-J. van der Woude, "Cartilaginous tumors: fast contrast-enhanced MR imaging," *Radiology*, vol. 214, no. 2, pp. 539–546, 2000.

[11] S. D. Weiner, "Enchondroma and chondrosarcoma of bone: clinical, radiologic, and histologic differentiation," *Instructional Course Lectures*, vol. 53, pp. 645–649, 2004.

[12] R. A. Marco, S. Gitelis, G. T. Brebach, and J. H. Healey, "Cartilage tumors: evaluation and treatment," *Journal of the American Academy of Orthopaedic Surgeons*, vol. 8, no. 5, pp. 292–304, 2000.

[13] M. Ryzewicz, B. J. Manaster, E. Naar, and B. Lindeque, "Low-grade cartilage tumors: diagnosis and treatment," *Orthopedics*, vol. 30, no. 1, pp. 35–48, 2007.

[14] C. Parlier-Cuau, V. Bousson, C. M. Ogilvie, R. D. Lackman, and J.-D. Laredo, "When should we biopsy a solitary central cartilaginous tumor of long bones? Literature review and management proposal," *European Journal of Radiology*, vol. 77, no. 1, pp. 6–12, 2011.

[15] B. S. Souna, N. Belot, H. Duval, F. Langlais, and H. Thomazeau, "No recurrences in selected patients after curettage with cryotherapy for grade I chondrosarcomas," *Clinical Orthopaedics and Related Research*, vol. 468, no. 7, pp. 1956–1962, 2010.

[16] R. Veth, B. Schreuder, H. van Beem, M. Pruszczynski, and J. de Rooy, "Cryosurgery in aggressive, benign, and low-grade malignant bone tumours," *Lancet Oncology*, vol. 6, no. 1, pp. 25–34, 2005.

[17] J. H. Schwab, D. Wenger, K. Unni, and F. H. Sim, "Does local recurrence impact survival in low-grade chondrosarcoma of the long bones?" *Clinical Orthopaedics and Related Research*, vol. 462, pp. 175–180, 2007.

[18] D. G. Mohler, R. Chiu, D. A. McCall, and R. S. Avedian, "Curettage and cryosurgery for low-grade cartilage tumors is associated with low recurrence and high function," *Clinical*

Orthopaedics and Related Research, vol. 468, no. 10, pp. 2765–2773, 2010.

[19] S. A. Hanna, P. Whittingham-Jones, M. D. Sewell et al., "Outcome of intralesional curettage for low-grade chondrosarcoma of long bones," *European Journal of Surgical Oncology*, vol. 35, no. 12, pp. 1343–1347, 2009.

[20] C. Aarons, B. K. Potter, S. C. Adams, J. D. Pitcher Jr., and H. T. Temple, "Extended intralesional treatment versus resection of low-grade chondrosarcomas," *Clinical Orthopaedics and Related Research*, vol. 467, no. 8, pp. 2105–2111, 2009.

[21] E. R. Ahlmann, L. R. Menendez, A. N. Fedenko, and T. Learch, "Influence of cryosurgery on treatment outcome of low-grade chondrosarcoma," *Clinical Orthopaedics and Related Research*, vol. 451, pp. 201–207, 2006.

[22] S. H. M. Verdegaal, H. F. G. Brouwers, E. W. van Zwet, P. C. W. Hogendoorn, and A. H. M. Taminiau, "Low-grade chondrosarcoma of long bones treated with intralesional curettage followed by application of phenol, ethanol, and bone-grafting," *The Journal of Bone and Joint Surgery—American Volume*, vol. 94, no. 13, pp. 1201–1207, 2012.

[23] A. Streitbürger, H. Ahrens, M. Balke et al., "Grade I chondrosarcoma of bone: the Münster experience," *Journal of Cancer Research and Clinical Oncology*, vol. 135, no. 4, pp. 543–550, 2009.

[24] L. H. L. De Beuckeleer, A. M. A. De Schepper, and F. Ramon, "Magnetic resonance imaging of cartilaginous tumors: is it useful or necessary?" *Skeletal Radiology*, vol. 25, no. 2, pp. 137–141, 1996.

23

The Oncogenic Functions of Nicotinic Acetylcholine Receptors

Yue Zhao

Center of Cell biology and Cancer Research, Albany Medical College, 47 New Scotland Avenue, Albany, NY 12208, USA

Correspondence should be addressed to Yue Zhao; alexanderyz@gmail.com

Academic Editor: Kalpesh Jani

Nicotinic acetylcholine receptors (nAChRs) are ion channels that are expressed in the cell membrane of all mammalian cells, including cancer cells. Recent findings suggest that nAChRs not only mediate nicotine addiction in the brain but also contribute to the development and progression of cancers directly induced by nicotine and its derived carcinogenic nitrosamines whereas deregulation of the nAChRs is observed in many cancers, and genome-wide association studies (GWAS) indicate that SNPs nAChRs associate with risks of lung cancers and nicotine addiction. Emerging evidences suggest nAChRs are posited at the central regulatory loops of numerous cell growth and prosurvival signal pathways and also mediate the synthesis and release of stimulatory and inhibitory neurotransmitters induced by their agonists. Thus nAChRs mediated cell signaling plays an important role in stimulating the growth and angiogenic and neurogenic factors and mediating oncogenic signal transduction during cancer development in a cell type specific manner. In this review, we provide an integrated view of nAChRs signaling in cancer, heightening on the oncogenic properties of nAChRs that may be targeted for cancer treatment.

1. Introduction

The nicotinic acetylcholine receptors (nAChRs) are of a family of ligands gated ion channels that are expressed in the cell membrane of all mammalian cells, including cancer cells [1]. In the nervous system nAChRs have high permeability to calcium, modulated by the extracellular calcium concentrations, phosphorylated by calcium-dependent serine/threonine kinases to regulate the release and activation of neuronal transmitters [2–5]. nAChRs are known to play several important roles involved in learning and cognition through regulating of synaptic plasticity, neuronal growth, differentiation, and survival [6]. The discovery of their expression on nonneuronal cells implicates their broad biological functions involved in cell proliferation, apoptosis, migration, and signal transduction. Recent findings suggest the imbalanced expressions of different subtypes of nAChRs in the cells contribute to the pathogenesis of diseases such as cancer [7].

Cigarette smoking or environmental tobacco smoke is an important risk factor for many types of cancers, including lung cancer, oral cancer, laryngeal cancer, oropharyngeal/hypopharyngeal caner, esophageal cancer, gastric cancer, liver cancer, pancreatic cancer, bladder cancer, renal cancer,

cervical carcinoma, myeloid leukaemia, and colorectal cancer [8]. Among the carcinogens presented in tobacco, nicotine acts on nAChRs in the central nervous system (CNS) and causes addiction to smoke [9]. And two of its metabolites, namely, 4-(methylnitrosamino)-1-(3-pyridyl)-1-butanone (NNK) and N-nitrosonornicotine (NNN), bind to nicotinic receptor with much higher affinity than that of nicotine [7]. Recent studies indicated nicotine is able to induce cancer directly via promoting proliferation, inhibiting apoptosis of cancer cells, and stimulating tumor angiogenesis. These findings suggest that nAChRs are the central regulatory module of multiple downstream oncogenic signaling pathways in mediating the cellular responses of nicotine and its derivatives [8]. And nAChRs mediated effects of nicotine function in coalition with the mutagenic effects of the cancerogenic nitrosamine derivatives and reactive oxygen species activated by intracellular nicotine to promote tumor development and progression in tobacco related cancers.

The nAChRs can either be composed of five identical $\alpha7$, $\alpha8$, or $\alpha9$ subunits (homomeric nAChRs) or consist of combinations of $\alpha2$–$\alpha6$ or $\alpha10$ subunits with $\beta2$–$\beta4$ subunits (heteromeric nAChRs). $\alpha7$-nAChR and $\alpha4\beta2$-nAChR are the evolutionarily oldest nAChRs predominantly expressed in

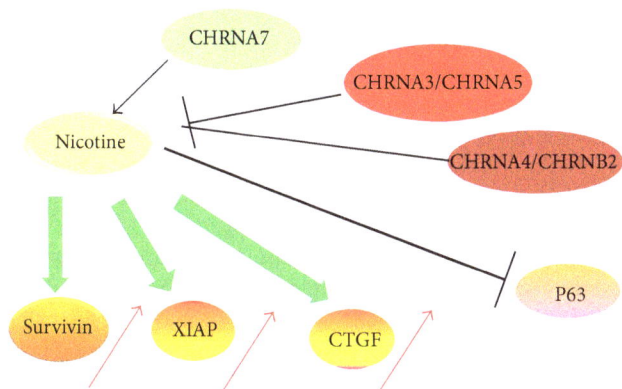

FIGURE 1: Differential effects of different nAChR subtypes on cell growth [21, 70, 96].

the mammalian brain [10]. α7-nAChR is selective for Ca2+ and other nAChRs allowing the influx of different cations (Na+, K+, and Ca2+) [11, 12]. α7-nAChR is the most growth stimulatory nAChR in cancer cells, whereas α4β2-nAChR is the growth inhibitory receptor. Under normal physiological conditions, nicotine binds to α4β2-nAChR with higher affinity than α7-nAChRs. However, in smokers chronic exposure to nicotine or nicotine-derived carcinogenic nitrosamines leads to the upregulation of all nAChRs and long-term inactivation (or desensitization) of the 2α4β-nAChR [11, 13]; in contrast, the sensitivity of α7-nAChR remains unchanged [13]. Thus chronic exposure to nicotine causes selective activation of the cancer stimulatory nAChRs in the cell (Figure 1).

The affinity of NNK for α7-nAChR is 1,300 times higher than that of nicotine, whereas the affinity of NNN for heteromeric α–β nAChRs is 5,000 times higher than that of nicotine [14, 15]. Thus NNK and NNN can cause displacement of nicotine from these receptors as a result of their higher affinity for nAChRs. Therefore nitrosamines may cause many of the cardiovascular, neuropsychological, and cancer-stimulating effects similar to nicotine. Thus, nicotine, NNK, and NNN bind to nAChRs and other receptors, leading to activation of the serine/threonine kinase AKT, protein kinase A (PKA), and other factors [16, 17].

Based upon recent discoveries in the field, an increasing body of evidence suggests the positive correlations between nAChRs signaling and cancer incidences related to cigarette smoking. Particularly, lung cancers, pancreatic cancers, and esophageal cancers are among the most commonly induced cancers triggered by cigarette smoking and nAChR signaling [8]. In this review we have special focus on the genetic predisposition and molecular pathogenesis of cancers originated from these three organs in related nAChRs.

2. Genetic Variants of nAChRs in Association with Cancer

Single nucleotide polymorphisms (SNPs) of the chromosome *15q25* region, which contains *α5-α3-β4* nAChR gene cluster (*CHRNA5-CHRNA3-CHRNB4*), is frequently associated with

nicotine- (tobacco-) dependence, chronic obstructive pulmonary disease (COPD), and lung cancer in genome-wide association studies (GWAS) [18]. The association of the SNPs of *15q25* genomic region with COPD and lung cancer could mediate by the combined effects of the oncogenic nAChR signaling and the neurological effects of nicotine addiction. Among these SNPs rs16969968 in *CHRNA5*, rs1051730 in *CHRNA3*, and rs8034191 are the most studied three SNPs of the region [18, 19]. *CHRNA3* and *CHRNA5* are arranged in a tail-to-tail configuration on the opposite strand of the DNA, and the two variants rs1051730 and rs16969968 are in a complete linkage disequilibrium [r^2 = 0.98 in samples of Europeans/Caucasians]. Similarly rs1051370 is in strong linkage disequilibrium with rs8034191; thus some studies report the results for rs1051370 only. Notably, Chen et al. reported rs1051730 is associated with larger tumor size at diagnosis of squamous cell carcinoma. rs16969968 is a G-to-A [aspartic acid- (D-) to-asparagine (N)] missense variant at amino acid position 398 of *CHRNA5* [α5 (Asn398) D398N] [20]. And 398N is less potent than the variant 398D in protecting cells against the nicotine α7-nAChR mediated signaling making cells more susceptible to proliferation and migration [21]. Consistently, risk allele D-Asparagine is observed to reduce the function of α4β2α5-nAChR [18].

Alternatively, polymorphisms in linkage disequilibrium with rs16969968 may modulate the expression of *CHRNA5* [22, 23]. Thus the expression of functional (α3β2)2α5-nAChRS may play an important role in regulating the homeostasis and integrity of bronchial mucosa under physical, chemical, and immunological damage. Depending on the balanced regulation of the nAChRs, bronchial mucosa may undergo repair and recovery or give rise to precancerous lesion or hyperplasia when these receptors are deregulated. Moreover, NKK induced bronchial cell proliferation and the susceptibility to the tumorigenic transformation were reported to associate with different variants of human α9-nAChR subunit protein (S442 as the most frequent) [24]. Thus polymorphisms in *CHRNA5-CHRNA3-CHRNB4* gene cluster may modulate the dynamics of the normal bronchial epithelium under stress conditions to influence cancer risks [25]. Similarly, these SNPs associated with varied activity of nAChRs may associate with enhanced invasiveness and metastatic capacity. Besides, the effects of the *15q25* polymorphism may impact on the neural behavioral effects on addiction to nicotine, resulting in an increased tobacco consumption, and so forth [26].

Interestingly Wu et al. reported rs8034191, rs1051730, and rs16969968 identified in previous GWAS are extremely rare in Asians, whereas they have identified four novel SNPs that were associated with significantly increased lung cancer risk and smoking behavior in Chinese population [27]. Particularly they have identified that rs6495309T>C considerably influenced the *CHRNA3* promoter activity, leading to higher α3-nAChR protein level and an increased risk of lung cancer. This seemingly contradictory observation could be explained as upregulation of (α3β2)2α5-nAChR in brain may dampen the nicotine responses mediated by α7-nAChR and consequently leads to reduced dopamine release upon nicotine induction [26]. Thus individuals with rs6495309C allele may need to consume more nicotine to reach the addictive neurological effects, leading to higher levels of exposure to smoking.

3. The Oncogenic Effects of Neurotransmitters Mediated by nAChRs

Stress neurotransmitters such as dopamine can stimulate the growth of cancer cells *in vitro*, which is in accord with nAChRs' role in regulating the release and synthesis of these neurotransmitters *in vivo* [13]. The effects are partly due to the facts that growth of nerve endings into the tumor microenvironment (neurogenesis) [28, 29] is necessary for the development of many cancers. The process is triggered by neurotrophic factors released from tumor cells to promote the nerve fibres growth into tumor tissues [30]. Consistently, α7-nAChR can promote neurogenesis by stimulating glutamate production whereas α4β2-nAChR can regulate neurogenesis by regulating Gamma-Amino Butyric Acid (GABA) synthesis and release [31, 32]. More importantly, the autocrine neurotransmitters of the catecholamine family play important roles in the carcinogenic pathways regulated by nAChRs. Thus under physiological conditions other risk factors also activate nAChRs to promote cancers in the body, such as psychological stress, and also activate the neuronal pathway through the activation of nAChRs and beta-adrenergic receptors [33].

Similarly NNK can stimulate the growth and migration of small airway epithelial cells through activation of β-adrenergic receptor which further transactivates EGFR through cAMP signaling [34–36]. β-adrenergic agonists such as adrenaline and noradrenaline triggered by nAChRs signaling are responsible for the development pulmonary adenocarcinomas (PACs). And adrenaline treated hamsters showed with significantly increased tumor growth in the NNK induced small-airway-derived PAC model [29]. Similarly noradrenaline plays an important role in promoting the growth of gastrointestinal cancer; it can mediate nicotine signaling through activation of ERK1-ERK2, cyclooxygenase 2 (COX2), prostaglandin E2 (PGE2), and VEGF [16, 37, 38]. Consistently, increased synthesis and releasing of noradrenaline and adrenaline are observed in colon cancer cells by nicotine treatment *in vitro*, an effect that is blocked by α7-nAChR antagonist [39]. Thus, the β-adrenergic signaling, transactivation of the EGFR, and releasing of EGF are the major contributors to the effects of tumor growth and angiogenesis mediated by nAChRs in colon cancer. Such an effect of nAChR signaling is also observed in many other types of cancers; for instance, the proliferation of mesothelioma cells is stimulated by nicotine through activation of the ERK1-ERK2 signaling cascade and nicotine also inhibits the apoptosis of the cell through activation of NF-κB and phosphorylation of BAD [40]. In bladder cancer cells ERK1-ERK2 as well as STAT3 is also activated by nicotine through nAChRs and β-adrenergic receptors [41].

Suppressive neurotransmitters such as GABA also played a role in regulating cancer cell, and they are synthesized and released by cancer cells in an autocrine fashion. Researches indicated NNK can cause the decreased GABA level in PAC cells and further leads to decreased GABA dependent

migration of PAC cells *in vitro* [42]. Desensitization of α4β2-nAChR is the major cause for decreased release of GABA in smokers and NNK treated hamsters [11, 13, 42]. Consistently, the RNA level of α4-nAChR has been observed to be significantly lower in PAC tissues than that of normal lung tissues [43]. Recent studies indicate suppressive neurotransmitter GABA can inhibit adrenaline induced migration of many types of cancer including colon cancer, prostate cancer, and breast cancer [44]. Joseph et al. reported the tumor suppressor function of GABA in lung adenocarcinoma [43]; similarly GABA can inhibit Gαi-mediated inhibition of adenylyl cyclase and further leads to the inhibition of isoproterenol induced DNA synthesis and migration [45]. These findings are in accord with the association between increased releases of stress neurotransmitters caused by smoking and increased risk of PAC, which is caused by upregulation of α7-nAChR and a concomitant desensitization of α4β2-nAChR induced by smoking.

4. nAChRs in Regulating Tumor Angiogenesis

The pathological angiogenesis of tumor growth and metastasis induced by nicotine has been firstly reported by Heeschen et al. [46]. The proliferation of Lewis lung cancer cells which do not have functional nAChRs was not stimulated by nicotine *in vitro*. In contrast, accelerated tumor growth was observed after systemic administration of nicotine in xenograft mouse model [46]. And a 5-fold increase of capillary density in the tumor nodules was observed after nicotine administration. These findings suggest nicotine promotes tumor angiogenesis rather than affecting tumor cell proliferation directly in the Lewis lung cancer model. Later work showed second-hand smoke increased tumor angiogenesis and tumor growth, an effect that is associated with elevated plasma VEGF in the Lewis lung cancer model [47]. Consistently, increased endothelial progenitor cells were recruited to the ischemic sites in mice after nicotine administration [48]. *In vitro* treatment of 10 nM nicotine to human endothelial progenitor cells increased the viability, migratory, and adhesive and vasculogenesis ability of these cells [49]. nAChRs antagonists mecamylamine and α-bungarotoxin can abolish the effect of nicotine on human endothelial progenitors [50].

Cholinergic angiogenesis is mainly mediated by α7-nAChR, which is predominantly expressed in the endothelial cell [50]. Other nAChRs modulate cholinergic angiogenesis through interacting with α7-nAChR. Notably, hypoxia can induce upregulation of α7-nAChR in endothelial cells. And ischemic hindlimb of the mouse expressed increased α7-nAChRs [50]. Consistently α7-nAChR antagonist α-bungarotoxin can suppress the increased endothelial cell migration, proliferation, and tube formation induced by nicotine *in vitro*. And the angiogenesis effects of nicotine are blunted in mice deficient with α7-nAChR [50]. Moreover, the effect of α7-nAChR on angiogenesis is further demonstrated by the α7-nAChR antagonist MG624 decrease of the angiogenesis effect of nicotine *in vitro* and in xenograft mouse model of small cell lung cancer. The effect of MG624 is probably mediated by inhibition of nicotine induced release of fibroblast growth factor 2 (FGF2) through activation of early growth response gene 1 [51]. Another research indicated that knockdown of α7-nAChR suppressed nicotine induced tubulogenesis of human retinal endothelial cells.

Other subunits of nAChRs are also expressed in the endothelia cells [52]. Interestingly, knockdown of *CHRNA9* in endothelial cells enhanced nicotine induced cell proliferation, migration, and tube formation [53]. The effect is probably caused by the compensatory increase of α7-nAChR on the cell membrane of endothelial cells.

The angiogenesis effect of nAChRs can function independently of exogenously added nicotine. Matrigel tube formation assay showed that nAChR antagonists have suppressive effects on angiogenesis [50]. Interestingly, antagonists of endothelial nAChR can also suppress the angiogenic processes of VEGF and FGF. These findings suggest pathways involved in nAChRs mediated signaling interact with the angiogenesis pathways of VEGF and FGF. And microarray studies indicated concordant transcriptional profiles induced by nicotine, VEGF, and FGF, which suggest angiogenic growth factors and cholinergic signaling pathways have close interactions [54]. In addition, endothelial cells can synthesize acetylcholine as an autocrine angiogenic factor [55, 56]. Besides acetylcholine, SLURP1/SLURP2 can also function as endogenous agonists of nAChR, and these proteins allosterically modify and activate nAChRs [57].

5. nAChRs Signaling in Lung Cancers

In pulmonary neuroendocrine cells (PNECs), nicotine or NNK stimulates the proliferation of PNECs *in vitro* through activation of protein kinase C (PKC), the serine/threonine kinase RAF1, the mitogen activated kinases ERK1 and ERK2, and the transcription factors FOS, JUN, and MYC. These responses are abolished by α7-nAChR specific antagonist, indicating that α7-nAChR is the primary mediator of nicotine and NNK signaling [58–60]. Similarly, serotonin and bombesin, the two autocrine growth factors, can activate the same signaling cascade *in vitro* [58, 59], whereas the effects of nicotine or NNK were abolished by a serotonin uptake inhibitor [59]. Nicotine or NNK induced DNA synthesis is effectively blocked by Ca2+ channel blockers [61]. In addition, NNK can cause ERK1-ERK2 dependent phosphorylation of m-calpains and μ-calpains and further promote the migration of small cell lung cancer (SCLC) cells [62]. The response can be blocked by ERK1-ERK2 specific inhibitors or RNAi silencing of calpains [62]. Furthermore, NNK can activate BCL-2 to inhibit apoptosis of SCLC cells, whereas PKC inhibitor staurosporine, ERK1-ERK2 inhibitor PD98059, or knockdown of *MYC* can block the effect [63].

The release of autocrine growth factors such as serotonin and mammalian bombesin is an important downstream response of α7-nAChR to stimulate the growth of cancer cells. In addition, several other autocrine growth factors of SCLC cells also activate the RAF1-ERK signaling pathway to cooperate with the α7-nAChR signaling cascade to stimulate the proliferation of cancer cells [64]. Consistently, inhibition of PKC or ERK1-ERK2 or upregulation of intracellular cyclic adenosine monophosphate (cAMP) can strongly suppress the

nAChR-stimulated responses of SCLC *in vitro* [65, 66]. The suppression is probably mediated by inhibition of RAF1 by cAMP-dependent protein kinase A [67].

Heteromeric nAChRs are also expressed in non-small-cell lung cancers (NSCLCs); however, in smokers the nicotine or NNK responses are generally mediated by α7-nAChR as a result of desensitization of heteromeric receptors. Nicotine or NNK treatment of NSCLCs stimulates the proliferation and inhibits chemotherapy-induced apoptosis through activation of PI3K-AKT pathway and nuclear factor-κB (NF-κB) [44, 68]. Consistently, constitutive activation of AKT is observed in NSCLCs to promote resistance of apoptosis in chemotherapy [69]. And nicotine induced AKT-dependent upregulation of survivin and E3 ubiquitin-protein ligase (XIAP) to mediate the antiapoptotic response of NSCLCs [70]. In addition, α7-nAChR also mediates the activation of β-arrestin and protooncogene tyrosine-protein kinase Src (SRC) to promote the proliferation of NSCLC cells [71].

In immortalized human bronchial epithelial cells the downstream signal pathways activated by nAChRs include ERK1-ERK2 activated transcription factors, signal transducer and activator of transcription 1 (STAT1), NF-κB, and GATA-binding factor 3 (GATA3). Interestingly, antagonist of α7-nAChR specifically blocked the stimulating effects of NNK, whereas antagonist of the heteromeric nAChRs specifically blocked the NNN responses [72]. nAChRs also control the release of growth factors such as proepidermal growth factor (EGF) in large airway epithelial cells; the effects are blocked by the selective antagonists of α7-nAChR through intervening with the Ras-Raf-ERK signaling cascade [73]. Thus the EGFR signaling pathway is incorporated into the nAChRs growth stimulatory effects in large airway epithelial cells.

The deregulation of nAChR subunits in primary lung cancer tissues is also evidenced by the epigenetic alterations of the nAChR genes [74–76]. Paliwal et al. reported that *cholinergic receptor, nicotinic, alpha 3* (*CHRNA3*) gene encoding the α3-nAChR subunit is frequently hypermethylated and silenced in lung cancer, and DNA methylation inhibitors can cause demethylation of *CHRNA3* promoter and reactivation of the gene [75]. Ectopic expression of α3-nAChR restored the protein level of the α3 receptor in H1975 lung cancer cell line and induced apoptosis [73]. They also observed a dramatic increase of Ca2+ influx response in the presence of nicotine elicited by knockdown of *CHRNA3* in α3-nAChR positive lung cancer cells, followed by activation of the AKT prosurvival pathway. Moreover, α3-nAChR depleted cells were resistant to apoptosis-inducing agents, underscoring the importance of epigenetic silencing of the *CHRNA3* gene in human cancer. Interestingly, they found *CHRNA3*, but not *CHRNA5*, is often hypermethylated and downregulated in cancer tissues, whereas a 30-fold upregulation of *CHRNA5* expression is observed in lung cancers compared with the normal lung [75]. Consistently, in a separate study α5-nAChR and α3-nAChR are identified as negative regulator of α7-nAChR mediated nicotine responses in human normal and bronchial cancer [21]. Knockdown of *CHRNA3* and *CHRNA5* in bronchial cancer cells and esophageal cancer cells leads to increased calcium influx induced by nicotine, which could be explained by the compensatory increase of the assembly of functional α7-nAChR on the cell membrane. Importantly, they have also identified downregulation of p63 after knockdown of *CHRNA5* or *CHRNA3*, which offered an explanation for the resistance to apoptosis in *CHRNA3* downregulated lung cancers. Moreover, knockdown of *CHRNA3* in A549 cells downregulates the cell-cell adhesion molecules and reduces the components of tight junctions (ZO-1) and adherens junctions (P120), analogous to epithelial cells undergoing epithelial-mesenchyme transition [77]. Together these findings suggest that α5-nAChR and α3-nAChR mediate the apoptotic responses and suppress the adhesion and migration of primary lung cancer cells and normal bronchial cells. In addition, the regulatory functions are mediated by the heteromeric (α3β2)2α5-nAChR rather than the AChR5 subunit alone.

6. nAChRs Signaling in Pancreatic Cancer

Cigarette smoking is most frequent risk factor associated with pancreatic cancer [78–81]. NNK can induce pancreatic cancer through the genotoxic effect of DNA adducts causing *RAS* gene mutations [40] but also has a hyperproliferative effect on pancreatic duct epithelia through β-adrenergic transactivation of EGF receptors [82, 83]. Recently, Al-Wadei et al. reported that nicotine and NNK promote the synthesis and release of adrenaline and noradrenaline to promote the proliferation and migration of pancreatic cancer cells [84]. And RNA knockdown experiments indicate the effect is mediated by α3-, α5-, and α7-nAChRs. Similarly, the process is coupled with increased β-adrenergic cAMP-dependent signaling and release of arachidonic acid in pancreatic cancer cell lines [45, 82, 85]. And the activation of CREB, ERK, SRC, and AKT pathways has been identified to mediate the oncogenic responses of nAChRs. Together these findings suggest nAChR mediated catecholamine synthesis, release, and transactivation of the EGFR signaling pathway promote the progression of pancreatic cancers.

Besides, nicotine/cigarette smoke promotes metastasis of pancreatic cancer through α7-nAChR mediated Mucin-4 (MUC4) upregulation. Chronic exposure to nicotine or cigarette smoke leads to increased expression of MUC4 in pancreatic cancer through activation of the α7-nAChR/JAK2/STAT3 and the MEK/ERK1/ERK2 signaling cascade [86]. And tobacco smoking induces chronic inflammation to trigger the development of pancreatic cancer [87]. The oncogenic effects of nAChR signaling in pancreatic cancer are also supported by the animal experiments, and N-nitroso compounds, formed from nicotine by nitrosation during the processing of tobacco plants, can cause pancreatic cancer in Syrian golden hamsters [88].

7. nAChRs Signaling in Oral and Esophageal Cancers

In oral and esophageal cancer, besides α7-nAChR, heteromeric nAChR composed of α3 and α5 subunits also regulates the responses of nicotine and NNK [15, 89, 90]. And chronic exposure to nicotine or tobacco smoke selectively upregulates α5-nAChR and α7-nAChR subunits in oral keratinocytes [55]. Similar to lung cancer cells [14], NNK preferentially binds to α7-nAChR with higher affinity, whereas NNN binds to heterometric nAChRs with higher affinity in oral and esophageal cancer cells. In esophageal carcinoma nAChRs mediated nitrosamine responses by activating signaling pathways such as Ras-Raf-ERK1-ERK2 and the JAK2-STAT3 pathway and NF-κB and in GATA3 and STAT1 to promote the growth and inhibit apoptosis of the cancer cells [7].

Consistent with the neurotransmitters' effects on cancer, nAChRs mediated synthesis and release of adrenaline and noradrenaline are important downstream responses of nicotine stimulated growth of esophageal cancers. Consistently, increased proliferation of esophageal cancer cells is observed by adrenaline treatment, which is mediated by activation of Ras-MARK pathway and transactivation of EGFR [91, 92]. The mechanism is similar to the signal transduction mediated by nAChRs in colon cancer and pancreatic cancer [38, 93].

Other nAChRs mediated oncogenic signaling pathways are also implicated in esophageal cancer. Arredondo et al. reported that secreted mammalian SLURP1/SLURP2 are cell endogenous allosteric modulators of nAChRs signaling that enhance the responses of acetylcholine and trigger proapoptotic activity in human keratinocytes [89]. The expression of SLURP1 and SLURP2 is reduced in esophageal cancers, and exogenous expression of SLURP1 and SLURP2 in esophageal cancer cells reduced the colony forming ability of the cells in the presence of nitrosamine, also inhibiting the growth of NNK transformed keratinocytes in mouse xenograft. Recent work done by our group indicated nAChRs also mediated the nicotine activation of the oncogenic YAP1 of the Hippo signaling pathway in esophageal cancer, we also found upregulation of YAP1 in esophageal cancer samples is significantly associated with the smoking history of the patients, and the effects are regulated by PKC signaling, as PKC specific inhibitor can abolish the activation of YAP1 by nicotine treatment [94] (Figures 2(a) and 2(b)). Besides, nicotine promotes head and neck cancer through activation of endogenous FOXM1 activity by loss of heterozygosity involving the whole of chromosome 13 and copy number abnormality (CNA) in oral keratinocytes (KC) [53].

8. Conclusion Remarks

An increasing body of evidence suggests that nAChRs stay at the center of regulatory pathways of cholinergic and nicotinic signaling to regulate the growth and migration of the cells, also regulating angiogenesis of the endothelial cells during physiological and pathological conditions. In accord with the findings of multiple GWAS which indicate that SNPs of the gene cluster *15q25*, which contains *CHRNA3*, *CHRNA5*, *CHRNB4*, are associated with increased risks of lung cancer and COPD as well as nicotine-dependence, recent cellular and molecular studies on nAChRs indicate that chronic exposure to nicotine or nicotine-derived carcinogenic nitrosamines upregulates the α7-nAChR and α9-nAChR and desensitizes the heteromeric α4β2-nAChR to activate the oncogenic pathways, promotes tumor angiogenesis, and inhibits drug induced apoptosis in multiple types

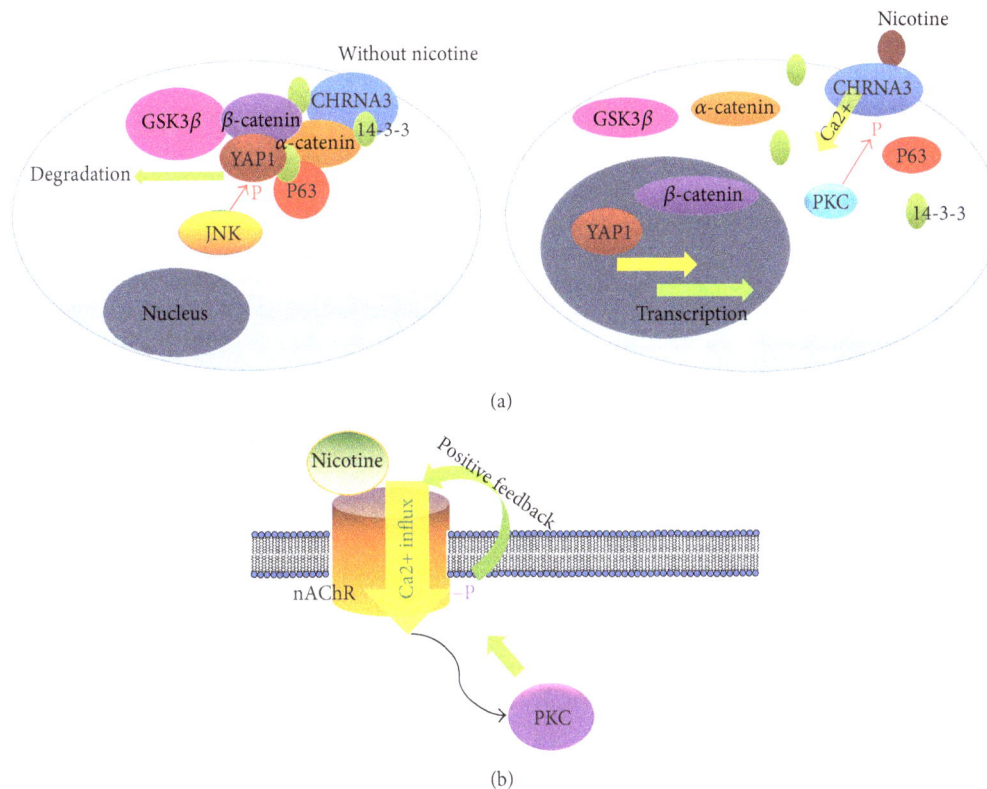

FIGURE 2: (a) Schematic model of nicotine action of YAP1 [94]. (b) Nicotine activates the positive feedback loop of PKC mediated phosphorylation of nAChR [97].

of cancers. Although α7-nAChR is the oncogenic receptor responsible for most of the oncogenic responses in cancer, α9-nAChR has been shown to be upregulated in estrogen receptor positive breast cancer cells, and α9-nAChR stimulates the initiation and progression of breast cancer in coalition with estrogen receptor [95]. Collectively, these recent findings suggest that nAChR mediated oncogenic signaling plays an important role in the initiation and progression of cancer, which functions in parallel with the mutagenic and cytotoxic effects of tobacco smoke to promote the growth and angiogenesis of the tobacco related cancers. Thus nAChRs yield as promising new targets for the prevention, diagnosis, and treatment of tobacco related cancers.

Conflict of Interests

The author declares that there is no conflict of interests regarding the publication of this paper.

References

[1] I. Wessler and C. J. Kirkpatrick, "Acetylcholine beyond neurons: the non-neuronal cholinergic system in humans," *British Journal of Pharmacology*, vol. 154, no. 8, pp. 1558–1571, 2008.

[2] A. Sobel, M. Weber, and J. P. Changeux, "Large-scale purification of the acetylcholine-receptor protein in its membrane-bound and detergent-extracted forms from *Torpedo marmorata* electric organ," *European Journal of Biochemistry*, vol. 80, no. 1, pp. 215–224, 1977.

[3] R. D. O'Brien, M. E. Eldefrawi, and A. T. Eldefrawi, "Isolation of acetylcholine receptors," *Annual Review of Pharmacology*, vol. 12, pp. 19–34, 1972.

[4] A. Karlin, "The acetylcholine receptor: progress report," *Life Sciences*, vol. 14, no. 8, pp. 1385–1415, 1974.

[5] J.-L. Galzi, F. Revah, A. Bessis, and J.-P. Changeux, "Functional architecture of the nicotinic acetylcholine receptor: from electric organ to brain," *Annual Review of Pharmacology and Toxicology*, vol. 31, no. 1, pp. 37–72, 1991.

[6] A. N. Placzek, T. A. Zhang, and J. A. Dani, "Nicotinic mechanisms influencing synaptic plasticity in the hippocampus," *Acta Pharmacologica Sinica*, vol. 30, no. 6, pp. 752–760, 2009.

[7] H. M. Schuller, "Is cancer triggered by altered signalling of nicotinic acetylcholine receptors?" *Nature Reviews Cancer*, vol. 9, no. 3, pp. 195–205, 2009.

[8] S. S. Hecht, "Tobacco carcinogens, their biomarkers and tobacco-induced cancer," *Nature Reviews Cancer*, vol. 3, no. 10, pp. 733–744, 2003.

[9] J.-P. Changeux, "Nicotinic receptors and nicotine addiction," *Comptes Rendus Biologies*, vol. 332, no. 5, pp. 421–425, 2009.

[10] G. S. Portugal and T. J. Gould, "Genetic variability in nicotinic acetylcholine receptors and nicotine addiction: converging evidence from human and animal research," *Behavioural Brain Research*, vol. 193, no. 1, pp. 1–16, 2008.

[11] J. Lindstrom, R. Anand, V. Gerzanich, X. Peng, F. Wang, and G. Wells, "Structure and function of neuronal nicotinic acetylcholine receptors," *Progress in Brain Research*, vol. 109, pp. 125–137, 1996.

[12] M. Gopalakrishnan, B. Buisson, E. Touma et al., "Stable expression and pharmacological properties of the human α 7 nicotinic acetylcholine receptor," *European Journal of Pharmacology*, vol. 290, no. 3, pp. 237–246, 1995.

[13] H. Kawai and D. K. Berg, "Nicotinic acetylcholine receptors containing $\alpha 7$ subunits on rat cortical neurons do not undergo long-lasting inactivation even when up-regulated by chronic nicotine exposure," *Journal of Neurochemistry*, vol. 78, no. 6, pp. 1367–1378, 2001.

[14] H. M. Schuller and M. Orloff, "Tobacco-specific carcinogenic nitrosamines: ligands for nicotinic acetylcholine receptors in human lung cancer cells," *Biochemical Pharmacology*, vol. 55, no. 9, pp. 1377–1384, 1998.

[15] J. Arredondo, A. I. Chernyavsky, and S. A. Grando, "Nicotinic receptors mediate tumorigenic action of tobacco-derived nitrosamines on immortalized oral epithelial cells," *Cancer Biology and Therapy*, vol. 5, no. 5, pp. 511–517, 2006.

[16] H. M. Schuller, B. Porter, and A. Riechert, "Beta-adrenergic modulation of NNK-induced lung carcinogenesis in hamsters," *Journal of Cancer Research and Clinical Oncology*, vol. 126, no. 11, pp. 624–630, 2000.

[17] V. Boswell-Smith and D. Spina, "PDE4 inhibitors as potential therapeutic agents in the treatment of COPD-focus on roflumilast," *International journal of Chronic Obstructive Pulmonary Disease*, vol. 2, no. 2, pp. 121–129, 2007.

[18] N. L. Saccone, R. C. Culverhouse, T.-H. Schwantes-An et al., "Multiple independent loci at chromosome 15q25.1 affect smoking quantity: a meta-analysis and comparison with lung cancer and COPD," *PLoS Genetics*, vol. 6, no. 8, Article ID e1001053, 2010.

[19] C. A. Wassenaar, Q. Dong, Q. Wei, C. I. Amos, M. R. Spitz, and R. F. Tyndale, "Relationship between CYP2A6 and CHRNA5-CHRNA3-CHRNB4 variation and smoking behaviors and lung cancer risk," *Journal of the National Cancer Institute*, vol. 103, no. 17, pp. 1342–1346, 2011.

[20] X. Chen, I. P. Gorlov, K. W. Merriman et al., "Association of smoking with tumor size at diagnosis in non-small cell lung cancer," *Lung Cancer*, vol. 74, no. 3, pp. 378–383, 2011.

[21] A. M. Krais, A. H. Hautefeuille, M.-P. Cros et al., "CHRNA5 as negative regulator of nicotine signaling in normal and cancer bronchial cells: effects on motility, migration and p63 expression," *Carcinogenesis*, vol. 32, no. 9, pp. 1388–1395, 2011.

[22] F. S. Falvella, A. Galvan, E. Frullanti et al., "Transcription deregulation at the 15q25 locus in association with lung adenocarcinoma risk," *Clinical Cancer Research*, vol. 15, no. 5, pp. 1837–1842, 2009.

[23] F. S. Falvella, A. Galvan, F. Colombo, E. Frullanti, U. Pastorino, and T. A. Dragani, "Promoter polymorphisms and transcript levels of nicotinic receptor CHRNA5," *Journal of the National Cancer Institute*, vol. 102, no. 17, pp. 1366–1370, 2010.

[24] A. Chikova and S. A. Grando, "Naturally occurring variants of human A9 nicotinic receptor differentially affect bronchial cell proliferation and transformation," *PLoS ONE*, vol. 6, no. 11, Article ID e27978, 2011.

[25] P. Brennan, P. Hainaut, and P. Boffetta, "Genetics of lung-cancer susceptibility," *The Lancet Oncology*, vol. 12, no. 4, pp. 399–408, 2011.

[26] J.-P. Changeux, "Nicotine addiction and nicotinic receptors: lessons from genetically modified mice," *Nature Reviews Neuroscience*, vol. 11, no. 6, pp. 389–401, 2010.

[27] C. Wu, Z. Hu, D. Yu et al., "Genetic variants on chromosome 15q25 associated with lung cancer risk in Chinese populations," *Cancer Research*, vol. 69, no. 12, pp. 5065–5072, 2009.

[28] A. Chédotal, G. Kerjan, and C. Moreau-Fauvarque, "The brain within the tumor: new roles for axon guidance molecules in cancers," *Cell Death and Differentiation*, vol. 12, no. 8, pp. 1044–1056, 2005.

[29] D. Palm and F. Entschladen, *Neoneurogenesis and the Neuro-Neoplastic Synapse. Neuronal Activity in Tumor Tissue*, Karger Publishers, Basel, Switzerland, 2007.

[30] F. Entschladen, D. Palm, B. Niggemann, and K. S. Zaenker, "The cancer's nervous tooth: considering the neuronal crosstalk within tumors," *Seminars in Cancer Biology*, vol. 18, no. 3, pp. 171–175, 2008.

[31] F. Zafra, D. Lindholm, E. Castren, J. Hartikka, and H. Thoenen, "Regulation of brain-derived neurotrophic factor and nerve growth factor mRNA in primary cultures of hippocampal neurons and astrocytes," *Journal of Neuroscience*, vol. 12, no. 12, pp. 4793–4799, 1992.

[32] S. J. French, T. Humby, C. H. Horner, M. V. Sofroniew, and M. Rattray, "Hippocampal neurotrophin and trk receptor mRNA levels are altered by local administration of nicotine, carbachol and pilocarpine," *Molecular Brain Research*, vol. 67, no. 1, pp. 124–136, 1999.

[33] H. M. Schuller, H. A. N. Al-wadei, M. F. Ullah, and H. K. Plummer III, "Regulation of pancreatic cancer by neuropsychological stress responses: a novel target for intervention," *Carcinogenesis*, vol. 33, no. 1, pp. 191–196, 2012.

[34] H. M. Schuller, P. K. Tithof, M. Williams, and H. Plummer III, "The tobacco-specific carcinogen 4-(methylnitrosamino)-1-(3-pyridyl)-1-butanone is a β-adrenergic agonist and stimulates DNA synthesis in lung adenocarcinoma via β-adrenergic receptor-mediated release of arachidonic acid," *Cancer Research*, vol. 59, no. 18, pp. 4510–4515, 1999.

[35] E. Laag, M. Majidi, M. Cekanova, T. Masi, T. Takahashi, and H. M. Schuller, "NNK activates ERK1/2 and CREB/ATF-1 via β-1-AR and EGFR signaling in human lung adenocarcinoma and small airway epithelial cells," *International Journal of Cancer*, vol. 119, no. 7, pp. 1547–1552, 2006.

[36] M. Majidi, H. A. Al-Wadei, T. Takahashi, and H. M. Schuller, "Nongenomic β estrogen receptors enhance $\beta 1$ adrenergic signaling induced by the nicotine-derived carcinogen 4-(methylnitrosamino)-1-(3-pyridyl)-1-butanone in human small airway epithelial cells," *Cancer Research*, vol. 67, no. 14, pp. 6863–6871, 2007.

[37] V. Y. Shin, W. K. K. Wu, Y.-N. Ye et al., "Nicotine promotes gastric tumor growth and neovascularization by activating extracellular signal-regulated kinase and cyclooxygenase-2," *Carcinogenesis*, vol. 25, no. 12, pp. 2487–2495, 2004.

[38] H. P. S. Wong, L. Yu, E. K. Y. Lam, E. K. K. Tai, W. K. K. Wu, and C.-H. Cho, "Nicotine promotes colon tumor growth and angiogenesis through β-adrenergic activation," *Toxicological Sciences*, vol. 97, no. 2, pp. 279–287, 2007.

[39] H. P. S. Wong, L. Yu, E. K. Y. Lam, E. K. K. Tai, W. K. K. Wu, and C. H. Cho, "Nicotine promotes cell proliferation via $\alpha 7$-nicotinic acetylcholine receptor and catecholamine-synthesizing enzymes-mediated pathway in human colon adenocarcinoma HT-29 cells," *Toxicology and Applied Pharmacology*, vol. 221, no. 3, pp. 261–267, 2007.

[40] D. H. Phillips, "Smoking-related DNA and protein adducts in human tissues," *Carcinogenesis*, vol. 23, no. 12, pp. 1979–2004, 2002.

[41] R.-J. Chen, Y.-S. Ho, H.-R. Guo, and Y.-J. Wang, "Rapid activation of Stat3 and ERK1/2 by nicotine modulates cell proliferation in human bladder cancer cells," *Toxicological Sciences*, vol. 104, no. 2, pp. 283–293, 2008.

[42] H. M. Schuller, H. A. N. Al-Wadei, and M. Majidi, "Gamma-aminobutyric acid, a potential tumor suppressor for small airway-derived lung adenocarcinoma," *Carcinogenesis*, vol. 29, no. 10, pp. 1979–1985, 2008.

[43] J. Joseph, B. Niggemann, K. S. Zaenker, and F. Entschladen, "The neurotransmitter γ-aminobutyric acid is an inhibitory regulator for the migration of SW 480 colon carcinoma cells," *Cancer Research*, vol. 62, no. 22, pp. 6467–6469, 2002.

[44] K. A. West, J. Brognard, A. S. Clark et al., "Rapid Akt activation by nicotine and a tobacco carcinogen modulates the phenotype of normal human airway epithelial cells," *The Journal of Clinical Investigation*, vol. 111, no. 1, pp. 81–90, 2003.

[45] H. M. Schuller, H. A. N. Al-Wadei, and M. Majidi, "GABAB receptor is a novel drug target for pancreatic cancer," *Cancer*, vol. 112, no. 4, pp. 767–778, 2008.

[46] C. Heeschen, J. J. Jang, M. Weis et al., "Nicotine stimulates angiogenesis and promotes tumor growth and atherosclerosis," *Nature Medicine*, vol. 7, no. 7, pp. 833–839, 2001.

[47] B.-Q. Zhu, C. Heeschen, R. E. Sievers et al., "Second hand smoke stimulates tumor angiogenesis and growth," *Cancer Cell*, vol. 4, no. 3, pp. 191–196, 2003.

[48] C. Heeschen, E. Chang, A. Aicher, and J. P. Cooke, "Endothelial progenitor cells participate in nicotine-mediated angiogenesis," *Journal of the American College of Cardiology*, vol. 48, no. 12, pp. 2553–2560, 2006.

[49] M. Yu, Q. Liu, J. Sun, K. Yi, L. Wu, and X. Tan, "Nicotine improves the functional activity of late endothelial progenitor cells via nicotinic acetylcholine receptors," *Biochemistry and Cell Biology*, vol. 89, no. 4, pp. 405–410, 2011.

[50] C. Heeschen, M. Weis, A. Aicher, S. Dimmeler, and J. P. Cooke, "A novel angiogenic pathway mediated by non-neuronal nicotinic acetylcholine receptors," *Journal of Clinical Investigation*, vol. 110, no. 4, pp. 527–536, 2002.

[51] K. C. Brown, J. K. Lau, A. M. Dom et al., "MG624, an alpha7-nAChR antagonist, inhibits angiogenesis via the Egr-1/FGF2 pathway," *Angiogenesis*, vol. 15, no. 1, pp. 99–114, 2012.

[52] J. C. F. Wu, A. Chruscinski, V. A. De Jesus Perez et al., "Cholinergic modulation of angiogenesis: role of the 7 nicotinic acetylcholine receptor," *Journal of Cellular Biochemistry*, vol. 108, no. 2, pp. 433–446, 2009.

[53] E. Gemenetzidis, A. Bose, A. M. Riaz et al., "FOXM1 upregulation is an early event in human squamous cell carcinoma and it is enhanced by nicotine during malignant transformation," *PLoS ONE*, vol. 4, no. 3, Article ID e4849, 2009.

[54] M. K. Ng, J. Wu, E. Chang et al., "A central role for nicotinic cholinergic regulation of growth factor-induced endothelial cell migration," *Arteriosclerosis, Thrombosis, and Vascular Biology*, vol. 27, no. 1, pp. 106–112, 2007.

[55] J. Arredondo, A. I. Chernyavsky, D. L. Jolkovsky, K. E. Pinkerton, and S. A. Grando, "Receptor-mediated tobacco toxicity: alterations of the NF-κB expression and activity downstream of α7 nicotinic receptor in oral keratinocytes," *Life Sciences*, vol. 80, no. 24-25, pp. 2191–2194, 2007.

[56] I. Wessler, C. J. Kirkpatrick, and K. Racké, "The cholinergic 'pitfall': acetylcholine, a universal cell molecule in biological systems, including humans," *Clinical and Experimental Pharmacology and Physiology*, vol. 26, no. 3, pp. 198–205, 1999.

[57] Y. Moriwaki, K. Yoshikawa, H. Fukuda, Y. X. Fujii, H. Misawa, and K. Kawashima, "Immune system expression of SLURP-1 and SLURP-2, two endogenous nicotinic acetylcholine receptor ligands," *Life Sciences*, vol. 80, no. 24-25, pp. 2365–2368, 2007.

[58] M. G. Cattaneo, A. Codignola, L. M. Vicentini, F. Clementi, and E. Sher, "Nicotine stimulates a serotonergic autocrine loop in human small-cell lung carcinoma," *Cancer Research*, vol. 53, no. 22, pp. 5566–5568, 1993.

[59] B. A. Jull, H. Plummer, and H. Schuller, "Nicotinic receptor-mediated activation by the tobacco-specific nitrosamine NNK of a Raf-1/MAP kinase pathway, resulting in phosphorylation of c-myc in human small cell lung carcinoma cells and pulmonary neuroendocrine cells," *Journal of Cancer Research and Clinical Oncology*, vol. 127, no. 12, pp. 707–717, 2001.

[60] A. Codignola, P. Tarroni, M. G. Cattaneo, L. M. Vicentini, F. Clementi, and E. Sher, "Serotonin release and cell proliferation are under the control of α-bungarotoxin-sensitive nicotinic receptors in small-cell lung carcinoma cell lines," *FEBS Letters*, vol. 342, no. 3, pp. 286–290, 1994.

[61] B. J. Sheppard, M. Williams, H. K. Plummer, and H. M. Schuller, "Activation of voltage-operated Ca^{2+}-channels in human small cell lung carcinoma by the tobacco-specific nitrosamine 4-(methylnitrosamino)-1-(3-pyridyl)-1-butanone," *International Journal of Oncology*, vol. 16, no. 3, pp. 513–518, 2000.

[62] L. Xu and X. Deng, "Tobacco-specific nitrosamine 4-(methylnitrosamino)-1-(3-pyridyl)-1-butanone induces phosphorylation of μ- and m-calpain in association with increased secretion, cell migration, and invasion," *The Journal of Biological Chemistry*, vol. 279, no. 51, pp. 53683–53690, 2004.

[63] Z. Jin, F. Gao, T. Flagg, and X. Deng, "Tobacco-specific nitrosamine 4-(methylnitrosamino)-1-(3-pyridyl)-1-butanone promotes functional cooperation of Bcl2 and c-Myc through phosphorylation in regulating cell survival and proliferation," *The Journal of Biological Chemistry*, vol. 279, no. 38, pp. 40209–40219, 2004.

[64] T. Seufferlein and E. Rozengurt, "Galanin, neurotensin, and phorbol esters rapidly stimulate activation of mitogen-activated protein kinase in small cell lung cancer cells," *Cancer Research*, vol. 56, no. 24, pp. 5758–5764, 1996.

[65] H. K. Plummer III, M. S. Dhar, M. Cekanova, and H. M. Schuller, "Expression of G-protein inwardly rectifying potassium channels (GIRKs) in lung cancer cell lines," *BMC Cancer*, vol. 5, article 104, 2005.

[66] S. H. Shafer, S. H. Phelps, and C. L. Williams, "Reduced DNA synthesis and cell viability in small cell lung carcinoma by treatment with cyclic AMP phosphodiesterase inhibitors," *Biochemical Pharmacology*, vol. 56, no. 9, pp. 1229–1236, 1998.

[67] J.-P. Pursiheimo, A. Kieksi, M. Jalkanen, and M. Salmivirta, "Protein kinase A balances the growth factor-induced Ras/ERK signaling," *FEBS Letters*, vol. 521, no. 1-3, pp. 157–164, 2002.

[68] J. Tsurutani, S. S. Castillo, J. Brognard et al., "Tobacco components stimulate Akt-dependent proliferation and NFκB-dependent survival in lung cancer cells," *Carcinogenesis*, vol. 26, no. 7, pp. 1182–1195, 2005.

[69] J. Brognard, A. S. Clark, Y. Ni, and P. A. Dennis, "Akt/protein kinase B is constitutively active in non-small cell lung cancer cells and promotes cellular survival and resistance to chemotherapy and radiation," *Cancer Research*, vol. 61, no. 10, pp. 3986–3997, 2001.

[70] P. Dasgupta, R. Kinkade, B. Joshi, C. DeCook, E. Haura, and S. Chellappan, "Nicotine inhibits apoptosis induced by chemotherapeutic drugs by up-regulating XIAP and survivin,"

Proceedings of the National Academy of Sciences of the United States of America, vol. 103, no. 16, pp. 6332–6337, 2006.

[71] P. Dasgupta, S. Rastogi, S. Pillai et al., "Nicotine induces cell proliferation by β-arrestin-mediated activation of Src and Rb-Raf-1 pathways," *Journal of Clinical Investigation*, vol. 116, no. 8, pp. 2208–2217, 2006.

[72] J. Arredondo, A. I. Chernyavsky, and S. A. Grando, "The nicotinic receptor antagonists abolish pathobiologic effects of tobacco-derived nitrosamines on BEP2D cells," *Journal of Cancer Research and Clinical Oncology*, vol. 132, no. 10, pp. 653–663, 2006.

[73] E. Martínez-García, M. Irigoyen, E. Ansó, J. J. Martínez-Irujo, and A. Rouzaut, "Recurrent exposure to nicotine differentiates human bronchial epithelial cells via epidermal growth factor receptor activation," *Toxicology and Applied Pharmacology*, vol. 228, no. 3, pp. 334–342, 2008.

[74] D. C.-L. Lam, L. Girard, R. Ramirez et al., "Expression of nicotinic acetylcholine receptor subunit genes in non-small-cell lung cancer reveals differences between smokers and non-smokers," *Cancer Research*, vol. 67, no. 10, pp. 4638–4647, 2007.

[75] A. Paliwal, T. Vaissière, A. Krais et al., "Aberrant DNA methylation links cancer susceptibility locus 15q25.1 to apoptotic regulation and lung cancer," *Cancer Research*, vol. 70, no. 7, pp. 2779–2788, 2010.

[76] J. D. Minna, "Nicotine exposure and bronchial epithelial cell nicotinic acetylcholine receptor expression in the pathogenesis of lung cancer," *The Journal of Clinical Investigation*, vol. 111, no. 1, pp. 31–33, 2003.

[77] M. Polette, M. Mestdagt, S. Bindels et al., "β-Catenin and ZO-1: shuttle molecules involved in tumor invasion-associated epithelial-mesenchymal transition processes," *Cells Tissues Organs*, vol. 185, no. 1–3, pp. 61–65, 2007.

[78] A. V. Patel, C. Rodriguez, L. Bernstein, A. Chao, M. J. Thun, and E. E. Calle, "Obesity, recreational physical activity, and risk of pancreatic cancer in a large U.S. cohort," *Cancer Epidemiology Biomarkers and Prevention*, vol. 14, no. 2, pp. 459–466, 2005.

[79] D. Qiu, M. Kurosawa, Y. Lin et al., "Overview of the epidemiology of pancreatic cancer focusing on the JACC Study," *Journal of Epidemiology*, vol. 15, supplement 2, pp. S157–S167, 2005.

[80] C. S. Fuchs, G. A. Colditz, M. J. Stampfer et al., "A prospective study of cigarette smoking and the risk of pancreatic cancer," *Archives of Internal Medicine*, vol. 156, no. 19, pp. 2255–2260, 1996.

[81] J. E. Yun, I. Jo, J. Park et al., "Cigarette smoking, elevated fasting serum glucose, and risk of pancreatic cancer in Korean men," *International Journal of Cancer*, vol. 119, no. 1, pp. 208–212, 2006.

[82] M. D. F. Askari, M.-S. Tsao, and H. M. Schuller, "The tobacco-specific carcinogen, 4-(methylnitrosamino)-1-(3-pyridyl)-1-butanone stimulates proliferation of immortalized human pancreatic duct epithelia through β-adrenergic transactivation of EGF receptors," *Journal of Cancer Research and Clinical Oncology*, vol. 131, no. 10, pp. 639–648, 2005.

[83] H. M. Schuller, "Mechanisms of smoking-related lung and pancreatic adenocarcinoma development," *Nature Reviews Cancer*, vol. 2, no. 6, pp. 455–463, 2002.

[84] M. H. Al-Wadei, H. A. N. Al-Wadei, and H. M. Schuller, "Effects of chronic nicotine on the autocrine regulation of pancreatic cancer cells and pancreatic duct epithelial cells by stimulatory and inhibitory neurotransmitters," *Carcinogenesis*, vol. 33, no. 9, pp. 1745–1753, 2012.

[85] D. L. Weddle, P. Tithoff, M. Williams, and H. M. Schuller, "β-Adrenergic growth regulation of human cancer cell lines derived from pancreatic ductal carcinomas," *Carcinogenesis*, vol. 22, no. 3, pp. 473–479, 2001.

[86] N. Momi, M. P. Ponnusamy, S. Kaur et al., "Nicotine/cigarette smoke promotes metastasis of pancreatic cancer through α7nAChR-mediated MUC4 upregulation," *Oncogene*, vol. 32, no. 11, pp. 1384–1395, 2013.

[87] U. A. Wittel, K. K. Pandey, M. Andrianifahanana et al., "Chronic pancreatic inflammation induced by environmental tobacco smoke inhalation in rats," *The American Journal of Gastroenterology*, vol. 101, no. 1, pp. 148–159, 2006.

[88] P. M. Pour, S. Z. Salmasi, and R. G. Runge, "Selective induction of pancreatic ductular tumors by single doses of N-nitrosobis(2-oxopropyl)amine in syrian golden hamsters," *Cancer Letters*, vol. 4, pp. 317–323, 1978.

[89] J. Arredondo, A. I. Chernyavsky, and S. A. Grando, "SLURP-1 and -2 in normal, immortalized and malignant oral keratinocytes," *Life Sciences*, vol. 80, no. 24-25, pp. 2243–2247, 2007.

[90] J. Arredondo, A. I. Chernyavsky, D. L. Jolkovsky, K. E. Pinkerton, and S. A. Grando, "Receptor-mediated tobacco toxicity: cooperation of the Ras/Raf-1/MEK1/ERK and JAK-2/STAT-3 pathways downstream of α7 nicotinic receptor in oral keratinocytes," *The FASEB Journal*, vol. 20, no. 12, pp. 2093–2101, 2006.

[91] X. Liu, W. K. K. Wu, L. Yu et al., "Epidermal growth factor-induced esophageal cancer cell proliferation requires transactivation of β-adrenoceptors," *Journal of Pharmacology and Experimental Therapeutics*, vol. 326, no. 1, pp. 69–75, 2008.

[92] X. Liu, W. K. K. Wu, L. Yu et al., "Epinephrine stimulates esophageal squamous-cell carcinoma cell proliferation via β-adrenoceptor-dependent transactivation of extracellular signal-regulated kinase/cyclooxygenase-2 pathway," *Journal of Cellular Biochemistry*, vol. 105, no. 1, pp. 53–60, 2008.

[93] M. H. Al-Wadei, H. A. N. Al-Wadei, and H. M. Schuller, "Pancreatic cancer cells and normal pancreatic duct epithelial cells express an autocrine catecholamine loop that is activated by nicotinic acetylcholine receptors α3, α5, and α7," *Molecular Cancer Research*, vol. 10, no. 2, pp. 239–249, 2012.

[94] Y. Zhao, W. Zhou, L. Xue, W. Zhang, and Q. Zhan, "Nicotine activates YAP1 through nAChRs mediated signaling in esophageal squamous cell cancer (ESCC)," *PLoS ONE*, vol. 9, no. 3, Article ID e90836, 2014.

[95] W. O. Lee and S. M. Wright, "Production of endothelin by cultured human endothelial cells following exposure to nicotine or caffeine," *Metabolism: Clinical and Experimental*, vol. 48, no. 7, pp. 845–848, 1999.

[96] H. Takeuchi, S. Kubota, E. Murakashi et al., "Nicotine-induced CCN2: from smoking to periodontal fibrosis," *Journal of Dental Research*, vol. 89, no. 1, pp. 34–39, 2009.

[97] K. Yamada, T. Yaguchi, T. Kanno, T. Mukasa, and T. Nishizaki, "Auto-positive feedback regulation for nicotinic acetylcholine receptors by protein kinase C activation," *Cellular Physiology and Biochemistry*, vol. 26, no. 2, pp. 247–252, 2010.

Permissions

All chapters in this book were first published in JO, by Hindawi Publishing Corporation; hereby published with permission under the Creative Commons Attribution License or equivalent. Every chapter published in this book has been scrutinized by our experts. Their significance has been extensively debated. The topics covered herein carry significant findings which will fuel the growth of the discipline. They may even be implemented as practical applications or may be referred to as a beginning point for another development.

The contributors of this book come from diverse backgrounds, making this book a truly international effort. This book will bring forth new frontiers with its revolutionizing research information and detailed analysis of the nascent developments around the world.

We would like to thank all the contributing authors for lending their expertise to make the book truly unique. They have played a crucial role in the development of this book. Without their invaluable contributions this book wouldn't have been possible. They have made vital efforts to compile up to date information on the varied aspects of this subject to make this book a valuable addition to the collection of many professionals and students.

This book was conceptualized with the vision of imparting up-to-date information and advanced data in this field. To ensure the same, a matchless editorial board was set up. Every individual on the board went through rigorous rounds of assessment to prove their worth. After which they invested a large part of their time researching and compiling the most relevant data for our readers.

The editorial board has been involved in producing this book since its inception. They have spent rigorous hours researching and exploring the diverse topics which have resulted in the successful publishing of this book. They have passed on their knowledge of decades through this book. To expedite this challenging task, the publisher supported the team at every step. A small team of assistant editors was also appointed to further simplify the editing procedure and attain best results for the readers.

Apart from the editorial board, the designing team has also invested a significant amount of their time in understanding the subject and creating the most relevant covers. They scrutinized every image to scout for the most suitable representation of the subject and create an appropriate cover for the book.

The publishing team has been an ardent support to the editorial, designing and production team. Their endless efforts to recruit the best for this project, has resulted in the accomplishment of this book. They are a veteran in the field of academics and their pool of knowledge is as vast as their experience in printing. Their expertise and guidance has proved useful at every step. Their uncompromising quality standards have made this book an exceptional effort. Their encouragement from time to time has been an inspiration for everyone.

The publisher and the editorial board hope that this book will prove to be a valuable piece of knowledge for researchers, students, practitioners and scholars across the globe.

List of Contributors

Nicholas A. Pease and Lisa Privette Vinnedge
Division of Oncology, Cincinnati Children's Hospital Medical Center, Cincinnati, OH 45229, USA

Trisha Wise-Draper
Department of Internal Medicine, Division of Hematology/Oncology, University of Cincinnati College of Medicine, Cincinnati, OH 45267, USA

Kentaro Kikuchi, Fumio Ide, Harumi Inoue, Yuji Miyazaki and Kaoru Kusama
Division of Pathology, Department of Diagnostic and Therapeutic Sciences, Meikai University School of Dentistry, 1-1 Keyakidai, Sakado, Saitama 350-0283, Japan

Toshiyuki Ishige
Department of Pathology, Nihon University School of Medicine, 30-1 Oyaguchi-Kamimachi, Itabashi-ku, Tokyo 173-8610, Japan

Yumi Ito
Division of Diagnostic Pathology, Tsurumi University Dental Hospital, 2-1-3 Tsurumi, Tsurumi-ku, Yokohama 230-8501, Japan

Ichiro Saito
Department of Pathology, Tsurumi University School of Dental Medicine, 2-1-3 Tsurumi, Tsurumi-ku, Yokohama 230-8501, Japan

Miyako Hoshino
Second Division of Oral and Maxillofacial Surgery, Department of Diagnostic and Therapeutic Sciences, Meikai University School of Dentistry, 1-1 Keyakidai, Sakado, Saitama 350-0283, Japan

Tadashige Nozaki
Department of Pharmacology, Osaka Dental University, 8-1 Kuzuhahanazono-cho, Hirakata, Osaka 573-1211, Japan

Masaru Kojima
Department of Anatomic and Diagnostic Pathology, Dokkyo Medical University School of Medicine, 880 Oaza-kitakobayashi, Mibu-machi, Shimotsuga-gun, Tochigi 321-0293, Japan

Anna Calleja, Frédéric Poulin, Ciril Khorolsky, Harry Rakowski, Michael McDonald, Diego Delgado and Paaladinesh Thavendiranathan
Division of Cardiology, Peter Munk Cardiac Center, Toronto General Hospital, University Health Network, University of Toronto, 200 Elizabeth Street, Toronto, ON, Canada M5G 2C4

Frédéric Poulin
Division of Cardiology, Hôpital du Sacré-Coeur de Montréal, University of Montreal, 5400 Boulevard Gouin Ouest, Montreal, QC, Canada H4J 1C5

Masoud Shariat and Paaladinesh Thavendiranathan
Division of Medical Imaging, Peter Munk Cardiac Center, Toronto General Hospital, University Health Network, University of Toronto, 200 Elizabeth Street, Toronto, ON, Canada M5G 2C4

Philippe L. Bedard and Eitan Amir
Division of Medical Oncology & Hematology, Princess Margaret Cancer Center, University Health Network, University of Toronto, 610 University Avenue, Toronto, ON, Canada M5T 2M9

Christophe Nicot
Department of Pathology and Laboratory Medicine, Center for Viral Oncology, University of Kansas Medical Center, 3901 Rainbow Boulevard, Kansas City, KS 66160, USA

Chuang-Chi Liaw, Hung Chang and Tsai-Sheng Yang
Division of Hemato-Oncology, Department of Internal Medicine, Chang-Gung Memorial Hospital and Chang-Gung University College of Medicine, Taoyuan 33305, Taiwan

Ming-Sheng Wen
Division of Cardiology, Department of Internal Medicine, Chang-Gung Memorial Hospital and Chang-Gung University College of Medicine, Taoyuan 33305, Taiwan

Franziska M. Ippen and Ekkehard M. Kasper
Department of Neurosurgery, Beth Israel Deaconess Medical Center, Harvard Medical School, Boston, MA 02445, USA

Anand Mahadevan
Department of Radiation Oncology, Beth Israel Deaconess Medical Center, Harvard Medical School, Boston, MA 02445, USA

Eric T. Wong, Erik J. Uhlmann and Soma Sengupta
Department of Neuro-Oncology, Beth Israel Deaconess Medical Center, Harvard Medical School, Boston, MA 02445, USA

George I. Lambrou
1st Department of Pediatrics, University of Athens, Choremeio Research Laboratory, Thivon & Levadeias, 11527 Athens, Greece

Apostolos Zaravinos
Division of Clinical Immunology and Transfusion Medicine, Department of Laboratory Medicine, Karolinska Institute, 171 77 Stockholm, Sweden

Fausto Pizzino, Giampiero Vizzari, Scipione Carerj and Concetta Zito
Cardiology Unit, Department of Clinical and Experimental Medicine, University of Messina, Azienda Ospedaliera Universitaria "Policlinico G. Martino" and Universita' degli Studi di Messina, Via Consolare Valeria No. 12, 98100 Messina, Italy

Rubina Qamar and Charles Bomzer
Aurora Advanced Healthcare, St. Luke's Medical Centers, 2801 W. Kinnickinnic River Parkway, No. 840, Milwaukee, WI 53215, USA

Bijoy K. Khandheria
Aurora Cardiovascular Services, Aurora Sinai/Aurora St. Luke's Medical Centers, University of Wisconsin School of Medicine and Public Health, 2801 W. Kinnickinnic River Parkway, No. 840, Milwaukee, WI 53215, USA

Panagiotis Papageorgis
Department of Health Sciences, Program in Biological Sciences, European University Cyprus,6 Diogenes Street, Engomi, 1516 Nicosia, Cyprus

Caroline Zimmermann
Graduate Program of Dentistry, Federal University of Santa Catarina, 88040-900 Florianópolis, SC, Brazil

Maria Inês Meurer and Liliane Janete Grando
Department of Pathology, Federal University of Santa Catarina, 88040-900 Florianópolis, SC, Brazil Stomatology Clinic, University Hospital, Federal University of Santa Catarina, 88040-900 Florianópolis, SC, Brazil

Joanita Ângela Gonzaga Del Moral
Hematology Service, University Hospital, Federal University of Santa Catarina, 88040-900 Florianópolis, SC, Brazil

Inês Beatriz da Silva Rath
Department of Dentistry, Federal University of Santa Catarina, 88040-900 Florianópolis, SC, Brazil

Silvia Schaefer Tavares
Integrated Multidisciplinary Health, Federal University of Santa Catarina, 88040-900 Florianópolis, SC, Brazil

Chirag A. Shah, Arun Karanwal, Maharshi Desai, Munjal Pandya, Ravish Shah and Rutvij Shah
Apollo Hospitals International Limited, Plot No. 1 A, Bhat GIDC Estate, Gandhinagar, Gujarat 382428, India

Jennifer Pasquier and Nadine Abu-Kaoud
Stem Cell and Microenvironment Laboratory, Department of Genetic Medicine and Obstetrics and Gynecology, Weill Cornell Medical College in Qatar, Education City, Qatar Foundation, P.O. Box 24144, Doha, Qatar

Jennifer Pasquier, Haya Al Thani and Arash Rafii
Department of Genetic Medicine, Weill Cornell Medical College, New York, NY 10021, USA

Antti P. Jekunen
Clinical Cancer Research Center, Vaasa Oncology Clinic, Turku University, Hietalahdenkatu 2-4, 65100 Vaasa, Finland

Amy A. Kirkham
Rehabilitation Sciences, University of British Columbia, 212–2177 Wesbrook Mall, Vancouver, BC, Canada V6T 1Z3

Margot K. Davis
Division of Cardiology, University of British Columbia, Diamond Health Care Centre, 9th Floor, 2775 Laurel Street, Vancouver, BC, Canada V5Z 1M9

Hina Khan
Department of Hematology Oncology, Montefiore Medical Center, Albert Einstein School of Medicine, 1300 Morris Park Avenue, Bronx, NY 10461, USA

Rasim Gucalp
Department of Oncology, Montefiore Medical Center, Albert Einstein School of Medicine, 1300 Morris Park Avenue, Bronx, NY 10461, USA

Iuliana Shapira
Department of Hematology Oncology, Hofstra North Shore LIJ School of Medicine, Hempstead, NY 11549, USA

Eugenio Zoni and Gabri van der Pluijm
Department of Urology, Leiden University Medical Center, Albinusdreef 2, 2333 ZA Leiden, The Netherlands

Peter C. Gray
Clayton Foundation Laboratories for Peptide Biology, The Salk Institute for Biological Studies, La Jolla, CA 92037, USA

Marianna Kruithof-de Julio
Department of Molecular Cell Biology, Cancer Genomics Centre and Centre for Biomedical Genetics, Einthovenweg 20, 2333 ZC Leiden, The Netherlands
Department of Dermatology, Leiden University Medical Center, Einthovenweg 20, 2333 ZC Leiden, The Netherlands

Rani Kanthan
Department of Pathology & Laboratory Medicine, University of Saskatchewan, Saskatoon, SK, Canada S7N 0W8

Jenna-Lynn Senger
Department of Surgery, University of Alberta, Edmonton, AB, Canada T6G 2B7

Shahid Ahmed
Division of Medical Oncology, Division of Medical Oncology, University of Saskatchewan, Saskatoon, SK, Canada S7N 0W8

Selliah Chandra Kanthan
Department of Surgery, University of Saskatchewan, Saskatoon, SK, Canada S7N 0W8

Nathan Haywood, Kyle Gennaro, John Obert and Paul F. Sauer Jr.
University of Alabama at Birmingham School of Medicine, Birmingham, AL 35233, USA

David T. Redden
Biostatistics Division, School of Public Health, University of Alabama at Birmingham, Birmingham, AL 35233, USA

Jessica Zarzour, J. Kevin Smith, David Bolus, Souheil Saddekni and Ahmed Kamel Abdel Aal
Department of Radiology, University of Alabama at Birmingham, Birmingham, AL 35233, USA

Stephen Gray, Jared White, Devin E. Eckhoff and Derek A. DuBay
Liver Transplant and Hepatobiliary Surgery, University of Alabama at Birmingham, Birmingham, AL 35233, USA

Nozomu Kawata, Kenya Yamaguchi, Tomohiro Igarashi, and Satoru Takahashi
Department of Urology, Nihon University School of Medicine, 1-6 Kanda-Surugadai, Chiyoda-ku, Tokyo, Japan

Apostolos Zaravinos
Department of Laboratory Medicine, Karolinska Institutet Huddinge, 171 77 Stockholm, Sweden

Robert M. Wolfson, Irina Rachinsky and Al Driedger
Department of Diagnostic Imaging, Schulich School of Medicine and Dentistry, Western University, London, ON, Canada N6A 5W9

Deric Morrison, Tamara Spaic and Stan H. M. Van Uum
Department of Medicine, Schulich School of Medicine and Dentistry, Western University, London, ON, Canada N6A 4V2

Eugenio M. Ferrer-Santacreu
Orthopaedic Surgery Department, Hospital Universitario de Mośtoles, C/Río Jućar s/n, 28935 Mośtoles, Spain

Eduardo J. Ortiz-Cruz
Orthopaedic Oncology Unit, Orthopaedic Surgery Department, Hospital Universitario La Paz, Paseo de la Castellana 261, 28046 Madrid, Spain

Mariana Díaz-Almirón
Hospital La Paz Research Institute (IdiPaz), Paseo de la Castellana 261, 28046 Madrid, Spain

Jose Juan Pozo Kreilinger
Pathology Department, Hospital Universitario La Paz, Paseo de la Castellana 261, 28046 Madrid, Spain

Yue Zhao
Center of Cell biology and Cancer Research, Albany Medical College, 47 New Scotland Avenue, Albany, NY 12208, USA